ARE YOU STILL MINE?

Westbank Community Library
1309 Westbank Drive
Austin, TX 78746

ARE YOU STILL MINE?

EESHA Mary Ellen Lukas

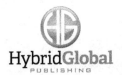
HybridGlobal
PUBLISHING

Published by
Hybrid Global Publishing
301 E 57th Street, 4th fl
New York, NY 10022

Copyright © 2020 by Michaelmas Publishing Company

All worldwide rights reserved. No part of this book may be reproduced or transmitted in any form or by in any means, electronic or mechanical, including photocopying, recording, or by any information storage and retrieval system, without the written permission of the Publisher, except where permitted by law.

Manufactured in the United States of America, or in the United Kingdom when distributed elsewhere.

EESHA Mary Ellen Lukas
Are You Still Mine?
LCCN: 2019918898
ISBN: 978-1-948181-95-2
eBook: 978-1-948181-96-9

Cover design by: Natasha Clawson
Cover art by: Chloe Clark
Interior design: Medlar Publishing Solutions Pvt Ltd., India

Disclaimer:
This book illustrates the fundamental beliefs of the Eeshan Religion. Contained herein, is information based on some of the teachings of the Catholic Church, which though presented in a discerning way, may be deemed to some readers unfavorable and/or formidable.

Please note that these, as well as other religions or scientific inclusions are interpreted and are wholly the beliefs and opinions of the Eeshan Religion and its members and are presented as such.

This book is not designed to convert, or pull one away from one's own faith base, but rather provide another path to God. You as a reader are responsible for forming your own opinions on what you want to believe and what is presented in this book.

Neither the publisher nor the author shall be liable for any physical, psychological, emotional, or spiritual damages to include any financial, or commercial damages; and is not limited to: special, incidental, consequential or other damages due to its contents.

This book serves as the primary teaching source for the Eeshan Church of Metta Spirituality and School of Enlightenment.

www.eeshanchurch.org

Contents

Preface . . . . *xxvii*
Foreword. . . . . *xxix*
A Note from the Author . . . . *xxxi*
Introduction and Guide . . . . *xxxii*

LESSON 1
What is Truth? 1
Understanding the Difference Between Religion and Spirituality

LESSON 2
Choosing a Religion or Spirituality 4

LESSON 3
Blinding Ignorance Does Mislead Us 6
Are We Guilty of Trusting in Humans More Than in God?

LESSON 4
Controversy Breeds Diverse Spiritualites 18

LESSON 5
Truth, Half Truths, and Ad Hominem 20

LESSON 6
A Brief Overview of What Religion Was Like in Jesus' Time...
...and the 'Word,' Words and Laws 27

LESSON 7
Understanding the Words Dogma and Infallibility 30

LESSON 8
The True Rock 33

LESSON 9
Eternal Consort and Wife: Twin Flames 37

LESSON 10
How God Worked Behind the Scenes 45

LESSON 11
Good People 51

LESSON 12
God Sends Another Guide 54

LESSON 13
God's Salvation Plan Continued 56

LESSON 14
A Step Towards a Hidden Identity 59

LESSON 15
Don't Let Fear Keep Us Apart 63

LESSON 16
How to Prepare for Enlightenment 67

LESSON 17
What You Will Find in the Eeshan Religion 69
The Use of Tones and Vibrations

LESSON 18
The Need for Repetition 73

LESSON 19
The Secret to Understanding Unfathomable Truths 75

LESSON 20
A Prayer 76

LESSON 21
Why Are We Like We Are? 77

LESSON 22
A Brief Look from Genesis to Revelation 80

LESSON 23
All Good Things Come from Above 84

LESSON 24
Strength from Above 87

LESSON 25
What Does God's Salvific Plan Entail? 91
    Lesson 25A *93*

LESSON 26
The First Kallahs 94

LESSON 27
The Resurgence of Mary Magdalen's Kallahs 96

LESSON 28
Why Do the Kallahs Have God's Protection? 100

LESSON 29
Peter's Constant Attempts to Sway Jesus' Attention Away from Mary . . .102
    Section II: Using Focal Points Introduction to: God, Free Will
    and Humankind *106*

LESSON 30
Focal Point: God 107
    Lesson 30A: Free Will *109*
    Lesson 30B: The Human Being *111*

LESSON 31
What Do We Gain by Finding Errors in Scriptures? 115

LESSON 32
What Traditional Scriptures Fail to Tell You We May Be Able to 118

LESSON 33
Will the Real Savior Please Identify Yourself? 121

LESSON 34
A Parent's Point of View 123

LESSON 35
Preserving the Old for Selfish Reasons 125
Section III: Women's Pleas for Equality Before God are Not Necessary, Their
Plea is Before Man

LESSON 36
And the Woman Asked Man 128
How Come Your Jesus is Not the Jesus I Know, Love, and Serve?

LESSON 37
What's Happened to Marriage 133

LESSON 38
Proof That Unconditional Love for God Exists 136

LESSON 39
Why Yet a New Priesthood 139

LESSON 40
The Love Between a Husband and Wife. 143

LESSON 41
Jesus is God—Not a Religion 145

LESSON 42
Section III: Why We are Plagued with Such Things as Illness, Suffering, and Sadness? Because We Have a Gross Physical Body 151

LESSON 43
Sacraments of God. 156

LESSON 44
What Do You Know About God's Love? 159

LESSON 45
Understanding Jesus' Sacrifice 164

LESSON 46
Parenting Lessons Meant for All Adults, and for Rearing of All Children. 166

LESSON 47
God's Timing 170

PART I

GETTING BACK TO THE TRANSCENDENTAL

LESSON 48
The Reason for God's Directive to Our Foundress. 173

LESSON 49
Why Does God Use Ordinary People to Bring About Vital Directives? . . .176

LESSON 50
God is Greater Than Human Error 183

LESSON 51
Heresy or Enlightenment? 185

LESSON 52
Is Anyone Out There? 189

LESSON 53
How God, as Jesus, Began the Age of Enlightenment, but Allowed for
Man's Free Will to Disrupt God's Plan of Salvation. 194

LESSON 54
What We Know About the Only Begotten Child of God. 203
*The Fruit of the Sacred Balance of Divine Male/Female and Who Jesus
and Mary Magdalen are*

LESSON 55
The Divine Becomes Human 207

LESSON 56
The Woman Who Was the Eternal Consort of Jesus 212

LESSON 57
Hidden Queen. 214

LESSON 58
Jesus Loves Mary, or Jesus and Mary Sitting in a Tree K-I-S-S-I-N-G . . .216

LESSON 59
Supramentalization. 222

LESSON 60
A Brief Description of the Eeshan Salvific Plan (Eeshan
Transcendentalism) and the Return of Ishvara. 225

LESSON 61
Repitition, Repitition, Repitition. 228

LESSON 62
Choice and Responsibility 231

PART II
BEGINNING YOUR JOURNEY

LESSON 63
Attaining Enlightenment 236

LESSON 64
What Did Jesus Focus On? 241

LESSON 65
The Soul 244
    Lesson 65A: Sin. 246
    Lesson 65B: Why Won't the Holy Eucharist Absolve Mortal Sin 250
    Lesson 65C: How Jesus Changed the Way We Look at God's Laws. 253
    Lesson 65D: How Sin Has Been Viewed Before Jesus, During Jesus'
        Time, and in Present Times. 255

LESSON 66
The Heart 258

LESSON 67
Spiritual Guidance and the Need for Renewed Trust in God 261

LESSON 68
Mercy 266

PART III

LESSON 69
An Exercise in Preparing to Walk the Path of Truth, Enightenment 269

LESSON 70
Finding the Key to Unlock an Enlightened Mind. 271

LESSON 71
The Master Key Jesus, God, Man, Spiritual Master 276
Door #1 Understanding Jesus' Method of Teaching How He Raised
the Human Consciousness to the Transcendental Level
    Lesson 71A: The Bread 282

LESSON 72
Door #2 The Rise and Fall of the Transcendental Life Experiencing
Phyicality in a Physical World. 288
    Lesson 72A: Tracing the Physical Back to the Transcendental 289

LESSON 73
Door #3 Jesus, the 'Way' to Enlightenment, and What Do We Mean that
Jesus is the 'Way'. 296
    Lesson 73A: The Genius of His Parables 298
    Lesson 73B: And Jesus Said, "…" ("Wait, What Did He Say?") 300
    Lesson 73C: "Therefore, See with Your Eyes, Hear with Your Ears;
        Understand with Your Hearts, and Turn, and I Will Heal You". 304

LESSON 74
Door #4 The Human Consciousness and its 'Far Reaching' Effects on
Religion and Loss of Spirituality to its Followers 305

LESSON 75
Door #5 Citing Disparities Between the Human Spirit and the
Transcendental Truth; The Things of God Labeled Heresy, to
Whom Belongs the Power and the Glory?. 307

LESSON 76
Door #6 New Age or New Knowledge 309

LESSON 77
Door #7 Who Has the Right to Decide Who Should Receive Christ and
Who Shoudn't, If Christ Welcomed Everyone, Even Women Who Were
from Shunned Cultures, Such as the Samaritan Woman 311

LESSON 78
Door #8 Faith 315

LESSON 79
Door #9 Jesus and Mary, Light of the World: Then, Now, Always. 318

LESSON 80
Door #10 The Ultimate Transcendental Experience 321
The Eucharist of the Marriage Feast: What Does it do and Why is it Necessary?

LESSON 81
Door #11 The Famine 325
The Cause and Fate

LESSON 82
Genesis 1:26-27, States the Elohim were Masculine and Feminine 330

LESSON 83
Is There a Hell? A New Revelation? 331
Heaven is Above, Hell is Below

LESSON 84
Door #12 Where Are You Going?. 338
That's Not the Way, Just a Random Path

LESSON 85
Door #12A Peter, Do You Love Me? 342
    Door #12B: Jesus the Young Savior. 344
    Door #12C: Sometimes God Allow Bad Things for a Greater Purpose 346

LESSON 86
Door #13 God's Use of Ordinary People as Prophets 352

LESSON 87
Door #14 God to the Rescue. 355

LESSON 88
Away from the Transcendental—Gender Identifiers Became Stronger . . .358

LESSON 89
Marriage is Defined by the Love Between Spouses;
Children are the Fruit of Their Love. 361

LESSON 90
Children 364

LESSON 91
Door #15 The Controversial Jesus of Nazareth: True God or True Man? . .370
If God, Why was He-Reimaged?

LESSON 92
Door #16 Water to Wine; Wine to Blood 375

LESSON 93
Door #17 Adam and Eve Knew About the Marriage Feast Eucharist. . . .381

LESSON 94
Door #18 The First Adam and Eve Begot Children: Human
Love and Natural Birthing. 384
*The New Adam and New Eve: Perfect Transcendental Love
and Back to Begetting Children*

LESSON 95
Door #19 From Famine to Feast 391

LESSON 96
Door #20 Living Forever Versus Eternity 397
 Lesson 96A 402

LESSON 97
Door #21 God Sends Another Helper. 406

LESSON 98
Door #22 When God Has Had Enough. 409

LESSON 99
Door #23 Wisdom! Be Attentive! 413

LESSON 100
Door #24 Genesis 4:1 Says: And Adam Knew His Wife and
She Conceived and Gave Birth to Cain, "I Have Gotten a Man
From the Lord" 416

LESSON 101
Door #25 The Philosophy of an Unguided and Spiritually Deprived
Mind Revealing the Cause and Origin of a Troubled Life. 421

LESSON 102
Door #26 Death 423

LESSON 103
Door #27 Death by Discrimination and Prejudice. 428

LESSON 104
Door #28 Conscience and Mind. 433

LESSON 105
Door #29 The Consequence of Assumption and Misuderstanding 435

LESSON 106
Door #30 Coercive and Persuasive Ideology. 438

LESSON 107
Door #31 "Unless You Become Like One of These" 442

LESSON 108
Door #32 The Eternal Consciousness .445

LESSON 109
Door #33 The What and Who Humans Are 447

THE EESHAN RELIGION AND SPIRITUALITY

LESSON 110
What is the Eeshan Religion. 450

LESSON 111
Quelling the Terror. 458

LESSON 112
'Repetitio' of Thoughts: A 'Kind' Disclaimer. 463

A SUMMARY OF EESHAN BELIEFS BASIC TEACHINGS

LESSON 113
Spiritual Teaching One: And God So Loved Us... 468

LESSON 114
Spiritual Teaching Two: Battling Hypocrisy 470

LESSON 115
Spiritual Teaching Three: Jesus Was Not Gender Conscious/Exclusive . . .477

LESSON 116
Spiritual Teaching Four: Love Thy Neighbor Continued 482

LESSON 117
Spiritual Teaching Five: God. 492

LESSON 118
Spiritual Teaching Six: Eternal Consorts and Their Love for
Each Other; Creation of Paradise and the First Human. 496

LESSON 119
Spiritual Teaching Seven: The First Transcendental Human. 499

LESSON 120
Sacred Writings of Eeshan Transcendentalism: What are
the Sacred Writings 501

PART I
MANIFESTING GOD'S DUALITY

LESSON 121
Section I: A Summary of the Creation of Adam and Eve
the First Human Marriage True Love .503

LESSON 122
Section II: The Key to Eternal Life and Eternal Love 506

LESSON 123
Section III: Eucharistic Beliefs. 516

PART II

TIMELESS LOVE

LESSON 124
Section I: Love: Originating from a Timeless God 521

LESSON 125
Section II: Becoming Man and Woman .522

LESSON 126
Section III: Law of Attraction, Law of Opposites 526

LESSON 127
Section IV: True Love Through, With, and in God;
And it all Began With a Kiss. 528
    Section IVA: The Sacred Kiss *529*

LESSON 128
Section V: Sacred Breath. 531

LESSON 129
Section VI: Spiritual Food for Eternal Life: Love Versus Sex 533

LESSON 130
Section VII: The Life With God in the Garden 536

LESSON 131
Section VIII: The Blessing, the Prize. 538

PART III

LESSON 132
Section I: Human Love Blessed By God. 541

PART IV

LUCIFER

LESSON 133
Section I: An Introduction to the Religious Corruption 544

LESSON 134
Section II: The Need to Destroy the Sacred Food and Drink 546

LESSON 135
Section III: The Legends and Facts Regarding This Being. 547

LESSON 136
Just a Reminder 550

PART V
THE CHURCH HYPOCRISY SATAN'S INFLUENCE

LESSON 137
Section I: Magic/Witchcraft Versus Mysticism 552

LESSON 138
Section II: Satan's Hatred of Love 562

LESSON 139
Section III: The Fall of the Heavenly Priesthood: Legend
or Endtime Prophecy? 563

LESSON 140
Jesus' Priesthood 565

LESSON 141
Section IV: The Emerald 570

LESSON 142
Section V: Satan Declares Himself God and Hell His Kingdom 573

LESSON 143
Section VI: Lilith and Eve 575

PART VI

LESSON 144
Section I: The Plan is Laid Out 582

PART VII
THE TEMPTATION OF ADAM AND EVE

LESSON 145
Section I: Satan Continues in His Plan 591

LESSON 146
Section II: Setting the Stage 594

LESSON 147
Section III: Spiritual Food 599

PART VIII
"THE APPLE"

LESSON 148
Section I: "The Apple" 604

LESSON 149
Section II: "The New Apple". 609

LESSON 150
Section III: True Love Through, With, and in God 613
*Understanding What Satan Was Up Against in Trying
to Destroy the Love Between Adam and Eve*

LESSON 151
Section IV: Spiritual Food for Eternal Life 615
Love Versus Sex and Wisdom Versus Knowledge

PART IX

LESSON 152
Section I: Time to Separate Soulmates. 620

LESSON 153
Section II: Without God, the Mind Fills the Gaps 622

PART X

LESSON 154
Section I: An In-Depth Look at the "SSSerpent:" By Far
a Very Complex Creature 631

LESSON 155
Section II: Comparing the Serpent with the Fallen
Human Consciousness and the Consequences that Led
to the Need for Salvation. 636

LESSON 156
Section III: Looking Past the Religious Tones
and Understanding Jesus, Master, and Teacher. 638

PART XI
LIFE AS THEY KNEW IT, WAS CHANGED

LESSON 157
Section I: The Story Adam and Eve Continues with the Choice for
Physical Life and Human Consciousness 647

PART XII

LESSON 158
God's Love and Mercy Brings the First Human Marriage 653
Section I: God Sets Guidelines for Physical Love

PART XIII
THE ORIGINAL SIN

LESSON 159
Section I: Who is Right, Human Man or God Made Man?. 656

LESSON 160
Section II: Adam and Eve Obtain Human Knowledge of
What is Good and Bad 658

LESSON 161
Section III: Insight into Sin 660

LESSON 162
Section IV: God of Love and Mercy. .666
Lesson 162A. 667

LESSON 163
Section V: What Did Jesus Teach?. 670

LESSON 164
Section VI: Changes in Our First Parents Lifestyle: The Beginning
of the Diversity of Human Beings 672

LESSON 165
Section VII: Where Did All the People Come From? 676

PART XIV
WOMAN

LESSON 166
Section I: What We Read, What We Seek, and What Jesus Meant 680

PART XV
MISTAKEN: BEING WRONG IN ONE'S OPINION OR JUDGEMENT

LESSON 167
Section I: False Impressions 685

LESSON 168
Section II: Building a Bullying, or Gossiping Mentality. 689

LESSON 169
Section III: Genocide, Euthanasia, Mercy Killing: Is There a Difference? . .696

LESSON 170
Section IV: Unjustices to Men/Women: How Can They Be Rectified? . . .702

LESSON 171
Section V: Mary and the Women Ministers at the Time of
Jesus and Today 706
The Beginning of Sexism?

LESSON 172
Section VI: The Women Who Loved God. 710

LESSON 173
Section VII: Da Vinci Decoded 2000+ Years Ago 713

LESSON 174
Section VIII: Where Have All the Women Gone? 717

PART XVI
THE OLD WINE SKIN AND THE NEW WINE

LESSON 175
Section I: What We Know. 721

LESSON 176
Section II: A New Priesthood 723

PART XVII
INTO THY HANDS, MARY

LESSON 177
Section I: Another Testament is Begun, Ishvara is Back. 728

LESSON 178
Section II: Peter's Path Versus Jesus' Way Who Was More Guilty Judas Who Thought He Was Doing a Good Thing or Peter Who Knew He Was Doing the Wrong Thing and Kept on Going. 739

LESSON 179
Section III: Don't Confuse Obedience to Man with Obedience to God . .744

LESSON 180
Section IV: Eeshans' Stance on the Reference to the "Bride of Christ" . . .746

LESSON 181
Section V: Enter Paranoia 750

LESSON 182
Section VI: Judaic Messiah, Christian Messiah, True Messiah[s] 756

LESSON 183
The Differences Between Christian and Judaic Messianic Beliefs 758

PART XVIII

LESSON 184
Our Eeshan Creed Explained 764

LESSON 185
Section I: The Imperfect Challenges the Perfect. 767

LESSON 186
Section II: Would Things have been Different? 772

LESSON 187
Section III: Men for Women. 773

LESSON 188
Section IV: Our Future 777

LESSON 189
Section V: Correcting the Consciousness of the World 778

PART XIX

LESSON 190
Spiritual Teaching I: The Return of the Wife of the Lamb 782

LESSON 191
Spiritual Teaching II: A Body Prepared for an Eschatological Time? 786

LESSON 192
Sacred Teaching III: Understanding the Fulfilment of Scriptures 791

PART XX

LESSON 193
Sacred Teaching I: Creation 795

LESSON 194
Sacred Teaching II: The Eternal Component of God
and the Human Factor. 798

LESSON 195
Sacred Teaching III: The Eeshan Versions: Of the Eternal Consorts
and the Creation and the Role of the Second Person of the
Holy Trinity 799

PART XXI

LESSON 196
Sacred Teaching I: The Story of Adam and Eve,
As Seen Through Eeshan Eyes. 804

PART XXII

LESSON 197
Sacred Teaching I: God Allows Bad Things to Happen
for the Sake of a Greater Good 821

PART XXIII
TRUE MEANINGS

LESSON 198
Section I: The Consequences of the Misinterpretation
of the Marriage Feast at Cana 826

LESSON 199
Section II: A Quick Review 845

LESSON 200
Section III: How the Holy and Sacred Transcendental is Greater Than
What Was Taught to Us 848

LESSON 201
Section IV: 'Try to Rectify Yourself Rather Than Blaspheming
the Nature or Activities of Others'. 853

LESSON 202
Section V: Metta True Charity/Love, Not Misplaced Compassion 857

LESSON 203
Section VI: Divorce 861

LESSON 204
Section VII: God as Human: To Live in a Vowed Marriage 867

PART XXIV
TRUE MEANINGS

LESSON 205
Section I: Symbols 875

LESSON 206
Section II: Translations: True and Fallacious 877

LESSON 207
You Are a Priest Forever, According to the Order of Melchizedek 879

LESSON 208
Section III: The Unfathomable Mysteries That You Were
Never Told Regarding Jesus' Role 881
    Lesson 208A: God Allows Another Wrong For a Greater Good
        the Order of Melchizedek 889

PART XXV

LESSON 209
Section I: The Culmination of Christ's Esoteric Life 896
    Lesson 209A: How Deep Was Their Love? 900

LESSON 210
Section II: Choosing to Live Only in the Physical/Material World
Obstructs Love. 907

LESSON 211
Section III: Mysteries, More Than Meets the Eye 909

PART XXVI

LESSON 212
Section I: God's Mystery Encrypted 915

WHERE HAVE ALL THE FLOWERS GONE?

INTRODUCTION 920

SUMMARY POINT 1
Reasons the Flowers Have Gone. 922

SUMMARY POINT 2 930

SUMMARY POINT 3 935

SUMMARY POINT 4 938

SUMMARY POINT 5 939

SUMMARY POINT 6 941

SUMMARY POINT 7
The Continuation of Supramentalization: Sacred Teaching 944

SUMMARY POINT 8
'I Will Help' 947

SUMMARY POINT 9
God in the Holy Eucharist and Loving Thy Neighbor. 949

SUMMARY POINT 10
Peter's Legacy Perpetuates 953

SUMMARY POINT 11
Our Lifeline to God Defined 955

SUMMARY POINT 12
The Vastness of God's Presence and Word. 957

SUMMARY POINT 13
The Celebrants of the Sacred and Divine Marriage Feast of the
Lamb and His Wife and the Divine Liturgy of Cana 960

SUMMARY POINT 14
Jesus Tried to Express the True Reason for His Coming,
His Marriage, and His Death to Peter .962

SUMMARY POINT 15
Peter 964
    15A 979

SUMMARY POINT 16
The Consequnces of Peter's Choice for a Rational Human
Consciousness Versus a Transcendental Consiousness 980

SUMMARY POINT 17
Jesus, the One True, but Dimidiated Messiah: The Revelation
of His Female Counterpart 985

SUMMARY POINT 18
Time Goes By So Slowly, and Time Can Only Do So Much:
Are You Still Mine? A 2000+ Year Reunion Sacred Teaching 991

SUMMARY POINT 19
From Cornerstone to Keystone: The Many Titles of Mary 997

SUMMARY POINT 20
A Very Profound Sacrificial Presence: Sacred Teaching 1004

SUMMARY POINT 21
Who is the Real Bride of Christ? What Are Her Responsibilities?
Sacred Teaching 1006

SUMMARY POINT 22
A Deeper Understanding of Divine Consorts Sacred Teaching 1010

SUMMARY POINT 23
The Human Consciousness and Early Church Rules Changed
to Suit the Need Sacred Teaching 1012

SUMMARY POINT 24
How Can One Believe in Supramentalization? 1019
*Connections of Religions to Deities with a Deeper Understanding
of Supramentalization*

SUMMARY POINT 25
Resurrection of the Body Sacred Belief 1021

SUMMARY POINT 26
Paul. 1027

SUMMARY POINT 27
Final Review of Foundational Beliefs 1032

SUMMARY POINT 28
Metta: God's Love, and How it was Meant to Play Out in
Human Love Sacred Teaching 1036

SUMMARY POINT 29
The Fullness of Time: Sacred Mysteries and Eternity 1039

SUMMARY POINT 30
The New Adam and the New Eve: Understanding Free Will 1045

SUMMARY POINT 31
Understanding Metta as Sacrificial Love. 1049

SUMMARY POINT 32
The Victim, the Altar, and the Sacrifice 1052

SUMMARY POINT 33
I have Died Every Day Waiting for You 1056

SUMMARY POINT 34
And in the End, the Love You Take is Equal to the Love You Make . . . 1064

SUMMARY POINT 35
You are Invited to the Sacred and Divine Marriage Feast:
The Lifeline of the Kallahs and the World. 1065

SUMMARY POINT 36
The End Time: The Holy Kallahs 1068

SUMMARY POINT 37
Metta: The Sacred Love of Eeshan Spirituality I am Meek
and Humble of Heart 1071

SUMMARY POINT 38
"You are no Greater than your Master" 1078

A Heartfelt Acknowledgement *1081*

Preface

It is said, *"Whenever a timeless mystery enters into time, the most powerful positive vibrations of epic proportion, brings a disruption of negative energies taunting these powers and causing change."*

That was especially true at the time Jesus began His public ministry. Often Jesus' followers forget that He and His Teachings were NOT immediately accepted. Once Jesus began making a case for not putting total trust into a human being, He saw the fulfillment of the prophet saying: "You will be met with a Rebellious People." He knew what He was teaching would go against the grain of the religion of the time. He talked about how He would be rejected by the Elders, the Chief Priests, and the Teachers of the Law, He tells how He would suffer by their hands and be killed. To this day, most followers of Jesus do not know that this "rejection" came as a result of His Teachings which made people aware of the True meaning of Love of Neighbor—second only, to Love of God. Though He taught the Truth, He also taught that human truth is based on human opinion, and this can always be altered, whereas God's Word cannot be altered; and this is where Persistent Memory comes in. The positive vibrations that brought about a disruption of negative energies that taunted the powers and caused change are present once again.

As the Word of God Himself was always subject to "tests" and always questioned, as was the Origin of His Authority, Jesus made it a point to differentiate how human interpretation will always be inconsistent and flawed. Being God His Words were perfect, timeless and unchangeable. Jesus did not borrow from the "Old Law" as often we are told, but rather, brought the true interpretation and meaning of the Law to God's People. Being Human, He experienced life in "all ways" even in marriage.

This mystery was and continues to be a source of contention even though we are told Jesus was truly human it is denied that He could have an attraction to a woman, fall in love, and get married.

Knowing human beings, He often warned of His Words being omitted or other words being added to His Teachings. He warned how His Words would be reconfigured to serve a meaning or law causing humans to lose track of the spirit, resulting in God's Law becoming inconsistent and flawed due to corruption. Why would Jesus address this? Because he knew that this was a common factor and means to sway the mind and guide masses according to an ideology, not necessarily to salvation. These powers are also present today.

What makes the Eeshan Religion and beliefs different is that they are being presented against this backdrop of traditional writings and scriptures, with teachings connected to the Ancient Perennial Wisdom, (meaning always TRUE), which when one is exposed, will resonate through God's people, no matter their race, culture, sexual orientation, religion, or spirituality, just as Jesus' Words did.

Our beliefs are our own. No one is expected to leave their religion and follow us nor will we turn anyone away from the celebration of our Marriage Feast Eucharist because they are not Eeshan. This is because it is our mission to fulfill the requirements according to Jesus' parable of the Wedding of the King's Son, which the King sent for those on the byways and highways to come and celebrate as those who were invited refused to come. It is however, necessary to become Eeshan in order to receive the other Mysteries/Sacraments of our Religion.

So, where do Eeshans get their authority to present these teachings as "true?" From the One who was married to Jesus Christ. For in marriage they are One and Jesus promised a Helper, in a sense that She brings to fulfillment the need and furtherance of God's plan for salvation in these end times. Through the process of Supramentalization, we now have the Helper and the "truths." It is up to the individual to believe, accept, and follow.

Foreword

With the obvious desolation of spirituality, it is no wonder why at this time in history—where there appears to be a tear in the fabric of humankind's heart, emptying itself of life—that we discover there is an outpouring of divine love coursing back through the tear—providing a spectrum of singular grace. Is it God? Of course it is. Who other than the All in All is wise enough to know what will bring comfort and peace of mind, body and soul, and use sublime love to fill this void?

God once again sends humanity 'the one' who 'is one' with the Divine Masculine to reveal the truth necessary to heal the deepest wound and mend the fascia of the heart, thus stabilizing and securing salvation.

The only-begotten Child who became our only begotten parents—came to restore what had been lost, and by their sacrifice would preclude such future errors designed to interrupt God's intentions and plan for their children.

In the folds of time, what was guarded and covered over by God—the Divine Feminine—patiently bided the time until the ideal moment had arisen allowing for the folds to be unfolded to reveal her name.

All that is required now is for one to desire and believe that all is possible with God.

Incarnation was a process which was used in bringing about the Divine Masculine presence into the world, in its being active in the undeniable marriage of the King's Son as Proof of God's unconditional love for us. However, in the case of Mary Magdalen, these present times supramentalization was used for the return of the passive Divine Feminine. Most definitely, however, first and foremost—we find that supramentalization serves to once again ignite the truth with the Divine Feminine now as the active Consort. But we would be remiss to not acknowledge that her presence originated and is grounded in the most intimate act between twin flames and soulmates—the love she and Jesus shared.

It is no wonder that the songs that tell of their love would be "Once Upon a Dream," which could very well have been "the dream" of Mary Magdalen during her suspended sleep and her response to Jesus when she was awakened.

The second most resounding language of the heart could, without a doubt, be found in Ecclesiastes, where the river flows to the sea and then flows back again. Their song "Unchained Melody" of today expresses the desire of a bridegroom nervously awaiting the moment he will be reunited with his bride in this world, with his heart filled with an innocence and anticipation that had been building over so long a period of time—a time where he was apart from his beloved. Because their love flowed like the river to the sea and they were never really uninterrupted from one to the other—they were never separated—a promise he made to her from the Cross.

Welcome back, Mary!

A Note from the Author

Though, without a doubt the central theme and foundation for the Eeshan Religion, is Christ's marriage to Mary Magdalen, or by their divine, eternal, and infinite component, the "Marriage of the Christs," the author feels it necessary to identify the unwritten yet entrenched thread of love that still divinely exists.

It is for this reason the TRUTH is told by the only One who can speak these words, namely the DIVINE FEMININE. Though the choices that our First Parents caused the deep wound between God and humanity, this bond remained unbroken; and it is this bond that is what unites our Begotten Parents to our souls. This unconditional love of God despite Adam and Eve's choice and those which have clearly demonstrated through the negligence of Peter and his successors for over two thousand years may have weakened 'our' love for God, but proves the steadfast love of God for us.

INTRODUCTION AND GUIDE

TO READING WITH A TRANSCENDENTAL VIEWPOINT

This book is written from a transcendental point of view. It is not meant to be read and absorbed like any other book one has read. In order to appreciate this transcendental point of view, one must in a sense, 'unlearn' everything one knows first. To do this we suggest that you try to remove all preconceptions, expectations, and as many frames of reference from your mind as you can.

Entering into a transcendental realm requires that you 'unlearn' in order to learn, thus allowing for new concepts, new theories, newly found information. Perhaps information once thought to be heresy will now shed new light necessary for your journey into the transcendence. As learning is the gathering and handling of all things outside of you in this the material/external world and encompasses things such as how to manage day to day affairs, your job, management of your time etc., unlearning is about letting go of the person you want others to see and exposing who you really are and what is inside you. These are those things that make up who you are as a person. As these things may not be obvious to someone else; however, they may be the very things you hide or suppress in order to present the person you want others to see, not the person you are or can become. In other words, you empty yourself in order that you may see yourself for the first time through someone else's eyes.

This is essential to point out early on, because in reading, the mind automatically begins to measure all the incoming information against what it/you have already gathered thus far in your life and against what frames of reference that have been placed in the mind through mental conditioning. All these things serve as 'reality checks' and 'evaluators' to the logical rational consciousness. These things find their expression in terms of personal 'likes' and 'dislikes,' personal standards, what one believes or doesn't believe. It's a phenomenon that is experienced on a daily basis in other activities besides reading.

This may happen when you find yourself suddenly encountering groups of people unfamiliar to you, or from another race or culture where an interior 'voice' instantly begins to generate various forms of commentary depending on what you have heard, learned, and how impressionable you are made by those daily experiences, and it begins to dictate what you believe and don't believe; it leaves no opportunity to explore and learn about those things which may seem foreign and unfamiliar. We believe the mind is a vast organ of files, and due to what we have been given as truth over the years, was merely the thoughts and opinions of only a few sources, and not necessarily from a God who is all-knowing, or omnipotent, omnipresent, omniscient and omnificent—whose words—though we are told are both living and vast—are written in ways that do not present this manner of thinking whatsoever.

God has been speaking into human history since the beginning of time, but without proper spiritual development, human beings have become increasingly deaf. They have been affected by the world around them, which poses rational/logic thinking especially in matters of religion and spirituality. Nowadays, we have a greater association with the gross physical body and are becoming more and more blind to the spiritual.

Over identification with the physical body and the senses essentially continues to move us further into a state where we live from the 'effect' of being, while, instead, we should be living from a state of 'cause.' That is, the human being has become increasingly absorbed by the power, force, and the experience of the sensation of the body, as opposed to being fully aware and transcendentally conscious—and is thus "out of balance" with the total human being God intended us to be. When this happens, the consciousness uses the 'body' rather than the mind as one's *personal vehicle* in everyday life in the physical world. It's amazing that though we appear to "think" more—we fail to "reason" properly. We fail to find just cause, explanation, or justification, and act mostly on the emotions of those we befriend, or who may have similar ideologies as we do. We have often chosen to trade our ability to form judgments by being open to concepts and opinions of others—to being brainwashed so subtly, that we become unaware of the many social, intellectual, and psycho-emotional methods that are impacting our innate intuition so often by using abusive language or key notes. In turn, it results in making one feel it is necessary to enforce someone else's will as your own. In other words, do you feel you need to be angry at something someone else is angry about to the point of dismissing what you know is right? Or are you finding it easier and easier to engage in a mindset that is fueled with anger and violence just to make "an impression?" Often those who readily engage in anger and violent ways start to find themselves going beyond normal pathways into rage, which is anger that is out of control. Often times, those in positions of authority who fuel such feelings are found to be and have been very unhappy people all of their lives—while their followers do not often have such deep anger but are fearful of being ridiculed.

Being aware of everything material, we somehow have never noticed we were blind and deaf, and totally unaware of why we feel such emptiness, loneliness, and are unable to find love and happiness. The answer is simply that this hole in our heart and soul is due to being deficient of the Wisdom of God, found only in the transcendental consciousness. As human beings become less spiritual they can no longer recognize the Wisdom of God, most notably *the Sophia Perennis* (the Wisdom Perennial), which permeates all of existence, but, instead, we get caught up in someone else's will. What happens next, is that you are under an illusion of a stronger, more independent free will, one in which you cannot see an opposing point of view because your mind has been conditioned to believe that any other opinions, or facts, that might seem contradictory are immediately warped by one's own mind to automatically be 'wrong.' In other words, no matter how much evidence is provided to prove the opposing reasoning as true, the person who processes a closed mind, as in a self-induced, or group-induced, so-called state of "brainwashing," will instead view and argue viciously that the people who don't agree with them are the ones deceived; and the evidence provided—which in fact disproves their thinking and/or conclusions—is not only wrong—but must be evil!

The further away we advanced from God, the less we are able to 'hear' and recognize God when that wisdom is spoken though a human agency. This Eternal Wisdom (or *the Sophia Perennis*) is exactly why God chose now for the return of the Divine Feminine, which is at the very foundation of the Eeshan beliefs found in this book.

Eeshans believe the absence of a morally formed and informed conscience, and lack of spirituality, is responsible for the decline of peace in the world.

The conscience is formed early in life, and yet that is one that is continually being groomed and refined further as a *morally informed* conscience, or even an *immorally informed* conscience. While it is the responsibility of the parent(s) to help shape the conscience when the child is young, it gradually becomes the responsibility of the young person to assume this responsibility for himself or herself up to and through the age of reason. The conscience is a guide which is consciously and subconsciously drawn upon in everyday life.

One way this method of formation of conscience can be described is through the Sanskrit terms *samskara* and *klesha*. There are a number of ways to approach the understanding of these terms, but for the present context, the following will suffice. A *samskara* is an impression made into the mind, a kind of "groove," that is created like rain water naturally flowing into an arroyo, so that when energy (*prana*) flows, it runs to this formed groove, or 'ditch' and makes it even deeper. This is how strong 'impressions' are made in the mind and in the conscience. This, we might see, is how our sense of 'values' is felt to us and sensed by us.

Secondly, there is the word *klesha*, which we could think of as a 'spur' in our heart-mind, an 'affliction' that is lodged in the forming mind and conscience, and which affects how we gauge and respond to pain from the point of the experience onward. A tragic situation or a loss, early on, for example, will shape the way pleasure and pain are gauged and how deeply they affect the person and his or her conscience. A *klesha* can be 'negative' in the sense that the experience leaves a 'bruise' in the mind which affects the way a person responds to various challenges, or discomforts, or pain in life; and a *klesha* can be 'positive' in that it becomes a sticking point for a person's frame of reference regarding happiness and goodness, so that the person is always measuring happiness according to that experience in the past, and so that it keeps them growing, moving beyond, recognizing, and appreciating the good that is happening in their midst. This phenomenon can be readily observed, and is useful in understanding the complexity of conscience formation, and how people come to understand what is good and what is bad, what is morally right and what is morally wrong.

This is where parents, teachers etc. guiding us through learning and experiencing life—whether easy or difficult—in a positive way is especially important. For example, how an adult reacts to, or the emphasis they place on, what is right and wrong will affect how the child sees life. This is especially true with the *favored* parent or teacher. If a parent displays such discrimination—this influences the child. If the favored parent is focused in an unhealthy way on eating, drinking and/or drugs—this will affect the child too, especially if the child is prone to a similar disposition because of inherited genetics.

The informed conscience is one that is researched and thought out through reason and logic is also enlightened by goodness, love and decency—which Eeshans would refer to as the *Light of God* that is the absolute gauge for all that is good and is what holds and bonds us together. Free will and interpretation may divide us, but *Absolute Truth* prevails. Without these, we cannot establish or discern what is good from what is bad, thereby creating a void deep within ourselves.

Though some may argue against the existence of an absolute truth, claiming human beings can only know 'relative' truths, it should be remembered that *Sophia Perrennis* is that *Light of God* that can be known through the heart-mind field and that is a human being's departure point from the limitations of the mind (which deals in the language of relative truth) and the launching point to the transcendental. The Truth exists independently of human beings and, indeed, in all things created. Its existence does not depend on human beings to conceive of it, or to believe in it; it is simply the original, primordial Truth and ground of being, from which all reflected forms of truth are derived.

Therefore, this simply means that to be more accurate in regards to the difference between the absolute truth and moral relativism, we need to truly consider our belief in God. If you believe in God, it is absolute truth; to not believe in God is moral relativism.

Again, Absolute Truth is based not on one's personal beliefs, culture, and historical circumstance, but rather on God's own revelation. As will be unpacked in this book, you will come to see that the Eeshan perspective is that while various cultures and religions all make the same claim, that God revealed himself, the problem of conflicting (or in fact, contrary) doctrines existing between them is due to the human tendency to superimpose human consciousness' egocentric pull, or tendencies, onto what God is said to have 'spoken' (revealed), thus creating apparent divergences.

We all need something to fill the void where a conscience and/or spirituality is lacking. We no longer have what we once embraced as the wisdom of God; so, we have now been turning to ourselves for guidance.

Today, we are taught that to be successful one must be focused; however, when we are more focused on ourselves, or what we are attempting to accomplish without balance, we choose our own selfish desires over the importance and needs of others.

This is known as a false ego (as opposed to a mind with healthy ego balanced by wisdom). This false ego, left unchecked, no longer allows one to feel the need to be accountable for one's actions, or to render to God or any Supreme Being for that matter, what is due them. This love and devotion for 'self' and 'self-gratification' is what the many of us in the world have made the center of all existence. This ego sees itself as larger than life and all that it evaluates—lesser than itself, to include the need for God. When the mind has nothing more than itself to which it is held accountable, it mediates between the conscious and the subconscious/unconscious mind and is responsible only for its own reality.

With a spiritually balanced mind, one would easily see why and how easy it is to discover what God reveals to human beings and thus enlightenment occurs. When one is enlightened, things muddied in darkness are wiped clean and the eyes can once again see truth—for no longer is the soul in a state of illusion and one can see the 'what' and 'who' of God and the purpose of all things created.

But spirituality requires a system of beliefs connected to the desires and directives of a loving God, which then embarks on a course of action requiring strength and courage. For to travel down this path, one can easily be derided, or looked upon, with skepticism and indifference, or even ridiculed by others as one's faith and belief in God dwindles; but to become the leaven for peace and love is well worth the sacrifice. Eeshans believe that the disbelief in God has its foundations in the hunger, pain, terror, and hopelessness we and our world are faced with on a daily basis. It is very difficult for those who do not believe in God to be converted, since their pain, and sometimes even a self-abasing attitude, turns them toward others who appear stronger, more confident, and who seem to be able to feel their pain.

These people, to whom they look, appear to be stronger as their solution is to abuse, fight, and/or attack the injustices of others, rather than finding solutions that are agreeable to both. There is one thing we must all remember: God's law cannot be changed. Saying that, one must also remember that God's law is the origin of all that is right and balanced. It is from here that we "will always" solve and find solutions to human mistakes and interpretations that hurt and destroy all that can make us happy. Without God's balance, there is always regret; whereas, with it there is never regret.

Each of us is given a soul with a natural predisposition towards *the Sophia Perrennis-Divine Wisdom*, which carries with it a transcendental consciousness. However, with the onset of the original sin we also possess a fallen nature—with a human consciousness attached to it. The conscience lies between the two.

The human consciousness includes the mind, body, and senses. It occupies a very limited range of consciousness, but is able to understand, through that limited mind and senses, very little. This is because it is so heavily wedded to the material energy; and so, the soul and intellect overly identify with the world of physicality, and eventually it is trained to think of the mind as basically the 'self.' This is the illusion.

The reality is, that God, being within a transcendental realm, is very present. God is not bound by any law physical or natural. In fact, God is the author of all law. This transcendental dimension is without limits, far above the limits of the material creation, but still accessible. In this way, God can speak through his creation, work through it, alter it, etc., but is not subject to it. So, it is safe to say, that from conception, we are still balanced because we possess the perfect transcendental, as well as the imperfect, human states of consciousness.

However, there are complications that arise after birth. This is due to the fall to the human consciousness. The human consciousness, via the human ego, is subject to being deprived of the Sacred Balance[1] and without guidance, can come to see its own existence as the *all in all*, and become swollen due to its saturation/identification with the physical body. The adult mind, however, always has a choice. We find today that more and more individuals are being led by their ego and cannot be but skeptical of the transcendental. Because of this, it minimizes the transcendental in proportion to what the ego thinks is necessary for its own survival. We are told that the ego-driven human consciousness, as a result, begins to advance rapidly, and continues to progress so that eventually it no longer sees itself as it truly is quantitatively—a spark from the fire.

The human consciousness on its own cannot accept such a reality except under certain very limited terms that are perceived as agreeable (and non-threatening) to the ego; and therefore, individually, or collectively, minimizes and relativizes God, in relegating *God* to a 'category' *of its own creation*, in order to be able to decide what '*God will be*' in relationship to itself.

This is because of the decision for a physical life resulting in the decline to a human consciousness which Adam and Eve made, along with the effects of entropy upon the body/mind/spirit interplay—through which human beings have felt the pull of illusion and of a physically centered/limited consciousness. This pull is so strong that individually, and as a group, human beings continue to choose to embrace this consciousness over and above the transcendental consciousness—since it is more familiar and has become easier throughout the centuries to do so, especially in the world today.

---

[1] Of the Divine Masculine and Divine Feminine. – Ed.

In the process, and increasingly so down through the ages, without effective, fruitful and balanced spiritual guidance, there has developed an ever-increasing communication problem between God and human beings. In lieu of this, it would naturally follow that human beings would develop, in turn, a communication problem between one another— *AS ABOVE, SO BELOW.*

The following are some basic principles based on the Eeshan perspective and an overview of some religions and spiritualities as they are directed via the human Consciousness with a 'prospective' view of what the Eeshan Transcendental Religion seeks to provide, which will also be presented and woven throughout this book.

LESSON 1

WHAT IS TRUTH?

UNDERSTANDING THE DIFFERENCE BETWEEN RELIGION AND SPIRITUALITY

Though many established Christian religions claimed to possess the truth and ignore those who have tried, and continue to attempt to present the truth—we believe in actuality they only possessed a truth according to the 'interpretation' of any one of many human, rational versions of what may be considered truth—not according to the transcendental, which is very different. Eeshans see that because humans teach from this perspective, *the onus probandi*—the obligation, or burden, of proof—is on us, and what we believe to be true will ultimately rest on how we assert what we present to you. Eeshans feel that we better understand, and see more clearly, what is necessary for others because we were there—we were victims of this propaganda also.

There are many religions throughout the world and though the word religion is used, few are transcendental. Being Eeshan, we hold Jesus is true God, true Man, second Person of the Blessed Trinity. He was, and is, the Master of spirituality; and we, as Eeshans, attest to this. Our religion is transcendental in its teachings and origin, and we believe Jesus' mission was to bring us back to the transcendental life God intended for us, while complimenting the human forms we were destined to have—via Adam and Eve.

We feel that because we lost (or better stated, were robbed) of so much of what Jesus, as the Divine Masculine Messiah came to restore, now more than ever we need to bring the truth, so that God may obtain the sacred balance that can only be restored by means of transcendental consciousness.

What happens when a religion relies only on a secular, rational, logical, perspective? The end result is that though professing a path to God, it does not teach with the transcendental overtone, and loses, or lessens the Divine quality of Jesus manifested in not just one facet but in endless facets—as God.

Though professing, they teach the true teachings of Jesus, which in fact 'if true,' Christian religions would have provided solutions for today's social and economic issues, but the *truth* is, they haven't come close to doing so. Deeply entrenched within their own errors, we find that the nondescript answers to these issues continue to filter down into the daily lives of God's people. Ironically, while church politics of this era encapsulate social justice, abortion, and gender equality over salvation, we see more evidences of divisive and sectarian undertones that capture a particular intended outcome with tremendous spiritual losses. In other words, they say one thing, but don't practice what they preach. Hypocrisy runs rampant.

This is a complete reversal to the outcome for which Jesus came. First of all, when he talked about love of neighbor, it was not meant to become the priority over loving God with one's whole heart, whole soul, and whole being. Secondly, it was not intended that we should only give from our overabundance. It was not an excuse to ignore indecency or immoral acts of one's neighbor out of a "love;" because this is not love, but rather a misplaced, misinformed, and willful ignorance that is confused with nonetheless than compassion itself.

Eeshans have witnessed as religion as falling under a 'formidable political' stance, yet most of what it is fighting would cease to be a problem had they followed Jesus' teaching the way he intended—by reprioritizing the transcendental, and by not allowing politics and secularism to become independent organisms within its walls, thus making it central to faith. God is, and always should be, central to one's faith.

The soul needs spirituality; and though you may have no spirituality, or are not seeking truth, you are ultimately responsible/accountable to provide it (the soul) with a spirituality.

Remember spirituality and religion are not the same thing. Spirituality may or may not lead you to a particular religion; and a religion may not provide you with spirituality. One thing is for sure, that two things are most important respectively: either or both should be at the heart of bringing out the best in you, and it should make you aware that you were created in God's image and likeness, and that your life was ransomed by Jesus Christ, as Eeshans do; or at least that you must answer to a higher loving and an Authority of goodness to whom you feel you owe your life.

Eeshans profess, that by understanding the sacrifice made by Jesus, Jesus' sacrifice was much more than the celebration of Christmas and Easter. What God did for our salvation is not something that can be boiled down to two holidays or holy days. There is an obligation due God which filters down to an obligation that we have to others. Each of us is not living alone in this world, and each of us has an obligation, therefore, to remember that all we have and have accomplished came directly from God and from the hands of others. Inherently, we should live as Jesus taught: Love God above all things and love your neighbor as yourself.

Both your religion and/or spirituality should make you thankful for your life, for it is precious—regardless of how you feel, or are made to feel about it. Whether you seek to thank God from whom all good things come, or whether you consider all things around you as good or not, do attempt to view each experience in your life as coming from God's hand, and with your best effort it will have a good result. If you are not happy with your life, perhaps you are missing why your life is disappointing. Perhaps it is the result of negative choices—so, make better ones. Perhaps you're missing the strength that God sees in you that if you look or tried hard enough, you can turn your life around to help others find strength in themselves.

Remember that the cause of much of our difficulties with God are the results of negative choices—ones made either by us or those who raised us. We don't have to turn out badly because our parents or guardians chose that path. In retrospect, God always forewarns us and if we miss the warnings, answers can be found and revealed in hindsight. What we consider as bad decisions can also have positive results if we correct them.

LESSON 2

CHOOSING A RELIGION OR SPIRITUALITY

If you feel grateful for certain people who were good influences on you and made you happy, be thankful that God put them in your life. It should not matter the age, color, creed etc. of these people, or if what they did was personal or something they did that affected your life in general. We are part of a family under God as taught by Jesus. What should matter, however, is if whatever your religion is professing, or the kind of spirituality that you are involved with, is making you a better person.

Be sure your spirituality is bringing out the best in you and for you. If you are searching for or embarking on choosing one, be sure it is what you're are searching for; and that it teaches decent and morally good beliefs, as you will be subject to living these teachings. Before you join, be sure that the belief system is not unbalanced, or that it supports any kind of immorality and violence, or is rooted in oppression, causes paranoia, exercises sexual discrimination and sexual favoritism, or abuse or anything that focuses on isolation, fear, or lack of respect of others, or of self. If it does, it is not from God. These kinds of beliefs are against both the laws of God and the laws of human nature.

Whatever the case may be, Eeshans strongly encourage you to approach spirituality as seriously and as effectively as you would medical/health insurance, etc. Be sure you are getting what you need and that the spirituality you live or choose satisfies your innate core beliefs and is leading you to peace of mind, heart and goodness, respect, faith, hope and love.

The failure or success of the communication between a religion/spirituality is the responsibility of both that religion/spirituality and the follower.

Persevering but not understanding the beliefs, or disagreeing with a belief system of any religion or spirituality, doesn't just lead to lack of understanding, it also potentially leads to disorder in personal as well as all human affairs to the point of chaos, conspiracy, and destruction of independent, free thought. These are instruments which virtually put an end to spirituality and create a distrust for any God-centered guidance.

LESSON 3

BLINDING IGNORANCE DOES MISLEAD US

ARE WE GUILTY OF TRUSTING IN HUMANS MORE THAN IN GOD?

Truth will set you free. The problem today is discovering truth. With everyone's version of the truth, and with the growing disbelief in God who is truth, where do disbelievers find truth? Religions and Spiritualities provide belief systems, but with the discovery of so many white-washed temples, we find that people are turning more to only trusting in their "gut." The fact is, truth can only be found in one who is good, holy, perfect, uncreated. Human sources apart from God may most likely be a perversion of the truth.

So, what about religion? You should not just accept a religion because you are told to or born into it. Not everyone believes the same things but what you believe should always be based on truth.

Christ's teachings are based on 'giving to God what is God's and to Caesar what is Caesar's;' but this requires that you know, love and serve God, and love your neighbor.

So, where do you find truth? God has always been considered the origin and source of truth. It's becoming more and more difficult nowadays because more and more people doubt the existence of God. If you aren't directed by divine guidance, you will not find truth—just the imperfect human version of truth. When this happens, a virtual truth is presented, which causes discovering the real truth practically impossible. With the faithful being let down with regards to their trust in the magisterium of the Catholic Church, we look to the past for the reason why and when it all began. First there is the blatant mishandling of the atrocious actions of its cardinals, bishops, priests and nuns by turning a blind eye to its horrifying cruel behavior of trafficking of women and children for sexual services in a mixed bag of corporal punishment involving great suffering over the centuries and stretching into the present times. With such revelations, the faithful and victim followers of Jesus see truth much differently and are not readily prepared to brush them off as the church proclaims this as a "time of healing," as if they wish to just expunge the memory of it and become better at concealing it.

This imperfect human version of truth resulted in faith being redefined and lost in translation. People are now sifting through the ashes of the burnt offerings once believed to have been presented on their behalf to God by the perpetrators who were once thought to mirror God.

As a result of this, the faithful now feel the responsibility that the church claimed to have is theirs; and, thus, the teachings of God are left in their hands. You can't serve two masters. Therefore, the laity feels they must preserve those teachings that they believed were as close to what Jesus taught as possible—against the backdrop of the "official teachings and practices." Presently it appears that all of these issues created quite a conundrum: either we serve our neighbor at God's expense or we serve God and all benefit; but what if serving God is becoming less and less an option? From these thoughts emerges a cry for a religion that satisfies and resolves all issues.

There are many who claim that secular religion is the way to go. Eeshans point out that the downfall of secular religion is when secular perspectives become the center point of religion. The transcendence quality and true intention of what and why Christ lived among us is forfeited, as it has been, and in what was always thought of, as His religion.

Though secular religions seem a reasonable alternative to some, without a balance we see from studying and observing, that what happens next is inevitable: suspicion, fear, and paranoia will rise to the surface as human logic and reasoning are finite. As humans become 'God,' wisdom and the infinite disappear. So, it appears that the Catholic/Christian faiths brought with them more of what a God-fearing (meaning respect for God) people needed for spiritual strength and love with secular religions falling short. What if these Catholic/Christian religions are also flawed? Would this then show that there should also be a greater emphasis on the spirituality of the Religion you are seeking? Perhaps this is true, if it is, indeed, one which is truly centered on God and on God's law and allows a personal relationship with God AS JESUS TAUGHT. What if by reasonable deduction the church was actually guilty by its own accord and thinking that it could (and did) lead people to believe their haphazard explanation of why women can't be ordained—and thinking that they would not eventually get caught? Another tall tale of theirs is that Jesus was human in every way and experienced all of what humans experienced and yet they would not accept he was married?

Throughout church history, as in present times, and as with all religions, there was the fear of losing power and followers. That is the nature of humans and dates back long before the beginning of church history and continues to present times. That is why, for centuries, any independent thought that was viewed as challenging to an established religion was often seen as threatening, or was even treated as a conspiracy. Being branded as conspiracy theories—any information or study that challenged "the truth" as it had been regarded, whether through discovery via science or private revelation was immediately deemed heresy—whether it made sense or not. These judgments were explained as protecting the sacred; yet one must ask, how can protecting the sacred and building a personal relationship with the sacred at its roots, can that lead to the criminally atrocious injustices launched against those who in their good faith were seeking to love God?

With religions that were established thousands of years ago, it is difficult to find their exact origins and foundational teachings. The Catholic Church claims infallibility and indefectibility with regards to her origin as beginning with the teachings of Jesus Christ in the 1st century AD and in the province of Judea of the Roman Empire. The contemporary church says it's a continuation of the early Christian community established by Jesus Christ,[2] which was based on the death, the resurrection, and the

---

[2] "Catholicism and the Jewish Story." Catholicism and the Jewish Story, Jack White, www.jewishwikipedia.info/catholicism.html.

ascension of Jesus Christ, approximately 30 AD. It did not successfully become established until 325 AD, when Emperor Constantine tried to unify it with the fragmenting of the Roman Empire.

Though to most, these facts are not important, they are important because she by proclamation, decrees that the church was instituted by Christ at His death and claims that she is the Bride of Christ protected by the Holy Spirit; and the gates of hell will never prevail against her. The Catholic Church is supposedly the institution of salvation until the end of time—via the succession of Peter and the apostles and their successors. Eeshans have found reasonable doubt to these claims and will present their case throughout this book.

Since the onset of Religion and spirituality, it has always been accepted that God gave Laws to a few and the masses had to obey them. There were always and always will be unanswered questions that confuse followers. One such conundrum is: how the Catholic Church says that the Jews are elder brothers in faith when both present opposing beliefs—one denying Jesus was the son of God and Messiah, while the other claims salvation only by Jesus. How then can we say that the leaders of the Old Law who denied Jesus are our 'Elder Brothers in faith'[3] when as elder brothers they rejected him, called him a blasphemer, and even though Jewish law expressly forbids a person from judging a case, especially if they are already negatively positioned against the accused, or the accuser,[4] and the charges were originated by the judges themselves? False witnesses were used at his trial in order that a conviction could be achieved (Mark 14:57 and Matthew 26:59-60). So serious was this foundational principle that lying in court was punishable by the death penalty.

---

[3] This is pointed out as an example of philosophical contrariness and hypocrisy on the part of the church authorities. What the Jewish people choose to believe or not believe with regards to their traditions and Jesus as the Messiah is between them and God; no judgment upon them as individuals or a people is implied in this discussion. Rather, in a civil modernity one would hope that there is room to agree to disagree and leave the rest to God. – Ed.

[4] "The Trial of Jesus." Bible Study, www.biblestudy.org/basicart/the-trial-of-jesus.html.

Another example of why the term "elder brothers" does not seem to be conducive to describing the connection is just how many times Jesus rebuked the Pharisees as is seen here:

Jesus said to the crowds:

> I will send Prophets and wise people and experts in the Law of Moses to you. But you will kill them or nail them to the Cross or beat them in your meeting places or chase them from town to town. That's why you will be held guilty for the murder of every good person, beginning with the good man Abel. This also includes Barachiah's son Zechariah, the man you murdered between the temple and the altar. I can promise that you people living today will be punished for all these things.[5]

And in John 5:45:

> Do not think that I will accuse you to the Father; that one who accuses you is Moses, in whom you have put your trust.

In both of these verses, Jesus' describes His suffering and death, as well as who the perpetrators are. But the Pharisees, or the Sadducees, are the only issue with the Catholic teachings. Evidence shows how a similar warning was given to another in whom the church bases its foundational 'rock' that it says the church is built on. Let's take a look.

The story tells how Jesus takes Peter, James, and John to a high mountain. Here on Mt. Tabor, we read about a very defining moment experience that Jesus allowed these men to witness. This was a moment in which the human consciousness that Jesus spoke against was being witnessed to, and at the same time that Jesus not only confirmed that Moses and Elijah knew and witnessed to Jesus, but that Jesus was a divinely sanctioned liaison between heaven and earth. That Jesus was standing between Elijah

---

[5] Cf. Matthew 23:34-36.

and Moses, and they were talking with him is very significant: for this event identifies him as the fullness of both Prophecy and the Law.

This is, however, from the Eeshan perspective, and is not the only reason Jesus had Peter with him on this day. One can't believe that this event was a surprise to Jesus. He wanted the apostles to be witness to this event also, as witnesses give testimony to the truth, and are usually required for confirmation. However, knowing human nature as a Master would, it was most important that his true identity was witnessed and confirmed before these three in particular (two witnesses are necessary, however in this case because of Peter's problematic disposition it was thus fitting that Jesus had two credible witnesses to the event taking place, and those two witnesses to what Eeshans believe in was Peter's lip service).

At seeing this, Peter's excitement rises, and he tells Jesus that he wants to build three tents. This moment in time speaks volumes, as Jesus stands before the apostles just as a voice from heaven says: "This is my beloved Son, whom I love. With him I am well pleased. Listen to him!" (Matthew 17:1-13). Without a doubt, his identity, indeed, is revealed.

There can be no mistaking now that he is the Son of God. All he taught, and would teach regarding his Father in heaven, and that he existed before Abraham etc., would lead back to this moment when they saw with their own eyes, and heard with their own ears—that He, indeed, spoke the truth.

Afterwards, Jesus tells them not to tell anyone about what they witnessed. Perhaps we will go a little further and look at Mark 8:27. On the road to the villages, around Caesarea Phillipi, Jesus poses this question to his apostles. "Who do people say I am?" They said, "Some say John the Baptist; others say Elijah, and still others, one of the prophets." Jesus then asks Peter, "But who do you say I am Peter?" Peter answers: "You are the Christ, the Messiah." Then he says, "This did not come from you who are flesh and blood but from God." Jesus tells them once again not to tell anyone about him. Then he continues to tell them that he will be rejected by the elders, the chief priests, and the teachers of the Law. He tells how he will suffer by their hands, and be killed, and after three days will rise again.

Jesus has now begun making a case for not putting total trust in a human being—even those closest to you, for he was proving Proverbs 146:3— "Do not put your trust in princes, in human beings, who cannot save;" Proverbs 118:8-9: "It is better to take refuge in the Lord than to trust in humans," and Psalm 60:11: "Give us aid against the enemy, for human help is worthless."

Soon after, Jesus taught about how he would be rejected by the elders, the chief priests, and how he will be put to death, etc. (Mark 8:31-38). Peter takes him to the side and rebukes Jesus by telling him not to go into Jerusalem. Jesus turns to his Disciples, and looking at Peter, says, "Get behind me Satan! You do not have in mind the concerns of God, you are seeing things merely from a human point of view, not God's." (Mark 8:33). Then He calls to the crowd, and to his apostles (again identifying the character of Peter), and says: "Whoever wants to be my disciple must deny themselves and take up their cross and follow me." (Here we present other purposeful reasons why Eeshans know that the person who Jesus would entrust the completion of his ministry to, and who would be leading his people back to him after he left, could only be his *wife*; for she was human, but by their eternal marriage was also Divine.)

Peter was not only just human, but with keeping this in mind, we find in end times, just as it was in biblical times, and in fulfilling Proverbs and Psalms, it would be necessary for God to once again be a human, and via his eternal Female consort, thus be completing Him. In the "Book of Odes of Solomon," found in the The New Testament, we find the words, "Clearly you,—His Wife, the Rock" are written. And we present here a saying that goes perfectly with warning the populous about Peter: "Be careful who you trust. The devil was once an angel."

By saying the Old Testament 'prefigured' Jesus does not make up for accepting the opposing views, or making the Old Law as acceptable to elders, when nothing changed in the Old Law afterwards, and until present times; for we know by virtue of the fact that He is still rejected in light of the Old Law, and for the most part his very name is still thought of by many as a curse.

As we continue on, you will find how, despite Jesus' directive "do not tell anyone what you have seen," Jesus was, more or less, telling Peter

He knew that Peter was going to reveal, and would continue to reveal, all of Jesus' mysteries to Jesus' enemies.[6] That was what was behind Jesus' teaching on "you cannot serve two masters:" keeping good ties with those Jesus talked about regarding his suffering and death, and telling Jesus how much he loved him. Knowing these things, was why Jesus would address Peter's love. When Peter was identified as one of Jesus' closest followers, Jesus revealed that he (Peter) would deny three times that he knew him.

Jesus would do this because Peter was so easily intimidated, even as he knew who Jesus was and why he came, and would come to see how Jesus' prophecies about his death were realized. Jesus told Peter in front of the others, he (Peter) was more concerned for himself than to pick up his cross and give up his life.

Throughout time, the church had always explained away any mystery or teaching whether understood or not—by saying that it 'fell under the blanket of faith;' for the alternative was to be considered insolent. How much of Jesus' teachings were used and how much were lost or deliberately mistranslated? Who now holds the truth, if indeed Jesus' words and teachings, that ended the Old Covenant and began the New Covenant, were intentionally changed for the sake of a political 'human consciousness agenda?'

We know that there are unintentional alterations in texts that account for a lot of Scribal changes—but there could well be *intentional* changes that account for thousands of corruptions. And, what does it matter in the scheme of things? For God becoming human in order to die, resurrect, and start a church or religion for sinners seems to lack depth, and is

---

[6] Which led to a confrontation with Paul. Even if the case were to be made that Peter was trying to 'build bridges' with the Jewish authorities, or that they proposed to do the same with Peter, Paul was known to have been concerned with "Jewish spies" spreading 'false gospels' or who were trying to gather information any way they could in order to disrupt and exploit the beliefs and weaknesses of the new messianic community. Is it possible that Peter, in his pride and foolishness, did not realize he was being used as a pawn and continued to betray Jesus even past denying him during Jesus' trial? Then, as well as now, 'The road to hell' could be paved with 'good intentions.' It is the benefit of the doubt, here, that they were good. – Ed.

just the tip of the iceberg when viewing a plan of salvation; to corrupt his word is quite another plan. To do this obscures the truth about this undivided, uncreated God—the most holy, sacred, omnipotent, omnipresent, omniscient, omnificent being—is who we are talking about.

Today, with the means of technology, we are finding confirmation of the above, especially with regards to studies and research, and with findings that are supportive of what transcendental teachers and mystery schools revealed as harmonious with what Jesus actually taught. We also see more clearly the problem and ramifications of scriptural alteration and corruptions. So, while the church claims it is a fact that all scriptures were inspired and inerrant, there is some gray area to be considered when one sees how scriptures were modified over time, sometimes revealing tremendously serious contradictions … or questions as to how much scripture is directly from God and how much is from man.[7] We suggest our readers check out Bible.org, or any sound and reputed biblical commentary, regarding Scribal Corruptions, especially with regards to the New Testament, for some insight. Though we may not agree with all points of view, and will at the same time present our own viewpoints, this is a very good reading with a perspective that may help you see 'more clearly' how the Sacred Books were edited in different ways, or contain texts used to 'clarify the meaning for liturgical reasons.'

Furthermore, we find how continued blind ignorance only proves how little Christians through the ages really knew about Jesus, his teachings, his apostles, and church history. Let's just take a look at some facts that religious people blatantly ignore and often deny.

Aside from what we have chosen to write about in upcoming sections, let's examine a few of the most terrible years the followers of Christ lived through. Did you know that during the time of the Inquisition, 1232, and, again in 1542, for the purpose of suppressing heresy, anyone professing a different understanding or questioning authority or church law, was imprisoned, tortured, or put to death? The Knights Templar were suppressed and accused of heresy with their leader condemned to be burned at the stake for refusing to confess to false charges of heresy,

---

[7] Especially when the latter has a political agenda to secure and further. – Ed.

while the fact was that the Pope, at that time, was in league with the King of France, who sought by treachery to obtain the wealth of the Templar Order.[8]

The infamous influence of the Borgias in ecclesiastical and political affairs, and their reputation, especially Alfons de Borgia who reigned as Pope Callixtus III, and Rodrigo de Borja, who was Pope Alexander VI, exhibits that the 'leadership' of the Vatican followed the same lifestyle that Jesus inflicted titles upon the teachers of the Law and Pharisees for, such as 'hypocrites' and 'white-washed tombs.'

Galileo's conflict with the church resulted in his being excommunicated for saying the earth revolved around the sun, building on Copernicus' theory to the point of proving it, and then it took 360 years for the Vatican to admit he was in the right.

During the French Revolution, the Carmelite nuns were beheaded for having a personal relationship with Jesus. So, it became truth or consequence as so determined by church law.

Scandals continued throughout the centuries. Many nuns were slaves to priests, or were providing children for their pleasure, but no one could stop these horrendous acts, due to the paralysis of fear of the church's power.

The point we are making here is that the teachings, which focus on the truth of what Jesus intended were not ever really lived by many of the religious clergy or teachers,[9] and most definitely was brought to the people even at its beginnings with the apostles. Without the help of God, through the private revelations of Jesus and Our Lady, by her use of public apparitions and private revelation throughout the centuries, we

---

[8] There was also the element of paranoia on the part of the church authorities over how powerful the Order was becoming not just because of their wealth, but also because of certain rumors circulating among certain church authorities about what they 'knew.' – Ed.

[9] That is not to say there were not true saints and sincere, good men and women among the priests and religious through church history. But it is also true that one abused child is too many, and it only takes one rotten apple to spoil the bushel. Those who truly lived in the light of Christ, are known by Christ. Those who did not, who were wolves in sheep's clothing, spread disease and damage far and wide, even if they were not publicly known. – Ed.

would have lost even more of the greatness of Jesus. This brings to mind the question of why the few Eucharistic miracles, which aroused the greatness of the Sacrament, were suppressed by the church and downplayed, rather than nonstop celebrations being held around so sacred an event, that were intended to inspire awe and reverence for the Divine? Even today, there are Cardinals and Bishops who are unaware of these miraculous events. Others just don't believe them. Those officials within the church tirelessly looked for ways to prove these to be contradicting to church law, teachings, and tradition—for they were given directly to the people outside of the normal channels of church authority, or at best, eventually downplayed the celebrations to a minimum until they ceased for lack of interest.

As to the results of these miraculous occurrences, whether it be of a private or public nature, and barring those found to be false or fake, there were and are those that proved truly miraculous. It is the acceptance of God using these methods in the Old Testament and Jesus' miracles where God employs this means to secure the people's attention, as did the church. Later, when the mindset of the church changed relative to financial gain and political power, the people were told that one must be careful, for it is not only God that uses such things, but the devil and other evil spirits who disguise themselves, who also perform these signs and wonders to take one away from God. After that, this became the platform for critical, reluctant, and very scrupulous testing which then took years to interpret, confirm, and explain. Of course, the faithful, now afraid, were conditioned to look for evil first, and the church has played the occult 'fear card' ever since. This resulted in the disbelief in miracles and supernatural occurrences, and despite efforts to preserve Jesus' approved legacy of miracles, this has caused unrest and confusion among Christ's 'rational and logical' faithful. Now, one asks if these could perhaps be explained using modern technology.

Any miracle, or supernatural experience, is doubted by most and especially by the church at large, mostly in an effort to discourage the 'old mindset' of 'grannies and naive people' who were raised to believe such 'nonsense.' The next generation after that which experienced apparitions of Our Lady around the world was seen as hysterical, or as overly zealous followers, trying to make a case for the supernatural. These were met with even more hostility as the church attempted to suppress the ever-growing crowds driven by their hearts, and the deep interior sense welling up in the people that something essential was being robbed from them, but yet God was bringing it back. The people, whether directly conscious of it or not, were putting Our Lady—the Divine Feminine—*above* the church authorities. That is why, to this day, anyone who had experienced apparitions of Our Lady, miraculous signs, or witnessed the Stigmata, will not deny what they saw and experienced. Yet believers, from all walks of life were pressured into silence. It became obvious that the heart consciousness was being awakened by what appeared to be a persistence of memory[10]—which the church could not suppress—identifying the connection between the soul and the realm of the transcendental.

Now it seems that God's people feel embarrassed about hearing or speaking of such things, but they still clamber to at least 'check it out' when they hear of 'something or anything' that just might be *real*, and to revive that connection with God. Without cause to believe, God's people feel further away from God. They seem to have lost the connection to the divine in the places where they should feel it most, such as at church, or mass, or even in receiving Holy Communion.

So, as few have continued to cling to God by raw faith, which was the only means one may have due to conflicting directives and divisive personal opinions by the clergy, Jesus is becoming increasingly outdated and outmoded; and by the time the priest pedophilia scandals broke, it appeared that Jesus too had become complicit from silence in the face of such horrific abuse within the church. It appears that some people had actually succeeded in diminishing the need for God and they no longer had a sense of Jesus' purpose and the need for salvation. Are we reliving those teaching moments with Christ though we had ears, but did not hear, and had eyes, but did not see? Have we placed too much trust in human beings and not enough in God? Have we outgrown Jesus or anything that has to do with the existence of God's law?

---

[10] Something that may be dismissed or disproven, etc., but yet still, for whatever reason, just "won't go away". – Ed.

LESSON 4

CONTROVERSY BREEDS DIVERSE SPIRITUALITES

It is clear, that throughout the establishing of the Catholic Christian sects, transcendental teaching was not the focus—power was.

Over time, and with less and less of the true and fundamental building blocks of the transcendental teachings of Jesus, the secular-minded spirituality, and the rational consciousness, which the world claimed as the truths of Jesus Christ, evolved into what we find today: a weak foundation. It is becoming more and more of a classic secular humanistic culture which only sees everything through the eyes of the world and what it believes:

A. that God—and all things related to God are obstacles for living; God is not necessary.
B. there was not or ever was, any need for incarnations.
C. there is no real afterlife.
D. there is no reason for salvation from a "God;" science, not religion, has the answers to the universe as well as,
E. there is no evil, just the need for sociology, psychology, and/or criminology.

Without the knowledge of how Jesus taught, or without his complete teachings, and because there was what Eeshans call 'a breakdown in the succession of apostles' and their leadership, one can find Jesus' teachings mirrored and spread out in different ways, religions, and beliefs. Today, because the church continues to teach what they say are the foundational teachings of Christ in the Mystery of the Mass and the Eucharist, Eeshans believe that God has brought the timeless back into time, and that is to teach the fullness of what Jesus' true mission and teachings were all about to all those who desire the knowledge.

Often in our search for spirituality, we are confused about what we want. Do we want a spirituality that is based not on God, but on human beings? Is there a God, and was there a Jesus? These topics, and the controversy that surrounds them, allows for the creation of many different religions and spiritualties, each claiming truths important to those of a like mind. Each centered on a particular platform they feel is more important than the last. Questions arise such as: Is transcendentalism by human definition more important and enough to guide humankind? Or, is the adeptness of secularism more realistic for today?

What if the best of the transcendental and the secular humanistic religions were combined? Guess what? It could work—it would work if we knew that what Jesus taught would, in fact, reveal both the mystery of God and the realization of personal potential to the betterment of humanity, through social works and ethical consciousness. You would see that the view of suffering, though not related to the spiritual but to human vulnerability to misfortune, illness and victimization, was what Jesus taught when asked by those who gathered around the young blind man, "Rabbi, who sinned, this man or his parents, that he was born blind?" Jesus, from God's perspective, answered, "Neither this man nor his parents sinned, but this happened so that the works of God might be displayed in him." (John: 9:3).

The fight for equality for all and the secular approach to the many sides of divorce and remarriage, ending poverty, promoting peace, and protecting the environment are more of the objectives that most secular humanists protest in favor of; yet, if given the true teachings of Christ, we would find that these were also revealed in what Jesus taught by how he lived and died.

LESSON 5

TRUTH, HALF TRUTHS, AND AD HOMINEM

You see, if using only the human rational consciousness, one would think that what they were fighting for was contrary to what Jesus taught. Jesus' teachings addressed the things of God, which were greater than the things of human beings—and yet he taught on their level so that he could lead them back to God. This was "the beginnings of his spirituality," which leads to everlasting life; thereby it's an eternal spirituality based on truth. Remember, Jesus is God; he is not a religion. You can love him without being part of a religion, or spirituality, HOWEVER, to have the fullness of a Christ-centered belief system, you need to have a connection to those things He commanded us to observe; and these things never change!

This is because the things of God are permanent, lasting, and never changing. In other words, there is no doubting, or room for error, as God is the same yesterday, today, and tomorrow. God is Truth. This is so, for God is not created but is infinite in Self. That is how Truth is defined. For as truth is truth, because of God, should anything about God change, or be found to be in error, then there is no truth.

Over time, people have become accustomed to using 'half-truths' as a way of life, both with themselves and others. Eeshans feel it is the result of confusion within so many religious institutions where a double standard seems to exist.

The acceptance of the secular, human, rational mindset that has become skeptical, easily becomes more dangerous than not working with truth at all, since it brings along with it the unfortunate phenomenon of manipulation of the human consciousness by means of corruption.

Thus, clarity and truth in communication is not to be taken lightly, because without the transcendental consciousness, truth as people know it is flawed.

One cause, which led to the dwindling, or loss, of personal spirituality today, is discovering that Jesus' words and teachings *were* changed, or revised, and slipped into other books or teachings. Again, if it weren't for changing the meaning and purpose of Christ's mission, one could excuse the changes, or omissions, if it harmonized with other texts of the same liturgical meaning. Sadly, they don't—as we find in Rev. 22:18-19:

> *"For I testify unto every man who hears these words of the prophecy of this book. If any man shall add to these things, God will add unto him the plagues that are written in this book. And if any man shall take away from the words of this book, God shall take away his part out of the book of life, and out of the holy city, and from the things which are written in this book."*

This citation placed at the end of the book was actually spoken earlier by Christ and can be found in the Book of the "Confessions of the Twelve," which is a book deemed "heretical;" but was it *heretical*, or was it taken away because it would change the outcome of the goal of those desperate to attain and secure success? Whatever the reason, it is important to see how other materials, such as Gospels, scriptures, and writings that show more of the teachings of Jesus, which when laid out proposed prophecies, and that, if heeded, would have saved us from ourselves—and even perhaps from war.

In the following, you will find that it is much clearer, and very prophetic, about what would take place with this "new religion" after Jesus' ascension. It reads something like this:

> *"There shall arise after you, men of perverse minds who shall through ignorance or through craft, suppress many things which I have spoken unto you and lay to Me things which*

> *I never taught, sowing tares among the good wheat which I have given you to sow in the world.*"[11]

Based upon our foundress' life, her personal experiences and teachings in both private and public engagements, and with the help of technology, after 30 public years of deliberation, we present that Jesus' words, as well as parts of his life, were indeed changed or omitted. The moment his mission was presented from the basis of the human consciousness, it was rendered incomplete, because it was blended with a purely natural, observable but redefined phenomena, holding only a limited and vague tie to the transcendental version of the Plan of Salvation really was with an incomplete theology of the Eucharist.

Knowing that if His (Christ's) words were altered, changed, or relocated, with additions of what he didn't say, deleting what he did say, or by using half-truths in order to omit/alter/destroy foundational truths, and by creating heavily edited, or falsified texts, the next question that should arise should point to the reasons 'why.' Would the answers prove certain that the texts were falsified in any way, and in these end times, would God deem it necessary, once again, for us hear the voice of Jesus, as did those who followed him 2000 years ago?

If one is seeking to understand the truth, which radiates from God, certainly half-truths, as well as corrupted texts would result in confusion and would cause the mind to substitute doubt in place of faith. Why? Because what we were taught is engrained in us that it can be thought of as part of the 'junk' of our DNA, and because of the link of the mind, body, and spirituality of a human being.

Lack of answers to questions cause the mind to fill the gaps with self-led guidance based on one's own capacity, and limited sources throughout life, to form opinions sans balance, due to lacking one or all virtues of faith, hope, or love.

As we said, God will always forewarn us, and, indeed, did during that teaching found in the Book of the Confessions of the Twelve, which, leaving his lips, became a prophecy for these end times.

---

[11] From the Gospel of the Holy Twelve.

There are many texts presented as truths today about Jesus that did not exist until hundreds of years after he returned to Heaven; even some of these have changed through councils. We find that during those centuries, where what are called 'Sacred Scriptures' were selected and Tradition was being formed, that there was tremendous turmoil in establishing which 'truths' were to be taught. Not too many people today know the history of the church, while others simply turn a deaf ear so as not to hear, and close their eyes so as not to see. As Jesus taught us: "You have eyes to see, yet you do not see; and ears to hear, yet you do not hear." Why? Because it's easier not to hear or see. Who wants to go up against Goliath, especially when one is told that this Goliath has rights over you, given to him by God?

What if Goliath was not given rights over you? Suppose the succession from Christ was not adhered to, and the "one" chosen to lead and teach was replaced by the someone who coveted this leading role? Would not this account for the break in succession? Would not God then reveal this grievous situation by bringing forward the one who was chosen? Would not that Person be revealed as the true initiating Spiritual Master, who is the manifestation of the Original, as are her disciples?

In the language of Yoga, it is written[12] that 'we accept both the universal spiritual Master and the initiating spiritual Master.' If at present we want to follow Christ's orders by accepting him as Jagad Guru, and we think we do not require an initiating spiritual Master, we will certainly face the doubt about how well we can follow Christ's orders. The Supreme Lord or universal guru delivers His instructions about the Absolute truth only through disciplic succession. If the instructions that Jesus Christ gave two thousand years ago do not come through disciplic succession, or if we have to sort them out from books, then perhaps we may create a blunder, a perversion of the truth taught in the name of Christianity. We may even come to accept something opposite from what he taught, thinking it is his actual philosophy. The initiating Spiritual Master is also

---

[12] The entire paragraph is drawn from the book Amrta Vani, Nectar of Instruction For Immortality by Bhaktisiddhanta Sarasvati Thakura Prabhupada, because the language in question so aptly expresses the point of view of the author. – Ed.

Jagad Guru because [She] is a manifestation of the Original and delivers the message through the disciplic succession.[13]

We have all heard about propaganda used as a psychological mechanism to influence and promote a point of view. We have seen and continue to see many forms of propaganda and fabricated narratives occurring throughout history. Since the time human beings first figured out how to utilize it for their own purposes, we have become a people who are comfortable not only being comfortable, but also with being lied to. We, in turn, also lie and use half-truths ourselves.

It's a sign of the times. Truth, as was Jesus, has been an offense. That is because without God, human truth is human opinion and this can always be altered; whereas, God's word cannot be altered. It is easier to get rid of God.

This lends witness to the fall and growing distrust and hatred of all organized religion and/spiritualties. Why? Because as lying and half-truths become the norm, suspicion and distrust follow—even though almost everyone lies. Truth, on the other hand, is always in accord with fact, reality, and in fidelity to the original[14] and authentic source, which is here and always being God. That is why in the court system we place our left hand on a bible, and with our right hand held high, we then swear that what we are saying is truth before God as our witness.

We have established that lying, or half-truths (which are still lies). Pose the arguments against religion/spirituality. What is worse than discovering the deprivation of Christ's gift of the transcendental to us, is realizing that it prevented His people from knowing him and thus leads to knowing Jesus only via the human consciousness.

There is adequate proof that:

---

[13] Jagad Guru here is Jesus Christ, for his influence on the world has the power to transform it. The word comes from the Sanskrit term "jagat," meaning world, earth, the cosmos or mankind; and guru means 'teacher' and spiritual Master—who was and is Jesus Christ. So the title literally means "Guru of the world"—and Mary Magdalen/Eesha is a manifestation of the Original Spiritual Master. – Ed.

[14] James. "Cults and Heresies." Jesus Israel, 2016, jesus-and-israel.com/cults-heresies/.

1. there appears to be deliberate distortions of the truth regarding Jesus' personal life and the complete reason why he came and the mystery surrounding the need for salvation. This points to the fact that,
2. this was done to hold a certain sway in the mind so as to guide the masses according to an ideology, not necessarily salvation. And there is one who is at the center of the use of ad hominem. So, what is and where does ad hominem fit in? Argumentum Ad hominem is a logical fallacy in which an argument is rebutted by attacking the character, motive or other attributes of the person making the argument or the claim or the persons associated with the argument rather than attacking the substance of the claim itself.[15] So, when the truth is recognized—rather than admitting to it—the person(s) bringing the truth is attacked. It's like killing the messenger. If the messenger is carrying a truth which in and of itself is powerful enough to alter the established/known intention and goal, it is quicker and easier to discredit the messenger(s) and kill the bearer of bad news from which the news came, who ultimately is identified as the reason for the bad news; therefore, in killing the messenger, the news will 'go away.'

Who is this person at the center of ad hominem, and why? The why and how can be traced way back to the different forms of propaganda used by those in religious sectors of power and influence, in order to set forward in a group of followers a particular belief, or set of ideas. and for the purpose of maintaining control and to continue to martial a desired action.

At other times, propaganda and fabricated narratives were used to prevent the masses from hearing a truth, which would threaten everything that had been built up over a long period of time. Many examples are found in the history of the Catholic/Christian religions. Take the case

---

[15] "Ad Hominem." Wikipedia, Wikimedia Foundation, 15 Dec. 2019, en.wikipedia.org/wiki/Ad_hominem.

of a document that was found being brought to public attention around March 2002 after being "lost" for 700 years in the Vatican. This document pardoned Jacques de Molay and the Knights Templar of their "alleged" crimes, and yet the church allowed the reputation of Jacques de Molay to be destroyed, turning a blind eye to his being tortured, imprisoned, and forced to confess to these alleged crimes. Before his death, he proclaimed his innocence before all who watched his execution. Why was the church silent about this for all that time?

Whether by fear or lack of faith, God's people have fallen victim to a new kind of propaganda—only this time it is the destruction of faith itself.

This carries a lot of weight, as we now have some people who have remained too comfortable, secure, or fearful etc., to challenge authority, especially a birth religion. Just belonging in name to a church, people believe this covers their duty and obligation etc. to their faith. Though they may neither believe in most of its doctrines, nor actively participate in its activities, younger parents restore, or see the need, for spirituality if only for the duty to comply with Catholic/Christian directives to send their children to bible study, or to the sacraments, even though parents, and adults at large, have been taught that the sacraments are the "efficacious" signs of grace given by Jesus Christ through the church; yet, we still see adults fall away with little to no guilt. What does this then tell us?

Well, it speaks volumes. Despite what you have learned, no matter how much or how little, it is safe to say that you are where people were at the time of Jesus. In other words, rather than living a fuller life with God, people have regressed from what Jesus intended and died for, and have gone back to the human consciousness, or retreated to "duty." So then, who is at the center of ad hominem? And why?

LESSON 6

A Brief Overview of What Religion Was Like in Jesus' Time...
...and the 'Word,' Words and Laws

God's principle for obedience, as taught by Jesus, is that one must "never" confuse obedience to man with obedience to God. This was exactly what was happening at the time of Jesus. At the time of Jesus, the Pharisees and Sadducees made up laws saying these laws came from God; yet, Jesus pointed out that many of the laws they taught were contrary to the original teachings of the Torah of Moses, but the people would obey them in fear of breaking laws that came from God.

The danger with such errors eventually leads to leaders, and to those in authority, who govern by imposing fear on the people; and such is not an uncommon occurrence in religions or governments. Those in authority, especially those who are supposed to speak on behalf of God, have used this technique for the retention of followers. Who would know? The only way the people would know is if God, or a consort of God, told them so. The Pharisees' and Sadducees' actions were consistent with making up these laws.

Yet, even though the laws of man became so scrupulous, (see the Book of Leviticus) fear of breaking God's law was first and foremost in people's minds. Those in authority knew this, and used the law to incite this fear. In this way, its members were required out of obligation to God to stay. The difference in God's laws vs. human interpretation of God's laws is that human interpretation will always be inconsistent and flawed. We are to obey human law except where human law violates God's law.

Jesus was consistent in his teachings regarding God's Laws and man's law.

On many an occasions, he pointed out that human laws can't save you. Humans will always let you down because they are not perfect.

We feel the aforementioned is important because our beliefs are being presented against a backdrop of some traditional writings, scriptures, and teachings that most Christians and Catholics have been exposed to, and have been taught and studied for centuries. With the intention of providing a transcendent pathway aligned with that of Christ, it was tremendously rewarding to find, just as we believed, that our religion connected with the ancient perennial wisdom (which was always true), and, in particular with those variants, once considered taboo by the church, which by themselves, without a context, may fall short, but collectively yet still comes full circle as eternally true. Thus, when studying Jesus and his teachings, seeing for oneself that he is the living, eternal Word, and as such, is vast, it is found that His truth has no limits, no restrictions, and his power is boundless. God's living Word cannot be stopped just because we don't want it. God's words should, and will, resonate through and by his people no matter their culture, religion, or spirituality, so long as these are grounded in wisdom and return to God in love, kindness, and goodness.

As Eeshans, we believe wholeheartedly what was made available to us in several ways, and in particular this definition (source unknown) is perfect in its meaning:

> *Whenever a timeless mystery enters into time, the most powerful positive vibrations of epic proportion, brings a disruption of negative energies taunting these powers and causing change.*

These powers are present once again. With truth comes responsibility and duty. As followers of Christ one would then expect that anything and everything related to Christ would be whole and bring about love and life. For wouldn't words that Jesus spoke be held to the highest standard, as he is "the Word?" And wouldn't this be true especially in those who claim they speak on his behalf?

The "Word" of God himself, was always subject to 'tests,' and his words were always questioned; yet, when questioned about his teachings, and where his authority came from, he very simply told them his authority came from God.

Being the Word of God made every word he spoke timeless, perfect, and unchangeable.[16] As we mentioned, it is by his words of transubstantiation that the most perfect alchemy turns bread and wine into his body, blood, soul, and divinity. However, this is only partly true. It may be true by the beliefs of the church of Peter, but in Eeshan eyes, the mystery is not complete—it is just the beginning of the salvation story.

That is why it is most important that when someone who is in authority speaks of or on behalf of God, that it be true and factual to be taken seriously.

The meaning of words must result in more than reconfiguring the meaning of a word, or Law, especially with regards to Christ Jesus. Often times, we see where error enters when humans lose track of the spirit, and, thus, the letter of God's law; and they thereby, find a need to create a 'safe secure'—meaning, a protection against questions regarding the validity of the authority.

---

[16] As in no need of change; perfect as they are, in themselves. – Ed.

LESSON 7

UNDERSTANDING THE WORDS DOGMA AND INFALLIBILITY

Let's begin by looking at the word 'dogma.' A dogma is a principle, or set of principles, laid down by an 'authority' as *not being up for discussion*. In the church, it is used to mean that it came from Jesus. All religions and spiritualities have a belief system. A dogma cannot be changed, or discarded in any way, since it is the basis of the primary belief system. If changed or discarded, it would affect and disrupt the entire belief system.

Then there's another term, and it is called 'infallibility.' Infallibility is a word that means whatever is *unable to be wrong*. In the church's case, infallibility means that, in virtue of the promise that Jesus made to Peter, the Pope 'is preserved' from the possibility of error. It reads, **"when, in the exercise of his office as shepherd and teacher of all Christians**, by virtue of his supreme apostolic authority, the pope defines a doctrine concerning faith or morals to be held by the whole church." The infallible teachings of the Pope must be based on, or at least not contradict, Sacred Tradition or Sacred Scripture. The use of his power is called Ex Cathedra ("From the chair of Peter").[17] *Most people have become confused and actually believe that 'anything' the Pope says is infallible. This is not true—it's only when he is speaking in exercise of his office as shepherd and teacher of all Christians.*[18]

This is precisely what happened at the time of Jesus and the reason he addressed it with the Pharisees. Without ever correcting the errors,

---

[17] "WikiVisually.com." WikiVisually, wikivisually.com/wiki/Old_Catholic_Church.

[18] "Papal Infallibility." Wikipedia, Wikimedia Foundation, 13 Nov. 2019, en.wikipedia.org/wiki?curid=21701253.

the Pharisees were steeped in the misconception that "everything" they taught, said, or did came from God.

It is questionable, especially over recent years, which the use of infallibility has been misused and that the people themselves were taken advantage of. The term Ex Cathedra was brought into existence in the late 1800's. This was done because the church was having difficulties retaining the faithful. Questions arose, and, by virtue of that fact, it was necessary to take control to curb the loss of followers.

Another interesting historical fact is that there was a time, and this is evidenced from Vatican documents, that there were four popes occupying the papal chair(s), each in separate buildings, with staff. There was a Pope Benedict XIV (1425), who rivaled Popes Benedict XIII (1427), Clement VIII, and Martin V (1429); and during 1347–1380 there were three popes and saints, such as Catherine of Siena, a mystic and theologian, who was canonized under the pope from two separate popes of the time; and from 1314–1316, there were no popes! The point is, what if each of these claimed infallibility, and Ex Cathedra but contradicted each other, then who would be right? So today, who can speak Ex Cathedra? Today, we have two Popes, both alive, though one resigned, but each is Pope. In fact, on March 16, 2016 Pope Benedict XVI, who is resigned, broke his silence and spoke of a deep crisis facing the church post Vatican II.

Why is this important? Because in Jesus' time, so many claimed to speak on behalf of God; back then there was the Torah and also oral law, which was accepted as the word of God, or dogma. The Talmud, which are a compilation of discussions, also was considered divine authority; and the High Priest, who was the one who supposedly spoke on behalf of God, along with the Pharisees, Sadducees and Scribes, who were the interpreters and teachers of the Law. Then came Jesus who was the actual Word of God. Could it be, that at the fullness of time, God felt it necessary to stop the ambiguity in the name of God and correct the falsehoods, the half-truths?

What if what has been happening for 2000 years with the church is what Jesus addressed with the High Priest, Pharisees, and Sadducees in his time? What if the church had continued to make 'any' desired teaching a dogma by virtue of the Pope's opinions? And what if it had been doing so since Jesus ascended back to heaven and it just continued to do these things because via the human consciousness it had claimed authority illegally? As we see by comparison, there is so much similarity with the present-day church and the Jewish religion at that time to the point where Old Testament books are used as writings that Christian consciousness must relate and conform to, fulfill, etc., and that it looks as though after Jesus' ascension, almost everything He taught was being reshaped to agree with the old ways of the status quo religion. Indeed, this would absolutely change the outcome of Jesus' plan. So, what does this mean? It means that the church's Dogma would be wrong as it came from *men*—and the terms of infallibility and Ex Cathedra, along with its doctrine of indefectibility, that says it will last until the time of Christ's return, and that it will always be the proper and true representation of Christ's church in its essential doctrines,[19] will be beyond reproach.

Today we see and feel the effects of the loss of the transcendental, and see how the powerful religious entity of the church of Rome now governs, not in the name of Christ but by the human consciousness, while saying it alone speaks for him, as though God's Word could be, and continues to be, subject to the human consciousness itself.

---

[19] "Punishment for Our Sins." Church of the Eternal God, Church of the Eternal God, 2016, www.eternalgod.org/punishment-for-our-sins/.

LESSON 8

THE TRUE ROCK

There are people who claim that the grace they received from being in the church helped them through terrible struggles; some say this is true even through tragedy. One might ask, was it the Catholic Church, or was it Jesus, in whom you put your trust? Jesus said to those who were healed, "It was your faith that healed you" (Mark 10:52).

We know that the church does not allow contraception. Did you know that the reason for their denial of use is "to protect women from losing control of their bodies?" Yet, interestingly enough, it was said that 1,200 women were sexually attacked by 2000 men in German cities on New Year's Eve 2017 'because the men didn't know how to control themselves when they saw the women.' And the Pope calls the pedophilia situation within the priesthood, which include bishops and cardinals, a 'leprosy.'[20] Indeed, in Pennsylvania alone, according to the official1, 356-page grand jury report of August 15, 2018, six dioceses were implicated in an enormous scandal involving approximately 300 priests accused through the years of molestation of more than 1000 victims, and nearly 70 bishops who were involved in their cover-up and this is only at press time. The numbers are expected to go higher; also, this is merely *one* state. Eeshans see this as a perfect example of what happens when the duality of God is ignored. In 2003, it was said that least 34 priests were suspended in a sex abuse scandal involving women, including twenty men from a single parish![21] Africa reeks with sexual abuse, especially sexual abuse reported

---

[20] www.dailymail.co.uk news

[21] "Catholic Church Sexual Abuse Cases by Country." Wikipedia, Wikimedia Foundation, 4 Dec. 2019, en.m.wikipedia.org/wiki/Catholic_Church_sexual_abuse_cases_by_country.

against nuns, and AIDS is at an epidemic high. So how sad it is that the women the church was concerned about...?

This claim and others such as "the reason women cannot be priests is because their bodies are different than Jesus'" is meant to end the discussion; however, it cannot. The ruling on contraception is absurd, since it blatantly exhibits that the patriarchal consensus is that women, as a whole, do not know what's good for them, and so they again try to end the discussion. This was the mindset back in Jesus' time.[22]

Catholics are told the Pope is the successor of Peter, and that he is the 'supreme apostolic and official authority.' In keeping with what Jesus supposedly promised to Peter, and being the supreme apostolic authority over all Christians, he defines doctrine concerning faith, or morals, to be held by the whole church.[23] How does this work with the disregard for gender equality, and how does it pertain to the many Christian denominations who do not acknowledge the Pope, or Peter, as the "rock," and whose doctrines vary in their opposition to the "official authority" of the Pope?

Most people believe that the Pope is a world leader because he holds this title and is the supposed head of all Christians; but, in reality, he is considered a world leader because of his governing position as Head of State of the Vatican, a sovereign city-state entirely enclaved within Rome,[24] but governed under its own laws.

Given that Peter's plainly accounted reputation of pride, arrogance, and cowardice deemed him least likely to be chosen to continue Jesus' work, what if it could be shown that Peter was NOT the one chosen by Jesus to be the 'rock,' as claimed, but another was? What if Jesus pointed out that Peter, whose name meant 'pebble,' would crumble. What if by pointing to himself he said that *he* was the "Rock of salvation," and that it would be *James*, not Peter, who was to lead his church, as stated by

---

[22] I.e., the people are ignorant and the authorities know better because they are more intelligent, educated, and informed, etc. – Ed.

[23] The Catholic Encyclopedia. "The 21 Ecumenical Councils of the Catholic Church." The 21 Ecumenical Councils of the Catholic Church, www.catholicbridge.com/catholic/21-catholic-councils.php.

[24] "WikiVisually.com." WikiVisually, wikivisually.com/wiki/Old_Catholic_Church.

Jesus' own directives.[25] In the *Gospel of the Confession of the Twelve*, lection XLIV: 4, (Jesus), said: "And what if I was his Wife who would be the Rock that he would continue to build My church," prophesying the future when knowing she would be rejected, that he said, "and the gates of Hades shall not prevail against it; and out of this Rock (Mary) shall flow rivers of living water to give life to the peoples of the earth." Jesus says, "All truth is in God, and I bear Witness unto the Truth. I am the true Rock; and the one who thought he was first, will be last?"

What if Peter was that "pebble?" What if that was the true meaning of his name, and what Jesus was saying was this: "There is no one but one who is divine that he [Jesus] could build upon—for a human will crumble—and the one who is the cornerstone will be rejected." We have been taught that Jesus was the cornerstone that was rejected. But Jesus would pick one who is equal to him to continue his work. One who is not just human, and though rejected, will not crumble, and this someone would be one in whom he would 'build upon.' This would be the "one who would crush the head of the serpent" as promised: "… For if the cornerstone is not exactly right, the entire building will be out of line." For that specific reason, builders inspected many stones, rejecting each one until they found the one they wanted. The builder would "use" the rejected stones elsewhere, but these would never become the cornerstone or the capstone. Wasn't this what happened with Jesus? Interestingly enough, the one to whom Jesus was referring, would be Divine, and would be rejected just as he was.

What if, for two thousand years, the church's authority had been used ad hominem—to attack anyone who would defend Jesus' future 'Rock'? What if others, or especially the person of whom it was most afraid, came to light? Who was Jesus' actual choice? And further, could Jesus' description of white-washed tombs be carried over into our lifetime and be those who falsified the truth and taught as though they were following Christ's directive? For his choice had to be for one like him and could not be 'just'

---

[25] Gospel of Thomas, verse 12: The followers said to Jesus: "We know that you will leave us. Who will become our leader? Jesus said to them: In the place where you came from, you will go up to James the Righteous, for who heaven and earth came into being."

human. Also, speaking as a builder, was Jesus' story of how the builder would go through many stones until he found the perfect one? As in allowing human free will to play out in many Popes, until the time of his prophecy was at hand?

If Peter was not to be the leader, what would God do? Perhaps that was what Jesus meant when he said, "and the gates of hell will not prevail against her," for this "Rock" was chosen by him? With all that has been found, how could it ever have been Peter?

It is now the fullness of time, and perhaps the fulfillment of the prophecy itself, is very much at hand. Has God awakened the one who was His first and only choice? Eeshans say: yes. As he was the prophetic "rejected cornerstone," Eeshans believe that Jesus identified his wife as the 'true Rock,' for she would be the 'rejected *keystone*.'

The result would be seen in a failed integrity of the whole structure, which depended on the stone which Jesus called the stumbling block to his work. As a result, today we see today the collapse of the foundation of religions founded in his name, largely because the one who usurped the authority of the 'true' rock was an imposter, and was only human, not divine, nor ordained by Christ to continue his mission, in his place.

As it happened, the keystone who was most closely aligned with him, who was divine and who was the only one able to continue the plan of salvation, and the only one capable of continuing the correcting of the errors and hypocrisies as Jesus had done, was in fact rejected. Aligned with Jesus in every way, to include the authority given by God, Mary was to be the one who would lead God's people back to the transcendental by encompassing her eternal Consort—who provides the Way, the Truth, the Life, and Light.[26]

---

[26] Light is included here because of Jesus' identity as Light of the World. She 'bears' he who is the Light, which makes her the enemy of the one who was originally called to this position but forfeited it. – Ed.

LESSON 9

ETERNAL CONSORT AND WIFE: TWIN FLAMES

The Eeshan religion, by its beliefs, sees that there is a definite need for restoration of the transcendental-right now. This is not an alternative to what Jesus taught and came for but it was the reason for his incarnation and death.

Transcendence is not a New Age term, nor is it outside what Jesus the Messiah came for. Rather, it was what He espoused. Unless you understand what the Plan of Salvation entails you will not have the understanding that is necessary to obtain the fullness of what God intends for you.

There are those who are within and outside the established church who are or have been struggling with one issue or another with the Catholic Church, whether they just stopped going to church, such as many family members have, or have been affected by the scandals, who are just seeking a deeper spiritual guidance, and cannot find what they are told they should feel, and have for the most part become self-instructed. There are those yet drawn to finding fulfillment in other religions, such as Buddhism, yogic meditation, the practice of Zen, New Age thought, or an experience of some form of the Transcendental. At one time or another, with an almost religious fervor, our soul will cry out for more. The call for answers regarding Jesus has caused a conundrum with linking Jesus to faith, Catholicism and truth vs. alternative measures, and the methods that would take one out of the purely physical human experience—whether with or without God.

It is with joy and gladness that along with the mandate of God to "go and seek all the truths about My Son"[27] and with the realities presented to us by our Eesha, that we present to one and all, those of all beliefs, race, and cultures, "The Eeshan Religion."

For God's mandate brings with it the whole unfathomable, fascinating Plan of Salvation, and the true meaning behind Christ's title, "the Way, the Truth, the Life, and the Light."

The Eeshan Religion gives to God's people the Life, the Light, the Truth, and the Way following Jesus by reversing, once again, those ties to darkness back to the light of the transcendental.

It was taught that Jesus was, is, and always will be the Way back to God's intended plan for us. It is what we were *not* told that takes away from the Truth and God's intent for us.

We know Jesus possesses a divine, human. and though not used in his description, a sacramental nature. By being God, Jesus would have to be Sacredly Balanced. Entering into the real truth about God's salvific plan for us, one would surely see that in order to accomplish his mission, he needed to be *married*.

Eeshans teach that being God, and that as the Second Person of the Holy Trinity, He too was perfectly and sacredly balanced in his divinity. In his humanity, in order to restore us to our original transcendental life, Jesus would come as the Divine Masculine and at some point, "in time," and that He would be reunited with his Divine Feminine consort. In order to complete the reconciliation of humans to God, their life would not follow the ways of the Mosaic religion, for God's plan was to bring truth and salvation to all humankind, and it was not to be found in his birth religion.

What does this mean? It means that Christ's life, especially his marriage, would have to mirror the first sacred marriage—that of Adam and Eve, with all its blessings and eventual sacrifices, and more. Jesus' marriage would not only ransom our lives BUT would become the spiritual food that was lost by the "fall" to the physicality of Adam and

---

[27] This mandate is unfolded and described throughout the rest of this book. – Ed.

Eve, by satisfying the light body and immortal soul housed within the gross physical body. so that we may return to life with God.

For what had been lost by Adam and Eve, was at that time, all about to be returned; for it was necessary to end the famine due to loss of this spiritual Food (who is the body, blood, soul, and divinity of the only begotten 'child' of God), and by revealing the Truth and guiding God's people back from the path of human consciousness to the Transcendental.

Who better to complete this plan other than by mirroring not just the beautiful created life of Adam and Eve, but also by the Sacred Balance found within all the Persons of God? The Second Person of the Trinity, along with his eternal consort, would then make their marriage the first human marriage, after Adam and Eve. His wife, known as Mary Magdalen, was the Female Consort of the Second Person of the Holy Trinity, in human form. It is she who is the Divine Feminine. Though it wasn't until their wedding night, by the kiss of her eternal consort, that she was awakened once again to realize her complete nature and for her to share in an earthly marriage, *it would be by a Sacred Kiss that their marriage would be consummated*. Though she was vital, Mary would take the passive role, since her husband would be the most visible and vocal at this time. This was so at the onset of their mission, as the culture of the time dictated it as such and made this necessary.

She, like her husband, would maintain her human nature until which time her consciousness would once again be suspended for the sake of God's plan. From the time he walked the earth, up to present time, they would sacrifice their love until God's plan for the salvation of humankind would be fully satisfied.

Eeshans believe that the prophecy of Christ returning for his Bride has been fulfilled in these end times, in conjunction with the prophecy of the Woman who encompasses the Man; thus, she now becomes the active consort and then Jesus assumes a more passive role.

That woman who fulfills that prophecy, lives under the title "Eesha" in this life. Eeshans profess that although the whole truth was hidden for so long, Truth be known, God's plans cannot be stopped, even though the consequences of man's choice, since Jesus, had to be played out; and this is: man proposes but God disposes.

The suppression of the truth of Jesus' marriage to Mary Magdalen serves as proof of a stubborn people, which began with the incomplete story of the life of Adam and Eve before and after their fall from grace. Eeshans present a two-part story regarding: 1) the cause and need for redemption, and 2) how the marriage of Jesus and Mary was the only way redemption and salvation was possible. We hope you will see how it was, and still is, vital for our understanding of the loving God we worship.

The first transcendental marriage is the revelation of Jesus and Mary Magdalen as being eternal *Consorts*. We revealed Mary Magdalen, as Jesus' wife, and last but not least the ever so intriguing title: Twin Flames.

Each of these proponents will be unpacked throughout this book, in order that you come to learn about this loving God that you have heard about since childhood, or perhaps feel drawn to know even more about.

We can begin by introducing you to the Who and What of God, the Sacred Balance of the Divine Male and Divine Female, and the love shared and expressed by the First Person of the Holy Trinity. It was by an extraordinary love that God the first Person, who was given the title Most High God, willed that the desire of love the Divine Masculine and Feminine shared brought about what is known as the begetting process. Through this begetting process no human conjugal relations were used but their extreme and endless love brought into existence without the organs and organisms needed by parent for reproduction were not present or necessary. The Child (the Second Person) just came into being. It was through their transcendental nature; whereas, to procreate by reproduction would require a gross physical body capable of producing organisms natural to the reproductive system. The begotten Child, being divine and infinite in nature and origin, is referred to as 'Only,' for there was no need for other "extensions" to satisfy God's desire to reverse the choice of the *created* being which would become fully human and fall victim to a choice (influenced by a lower being); and thus losing the transcendental life created for it.

The triumph of love by the first created being, which when separated, experienced the mirroring of its Creator's love. The transcendental marriage of the first being which was separated into two to experience a reciprocal love different than that as one would now become known as Adam and Eve—representing the One.

Hidden away was the truth that by a *mutual desire to love apart from their true nature*, the couple risked, and, thus, lost their transcendental life.

Because of their choice they were subject to live out their days as physical beings, such as we, with daily challenges, temptations, heartache, and pain, which together they could overcome and develop a relationship with God. Salvation for them and their children would eventually come, as God promised a savior who would restore what was lost. Without ever losing faith or hope in God, our first parents, though weak-natured, lived their life apart from the transcendental. You will see how because of Jesus' marriage, humans were once again capable of proving that love overpowers everything.

As Mary Magdalen's role becomes clearer in God's plan, the title of Twin Flames was mostly unknown, and if known, was not thoroughly understood. Twin Flames are also called "twin souls." We are said to be the other half of our soul. It is said that we each have only one twin, and, generally, after being split, the two went their separate ways, incarnating over and over to gather human experience before coming back together.[28] This is not the same as a soulmate. Soulmates are said to be perfect matches. Twin Flames, on the other hand, are our perfect mirrors. These statements can be found in an article from Thoughtcatolog.com titled "Signs You're Experiencing What Is Known As A 'Twin Flame' Relationship." We like to use references and texts that are familiar to readers in our book to help bring about other perspectives that we think people may find easier to understand when it comes to some of the more unfathomable mysteries, which if we had to write and describe to completion, it would take volumes of books. This way we can draw out some of the similarities used in other texts and references by other authors to show their special gifts in, perhaps, not the fullest, or best, explanation, but one in which assists us in our teachings and serves our best purposes.

---

[28] Antera. "What Is a Twin Flame?" Twin Flames, Introduction by Antera, 2007, www.soulevolution.org/twinflames/twinflames.htm.

Also, these references, guides, and manuscripts etc. are available for you to go back to and reread.

Written in this account regarding Twin Flames, we find very similar details that will better clarify Jesus and Mary's personal relationship, and through which came to earth to become human, and the role theological and scriptural accounts played in and through their lives, as designed by God; yet, which were still, wholeheartedly, lived out of free will. We will use what is true concerning Mary Magdalen, as Jesus' intended, and some detail to help understand their human experiences throughout their life together and apart.

Given their Divine natures, Jesus and Mary Magdalen this entitles them to the privilege of both time and eternity. [**Perhaps while trying to gain enlightenment we should remind you that you must try, and not limit your understanding to just the 'letter' of the word, but instead to try to decipher, and gain understanding through the *spirit* of the word. Words alone are stepping stones but are rather useless if you can't see beyond them.**] Man's words are very different from God's 'Word' because we tend to define the meaning of a human's words through human consciousness and human reasoning. That is how so many missed what Jesus was talking about regarding the transcendental meaning and life. God said, "My thoughts are not your thoughts, and My ways are not your ways." These words clearly provide the explanation as to how our thoughts and words are finite and limited to the human thought process and flawed reasoning; whereas, God's words are infinite with vast meaning.

Throughout their relationship, Jesus and Mary Magdalen (through to Eesha) experienced ongoing separation. This was true though they were never really separated. As you continue to read on, you will come to see how being Twin Flames is truly revealing the 'what' of these two individuals, and allows a closer look at the 'what and how' of an unfathomable mystery. Even with all the efforts and means used in this book to help you come to an awareness of terms and words that helps you on the way to enlightenment, you will still find yourself questioning, or misunderstanding, the transcendental meaning of these words and boundless natures of God. This is because you are subject to a fallen nature and limited by human reasoning; therefore, these are all you have to rely on in your translation of the matters of God. Don't worry, however. Once the effort is put forth that the divine nature of God, will by grace and Spirit, assist you in surpassing the human, it will elevate your being towards the infinite, and, thereby, ease your soul.

Getting back to understanding the meaning of twin souls, with regards to Jesus and Mary, his wife, we align this writing with many instances to substantiate, as best we can, examples of what we are discussing throughout. A few examples of the above text are used to show how, by taking on human forms yet being fully divine, all that the couple experienced was by free will, which made their sacrifice of love a continual one linking all ages, so that no one is left without hope and salvation. For example, when Jesus and Mary met in the marketplace as children, they may have played but did not really have opportunities to become friends. Yet, seeing each other as they were coming of age without a doubt caused an attraction between them, even though both were subject to their parents/guardians. The horrible incident that occurred when Jesus was seventeen and Mary was going on fourteen brought them together. Providence separated them again when Jesus left for the Himalayas. Eleven years later, he returned in search of his bride. They married, and Jesus began His work.

Jesus' death separated him from his 'timestamped' human form. The generating of his glorious body, being necessary to return, indicated that there was to be another separation of the couple. Though by their divinity were never separated, Jesus went back to heaven, while Mary lived out her life here. Upon Mary's death, Jesus raised her body, and her consciousness was secured, until which time a new body was prepared, which would house it, in a new age, becoming the vehicle which will encompass the couple—this time as one. While both embraced humanness once again in a different way, they are One but are also uniquely bound within the promised Sacred Food by an unfathomable mystery, called Eucharist, meant to be the 'leaven' of which Christ taught that provided the means for all those who believe to return to heaven. So, this is how, as Twin Flames, they were destined to come in and out of each other's lives. Each time they came together they experienced a passionate love, but when separated, they suffered excruciating pain. Truly in every way, they were, indeed, "One." They were, and forever will be, Yin and Yang, just like the Father and Virgin Mary!

This however, was a necessary act of God's extreme love and mercy for us. If humans had been blessed to have heard the true story of the fall from the transcendental life and grace, this merciful act of love would've reflected God, as parents right from the start, and not a punishing God; but a 'Father and Mother' demonstrating unwavering love.

On your journey to enlightenment, you will come to understand why a human being is flawed, why it was necessary for one who was both divine and human to provide the Way, the Truth, the Light, and the Life back to heaven. You will see how One became two, and how they would become two and one again. You will see how marriage reflects the creation of Adam and Eve, how a sacred *marriage* was used to reverse the consequence of Adam and Eve's choice, and how it was used to provide the 'Way' back to our original transcendental state, but only better.

LESSON 10

HOW GOD WORKED BEHIND THE SCENES

To accomplish this, it was necessary for an only-begotten Child to sacrifice and provide what was lost because the created child of God (even though Adam and Eve's life was transcendental, it was still created), and it would now take one who was begotten, uncreated, and divine to bridge the gap.

By this plan we would not only be restored to our original transcendental life and consciousness where we share in God's plan, but we are actually grafted into God in a way which not even our first parents experienced.

Over time, by man's hands, (and we mean, 'men's') we were made to believe that woman *caused* man to fall, through which we lost all standing with God, and we were doomed to suffer and die. We were made to see a God who, despite sending us a Savior, doesn't seem to want to help us, but rather seems to still want to punish us with suffering because 'he' was so hurt and offended. Because of woman, humans are destined to live out this very sad and miserable life, with little joy that we find by our own means, which we also owe to God. Our free will is not free, nor does it provide freedom, but, rather, it appears that one's life carries a hopeless *fate* rather than a promising *destiny*, since the life here in this world allows little hope for those who live a life of pain, suffering, hunger, and oppression etc., simply because they were unfortunate to have been born under these conditions as God watches. If not for men, we would have no connection. Women can, however, accept a subservient role, and work for the good of the church in Christ's name, by doing a lot of the grunt work, or by supporting one, or more, priests by doing office work, cleaning, wining and dining, sending them on vacations. The same was applied to bishops, cardinals, etc., and these women are viewed as "privileged" to work for them. Of course, it is to be understood that not all priests fit this category, but over the years many have taken advantage of women's good nature and love for Jesus.

There would be no value to our moral fabric and our value of life if we believe that God looks to punish all of humankind. If God abandoned us this would be true. As Jesus asked, "If your child came to you asking for bread would you give a stone instead?" So as Jesus identified us as children of God, then with God as our parents,[29] despite Adam and Eve having *mutually* chosen this path, God is still there to guide and provide us with a "Way" back; and believe it or not, God wants us to be happy, even when things go wrong.

God loves us with an unconditional love, and does not enjoy watching us suffer, hurt ourselves, or each other. God's love is without fault, and that is why the intense love of the first Person of the Holy Trinity actually brought into being, without a beginning or an end, the Only-Begotten Child. So perfect is the love of God, that this amazing manifestation (or Promise) came into existence to give us not just hope of eternal life, but eternal life itself. As an added bonus, this Child disclosed that God is our Father and Mother and as children of God, we are heirs to even more than all that Adam and Eve were given.

God is loving, and no doubt sees the evil of those who were, and continued to be, responsible for fabricating the traditional story, that not only changed salvation history but also solidified in God's name the inequality of genders; thus, negating all of what Jesus as God and Man, Divine and Human, came to correct. Eeshans believe that by the misogynistic and strongly prejudiced leadership against women from Peter on, everything once again reverted back to the time before Jesus, without Sacred Balance, without guidance to the transcendental way of life, almost as though it took upon itself the desire to make women suffer so long as they live as payback. Why? Because the human consciousness, and its reasoning,

---

[29] Divine Masculine and Feminine. – Ed.

is flawed. As man could justify his actions as long as he, being made in God's image and likeness, felt obliged to carry out the punishment for what He felt was equal to what man lost or what man fears. Knowing the truth this would not have caused this set of attitudes. Perhaps, that is why Jesus' trial was handled the way it was—more on that later.

Those that came before Jesus were comfortable with lying to achieve a goal. After Jesus, those who feared Him used lies, and those in charge of carrying outside the law would eventually use the law to aid in corruption and discrimination. This, observed in hindsight of what is found after Peter, would represent those, who for one reason or another, would find justification in denying Jesus and/or his teachings out of what they feared they would lose. These leaders refused, and continued to refuse to turn away from the human consciousness to avoid whatever it was that they don't want to deal with or be associated with, unless or until there was guaranteed success and self-gratification, found only in compromise.

Being a rebellious people, especially today, we don't seek stress or confrontation, and we certainly don't want to be considered wrong, especially according to what others think of us. This is pure human consciousness and this is what would ultimately make it necessary to bring to completion Christ's mission to successively guide his people back to the Way of the transcendental consciousness. It is now time for this occur. It is now a time to change the consciousness of the world we live in. It is time for an Avatar, one who is a part of Jesus, because she is his consort in the Sacred Balance.

Understanding this, we find the keystone, the she, whose place with Jesus Peter resented and despised. The consciousness of Mary Magdalen has returned in these end times, and Mary Magdalen carries the title: *Eesha.*

The Eeshan Religion, by the authority of Christ, welcomes Mary back, because she is the one who presents the truth Jesus taught when they lived here on earth, as one among the female counterparts of the three Persons of God. She is the Shekinah—the dwelling and setting of the feminine aspect of the Divine presence of God. Just by her presence the world itself is sustained by the flow of divine energy. To hurt the

Shekinah is to bring God's wrath; whereby, all peace will be forfeited, since she loves and wishes for peace, but is also the witness to the Spirit of God, who listens to her.

The Divine Feminine aspect, along with the findings and prophecies are re-presented for this the age of Enlightenment as the foundation of the Eeshan religion.

Could Peter, who was not only an imposter but was a leader who didn't just covet the place of Jesus' Wife's, but he also assumed it. He additionally was someone who revealed Christ's mysteries to His enemies, playing out his role as Jesus referred to him, as the 'stumbling block' to his work? Unlike giving Jesus a kiss, as did Judas (who died of remorse), was Peter's alleged inverted crucifixion a warning to us of Satan being on the seat of Peter?[30]

We as Eeshans feel that, if this is true, perpetuating this corruption is worse than Judas' betrayal, especially as Peter's successors continue in this maligned agenda; thus, allowing corruption to enter into God's plan of salvation, and cheating humankind of the truth of veritable spiritual sustenance.

The loss of the transcendental aspect does not provide for the Sacred Balance to be restored, but it appears that a rather distorted secular version of spirituality, where love of neighbor has become more important than love of God, has filled this vacuum, and where social injustice and oppression by discrimination prevails, do we see proof of that loss.

To describe the Eeshan religion as reflecting a version of a humanistic religion with a thealogical[31] and theological overlay does not come close. Our religion is a transcendental, "ancient," mystical, beyond Merkabahalic[32] and Kabbahlic religion, brought back into sight because of the love of God; it is not just presenting new doctrines of Jesus, but is *re-presenting* what Jesus Christ originally taught, fully and unabridged,

---

[30] The inverted cross has always been understood as a principle satanic symbol. – Ed.

[31] Thealogy, with an 'a,' should be noted as referring to the Divine Feminine. – Ed.

[32] From Merkabah (meaning 'chariot'): the Heavenly Throne. See the full description in Jewish Encyclopedia. – Ed.

against what may be defined as a two-thousand-year ad hominem belief system. This means that under our belief system, one can no longer turn a blind eye, or deaf ear, to the countless, tireless works of those fearless and daring individuals among the chosen who have demonstrated courage in seeking the truth and not giving in to negative and high-pressure influences. To those we say:

> *"fear not those who can kill the body, but fear the One that could kill both the body and the soul. Do not fear the path of truth. O all those who realize the injustices against Mary Magdalen and her marriage to Jesus Christ, do not falter. For the prophecy of Jesus returning for his bride has come to pass. Don't hide—but know Jesus has provided a refuge for you"*

The Eeshan Religion gives you the freedom to know the Mysteries of God and enter into the transcendental realm, where you can once again hear the Word of God's 'voice' through the only person with the authority to speak with the same organic voice. To hear again Christ's words through the voice of the Shekinah is to feel the peace that only Jesus can bring. Only the voice which shares totally in Jesus' body, blood, soul, and divinity can speak his words. Over the years thousands have been drawn to hear once again the words and teachings of Christ and to witness his presence, one in which has been so desperately lacking against the backdrop of what some say appears to be "a finite or expendable set of laws" left behind by Jesus that don't relate to so many modern-day issues.

May you feel freedom to experience the real transcendental spirituality as originally brought to God's people by Jesus Christ; and with the supramentalized—consciousness of the Wife of the Lamb, who with the real and authentic God-given authority, will break down the sectarian based stigmas and heresy labels placed on those who have fought to bring to light the truth. Examples of these include those who suffered at the hands of religious teachers who claim the right to expel or excommunicate anyone who does not support the claims made over 2000 years; or had the audacity to question their orthodox beliefs or hypocritical practices and behaviors, especially when knowing that they will 'certainly' be viciously marginalized by those who are afraid to think outside the box, and aren't afraid to embrace their own spiritual powers from God. However, what about the good people: the holy saints and priests, teachers, friends and family?

LESSON 11

GOOD PEOPLE

When discussing errors in teachings and victimization of people, we want to be clear that in no way are we grouping together every individual or religious, but rather those who were trusted to bring the truth and failed to do so. It would be like damning a whole nation of people for the errors and actions of its government.

Throughout our lives, we have and always will find people, really good people, who have impacted our lives. There are even those who seem to be sent by God to bring joy and laughter whom we don't know but whom we follow on TV, the news, social media, etc. These may well be truly genuine, decent, and wholesome, and in their own way, loving and kind people. You will find that these have an intuitive sense of Jesus, his teachings and life, and regardless of age, are genuinely trying to be a good example. These live their lives, NOT always as followers of an organized religion but by wholesome standards found within themselves or in how they were raised. Then there are those who are naturally inclined or guided by Providence, and are unaffected by most things, and avoid those things that might affect their love of God.

Others find their way by staying close to God despite issues happening within the established religions. Some live according to what they have been taught pre- or post-Vatican II in the Catholic church, or some other religion. Regardless, we respect their religion or spirituality. Some in our lives have no spirituality, nor do they go to church, but still live by a decent code of ethics. That is where decency, kindness, love, etc., make them admirable character examples to us.

In Christian circles, since their inception, we also find the very good, kind, even holy priests, ministers, presbyters, evangelists, etc. who have believed that what they taught was true and that they remain true to it, and live it. These who are genuine in their love for God, and who are wonderful examples of strength in spirituality.

It is when those in authority, or members, who judge, or attack, others for their beliefs and do not live what they preach themselves, or worse, use Christ as the battering ram, or a stick to hit others with, makes one wonder what it is that precipitates them to think that what they are doing will cause others to *want* to believe in Christ? The fact is that these are often the reasons why Catholics and Christians are not liked or respected. Hate crimes against gays, or the trend surfacing in the 1990's of killing abortion doctors, are just two examples of actions against Christ done in Christ's name. Then we have outright discrimination against age, color, creed, culture, sexual orientation, and political affiliation; and the list goes on and on that serves as reasons for humans to hate rather than for reasons to love. The downside is that it is virtually impossible to have role models, or heroes, without they themselves ruining their reputation, or those who MUST discourage any good that others do. In the eyes of the world, a person cannot go from bad to good, experience conversion, and then will remain guilty, even if proven innocent.

Anyone who wholeheartedly lives their faith as they know it, so long as it builds a foundation to know, love and serve a loving God, is to be commended; for they have lived as their heart and soul dictated.

The Eeshan Religion is founded on a mandate from God which was to our Foundress to go and find all truths about Jesus. What was revealed in that mandate was that she discover who she was, and what was her own role and identity. What she found was twofold. First, she found the missing transcendental love brought into this world by Jesus Christ the Divine Masculine of the only Begotten Child of God, with whom he shared with his Divine Feminine consort, and who she was. Secondly, she saw how this transcendental love had been denied to God's people from earliest times. Eeshans believe that this knowledge was heralded into being by all those who, in their hearts, kept vigil, and awaited the return of Mary Magdalen, the Bride of Christ:

- by the promise and hand of her Husband;
- and who was to have been the guide for all those who followed the true teachings of Christ, with the desire to hear, once again, his words as he taught them.
- She was to be the Avatar and who by love avenges all those whose morals and character had been attacked, and those who have been victimized for trying to bring the truth to God's people; only to be met with vicious condemnation by those using logic, and not wisdom, along with a corrupted reason by using ad hominem arguments against the innocent, yet are guilty of this very grievous sin themselves.

LESSON 12

GOD SENDS ANOTHER GUIDE

While we mention throughout these passages the reasons why our Religion and Spirituality has come 'back' into existence, we also feel we should make it clear to all that it is not intended to try and turn you away from your religion, or spirituality, of choice.

Also, we do not expect or ask those who are loyal members of the Catholic/Christian denominations to justify their reasons for believing what they are taught. Again, we are addressing religious leadership—not those who have lived their faith to the letter out of love and trust in God. These are the innocents, and as Jesus says, "There will always be innocents."

At the same time, we do feel it necessary to present the reasons behind *our* objections to what has been presented as truth regarding Jesus Christ, and to outline reasons why we disagree with foundational doctrines of the Catholic/Christian origins, in order to show those errors that we believe caused a collapse of faith. We do not feel a need to apologize for what we believe.

It is with joy that we introduce back into the world what we believe was given to God's people originally for richer, fuller lives.

It is often times said, the ways of humans often reflect the shadows of things to come and not necessarily the image of things. The things of Jesus were for our edification which, when properly taught, should reflect truth so that we may have hope.

This brings us to point out those things which, in light of the way the story of Adam and Eve has been told, presents no hope for women in terms of equality to men. As with any Divinely inspired book, we ask only that our levels of interpretation of what Jesus taught, and what we are passing along from our foundress, be recognized as an expression of God's constant interaction with his people, even today.

God is multidimensional and multifaceted. God is not bound by humans or their laws. God is not limited to the Old, or New Testaments, but rather is continually teaching his children and guiding them to truth. To believe that all knowledge of God, the Trinity, the Mysteries, etc. has already been written, or taught, and there's nothing more to say about it is to put God within the confines of our control.

The Eeshan religion goes beyond those things that many of God's people have come to believe are the limits and only truths deigned by God, as all that is needed. Not so. God causes the heart to seek and search for truth through all ages. Today, we have the ability to learn more, understand more, seek more, and love more. Not unlike David in his going up against Goliath, the Eeshan Religion is based on faith in, the strength of, and love of God; and though we may be ridiculed and persecuted for his sake—so shall it be. It is written that our battle with the giants in our lives will result in victory if we cling by faith to God's power. Though the world will not accept what it can't see, we believe God sent Jesus' consort, who we *can* see and will help *us* to see.

LESSON 13

GOD'S SALVATION PLAN CONTINUED

THE WORD...

What if it was not Peter who was to be head of the church, or the one that Jesus gave the authority to? How would it affect you? What if you found that everything you believed about the beginnings of the church was not true? Would you be angry at the messenger, or the fact that you were lied to? This is not impossible, for over the years you also believed that a priest, or nun, could never hurt your children and grandchildren, and it was an honor when the priest wanted to spend a lot of time together with them.

Eeshans believe that Mary was in fact the Wife of Jesus. Despite what has been declared by the church, we believe she was the rightful authority, and along with James, the others were to look to them for guidance and leadership.

What if history is repeating itself but this time Jesus is sending 'his wife' via the supramentalization[33] of her consciousness and returning as the Co-Messiah she was? And suppose she is to do as he did? Like Jesus, her presence and teachings include addressing modern day Pharisees and Sadducees who, as back then, made up laws to impose on people, saying they came from God. What if today this same Jesus may be pointing out that though many of the laws the church has taught since Peter are said

---

[33] This term is not one which could be clearly and adequately defined in a sentence or two. Suffice it to say for now that this is a divine process which will become clearer to the reader, like a traditionally developed photographic image, as its spiritual context unfolds throughout the book. – Ed.

to be from Jesus, they are by nature of the human consciousness, and contrary to his original transcendental teachings. In other words, they are from those who seek the things of God but are just from the higher reasoning of humans.

Words are important. When words are changed, omitted, or destroyed, especially God's words, from original teachings, we are all affected. As a whole people, we suffer. Eeshans found that there were more truths from Eesha's teachings some thirty years ago that are just now being discovered and unearthed than those from the church taught for over two thousand years.

As a result of her teachings, we find more and more people have continued to seek out spiritual direction on their own out of dissatisfaction found within the four walls of their churches. As the Divine Feminine entered the world, it became obvious that what was once before considered to be one's heart keeping one in church, is now revealed to have been conditioned thinking, and not faith. Left behind are empty pews, for the Divine Feminine has truly awakened hearts, causing people to think for themselves and to act on what their heart has been telling them all along. Where before many felt they couldn't go against what they 'thought' was their heart, now in the 'light' find that what God has revealed to them was that it wasn't 'their heart' after all, but it was actually their *conditioned mind*. Before, they were merely being told what to think and feel, and suppressing what they knew or suspected all along was wrong or didn't make sense. This can easily be confused, especially when a conditioned mind is made to look like it is the heart. Out of fear that their spirituality was being taken away from them, hearing and learning about the Eeshan Religion brought with it once again, a desire within people's hearts, to hear more of what has been taught about God over the last thirty years of our Eesha's private and public teachings.

As Eeshans will continue to unpack what has been removed, omitted, or destroyed that filled in the 'missing pieces' to traditional scriptural writing and completed verses, it will provide a rise of excitement for an even greater appreciation of Jesus' Life and Ministry.

Eeshans find that as truth was manipulated for alternate goals, God's plan for Mary Magdalen's work could not be stopped; but by God's design, it was just delayed until end times.[34] Perhaps God knew it would then serve the people better.

We find these times are called, by some, "eschatological" times, because people sense that we are in the last, end, or final days. Well, if that is true, then it only strengthens God's reason behind bringing about that which was once stifled, bringing forward with the power of the Divine Feminine a demonstration of God's love. Though human beings often make efforts to change God's plan for selfish reasons and goals, God's love endures. Always remember, though there are times when it may look like evil has succeeded, God's plan will prevail with seemingly no interruption.

We welcome you to take a look at this transcendental Eeshan Religion and School of Metta[35] Spirituality and see what we are all about. Being mystically and transcendentally immersed in what we believe, we feel we offer a complete spiritual journey through the teachings and life of Jesus Christ—as you have never experienced before. Let's now take a brief look into the Eeshan Religion.

---

[34] While the expression "End Times" may have several meanings, depending on how it is used and by whom, the context here could fittingly be directed to the "end of the great Lie." – Ed.

[35] The Pali word for "loving-kindness," but in the present context should be understood as God's own love, which is unaffected by the modes of material nature, is transcendental and unconditional, and which is, once shared with humans by God, may then be shared, or extended, to others as the very love that comes from God. Metta is different from human love arising from purely human experience and emotion, no matter how noble and unselfish. – Ed.

LESSON 14

A STEP TOWARDS A HIDDEN IDENTITY

In approximately 2010, through Divine Revelation, our foundress, Eesha, was commissioned by God the Divine Father, to "go out and find all the pieces of truth about My Son." And so, she did. With her uncompromising love for almighty God and deep devotion; yet, still unaware of her true consciousness, she began her mystery school, which later evolved into the School of Enlightenment. With a few chosen companions, she began her work with what she knew best, which was her own personal relationship with the Divine. What happened was nothing short of a miracle that opened hearts and immediately began to unfold the deepest, most mystical and unfathomable mysteries of God; and it was once again being revealed by someone who would have the authority to teach the way Jesus did, both on his level and by his standard.

Already known for having the Stigmata, and her ability to heal people who were turned away by the medical professions because their cases were terminal, she would go quietly into towns, and left without notice, leaving behind a greater awareness of God's love for her and for those she tended to.[36] Usually in the public spectrum she would try and preserve her privacy and always refused interviews, requests for TV appearances to include *Oprah*, and would often deny her identity. At public appearances, however, she rarely left early, often spending time with crowds, hours after healing services, except if she had scheduled time set aside for private gatherings for those who had the rare chance of scheduling to

---

[36] The Stigmata, in Eesha's case, far from being an unexplainable phenomena to attract, test, or provoke curiosity of other people, or even to 'prove' God's existence and Jesus' presence to others, was actually primarily a manifestation of Jesus' love for *her*. – Ed.

see her while she was available in town. It should be said that a person or child didn't always need a personal touch, or her presence to begin, or to attain, healing. Often, she did so from a distance. It should be noted however, that she is known for turning people away; for as she said, she does only what God wants her to.

Whether you believe or not that God can, has, or continues to work outside of the church, i.e., apparitions, saints etc., we have witnessed tremendous phenomena, including even levitation. By our faith in God, we do believe that there are many ways Jesus healed those who came to Him, but faith was the number one cause of healing many experienced. Jesus' techniques, when studied, showed that as God, and though he embraced his human nature, he was pure energy; and that by his divinity, he could transfer positive energy by his transcendence, which caused the recipient to absorb the vibrations and energies (grace) of the Sublime. Thereby, one surely gains a degree, if not a greater degree of enlightenment than ever expected. Spiritual healing is always the ultimate healing. That is why those healed spiritually were not usually witnessed by others, and physical healing was most sought after. This was revealed by the healing of those who were healed at great distances, and those who were close enough to touch his garment, as in the case of the woman with the hemorrhage. Jesus used many techniques to heal, including his word, "Go, your servant is healed."

Though our foundress demonstrated these same techniques, finding faith today is another issue. Today, her greatest desire is healing the faithless, the hopeless, and the loveless by reintroducing God/Jesus, back into people's lives. This is to heal by love and awareness that God exists. Though physical healing is still what most seek, if Christ does not heal the person, it does not mean that the 'healer' failed, or is a fraud, it just may mean that this is one of those times that God knows the better outcome. Under the human consciousness we might think that if the person is healed it is an answer to a prayer, where God knows that it would be detrimental to the soul of the person, or someone, or others close to the person. One time there a was wife who went with her ailing husband to a healing service, and afterward he remained sick. Later the woman claimed that she was the person healed. She realized that the ailments which kept her husband home kept him from cheating on her.

The Eeshan religion teaches enlightenment. It is also here to help correct the wrongs of the many errors brought about by the fallacies of misaligned teachings prominent in today's world. Being the primary reason for the return of the Divine Feminine, this religion delights in bringing back faith, hope, and love, beginning with teaching truth, and correcting the misconstrued story of Adam and Eve, what they lost and why, and God's 'real' Salvific Plan, in order that one can truly attain the fullness of God's promise.

In order that you receive all that God intends for you, you must first attain spiritual knowledge and insight. This kind of knowledge is an *awareness* that frees you from all those things that imprison you within the material, logical, human consciousness, and discourages any happiness, or hope, resulting in your existing in "not living" the life God intended for you. It begins with giving you the strength needed to allow you to experience Jesus' teachings apart from the limited knowledge that the world claims or finds outside the human heart, rather than within it. The greatest knowledge focuses on living words which live through eternity, not those that are spoken by humans. Yet, too often those words, or quotes, that we find that the world claims are pearls of wisdom, were often derived from what Jesus taught! People claim that they choose "reality" over superstition when they choose to turn away from teaching their children about God, or keeping them from learning about God. Remember however, that all the world can offer is a flawed "finite reality." God's reality is perfect and infinite.

Sadly, the world is also responsible for taking God's word and revising it. For example, in the past, in trying to translate the "what" of Jesus, the only common description of the day would be 'Logos.' This word was used in an effort to bring both the Jews and Gentiles to a common ground denominator in an attempt to unite these two very different cultures. You will see later why. So, calling Jesus the 'word' or 'logos' was meant to bring the Jews to their understanding of the word, which was the "personification of God's revelation." To the Gentiles, the 'word' or 'logos' meant that Jesus was the link between God and humans—similar, but different. Each culture had enough familiarity with this word to at least bring them to the table to talk. But that is wrong. Where it was supposed to present Him as being the Messiah, it caused distress seen in their differences of opinions on what the Messiah would be like. Even here, as attempts are made to show similarity, it is obvious that the Jewish Messiah and Gentile Messiah had one very glaring difference. One couldn't be God. Enlightenment is the tool which allows one to bridge the meanings discovering when, put together, the two become one. Only through enlightenment does one see that God and love are the only things you take with you after you leave this world. Everything else from this world remains behind. Enlightenment breaks the barriers of fear-invoked teachings and useless/groundless information.

LESSON 15

DON'T LET FEAR KEEP US APART

'Don't be afraid,' and 'Fear not,' are probably the most used salutations mentioned whenever we read or find stories of God, Jesus, or the Virgin Mary interacting with humans. Why? To put the person at ease, of course, but also to acknowledge that humans become frightened when having to face things, or moments, unfamiliar to them, or whenever they encounter those things that are 'supposed' to be bad or not normal.

At this time, let us say to you, "Salutations! Don't be afraid." Just like in the song,[37] where Jesus is saying, "Don't let fear, keep us apart. Long have I waited for your coming home to me and living, deeply our new love." Perhaps your soul was waiting for this moment. Perhaps it is crying out to you, who may be the only one who could help ease its journey.

In order to understand the Eeshan mindset, concepts, and point of view, you will find we incorporate many methods to assist you in acquiring a transcendental perspective, leading to enlightenment. You are going to read about many terms which are linked to, or identify with, things once deemed as 'heretical,' or even 'evil' by the church, but only because the church would not allow anything, or any sciences, that would not conform to its agenda and claimed its own stance was out of protection for its teachings and scriptures. While consumed in fear that the works of such geniuses contradicted its authority, scientists, mathematicians, and astronomers, such as Galileo, Copernicus, Newton, and DaVinci (who studied secretly), are now hailed for their work and advancements.

---

[37] From the hymn, "Hosea" by Gregory Norbert.

We are finding today, through scientific studies that continue on, there have been advances in treatments for disease, and a much greater understanding of the human body. They have now discovered, and are studying photons, which are elementary particles and the quantum of all of forms of electromagnetic radiation, including light. It is by light that we can find cancer, etc. Discovery of the photon has led to understanding of how important light is, and what it is capable of; thus, we better understand why Jesus' use of the word 'light' was so important, especially in his identity as "I am the Light of the world"! Discovery brings truth and discards darkness—just as he said.

The many things we reveal from our studies within our Mystery School have been used throughout history predating Adam and Eve. Seeking enlightenment is important to truly understand God's ways and the person of Jesus. As you begin to become enlightened you will see how spiritually locked down you really were in your thinking and living. As you will find that a lot of what angers you about people or the things you hated, or were told to hate about people and their views, are baseless. Being more enlightened may help you find these same people more interesting, or you might understand what makes them feel like they do and why, but in doing so, you may well see these things all in the positive, and not totally in the negative, as perhaps you did before.

Don't panic over the words zodiac, vibrations, or constellations, for these, as well as sacred geometry, were all of which that was used by God. If one is intuitive enough, one should be led to a level of spirituality where the mysteries of God and truth are realized in actual and physical form in these mysteries. Ignorance should not rule your life, whether voluntarily, or involuntarily. Remember that the nationwide panic that occurred when people heard on October 30, 1938, H. G. Wells, *World of the Worlds* on the radio, or, more simply, the fear of going into one's own basement?

Though our focus is first and foremost Jesus, it is important to understand all you are about to be exposed to. Through enlightenment, you will learn not to fear these once banned and suppressed studies, or worry that they are evil, or will take you away from God. Topics such as, crystals, stones, chakras, and vibrations were all used by God and for God's purposes. Today minerals, supplements, and treatments using these are being investigated, and ancient methods of healing are being studied. You will find the very importance of the use of vibrations in the Gregorian chants, which without them caused a disconnect between humans and God, since *the solfeggio* tones connect with how God put our body together so that sacred hymns kept us close to the divine. Medicine is now used in dealing with many forms of autism. Helen Keller learned to read via vibrations.

Another very interesting fact is that if you look closely at your zodiac sign, it can tell a lot about your health history. Yes, with your Zodiac sign and blood type, and even with your name, you will find a lot of information about yourself by God's design, just like in DNA tests today. In particular, you may be surprised at what ailments and physical maladies are common under your sign, and you can see how your name, birthday, and day of the week you were born were not by chance at all, but were all in God's plan. That is why Jesus said: (Matthew 10:29 & Luke 12:6).

> *"Are not five sparrows sold for two pennies? Yet not one of them is forgotten by God. Indeed, the very hairs on your head are all numbered. Don't be afraid, you are worth more than many sparrows."*

So, pace yourself and try and patiently continue reading without cause for alarm, and we guarantee you will find these things are NOT EVIL, at all, but are actually used today, and taught to treat many physical and mental diseases and maladies. These studies will dismiss the irrational and misunderstandings governed by fear that invoked methods to sidetrack one from actual demonstrations of the supernatural, such as Jesus' miracles or his walking unnoticed through the crowd, etc.

Did you know Jesus would pray unceasingly, throughout the day and night? He would chant and sing, teach worship services and scriptures. He would seek solace in meditation upon facing difficult times—in a desert setting, or on a boat, or in a cave. He loved spending time by water. This, along with his wife Mary, brought him comfort and strength. Later, you will find his connection with water and the meaning behind his use and how important to him was the symbol of his own wife's zodiac sign, blood type, and name. That is why we tell you that your zodiac sign, your blood type, and your name, all make up who you are in a very scientific, yet spiritual, awakening.

Remember that nothing we teach is intended to take you away from God, for this would be contrary to our beliefs and to the person of Jesus Christ as God and Man.

So, let us reiterate here, once again: that in order to understand Jesus' life, death, and resurrection, you must first suspend all the interiorly accrued mental machinery of evaluation and analysis based on former experience, education, and social conditioning, in order to enter into, or that you at least have an open heart and mind to, what we believe. Unless you try and suspend all that you have learned on your own that makes you feel confidently knowledgeable about this subject, it will be your own consciousness that will lead you rather than the Holy Spirit of God's consciousness. Everyone has ears to 'hear' what is being said by a speaker, or an author, but understanding and listening is done by choosing to do so consciously. Also, you would be surprised at the degree of learning one absorbs subconsciously, and that is why attention to what is being taught is important.

If you don't pay attention, even though you have 'eyes' to see, you will not 'see.' Thus, what are deemed as core teachings within our spirituality can be mistranslated into what was once considered 'New Age,' or other heretical notions, in your mind. We don't want you quitting before you begin what we feel will be your most enriching journey. Putting God first is vital, since that is the first command of God.

LESSON 16

How to Prepare for Enlightenment

Before entering into any spiritual writing, book or exercise in your search for enlightenment, it is highly recommended and ideally helpful if you engage in some form of prayer and/or meditation before you begin—just as Jesus did. You want to remove distractions, concerns, irrational thoughts, fears etc., so that you can not only concentrate but enter into a state where you can be refreshed, gladdened, strengthened, and calmed.

A spiritual exercise may be as simple as chanting a very personal mantra consisting of a syllable, word, or phrase—something as simple as Jesus' name or "help me Jesus," etc. Believe it or not, this strengthens your resolve as you take time to spend with God. It will also give you courage to leave your safe place and journey beyond the familiar in seeking enlightenment. Breathing is also an excellent exercise.

So, begin by clearing your mind and clarify your intention to open your Heart, giving way to the possibility of learning something truly brand new, or simply to have the ears to hear beyond the ordinary into the sublime mysteries unlike you have ever imagined.

Understand also that the Eeshan Religion and Metta Spirituality is *intended to enrich your faith*, not to create within you a sensitivity that is contrary to your own religion or spirituality. Within this spirituality, the excitement you shall find should fill you with a sense of duty and obligation to reveal and re-present to others, what we wholeheartedly believe has been omitted from Jesus' life, passion, and death according to the accepted Gospels of which everyone is familiar.

Approach your reading as if your soul is in communication with your heart. That is why you should use meditation and prayer to clear the mind of all the obstacles that cause most forms of dysfunction that interfere with your spiritual concentration. It could be as simple as promising yourself that all you read will be read with a positive attitude.

While not an easy practice, if you have never done this, it is something you should do for yourself each day to relieve stress, knowing that "Someone," the Spirit of God, is there and listening. You are not alone. People really don't understand prayer. We were always taught that prayer was a solemn request for help, or expression of thanks to God, or words used in worship services. The prayer we are talking about is an 'actual *conversation*' between you and God. The revealing of your true self with those weaknesses and faults which may cause you distress, is important to be honest about; in turn, you desire God's help in resetting your priorities.

It does take work in the beginning. It requires you to dedicate your attention to God without allowing your mind to take over and wander. Steadily, a little bit each day, and with practice, one gains a foothold on the wayward tendencies of the mind and eventually can experience the things of God.

The simple principle of repetition, i.e., a prayer or mantra, helps to stabilize the attention so that one's *intention to be enlightened* is carried out.

As an experiment to see where your own capacity is for attention and clarity in understanding and exercising control over the mind on your journey to enlightenment, you may try to focus on a mantra, or brief prayer, or devotional phrase, and repeat it until you become distracted. For some this will happen quickly, while for others perhaps it will take just a bit longer before they become distracted—and by distracted, we mean as soon as the mind drifts and takes the consciousness away from the object and person of focus in the prayer or mantra. Even as simple an exercise as closing the eyes, relaxing the body and counting the breath up to ten, without becoming distracted, can feel like a Herculean feat.

The point of this exercise is just to see how blocked the "filters" (described above) are to the chakras, which are energy points in the subtle body, and not in the physical body. They are aligned with the spine, starting with the root chakra, at the base of the spine, up to the crown chakra, which is located at the top of the head.[38]

---

[38] Michaels, Kim. "You Are Here to Build an Upward Spiral." Ascended Master Light, 2005, www.ascendedmasterlight.com/ascended-master-light/authors/13-mother-mary/54-you-are-here-to-build-an-upward-spiral.

LESSON 17

WHAT YOU WILL FIND IN THE EESHAN RELIGION

THE USE OF TONES AND VIBRATIONS

When one enters into the Eeshan Religion and Metta Spirituality and School of Enlightenment as an inductee, or simply come to or live steam our many worship rituals, you will find a great emphasis on music. Music is powerful and through it we express our feelings and emotions, memories, dreams and fantasies.

Our prayers and reflections are often used in the background; just like our teaching and course studies are apt to use harmonious tones, and vibrational chants, which should not be unfamiliar to you, since music has always been part of religious ceremonies, especially for Catholics and Christians, and of most world religions sans a few. Included, however, you will find that Eeshans use a variety of music, such as soul-satisfying love songs, fun songs, and deep and light melodies honoring the love shared between the soul and its Creator but most honoring the love between Jesus and his Wife. This music may be selected for daily worship, as well as for celebrations, often to bring the mind to imagine the relationship shared by Jesus and Mary Magdalen, since it not only allows one to share in the most incredible love story this world has ever witnessed, but in doing so it helps one to stay focused on the love of God has for us by hearing and reflecting on Christ's love for his bride, and the soulful love expressed as they speak to each other with memories they shared and that which reflects their continued love story today; but it offers a genuine heartfelt realization of the Christs'[39] love for us.

Eeshans have always used a variety of music—as music can elate the heart, comfort and still the mind, and heal the soul. As music is also a personal choice, when you enter into meditation you should choose music that keeps your heart and mind united and focused. If you sense there is something blocking your path, then it is always suggested that you listen to vibrational chakra chants for healing of your DNA in balancing the chakras. If you remember, the chakras are the energy points that line the spine from the base of the spine to the crown of the head.

'Source vibrations'[40] download provides an excellent background music for all forms of prayers, meditation or prayer/worship services, but there are many others.

A bit of history! The Solfeggio Frequencies, which make up the ancient 6-tone scale, were at one time used in all sacred music such as the Gregorian Chants. These chants, and their special tones, were believed to impart spiritual blessings when sung in harmony.[41] You probably hear elderly people talking about when they were younger how the *Mass used to feel*; or, perhaps, you even experienced these feelings when you were growing up in songs you learned in religion class, or sang in the traditional mass before the 1960's.

Though many of these tones are still used in the Eastern Rites, i.e., Byzantine and Orthodox rites, since a greater number of Catholics were more familiar with the Traditional Mass, most remember the Communion songs and many still remember the words. What happened? Was it the changing to modern Christian songs, or was it the guitar music that drove a wedge between what the older congregations liked versus the younger? We don't think so; but for a better understanding of

---

[39] Both Jesus and Mary are to be considered in this context a "Christ"—together—in human form because of their marriage. – Ed.

[40] Source Vibrations, Solfeggio Harmonics, Vol. 1.

[41] Mowry, Scott. "LIFE TRANSFORMATIONAL TOOLS #9: The Ancient Solfeggio Frequencies—'The Perfect Circle of Sound.'" The Solfeggio Frequencies ... Miracles & Inspiration ... Change Your Consciousness, Change Your Life, 2009, www.miraclesandinspiration.com/solfeggiofrequencies.html.

the continued spiraling of spirituality from the transcendental, despite God's efforts to connect and guide humans through their poor choices due to the human consciousness, we suggest you read 'Soma energetics' website.[42] It says:

> *"The origin of what is now solfeggio, arose from a Mediaeval Hymn to John the Baptist, which has this peculiarity: that the first six lines of the music commenced respectively on the first six successive notes of the scale, and thus the first syllable of each line was sung to a note one degree higher than the first syllable of the line that preceded it. By degrees, these syllables ended in a vowel. They were found to be peculiarly adapted for vocal use. 'UT' was artificially replaced by 'Do.' Guido of Arezzo was the first to adopt them in the 11th century, and Le Arie, a French musician of the 17th century added 'Si' for the 7th note of the scale, in order to complete the series.*
>
> *After the death of St. Pope Joannes the scale was changed, and the Master Composers were told not to use it anymore, and changes such as "si" later became "ti," which then significantly altered the frequencies sung by the Masses and for the masses. It was found that the alterations weakened the spiritual impact of the Church's hymns. Because the music held mathematic resonance, frequencies capable of spiritually inspiring mankind to be more Godlike, the changes affected alterations in conceptual thought as well as further distancing humanity from God. "In other words, whenever you sing a Psalm, it is music to the ears. But it was originally intended to be music for the soul, as well as the secret ears. By changing the notes, high matrices of thought, and to a great extent well-being, were squelched."*

---

[42] Somaenergetics.com

Each Solfeggio tone is comprised of a frequency required to balance our energy and keep our body, mind, and spirit in harmony.[43]

A transcendental consciousness is not the same as the thought processes of the mind, and the chakras play a big part in the enlightenment process. Since the consciousness we desire here is not bound by material or earthly things, but has an openness to the beliefs of others, we want to be sure that we implement the method of prayer and meditation used by Jesus. Being enlightened does not necessarily mean 'the acceptance of everything you hear or read,' *but rather the patience to hear and read through those facts presented to make their case.*

By heeding these suggestions, you will help prevent the interference of the conditioned mind and the ego (which is attached to the materially-centered mind and senses for its sense of identity).

---

[43] Mowry, Scott. "LIFE TRANSFORMATIONAL TOOLS #9: The Ancient Solfeggio Frequencies—'The Perfect Circle of Sound.'" The Solfeggio Frequencies ... Miracles & Inspiration ... Change Your Consciousness, Change Your Life, 2009, www.miraclesandinspiration.com/solfeggiofrequencies.html.

LESSON 18

THE NEED FOR REPETITION

Please keep in mind that repetition strengthens connections in our mind, making it easier for our brains to access information—and it also includes an emotional implication along with it. It is this emotional tie that actually allows for the consciousness to rise up, while the mind disengages during the enlightenment process. How this works is like this: when one reads new information for the first time, it can easily be forgotten. If not read again, even the translation changes since one does not remember exactly what was read. This then allows for other information to possibly be considered—perhaps the insertion of an opinion by the person repeating what was read. New information added changes the end thought from the information first read.

You will find that repetition of what you previously read solidifies the information and it is no longer 'something' of a new or desired point, but becomes part of your thought process, and your brain accepts it as infused knowledge. You will find that some fundamental ideas and concepts will repeat and weave throughout this book. This serves to represent our point of view thoroughly and with the perspective needed to tie together a specific belief, or its connection to a prefigured link, or even a present time discovery, or a future revelation being fulfilled in one's midst.

You will find that the more our beliefs are repeated the more confident you will become in your understanding of our transcendental point of view. A close friend showed me a cute little blog that they felt backed up the Eeshan view on repetition that is called, "Intellidance.ca." This simply exhibits how the more you use the application of repetition, the more you will find that your brain will begin to function at a higher vibration, and be more receptive to new information presented—and thus allow for the brain to disengage and operate on a very subtle wavelength.

LESSON 19

THE SECRET TO UNDERSTANDING UNFATHOMABLE TRUTHS

Exploring the transcendental brings with it concepts—though mentioned, touched on or alluded to—that are certainly not discussed in as much depth as in mainstream secular religions. The transcendental focuses, primarily, on the mystical and is centered on terms that were once labeled 'New Age;' this is so, frankly, because these are the only terms that best describes what goes beyond the limits of ordinary experience. These defy the human consciousness, allowing entrance into the deepest mysteries of God, since neither Jesus nor his teachings were ordinary—because he is the Son of God.

It is known among mystics, that when one encounters unfathomable truths, one experiences the arousing of a kind of blissful, or synesthesia effect, where the heart, mind and spirit, and will, while becoming united, evoke a kind of clarity to the conscious mind.

Achieving this clarity will present to the conscious and subconscious mind a powerful awareness—thus, bringing with it a kind of euphoria known to happen to the ancient prophets, holy people, and authentic gurus and yogis.

Guidance is key to an enlightened path. That is why those who have lived at the time of Jesus, and were taught by him, continued to follow him despite the ramifications that came along in their pursuit to "do whatever he says."

LESSON 20

A Prayer

May God bless you with enlightenment and spirituality. May God pull from within your heart the "values" that identify with the best part of you. May you always strive and seek to be the best version of yourself, and not just the better.

In doing so, may we obtain together, the world that God intended for us, despite being imperfect ourselves.

May God, Divine Masculine, and Divine Feminine, bless us with the Sacred Balance so sorely needed in this world and fill us with truth, love, and happiness that we may stir within each of us a profound desire to share with one another.

LESSON 21

WHY ARE WE LIKE WE ARE?

Life before the fall from the transcendental was much different than life after Adam and Eve's choice for a physical life. We know for sure that what followed their decision naturally negated those things the couple would normally have at their fingertips, including a strong love, with no desire for anything outside, or apart, from God. Needless to say, as Adam and Eve continued to drift further and further away from the transcendental, they moved more deeply into their human nature until they became subject to all that entropy brought with it. This began immediately after they were put out of the Garden, until the One promised would come. That 'One' was always taught to be Jesus.

The sacredly balanced spiritual mindset, which was sustained by Adam and Eve's unified relationship with God, became more and more weakened outside God's garden, and the lack of Spiritual Food and Drink necessary, to maintain a transcendental marriage was no longer available to them. This left them with only the bread made from the wheat grown—by Adam's hands, which nourished their bodies, but offered little to strengthen their resolve in dealing with their separation from the transcendental world. Contact from God was only when they were in dire need for help and guidance; and it was by their pleading and effort that God answered. This is not to say that God wasn't present—it was only to allow for the couple to realize what they had chosen and what they had lost.

What were the effects of the loss of this "Manna/Bread and Drink?" As one can deduce, the couple mutually stood before God as guilty for their misuse of free will, but certainly did not expect the consequences of their choice. When God spoke of death, being unfamiliar with all that went with that, what happened as time went on required God's assistance. Life as humans continued to wear them down. They witnessed how their transcendental thought process was not available to them. They were now subject to minds governed by a purely human consciousness which, more often than not, filled them with a sense of helplessness. This new rational awareness continued to force the couple to seek answers to daily struggles that they were constantly faced with. Ongoing changes in their bodies forced them to make adjustments while the understanding and the handling of these differences now plagued them. Their previous bodies were sustained by light; whereas, their new gross physical bodies, with an obvious weakened spirit, needed sustainable, organic food, which was now not readily available to them as it was in the Garden.

As time now entered the picture, and with no regular contact with God, and nothing to nourish their souls, we find yet another change taking place. Evidence of today's male behavior shows how the linear male mind started to become more developed. For without the influence of the Sacred Balance, Adam now began processing everything through a more limited (as in tunnel vision) way of looking at things, causing a diminishing sensitivity to Eve and their surroundings.

The directive from God to Adam to work the soil played out first in the male mind as different and foreign, but as time went on, we find how this change actually caused the male to become more task-oriented. Unfortunately, as Satan continued to be allowed to be the negative driving force, man fell victim to his fallen nature, and his use of free will was challenged with trying to be positive under decisions that would seem to create a darkness that would bring confusion to Adam. With the ongoing and continued loss of his transcendental consciousness, the male began experiencing feelings drawn from ego. Filtering down was feeling of 'a kind' of superiority over the woman, since, again, his physique was stronger. Without the spiritual nourishment he relied on in his past life, his physical body became testosterone-driven. The setting in of this hormone began replacing the love hormone oxytocin, and created within the male a more sensual drive. Thus, we see a more aggressive and possessive side developing—one which didn't possess a tremendous need for relationship maintenance.

The woman, having more white matter of the brain, found it easier to transition over to physicality, and still possessing more oxytocin, she was more relationship-oriented. She felt desire and the need for kindness and affection. Together, by God's design and command, the male and female would eventually balance each other through sacrifice and love.

LESSON 22

A Brief Look from Genesis to Revelation

Some think that after Adam and Eve chose the physical life over the transcendental life, Satan had completed his goal. This is not true. If this was true, there would be no evidence of his existence today.

His plan was first to destroy this human relationship with God, and then to destroy the couple's relationship with each other, which was blessed by God. Both could be accomplished if he could turn the couple away from God through their misery and suffering, and cause each to turn on the other through loss and blame.

The sole purpose of Satan's plan was to regain what he lost, and this was God's blessing. One sure way to once again obtain this blessing would be to have a child, a first 'born' male, who would rightfully receive the blessing. His efforts were eventually realized through delusion in the child Cain, but you will see how love conquers all.

We also find that if we accept the language of man in the traditional story of 'the Fall,' the above would seem rational and logical, since it solidifies what has been taught as true, which is male dominance over woman, and since it is written that 'man' was made in the image and likeness of God. Decades of denial (claiming the word 'man' is 'inclusive' and was meant to mean men, women, and children) is not reflected in the end result. It clearly reflects the contrary, which puts man above woman. One needs only to read the doctrines and laws to see how they were written to support this belief.

As Satan continued to position himself as a wedge between the couple, since he just didn't go away, it wasn't long before Eve began to notice the deterioration of the love that she and her husband once shared. Adam, tired from working the soil, and experiencing the wear and tear on the physical body and the constant mental idleness that made him a prime target for Satan's methodology, found himself thinking more and more of what he had lost and questioned if there was, mutuality of their choice. Though both tried to balance each other, it was obvious that the two both suffered from their choice. Eve would continue to show patience and kindness towards Adam, but she began feeling inadequate to satisfy him. Adam would make the effort to try and be more sensitive to Eve, despite the constant feelings of loss and failure. Eve suffered her own pain, since she, too, began to pick up on Adam's conflicting thoughts. There seemed to be more focus on human failure and loss than on their love. Both lacked the joy of sharing in each other's love.

One constant with the couple was their determination to appraise their daily problems and regrets and pray for God's help. In their frustration, and as they lost the desire to share love, Satan's efforts of preying on the couple's newfound inadequateness and incompleteness would pay off. One night Satan appeared to Eve as a beautiful being, mirroring himself as a son of God, shrouding himself in a glorious light, and he told her of God's desire for her. Hailing her as favored by God,[44] he entertained her with music, causing an intoxicating sensation to come over her, and he seduced her. Awakening from the slumber, however, she found Adam by her side awakening also.

Eve told Adam what she experienced. Though neither understood the experience, Eve continued to feel very much blessed by God. Thus, when the time was at hand and the child was born, Eve exclaimed to Adam, "I have gotten a man child from the Lord."[45] And thus the first male child was born into the world. Adam praised God, and together

---

[44] Cf. The angel coming to Our Lady and announcing that she was "highly favored" by God, making it the necessary reversal and correction of the original encounter between Satan and Eve. – Ed.

[45] Gen. 4:1.

with his wife, they shared a newfound love. Shortly afterwards, the love of the two brought Abel into the world.

The child that Adam and Eve thought she conceived by God, was in fact conceived by the seed of the evil one, which God spoke of when he said to the serpent, saying,

> *"I will put enmity between you and the woman, and between your offspring and hers; he will strike your head and you shall bruise his heel."*[46]

Eeshans believe that when God told Satan that there would be enmity between Satan's offspring and the woman's seed, the offspring of Satan would appear to be linked to the line of Cain. According to the story of Cain and Abel, this would seem to be the outcome for all those who deliberately reject God. For God warned Cain about the sin crouching outside the door, meaning Cain's jealousy was getting the better of him. God told Cain that all he had to do was what was right. God was giving Cain every opportunity to give generously from his heart, and not give only what he felt was good enough, expecting to receive praise for it. Satan too had turned his back on God out of jealousy of God's love for the created beings. In his jealousy, he seduced Eve.

Today many men who feel that because they have a God complex, due to money and power, think they can abuse women. These are those who seduce and use women as a trade-off for their dreams. These will feel the hatred of God through their emptiness due to loss of God. Like Satan, they want to be worshiped and feared, so they feel they have a right to take what they want.

It would take the only-begotten Child-beginning with the birth of "The divine Masculine of God," born of the Virgin Mary *who, through his marriage* to Mary Magdalen, will bring forth a Child in end times, who is the One who is like the Son of Man, and who will be born of the Woman in the wilderness. This will be He, whose head is in heaven for He is the

---

[46] Gen. 3:15.

Spirit of God; yet, being a human will rule using an iron rod, which is symbolic of a shepherd who uses a staff to protect his flock. As a shepherd. He will protect the new transcendental life, the new earth, filled with those who are ransomed through Jesus who conquered death, which is the opposite of the death brought about by Cain's father.

LESSON 23

ALL GOOD THINGS COME FROM ABOVE[47]

We have always been taught that all good things come to us from above. Indeed, this still stands true to today. 'God's example' is important and relative to social issues today. Has 'man' altered the focus away from the greatest and truest form of human love: Marriage? We believe so. Though the greatest love is that relationship that one has with God, *'true love' between humans has a 'divine' quality*, that when centered on love of God, possess that inexpressible love in which two human beings go beyond what the human consciousness can rationalize or explain. This is the love that, even after the fall, we witness and through which we see the totality of God's tenderness and unconditional love shine, since even though the first humans fell to physical love, human marriage received God's blessing. It is in marriage that this reaches the *agape* love that is mirrored in God's love for us and us for God; and because of that divine quality, that true love is shared between humans who are capable of sharing it.

The most important purpose and lesson behind the "Fall," as Eeshans teach, is to show how love, through the sacramental marriage, the blessed union where there is sacred balance, serves to contain within itself everything that is needed for the rest of one's life. In other words, we as males and females, who share in this extraordinary love through the Sacrament, can get through any difficulty, and experience a far greater love than imagined. That is why Jesus says, "love conquers everything." Though it is

---

[47] Cf. James 1:17.

difficult to imagine, the love and sacrifice which is shared with another human being in this union is capable of turning anything that is sad and hurtful, into many *ha-ha* moments. We find a greater appreciation for the life we have by loving one another, and ultimately witness true love of God's people and God's love for us. Jesus brought humankind back to perfect love, which he witnessed to daily; however, when one does not want change, and is satisfied with the status quo without any accountability, things won't change.

These same results occur when we find within ourselves anger and disdain for anyone, and everything just for the sake of feeling contempt, often with no valid reason. Hate will take on a life of its own and today it has become a natural way of life. When in marriage one no longer desires to give, feel, or express kindness and love towards the other person, the connection is lost, and each is vulnerable to selfishness, insensitivity, frigidity, and hatred can begin to grow. If these hurts could be found in a union of such strength under God, it's no wonder how it can be responsible for causing a breakdown in all relationships.

How often do we see people who look to be good examples for others, especially children? Personal examples evidencing manners, good habits, and kindness, expressed through civility, have become fewer and far between. According to the Vedic point of view in relation to the Yugas, or periods of the division of the Ages from a distant ancient past into the present time, and ending in the not too distant future, humanity steadily degrades itself, much in the same manner as captured in Isaiah 5:20:

"How terrible it will be for people who call good things bad and bad things good, who think darkness is light and light is darkness."

One needs only to observe children's shows, cartoons, and board/video games to see how bad things have gotten when fecal waste "poop" has become central to so many of these means of entertainment and pastimes. Everyone knows it's a normal body function but look what's happened!

Few feel the need to be honest, loyal, courageous, and honorable. It shouldn't matter who is against you no matter if it is religious teachers, politicians, or even the whole world! What should matter is how God sees our behavior, and if we are strong and courageous enough to think on our own principle of justice, goodness, kindness, perseverance and valor in order that we can make the world a better place. Believe it or not, the origin of such strength and balance of principles and morals should not only be found in marriage but should be actively sought after.

LESSON 24

STRENGTH FROM ABOVE

Eshans believe that because we can't seem to succeed in stopping inequality regarding genders, we must at least start by using every effort to reach a clear understanding of how this happened and 'why' we can't correct this. Being staunch believers in 'everything happens for a reason,' we inflected this reasoning when seeking out what it is/was that caused this divide. We know how things should fit together and when the facts point to more confusion, then we have to begin as far back as we can to discover when it all began.

Many have come to believe that what has been used and taught in Christian/Catholic circles, DOES NOT complete a picture but rather leaves us with fragments of parts of a puzzle that never really made sense or came together. So, we kept searching and moving the pieces until we found that what we were given were the *wrong pieces*, and, therefore, this puzzle would be impossible to solve.

What we found was that despite the fact that Jesus upheld women with the greatest of dignity and respect against the backdrop of other established religions, cultures, and mindset, his example and teachings in this regard didn't carry through the ages. In fact, it didn't go past his Ascension.

What was handed down were those same beliefs and improprieties that existed even 'prior' to his birth religion, since in other cultures, and/or mystical books and writings of patriarchal origins, this would inevitably be reflected among the fears and charges, which were also among the reasons he would be killed.

Once Jesus ascended into heaven, some of the apostles under Peter, who suffered from the weakness of man, took what they felt would cause them retribution, and so it appears it became a bargaining tool with religious authorities at that time. We presume it wasn't hard to instill into Peter thoughts of what his life was like prior to Jesus; and as a result, what Jesus taught was regressed back to what was easier, or perhaps safer, for those who felt as Peter did. We have found convincing evidence which seems to indicate that Peter succeeded to continue a spirituality that was a *blend* of old and new religious ways. Though that was the beginning of the early church, that of which we speak coming after Jesus, the end result proved to be the comparable actions of Peter's successors. On this same subject, what we ended up with leaves little to doubt. As they say, actions speak louder than words. Among those teachings that were lost were rights that Jesus had given to women. What we find is the same mindset of men, very much mirroring the culture of the time.

What we have knowledge of, and have found throughout the Old Testament, but especially at the time of Jesus, was that that there were none stronger than those women who loved Jesus and stayed near him during his passion, death, resurrection, and ascension, who unlike his male apostles, never feared for their lives. Unlike those male apostles who denied, or ran for fear of their lives, these women stood with Mary Magdalen and Jesus' Mother at the foot of the Cross. These women would, henceforth, continue to do what He taught them, and teach how He taught them, until eventually they were forced to stop or were killed. This is strength from above! The few men who stood by these women, and wrote accordingly, i.e., James, John, Philip, and Thomas, accepted these women as equals before God, who wondered who *among them* would dare to question Jesus or his wife? Only those who had not transcended, or gave Jesus lip service, would dare do that. Those who had transcended were like the 'seed that fell upon good fertile soil.'

Throughout the 'persecution,' women would remain loyal to Christ's teachings. Without Jesus being the power to be reckoned with, fear of being arrested, and killed, was, and continued to be, the method of choice to maintain the status quo.

A lie is not easy to admit to, so often times a weakness will use blame as the tool of choice to censure, or hold fast to a source, be it true or false. Deflecting charges is easier than taking fault, allowing oneself to stand with the strong, or not be included with the guilty. Making negative statements regarding an individual or group for his/their actions, respectively, when viewed as socially or morally irresponsible, especially against the backdrop of claims that what is being proposed, is against God's law. Here the oral law, as well as the Torah and Talmud, were, in effect, understood commonly as 'God's' law. Jesus, by virtue of the fact that he was and is God, had/has the right to end any part, or even the whole of the Old Law, and replace, or correct it with a New Law; and no human has the right to question, or change, what Jesus put into words and actions himself; since He is beyond reproach. Further, it would be expected that those followers, especially those closest to him, would have at least an inkling about what Jesus was doing, wouldn't you think? Wouldn't they also continue to live and teach following what he put into action after he left them?

Therefore, as we pointed out: if Jesus was God, and as he spoke, taught, and lived equality of gender, taught women, and used them in his parables, so when he was questioned about divorce, did they not see what he was saying? Jesus reminded them, "Haven't you read, 'that at the beginning the Creator made them male and female?'" He did not refer to the other story that says woman was formed from Adam's rib, which he could've pointed out. Instead, he used the version which indicates he saw that Adam and Eve were equal. If both made a decision to become human then both are responsible for the outcome; and if both were the cause of losing the transcendental, well, then, *both* would have to be represented since *both* were to be restored; and the only way back to God would be by a transcendental (yet, also human) marriage.

The marriage of Jesus and Mary was the example of the precious life two individuals shared as one before God, and the meaning of marriage was exalted. This means, if Adam and Eve were both joined in a transcendental marriage turned human, it would take a human marriage turned transcendental to accomplish this, with the exception that the latter have a divine component. Again, we derive strength from above.

What we are proposing here, is that Adam and Eve's human marriage no longer had a connection to the transcendental life, which means this 'new' human marriage of theirs lacked the divine element, which the transcendental marriage, indeed, possess, and this was the greater part. Also, because of Jesus' marriage to Mary Magdalen, their divinity completed the human marriage, and it would reap the greatness of a transcendental life *during its lifetime.* This is what Jesus taught and prophesized regarding his own 'marriage' when he said, "Greater is the love that one would lay down one's life for a friend." As they live, so shall they die; and as they die, so shall they be Resurrected. Being the epitome of human love, we find a perfect example of God making human weaknesses our strengths. The Son of God, the Divine Masculine of the only begotten Child, was revealing the most powerful love of all by restoring and bringing the love of God to human marriage, since this is enduring love which derives its strength from God and trumps all other loves. That is what He accomplished by his transcendental marriage. But why is this important? Because it boggles the mind that no one figured out who, and what, Jesus was, let alone why he came. He may have taken on sin, but this was not the reason, as one is led to believe, it was a means.

LESSON 25

WHAT DOES GOD'S SALVIFIC PLAN ENTAIL?

For success of God's plan everyone is taught that Jesus Christ had to be the altar, victim, and priest; but what is not taught, is that God's plan required 'two humans:' a Male and a Female. Jesus reiterated this when asked about divorce. He taught, "In the beginning, God created 'them' male and female." Therefore, if both disregarded God's directive, then both are guilty. It would then take two 'Eternal' Consorts. The human Jesus would have to be married, and live transcendentally in a human marriage, to bring a richer and deeper, and divine sustenance to be a salvific plan, and to restore the divine component in the sacrament. By introducing his human wife to be equal to Him was an outward sign of their oneness and equality. By their marriage both were subject to each other; and, as God, he showed how both were called to love, serve, and worship God.

Jesus did not just enjoy the company of his wife, but prayed with her, taught her, and shared everything with her. He also included her in all aspects of his work, and Mary did the same. The love and relationship between God, the Father and the Virgin Mary was always reflected in the relationship between Jesus and Mary, since it accompanied with it the reality that all that is good comes from God who is above us, and which filters down to us and infiltrates each cell in our body. Thus, from this sacrificial love we then are supposed to be the leaven of which Christ spoke, bringing love and mercy to each other. The eternal marriage of Jesus and Mary Magdalen was meant to bring back this Metta.[48] Their marriage

---

[48] Suffice it to say for now that the term "love" as human consciousness can comprehend it is inadequate to describe Metta. The term should invoke the image of a love from a transcendental origin or divine element; whereas, the divine element was slowly

exhibits the remarkable, undying strength of this human bond and its endurance through suffering and pain. Each manifested a love so strong that, without question, each would die to save the other. Their love was the altar on which they laid their cross. They were the High Priests who offered their love in exchange for God's love for us. They were the victims who laid down their life in order that we could live.

Both, as one, sacrificed their marriage and life together to save us. We are their begotten children—human by a choice, made by Adam and Eve; divine by the New Adam and Eve's choice. But it couldn't end here, *for it was a salvific plan.*

---

drained from Adam and Eve's human marriage and brought back through Jesus and Mary's human/transcendental marriage. Their marriage bridges the threshold from the human to the transcendental, between the earthly and heavenly realms, as in the beginning of marking a new life, where the bride and groom cross over the threshold, "As above, so below." Note also in this connection, that as the Groom traditionally carries the Bride across the threshold, it reflects Jesus holding up the Divine Feminine out of love and respect, and allowing her to precede him into the heavenly realm. Cf. Coomaraswamy, Traditional Art and Symbolism, p.8 – Ed.

Lesson 25A

Jesus had a limited time to bring people to the awareness of why there was a need for a Messiah and what was going to be accomplished. By Mary's presence, he showed a wife's place; by his defense of her, he showed truth; and by keeping his wife close to him, he showed their oneness in what God had put together. Jesus talked about marriage and with the parable of the King's son, Jesus outlined, almost as a prophecy, things to come as he witnessed the obstinacy of Peter, and others, towards her constant inclusion at their gatherings. Maybe he used it all knowing how it would be played out in the future, as he was coming to the end of his public mission with his Bread of Life discourse.

Just as it was no accident that he would use Melchizedek's example one day when he was speaking to the crowd who came to hear him, and then distributed bread and fish to a great number, often said to be 5,000 people. Melchizedek was known for having a tent where weary travelers could come and rest. First the King would wash their feet; and then, and only after he talked to them about God, would he give them bread and water.

LESSON 26

The First Kallahs

The women closest to Mary, who lived with her and Jesus, were the first to experience Jesus' private teachings, and when it came time for their public mission, the men would be chosen. It was these first women who participated in prayers and who Jesus taught. They learned techniques for worship services; and along with him practiced privately. This was necessary, as, again, women were not familiar with religious ceremonies, except for what they heard, or witnessed during the preparation and serving of food, or in other instances, or what their husbands told them.

With the growing number of women who would eventually join them, it would be these women of Mary Magdalen, that would bring alive the many stories and teachings of the marriage of Jesus and Mary and its most intimate nature.[49]

Jesus was the best thing that ever happened to women. From the moment he became public, women were made to feel special by him and loved by God. Even though it is written, 'Husbands love your wives, just as Christ loved His church, that he gave Himself up for her', Eeshans know that it was Jesus' intention to have his wife fulfill His desire to continue His work which would disconnect the error of the Old Testament meaning. For it would be for her, Mary, that he would give up his life, and to our benefit. Why do we say this? We say this because his mission counted on it.

---

[49]Today interesting and compelling evidence has been found with regards to this with the excavation of Mary Magdalen's altar on which their names were carved.

Though we are told that his last words were: "Into Thy arms I commend my spirit," His last seven words were to His wife, "Mary, we will never be separated again." It was from the cross that He together with his wife declared, "It is finished."

With those words, the "curse" was lifted. The two were linked together—from eternity to eternity. Because of their unconditional love of God and each other, even in their temporary human life, together they became victims to death, and once Christ was resurrected and death was conquered, death only became temporary.

Even though they knew Jesus was the Messiah, and were very much aware of His impending suffering and dying, Jesus was, nevertheless, preparing them for the future, since their present time with Him would be short lived.

Under Mary Magdalen, there were a group of women who lived with her, which in time would be called Kallahs. Kallah means 'timeless brides.'[50] These were the first women apostles/priestesses, of whom nothing was ever said or written. These were the first to have received the sacred words of alchemy, which is necessary for the transubstantiation of the human gifts of bread and wine into the greatest of all alchemical wonders.

What happened to them? After Jesus ascended, Peter forced the women out of their roles, by making them subservient. After he had enough of Mary Magdalen's claims that Jesus was instructing her, he had others force her into exile in hopes she would die aboard a boat with no oars. Others who would not be subservient would be, by "God's Law" (but in reality it was by '*man's law*'), arrested or put to death. Along with them, any evidence, or memory of them, was destroyed or suppressed; and like Mary's Consciousness, their consciousnesses would lay in a suspended state, until brought forward via the Divine Feminine, once again, in these end times.

---

[50] "Kallah" in Hebrew means "bride;" "Kala" in Sanskrit means "eternal time;" Eeshans consider it fitting to employ the meanings of both words in their respective languages in the one term. The sense of meaning of the term as employed by the author continues to unfold. – Ed.

LESSON 27

THE RESURGENCE OF MARY MAGDALEN'S KALLAHS

On October 23–25, 2013, Eesha, once again, introduced to the world, in an exceptionally mystical and emotional ceremony, the resurgence of Mary Magdalen's Kallahs (Brides) of Christ. Hence, this solemn occasion would mark the beginning of the Age of Enlightenment, or Final Testament, second only to the supramentalization of the consciousness of Mary Magdalen by the hand of Christ Himself.

These women, whose 'recent' presence was prophesied, have been conferred with the Sacred Mysteries and endowed with the mystical powers of the Sacraments. They were brought back by the divine feminine, in these end times, to be the guardians of she who has been awakened to continue Christ's mission. How do we know that these were the original women who have been awakened by the consciousness of the Divine Feminine to present time? With yearning hearts and a predestined calling, Mary, and her Kallahs, trusted in her belief, and promised that they would always be together; and once Jesus and Mary were reunited, it would be necessary for these women to propagate the Eeshan Religion. These women will assist the divine feminine in her efforts to complete Christ's salvific mission, alongside her once again! Eesha would recognize who they were, and they would recognize her.

With Mary's encrypted identity finally realized, her title as Eesha can now be claimed. The Kallahs' true identities were also hidden, and their life as they knew it, was obscured. The reason for this is the prophecy of the Seven Women to be raised up in these end times, and that the peace Jesus brought into the world quite possibly may resound once again.

These words were prophesized as Isaiah 4:1. Taking the prophet's word in the manner in which it not only predicts the Kallahs of Jesus' and Mary's time, but for present time, he says:

> *'In that day seven women will take hold of one Man [Jesus] and say, "we will eat our own bread and wear our own clothes, only let us be called by your name; take away our reproach* (by men)!*"'*

And he did.

Each Kallah is married to Christ and enjoys the ancient, Kabbahlic, Merkabahalic, mystical marriage of the Lamb, and his Wife in their priesthood, and shall be pundits,[51] having a positive effect on all those who will listen. They share in the sacred union, unlike one had ever experienced before. They are Kallahs to Eesha, the hidden queen, who carries the consciousness of Mary Magdalen in human form. As extensions of her, they shall be guided by her wisdom; and prayerfully, and with love, she will assist her Kallahs in bringing to an end the cries of injustice.

The Kallahs are likened to the seven golden stars mentioned in Revelation with respective golden lampstands. Though difficult to comprehend with a human consciousness of rational, logical thinking, in this age of Enlightenment, by the hands of the Divine Feminine, the Kallahs are once again brought back into time. One must remember:

> *'When a timeless mystery enters into time, the most powerful positive vibrations of epic proportion brings a disruption of negative energies—taunting these powers and causing change'.*[52]

These moments, or mysteries, are not always easily accepted. People had a difficult time accepting Jesus also. Some who profess loyalty to

---

[51] From the Sanskrit word 'pandita,' meaning learned, denoting a learned person or teacher, one who gives opinions in an authoritative manner. – Ed.

[52] Source unknown. – Ed.

Christ and his Wife,[53] may yet find the resurgence of the Divine Feminine and the Kallahs difficult to accept. If you believe in the transcendental, or have experienced supernatural incidents, it may come a little easier, but we still suggest you continue on in your reading.

It is written in Revelation 2:1-29:

> **To the angel of the church of Ephesus writes: The words of him who holds the seven stars in his right hand, who walks among the seven golden lampstands, "I know your works, your toil and your patient endurance, and how you cannot bear those who are evil, but [I] have tested those who call themselves apostles and [they] are not and [I] found them to be false. I know you are enduring patiently, and bearing up for my name's sake, and you have not grown weary.** *[the warning:]* **But I have this against you** *(who continued to ignore my teachings and change my directives),* **that you have abandoned the love you had at first.** *[For to ignore the Kallahs and love only the co-redeemers is to not believe or trust in the co-redeemers' directives, which denotes that you have fallen away from what you first professed—and this is to doubt or worse: deny the spirit of God is within them through their ordination—or think these cannot or should not have the co-redeemers Christed bodies—or that they are substandard to males.]* **Remember therefore, from where you have fallen; repent and do the works you did at first.** *[Go back to where you professed to do whatever God asked of you, despite the lies and tribulations of what you once believed and thus invested your love and continue on the path of the*

---

[53] The expression Christ and his Wife is used to denote Jesus and his wife Mary, who are, together, both a part of the 'what' of Christ. The reader will see in subsequent descriptions the expression 'the Christs,' which denotes both Jesus and Mary as a part of the Second Person. This Second Person is revealed as two together and as one in mutual self-offering, being both Divine Masculine and Divine Feminine. – Ed.

transcendental. Do not grow weary] **If not, I will come to you and remove your lampstand."** *[and you will no longer see the Way—who is Jesus—unless you repent.]*

These verses are interpreted to be for end times.

The Seven Lampstands are Christ's seven Kallahs (priestesses[54]) who are created by God's design, and the stars are the Christed Bodies of Jesus and Mary (co-redeemers) within their bodies. These Kallahs offer on earth the Marriage Feast of the Lamb and His Wife, as celebrated in heaven, which is the Marriage Feast described in the Book of Revelation 1:7.[55]

To those who have accept and believe in Christ's Wife, and feel that they fought the good fight against those who persecuted her; yet, cannot accept with love these seven extensions, these ordained women priestesses for whatever reason, must repent, for this, too, is true. So, as you see why we believe and fight to have Mary Magdalen vindicated, as it was in the beginning is now and ever shall be our goal for women/females, since no trickery gets past Jesus, because He knows all, sees all; since He is almighty God.

---

[54] While it is common to hear the term 'women priests' in modern parlance, the Eeshan perspective will, henceforth, employ the term "priestess" when referring to women who function in the priestly role of Kallah, as the term is now gender appropriate. It would be a misnomer to refer to the Kallahs' service in this capacity with language denoting male roles. Formerly the term 'priestess' may have been considered 'uncomfortable' by some, especially in traditional Christianity, because it would seem to evoke a 'pagan' image of something impure or unclean; nevertheless, the proper term 'priestess' will, henceforth, be used pertaining to the female, while 'Chatan' will be used for males who are priests. – Ed.

[55] Commentary: which is the return of Jesus to earth with his Bride, and the armies of heaven to establish the Throne of Jesus upon the earth which will bring a new time. Perfect union with Him and participation in his holiness at the marriage feast of the Lamb she becomes his wedded wife. It is in this time the Bride of the Lamb: Mary Magdalen is to be known. She is the wisdom Christ Sophia sent forth from the beginning of time with her companions to bring a new hope, faith, and truth into the world desiring unity with a light and spirit of Jesus. Now the Bride can be with the Bridegroom, united, to never be separated, for all eternity. She is seated beside him and suffered with him as he did on earth. She is set above all creation as wife to the Divine Masculine of the only begotten Child of God. She will always be beside him for all eternity.

LESSON 28

WHY DO THE KALLAHS HAVE GOD'S PROTECTION?

The Lampstands we are talking about here, are the Alchemical Words of Transubstantiation that each Kallah possess today, and are those which are used in the ceremonial Sacred and Divine Marriage Feast of the Lamb and His Wife. This is likened to the turning of basic foods into living gold, which includes the fire of life through the marriage of Jesus and Mary and the fruit of their marriage; the first born of the first born, Emmanuel, truly Divine, androgynous, fully human and already present in these end times.[56] The benefits of the marriage feast are then passed on to all human beings who believe.

We possess an immortal soul, and, by our physicality, we have DNA which contains within it light and evidences a light body. The Eucharist of the Marriage Feast is the sacred presence and totality of what was lost and now regained. This Eucharist is the spiritual food necessary for eternal life, fulfilled "only" through the Marriage Feast of the Lamb and His Wife, being the final mystery, the Final Testament.

The Kallahs honor, surround and protect the Eesha in these eschatological days. They are pure in heart, and though they hold a place of great

---

[56] The mystical body of Christ and his Wife—who, in end times, is the woman in the wilderness, and, who, on earth, will bring forth a man child as foretold in scriptures as being One who is like the Son of Man. Clothed with the sun, she is the woman with twelve stars upon her head.

honor, they themselves function in a world of rebellious people. They do, however, value the kindness extended to them from those who follow Mary Magdalen, and "exhume"[57] Metta, which is unsurpassed loving kindness to whomever they encounter.

---

[57] In line with the Eeshan perspective, the word "exhume" is deliberately used here to convey the sense that Metta, God's love, was 'buried away' so that it would not interfere in the plan of furthering the objectives of the human consciousness. – Ed.

LESSON 29

PETER'S CONSTANT ATTEMPTS TO SWAY JESUS' ATTENTION AWAY FROM MARY

How many of you remember when women were not included in men's discussions about business, politics and other issues? How many know of the threat of men losing their jobs, or status, should they promote such a thing?

This was the reality of thinking before Jesus and continued within the church as early as found in 1 Corinthians 14: 34-35, where it is said that St. Paul wrote, "As in all the congregations of the saints, women should remain silent in the churches. They are not allowed to speak, but must be in submission, as the Law says. If they want to ask a question, they should ask their own husbands at home; for it is disgraceful for a woman to speak in the church." (vv 35-36). Then he contradicts himself in chapter 11, when he said women could pray in church, and prophesy, if in the proper attire. Well, something went wrong with Paul's first comment, unless he was following Peter's witness as Leader. Perhaps later, he witnessed the words of those who listened to Mary Magdalen's teachings and instructions given to those who followed Jesus' example regarding women.

Later in the texts you will see what we mean by the human consciousness and Peter's continued link to the Old Law.

Because women, especially Mary Magdalen, could not participate in worship services in the same way men did, especially in the temple, so that Jesus used the outdoors as his synagogue. This gave him the freedom to introduce women in this capacity. Eventually women disciples from several places and cultures joined the group, and began to travel with them and pray with them. In time, this would become the underlying growing rage of the religious leaders and teachers of the time. Paul was brought up according to the strictness of the Law; and, thereby, evidences this in his first statement, especially if not all of Jesus' apostles were on board with this 'new' teaching. Eeshans believe that what he heard about Mary Magdalen's teachings is the reason his opinion was changed in his second statement.

We are not exempt from the difficulties Mary and other women ran into in biblical times, because they are mirrored today. We won't find too much in scriptures either for obvious reasons, and, what we do find, lacks details, or changes, that caused the truth to be obscured.

In Matthew 7:2-5, we find many teachings where Jesus would make use of public forums to rebuke Peter and the others who had serious difficulty with Mary and other women being present at conversations that Jesus was having with the men. One specific time (as seen in the Gospel of Thomas, Logion 114, which was omitted from the official canon of scriptures), Peter requested Jesus to remove Mary from their private gatherings with those males who were present, "for women are not worthy of life." Jesus responded: "This is how I will guide her so that she becomes male. She, too will become a living breath like you men. Any woman who makes herself 'male'[58] will enter into the Kingdom of God." He continues addressing this issue in Matthew 19:12, that there are all kinds of people born differently than what was considered the 'norm' at that time for males and females. Whoever can accept what Jesus said should be allowed to accept it (here you will see how the words were changed only to reflect *eunuchs*, but he also meant all people), and making the point that the one who can accept this should accept it. He further addresses Peter's statement in Matthew 7:2, when he says, "For in the same way you judge others (to include Mary and any woman), you will be judged;" and Jesus continues in Matthew 7:5, "You hypocrite! First take the plank out of your own eye before you attempt to remove the speck from your brother's eye." (This was intended to tell Peter to stop trying to influence Jesus.) Instead, Jesus rebuked him and continued in

---

[58] Few consider the possibility that Jesus was employing sarcasm in response to Peter, much in the same manner as he would rebuke the arrogance of the Pharisees. – Ed.

1 John 4:20: "Any man who says, 'I love God,' and hates or insults [(my wife) or any woman, (and this can most assuredly be applied again for today adding): especially a woman who loves and serves her God (especially one who is a Kallah)], is a liar. For how can you not love one you can see, and say you love one whom you cannot see" (meaning God)? Here he was calling them to see that in his eyes, his wife, or any woman, as well as any person who came to hear him at the time, had equal rights to hear what he had to say and teach.

As Jesus is the living and eternal Word, his words are for *all* ages, and rest assured, He was addressing all those in his day and in present times, who rejected (or now reject) His eternal consort, and those women who stood by His side then and in the future who carry Christed Bodies. To attack or insult his wife [or any woman at that time, especially a Kallah (a woman priestess/follower) becomes that person's problem, and he warned them to consider the reasons why. Perhaps it comes down to the male rejection of any female in equal place with a male before God or pre-Jesus man-made laws. For Peter, it was two-fold: he could not let go of his birth religion; and, secondly, he wanted Mary's place with Jesus, since he as a man felt entitled.

Eeshans warn that Peter's difficulties regarding Jesus and Mary's equality could be judged as an attack on the Spirit of God. By his ignoring Jesus and Mary's oneness by their marriage, thus dismissing Jesus' private and public teachings to include his identity as the Son of God, was he judging the spirit of Jesus as God? Was Peter capable of the unforgivable sin, which is the eternal sin that Satan committed? IF he knew who Jesus was and doubted Jesus' word, maybe.

Could Peter have had personal problems which would present an issue with the law if discovered? Whatever the reason, we know he was motivated by cowardice. We also present this: in following the old ways and laws, could malcontents, out of fear, continue to put down alternate gender relationships and condemn them in order to keep their own issues secret?

Peter was always 'concerned' about Jesus' safety. Why? Did he not remember how he exclaimed that Jesus was the Messiah? Could Peter have given others wrong impressions of Jesus? Could he have voiced concern over Jesus' marriage to a woman who was rumored by men to be a prostitute? Could Peter have been lax in keeping his own issues private, and questions were arising regarding his overly possessive interest in Jesus, because Jesus never condemned different gender relationships? Could this be his concern? Could he have sinned against one of God's laws as listed in the book of Leviticus? Or because the Pharisees had already committed the eternal sin by proclaiming that Jesus was a sorcerer, and the source of Jesus' miracles was Beelzebub, could this then make Peter afraid that they would judge him, too; so he played both sides of the fence?

SECTION II: USING FOCAL POINTS INTRODUCTION TO: GOD, FREE WILL AND HUMANKIND

At this time, we would like to introduce some center points which should begin a kind of *data that will continue to run in the background of your subconscious*, which your brain, in attempting to deal with this, may use as anticipation and prediction, as well as cause and effect.

This means, that if you come to recognize these points, as you come across certain texts, these words, or verses, will be in the background of your mind, giving you a quick reference point to keep your mind from venturing back to the human consciousness, while you continue to grow into the transcendental consciousness. These focal points about God and humankind will allow this quickening access and expand your awareness. Knowing and understanding the following will help in the understanding of the Christs' mission, which was the restoration and means to attain the transcendental life, as once enjoyed by Adam and Eve and their offspring before they fell to physicality.

They will also give you some examples of some similar common threads, as well as providing the very distinct differences between the Eeshan Religion and other more traditional religions.

LESSON 30

FOCAL POINT: GOD

When we think about God we think only about those things we were taught which define a being with one gender. We are taught that though God is to be seen as genderless, for the sake of a relationship with humans, God is labeled male, even though all that was created by God carries a masculine, feminine dynamic. Also, when questioned about God as being female: we are told 'He' has feminine attributes. Yet attributes defined is resulting from a specific cause. Wouldn't the cause here be a feminine nature? We don't realize the vastness of this incredible Being of God. In other words, we think about the Who of God, but forget there's the What of God.

The following gives you some insight into the "what" of God, and, in particular, it should help you on your journey to enlightenment. Let's take a look at a couple things that will enable you to see more clearly and transcendentally the true wisdom behind God's perfect parental love, what it is and how it continues to be the origin of our parental love for our children. You should begin seeing how it mirrors exactly what we go through with the raising or rearing of our children as well as the children of others. Let's try and remember these four things about God, which will help in seeing the difference between God the Creator, Redeemer, and Sanctifier in comparison to the *created beings* that *we* are. This is important, since we tend to forget that God made us; and, therefore, we are not on the same level. This is where Lucifer made his deadly mistake in thinking he was equal to God; and, therefore, he could expect to be seen and adored by those who, too, were created. God is:

1) *Infinite* with no beginning and no end, meaning that God was not created.
2) *Sacredly Balanced.* This refers to the what of God. The sacred balance is comprised of two energies, Divine Masculine and Divine feminine. This is the heart of the Yin/Yang dynamic of inter-penetrating and mutually supportive/nurturing energy playing out as positive and negative polarity; or masculine and feminine energies expressed through personhood. *In other words: as we consider God as being beyond all conception and human ability to imagine, or define at the same time, we do know that God is, indeed, perfectly balanced and purely reflected in the created order. This means that every person created has a yin-yang dynamic of male and female operating in their being.*
3) *Both unlimited power and energy, and is also unlimited in Personhood; that is, God has both an impersonal aspect and a personal aspect.*
4) *Trinity, three persons, with actual feminine Consorts; but also, together one God.* In each person of the Trinity, the Creator, Redeemer, and Spirit is a manifestation of pure consciousness, which is divided into two aspects, neither of which exists without the other. Each requires the other in order to manifest its total nature. As there is a shared Divine male and Divine female aspect which precedes Christianity in many other religions, Eeshans feel the result of God's Dual identity was played out in the world prior to Christ's incarnation, by all Persons of the Holy Trinity, beginning with the First Person.

Lesson 30A

Free Will

There is one fact that has been taught for thousands of years: life was different before Eve coerced Adam into eating the apple of the forbidden tree.

Eeshans believe that the committing of the Original Sin was not a deliberate transgression of the law of obedience, meaning that Adam and Eve did not want to hurt God; however, they did not weigh what their God told them as opposed to what someone who falsely indicated that he was God told them. This being the case, Adam and Eve's choice was abetted by one we have come to know and identify as Satan, who is a being and a perverse hyper-grace teacher.[59]

Most people are under the assumption that the story of the "Fall" was the greater of the two-part story, of which the first part gives us very little detail with regards to Adam and Eve's life before the 'curse' and emphasizes more of the second part. Eeshans feel the need to show how the traditional story, minus the details of the first part, of Eve's coercing Adam deludes one into basing Christ's suffering and death on a very misleading premise and makes lovers of God look like fools.

Eeshans feel that they had a need to compare the traditional story of the 'Fall' with what they believe was not just a vague superficial and unsound reason for God to take such drastic steps, since He is also having his only-begotten Son, suffer, and die.

It appears to be a fallacy upon which the argument is based against women, and all humans, that was, indeed, contrived by humans; whereas, Eeshans view that what took place was not solely contrived by either Adam or Eve, but was the result of the cunning, overwhelmingly delusional mind of Satan and the corrupted 'facts' that he presented to them.

---

[59] Referring to a way of teaching with emphasis on the grace of God to the exclusion of other vital teachings. – Ed.

Once this occurred, a weakened spirituality, along with corrupted reasoning and logic, left them vulnerable to the One of whom Isaiah 14:12 says:

> How you have fallen from heaven, morning star, son of the dawn!
> You have been cast down to the earth, you who once laid low the nations!
> For you said yourself, "I will ascend to heaven, and set my throne above God's stars. I will sit on high. I will preside on the mountain of the gods' away in the north."

Adam and Eve were strong, and Eeshans believe that it took tremendous 'convincing,' and with the frequency of planned occasions and deliberate attempts to keep the couple from being in God's presence, since in doing so Satan could, thereby, demonstrate the logic and reasoning necessary to encourage the couple's misuse of their free will.

The choice of Adam or Eve was not impulsive, but occurred only after lengthy deliberation, even though Satan was the master of reasoning. Satan waited for wisdom to fall to logic, and downplayed the consequences God presented to the couple. In doing this, it did not seem or appear from the start to be a serious offense, after hearing his provocations. Temptation under a broken will, due to the bombardment of logic, seems to be what ended the strong tie the couple had to God.

It took tremendous effort on Satan's part against the transcendental humans to the point where they ate the apple. This poisonous fruit brought with it death. In order to get them to eat the fruit, it was enhanced in beauty, and carried with it intoxicating effects. This mystical fruit, which was the final act that ultimately caused the fall from the transcendental world, caused Adam to see Eve more beautifully, as well as Eve more desirous of Adam in ways she never experienced before. What then was the end result? They kissed. They kissed in a very strong sexual way.

So, were they *punished*, or did they merely have to live out the consequences of their choice?

Lesson 30B

The Human Being

In human beings, there can be one nature that is dominant, while the other is recessive, or there can be a neutral energy where both energies seem to be prominent. Through the window of the physical body, there are various expressions of these combinations of male and female in relationship to one another. These comprise the different genders with which we are all familiar.

The body is a covering and is necessary for being here in 'this world'. By virtue of the fact that it is the result of the choice made by Adam and Eve to engage in physicality, it is flawed and broken, but necessary for life and serves as the vehicle for the soul. The body is *not* the self.

Through emotion and the endocrine system of the physical body, the basic forms of physical gender are called male and female. This is due to the predominant expression of that masculine/feminine energy. Then there are various combinations of that energy interacting in the physical body, and this interplay and mutual complimentary energy flow from this yin/yang, male and female relationship; BUT it is through the heart-mind complex that the male/female expression of the person shines forth. In balanced polarity, there is relationship and communication, harmony and balance. When these are disturbed, we are left with friction and chaos.

The first humans were creatures created by God who once lived in a transcendental world, who ended up making an imprudent choice, having exercised their free will under duress. Every day we have to make decisions. These are made in much the same way. Under duress, we can make imprudent choices; when we are clear minded, we make prudent choices. In having a relationship without God, the chances of making an imprudent decision are greatly increased. It is possible to make wrong choices even with a relationship with God, but the difference is that with God's presence in our life and nourishing our soul, we can accept the result of a imprudent decision, and chalk it up to God closing a window and opening a door.

Without proper guidance, or perhaps to give us what God desired, a free voluntary love, he taught us, by our first parents' mistake, how by staying close to God and being nourished, we will make better decisions. The consequence of not learning from Adam and Eve's experience can alter our 'destiny' and become our 'fate' too.

God is not rigid but being "all good," and our Father and Mother, as Jesus told us, since it is time we realized the efforts we must put behind being the best we can be.

The story of Adam and Eve gives us proof of God's existence, what true love is, and rules for parenting, allowing us to appreciate God's gifts. We know how true this is for it is said, "We don't know what we had, nor do we appreciate it, until we lose it."

If God wanted the best for us, and to share in all things in God, we know that it was important then for Adam and Eve to come to this realization—not by force, but by choice. Making choices defines who we are and what's important to us. Adam and Eve had everything. Did they know what they had? They obviously did not.

We can look at free will as the one imperfection God built into Adam and Eve; or we can look at their decision as presenting a choice to listen, or not to listen to one who is experienced, or in this case, one who is all-knowing. What was apparent in this situation, is that apart from what God tells us we need, our free will is susceptible to being deluded into thinking that 'we know better.' This is when our already fallen nature becomes subject to all the imperfections we 'all' have, and we find ourselves lost and on our own. Having God in our lives is the best way for us to find "real happiness;" since despite our not wanting to admit it, God is the one with all the answers. What would serve us to better appreciate what God has given us, and to love genuinely, are examples of those things, or people, which simply show us what and how life would be without God.

Eeshans can't imagine how the traditional story of Adam and Eve could ever be accurate in the face of all things that relate to us who Jesus is. When you consider all He taught, and then try to apply it to what was taught about Adam, Eve, and God, there are glaring differences between how Jesus talks about his Father, and the 'punishing' God in the story.

Being disobedient to God, as described in this book, seems to define 'free will' as exercising a not-so-free a will, at all. It does not give way to learning how God is there for us in good times and bad. It just doesn't allow for seeing *how we need* 'Him,' discovering true love, and working, living, and dying for that love. It is curious how everything about Jesus shows *these things* in how He lived what He preached, and more. In fact, it shows how he sighted and addressed the 'wrong' impressions the people had of God with stories like the 'Prodigal Son,' and how we are to call God "Father," and how the Virgin Mary was not only his Mother, but our Mother (thus, making the two married, and truly His Parents).

What we were told regarding Adam and Eve's fall set the platform and agenda for those who speak on behalf of God, assuming the right to punish and abuse, render their opinions regarding social injustice towards all genders, cultures, and God-centered belief, but not have to live what they preach and threatened those whose hearts spoke differently about these issues.

Over time, the exile of the couple from Paradise, since the reason of being "disobedient" to God's law has been significantly responsible for creating the collateral damage of an imbalance of soulmates, heavily influences the development of the human mind and heart towards discrimination throughout the ages.

If the truth had been revealed that Adam and Eve were both soulmates and twin flames, we would see that the purpose of their life was God's desire for them to share in the kind of love the Divine Masculine and Divine Feminine shared as One. After their choice (to leave the transcendental) to embrace the physical, being 'outside' of God was not balanced automatically, as when they lived their transcendental life, they now had to put effort towards loving each other under very difficult circumstances. They had to work together and keep each other spiritually strong. They realized, through sacrifice, that they were accountable for their decisions, but attained a deeper, richer, and more abiding love, despite the trials, tribulations, and just the everyday hard hits of life, which would be reflected in the love of the divine consorts that would come as the Messiahs, as promised by God to end the affliction Adam and Eve's choice caused their children.

Learning about Adam and Eve before the 'fall' we realize how God actually saw them. Just as parents with children, God wanted to give them everything. Doesn't God's response to the couple's decision reflect how we handle situations with our own children? God wanted Adam and Eve to have everything! This was to include no pain, no suffering, etc. All that was desired for them was for them to love, appreciate, and be thankful for what God had given them. Don't we try and make things possible and easier for our children so they don't have to work as hard as we did, and that they could have everything of which they could possibly dream? And, do we just want them to see what we sacrificed so that they could appreciate what they have been given out of our love for them? Sometimes however, when we find that what we gave them is not appreciated and they want to do things 'their way,' despite our efforts, and they fail, we exercise tough love, even if it means they must lose everything? Why then do we then expect God to overlook what may serve to make them better people, by not giving in to our pleas? Where we may slip back from 'doing what is right' to thinking we are too hard on them, or that they may have suffered enough, that even maybe God is showing them how working and sacrificing makes one appreciate more of what was given and earned. God does not give in to children's, even 'adult' children's, temper tantrums. If this happened they will never go out on their own. Seeing our children happy and handling life's situations is a parent's greatest accomplishment and joy. It's God's, too.

Though it is taught that 'disobedience' was the 'punishable offense,' Eeshans believe differently. It was the continued delusional, or fixed *false* beliefs, which were projected on the couple, that though were caused by Satan, were, in fact, they were allowed by God. It was allowed for God's will not to impose on free will, even at the risk of losing the transcendental world. To do this would negate the true meaning of love, since to love is a choice and often requires 'sacrifice.'

LESSON 31

WHAT DO WE GAIN BY FINDING ERRORS IN SCRIPTURES?

Challenging scripture's veracity is the only way we can preclude the continuation of the lack of change which was never intended for humankind. What we want to see is the return of faith and hope. No longer should the traditional story of Adam and Eve be a foundation for disappointment and sadness, misery, and pain inflicted upon God's people, by a very angry, merciless, and intolerant, God. Even though there is a promise of hope there, because of a flawed human consciousness, the totality of love and mercy was not realized through the greatest gift we received from God—Jesus.

Not being consistent with the God Jesus taught us about, we as God's children can be confused and resort to the Old Law, and that being an eye for an eye, as a factor in promoting any agenda that persuades people to see other people as anything less than human.

The traditional Adam and Eve's story witnesses to major scriptural inconsistencies, that prevents God's people from walking and finding the true *Way* back to the reality of *Metta* (God's love). Unless this is corrected, the 'luminous' teachings of the 'Light of the world' will continue to witness to a world engulfed by darkness. How dark is this world? It is so dark that the continued cries for a Messiah are heard these two thousand years after Christ and his wife walked the earth?

Still, despite the errors of Peter and his successors, the promise of a Savior is still resounding in the ear of God, because of the negligence of religious leaders regarding standing steadfast to the truth. Though the truth of the Divine Masculine Messiah is recognized in the hearts of those who love him, it is still only *half* of God's plan. For if the truth were known, there would not still be those praying for the true Messiah. For those who are waiting because of false teachings, this Religion has reappeared. Seeing the need for one to come who will enliven love for God and neighbor shows that we have, once again, reached the fullness of time.

There are many versions, none of which seem to agree, whether the Savior will be a man or woman, unlike in biblical times, where it was assumed that it would be a man, or just as the words regarding who will crush the serpent's head has been changed back and forth as 'he will crush and she will crush.' One thing is for sure, however, it is time for these prophecies and/or promises to be fulfilled!

With the demands of God's people for proof of God's existence and help, Jesus' accomplishments continue to pale when all we find in this world are division, inequality, chaos, and death.

Of course, God knew that Adam and Eve had to learn to rely on each other in life, and this would teach them empathy. It would also provide a kind of penance and reparation played out in the form of sacrifice. Though it looked as though they were on their own, the Word of God was ever-present to them when called upon for help.

With truth, and with the guidance of the Divine Feminine, we too could gain back what God wants for us with a love and a greater appreciation for each other.

It would certainly attest to what can be accomplished when male and female energies bond in true love. In the case of Adam and Eve, imperfection certainly would not cause God's anger and punishment, but rather it would bring about God's unconditional love and mercy. Like good parents, these lessons in life, and the responsibility we have to having free will, should bring along the desire to have the Eternal Consorts as their sustenance, guide, and example throughout life. One would not be aware of these life lessons by reading only the traditional scriptures, as they were handed down.

What if the couple had turned against God in such a way that they became angry towards his spirit, by thinking that God *led* them to this act of disobedience? If this happened, they would have committed the unforgivable eternal sin, which would be to say that God's Spirit could do *evil*. That is why the sin that Satan believed himself to be God, and not see he was created, and thus refused to worship God, marked his fate with eternal damnation. *This was not the case with Adam and Eve, since they did not give up on counting on God for help*, but did suffer from deep and painful regret for their wrongdoing.

The mere fact that traditional scriptures were interpreted and taught with compunction, is yet another example of cogent evidence that what was given to God's people fell way short of love of God.

God, as our parents, saw how logic played a role in the couple's imperfection and weaknesses due to how excessive temptation was responsible for their decision for physicality; however, before you find fault with God, remember that if they in fact had remained close to God, and had been nourished spiritually, the taunting effects would have been minimized. Instead, they became subject to Satan's tremendous delusions.

LESSON 32

WHAT TRADITIONAL SCRIPTURES FAIL TO TELL YOU WE MAY BE ABLE TO

Without spiritual nourishment, Adam and Eve's weakened strength caused a blurring of good and evil. This of course, was the intent behind the evil one wanting Adam and Eve to see him as God and exercise free will against God's directives. How did this happen? To begin with, Satan was sure to occupy more and more time with them. The more time with him meant more time under his influence and less time with God; and though in the beginning they could handle the conversations and innuendos without being affected, time away and not being nourished as necessary for immortality, they began guiding themselves. Soon they concluded that it was not necessary to bother God, and that resulted in their replacing wisdom with logic. Haven't we all, at one time or another, thought that even though we are bothered and uneasy, God had more important things to worry about without us bringing things to him which we should be able to handle?

Where they were once strong in the Spirit of God, they were weakened by the constant returning visits of Satan.

After their 'fall,' being good parents, God deemed it necessary for them to live out this life they chose with the consequences that went along with their choice. Unfortunately, though Adam and Eve regretted their decision and were sorry for what they had done, they made their choice and had to live with it. You see, as they had changed and gone from the transcendental consciousness to a human consciousness, they no longer had access back to their previous life. The means to facilitate what they wanted to have again was no longer available to them, since everything about them changed. They were now human beings, not transcendental beings.

No longer was the presence of God, which they took for granted, available in the same way to them; and the lack of the spiritual food that fed their light bodies, and kept them close to God in a very unique way, left them with a hunger and an insatiable thirst—an emptiness which was only satisfied by God's presence and nourishment. They were now subject to only hearing God's voice, on occasion, and eating only that food which would sustain their bodies. They did not have the understanding and wisdom they once had. Life as they knew it was over, and this life paled by far to what they had before; and it would remain this way until the fullness of time was reached, and God felt they had learned their lesson and then the journey home could begin.

Of course, in order to achieve salvation, one needs a savior. Why was a Savior necessary? Most people believe that because they were sorry that they should be seen as antinomians, meaning, because of grace, and the fact that they were sorry, they should have been released from the obligation of observing the moral law, finding this mindset rooted in the human consciousness. But, as *it was against God's directive*, there must be atonement which, in this case, was played out by living as human beings in the material world, which was subject to entropy,[60] and awaiting a Savior, who was the only one(s) who can 'save' them from the grips of the worst possible reality, which was eternal death.

The consequences from choosing this physical life style immediately came into play. Their soul was marked as finite, or subject to death, the difference being as the body experiences death because of entropy, the soul being immortal also experiences death in a different way; since without a Savior to eradicate the consequences of their choice, salvation would be impossible.

Filling in the gaps with Eeshan teachings explains how Adam and Eve's descendants, henceforth, would have to struggle against a fallen

---

[60] Entropy, in this context, refers to the effects of time and gravity—in a spiritual and material sense—on the mind, body, and soul. The meaning of this term will be increasingly made clear as it unfolds throughout the book. – Ed.

nature that inclines one to bend towards toward the human consciousness rather than the transcendental consciousness. God's creation reveals this tendency in the sunflower: the flower bends towards the earth until the sun comes up, at which time it lifts it head and faces the light.

This means that all their children who were born into this world, up to and including us, and our descendants, would be subject to this fallen nature with only a human consciousness, with no passage to the eternal life, unless we accept the Savior sent by God.

LESSON 33

WILL THE REAL SAVIOR PLEASE IDENTIFY YOURSELF?

How does one identify the Savior(s) sent by God? First the Savior is known by self-identification. Then the Savior fulfills ancient prophecies with miracles that attested to the Messianic Mission. The Messianic Mission, however, would not be the freeing of God's people from the slavery of government, tyranny, or political oppression, but would be the freeing forcer from the slavery to/of the *human consciousness*. These salvific features were perfectly manifested in Jesus and his consort. *SO WHAT'S THE PROBLEM?* Graced with God's presence here on earth, these most powerful and positive vibrations of epic proportion caused a disruption of negative energies, taunting these powers, and were the catalyst for change. Identifying Jesus as the true Messiah left a lot to be desired at the time Jesus walked the earth, and, that and the omission of his eternal consort, added to "present time" issues.

What happens if half of the people accept and half don't accept a Savior? Where are we then before God? Eeshans also pose this quandary: what if the actual Savior(s) was/were reimaged by religious authorities to suit another agenda? What benefits, if any, were found?

As a people, if we continue to choose to live apart from God, and refuse to accept the gift of a Savior(s), the end result is living a purely human life, with a human consciousness devoid of accountability to a higher being. Of course, then there would not be a need to have contrition for any transgression, which denotes no need, or desire, for forgiveness; thus, what results is a judgment according to the standards of man's imperfect and finite laws, subject to all human factors, which originate from a flawed, limited consciousness and mind.

These judgments would indeed be without mercy; since without a divine connection, you would not know mercy, since mercy is driven by love. Also, Jesus warned of self-condemnation. Being God's child, we have to allow for God's opinion of us. Believe it or not, self-condemnation is wrong. There is a difference in knowing when you should have done something and you did not, and condemning yourself because you can't be like someone else. You know what I mean ... the "I'm nots;" "I'm not good enough;" "I'm not smart enough;" "I'm not pretty enough;" and there's also "I'm not lucky" and "I'm cursed." Hiding your talents because you deemed yourself a 'loser' before you even get started, or being afraid that people will find something to hurt you, is not healthy. If you look at all of these, take away the 'not' and put before them, "God thinks I am ...," then you have the truth. God did not make you the first mistake of Creation. God does not want you sad, self-condemning, or to be a defeatist. On the contrary, besides, by condemning, as opposed to critiquing, you are saying that you know better than God, or that He lies, cheats, and is discriminating, etc.!

Rather, just address your issues with solutions. Talking about what you 'should do' should be countered by really 'doing it.' God is most likely saying to you, "Why did you, or why didn't you"? God does not have a fallen nature; therefore, all the talking going on in your head, if it is positive, is from God, while if it is negative, it is not. Most likely, it is coming from self. We don't see the need to blame Satan or the devil, whatever you want to call him, for everything negative in your life. Since if you naturally think these things, there is no need for him to torture you, and you are probably doing a great job on your own.

When you think positively then you are actually abiding by Jesus' directives. Jesus teaches that in order to enter into the transcendental life, which is necessary to be saved, *believe* him. In 1 John 4:16, the verse is written: "God is love, and whoever abides in love abides in God, and God abides in him."

LESSON 34

A Parent's Point of View

As parents, Adam and Eve's soul was destined to carry the indelible mark of "original sin." Though this is not what Eeshans call it, it is the term that most people are familiar with. Whatever the case, whatever the term, there is a mark that is stamped on our soul. It is to identify it as being finite. This, too, is part of the consequence. What this is, is the Divine's way of marking the change from a transcendental body to a gross physical body. Where the body Adam and Eve had been created with used the begetting process, the gross physical body would not be able to reproduce in this way. All of their children would now have to be 'born,' using physical organisms. In birth, there are hormones involved, implantation, and gestation. At the time of birth, the amniotic sac bursts, and the fluid is released by the rupture of membranes. The body then begins the process of moving the child towards the birth canal, and, finally, with the mother's help in normal cases, the child is pushed out of the mother's body. The infant's body has been prepared to breathe air and eat food. Birth through this gross physical body made way for the soul of the child to be subject to the mark of original sin, also. This mark carried with it the origin from where it acquires it's life, which is that it was 'born,' not 'begotten.' A begotten child is formed by light, and this light emerges from the transcendental being as capable of eating vegetation that provides light. There is no labor, nor is there anything that resembles a 'human birth,' except for the fact that a being is formed and alive. The child formed and born of the gross physical body was marked, or "time stamped," meaning that the soul did not come through the transcendental light body. This means that a soul within the fallen human nature is likened to manifesting an inherited disease in which a kind of mutation, that is 'Original Sin' in this case, and is present on both souls of both parents, and through birth, and acts like a diseased chromosome that is found in one or both parents, and then passed on to their children. That is why the children they had begotten, having light bodies, were unaffected, even after the fall; and, thus, having no mark upon their souls, they could continue to travel back and forth to Paradise. Did these children understand entropy? Did they understand, or wonder, why their parents had new bodies? Did they wonder why their parents had to leave the Garden? No, but these will be a story for another time.

As parents, Adam and Eve did have feelings. They just didn't think about *themselves*. They suffered knowing they had disappointed God, and had to leave their transcendental children behind, whom they loved, and now made life less than perfect for their 'birth" children and their children's children.

What kept them from despair was the hope of having this mark removed and regaining what they lost. They thought of how long it would be before the fulfillment of God's promise would come.

Of course, they didn't live to see the one who would come to restore their transcendental lives; but they eventually did see Jesus, when, after He died, He went to them, and ignited their light bodies, so they could return home.

LESSON 35

PRESERVING THE OLD FOR SELFISH REASONS

SECTION III: WOMEN'S PLEAS FOR EQUALITY BEFORE GOD ARE NOT NECESSARY, THEIR PLEA IS BEFORE MAN

In the traditional story, as handed down, the couple was charged with "breaking God's law" by the hand of Eve (Genesis Chapter 2), and, this, therefore, caused generations of collateral damage to women. This laid the claim that it was God's plan from the moment she (Eve) was created, and it would continue, through selfish reasoning. In turn, women would become the cause of man's losses, pain and suffering, until the end of time, because time came into being because of women. Now we know how, and where, the origin of this misinterpretation and misaligned, unbalanced, human consciousness came about and from where.

Eeshans know that Adam was a greater man than that, and if not for the fact that he was both soulmates and Twin Flames with Eve, he would not 'throw Eve under the bus before God.

Research within mystery schools show that under ancient patriarchal religions, in order for man to be in control and master of all, there had to be a solid reason for a woman to be of lesser worth. We present that this is exactly what took place with this story. How better than:

1. by God's design, make woman's reason for living to serve man,
2. make her feel she was responsible for the first sin, which caused God to become an angry God seeking retribution right from the beginning,

3. make women servants to the gender who considered the male alone was imaged, and likened to God himself?

Putting women in a very subservient and compromising light was not a new concept since it was in both the oral and written law of the time, long before the Old Testament, and in other patriarchal cultures, as in this story, and those similar stories found in said cultures.

Yet, as educated as we have become, we have been conditioned, and choose to live as though these teachings have always been correct. We lived as though what dissatisfied us in these stories didn't apply to life as we know it. Faithful as women have been in loving Jesus, women find solace in the fact that they are accepting these claims and carrying them out for Jesus. It is no wonder why women's charges and concerns have fallen on the deaf ears of those who claim they hold the authority of God, especially when they have Adam and Eve's story to back up these outrageous and wildly exaggerated assertions. Even though it is perfectly clear how this can be the cause of the loss of eternal life, it is used in a way that cannot be disputed or doubted or questioned.

Over recent years, women who tried to change this mindset were vilified, ostracized, and, silenced, and not just by men, but by women alike. The men, and few priests, who supported these women were declared anathemas because of how vehemently disliked they were. Needless to say, there is always a pope, or council of the church, who excommunicated one of these for *denouncing a doctrine.* Yes, there is a doctrine, more or less, that claims anyone who stands with these women contradicts *Christ!*.

Are we still a people who do not have eyes to see or ears to hear what Jesus desired for all to know, love, and 'serve' God? Over time, the deliberate ignoring of women's love for God is what allows for the injustices, not just for women, but for different expressions of gender, cultures, and nonviolent religions that were influenced by God's love for all, and apparently is a doctrine that costs them dearly. Often a priest is punished by being placed on administrative leave to 'pull it together,' or his faculties have been denied him, or permanently taken away.

Other spiritualities that did not oppress women, or other genders, were more in line with what Jesus taught than what has been considered from "his" own religion. Over the centuries, it is the love of Jesus where woman has drawn her strength; and it was always because of her love for Him that she accepted this wrongful mindset, since, again, women up and until they were allowed to be educated believed they had to rely on what they were told, since it was man who was given the authority to dictate and interpret God's word and law.

A woman's love is what often imprisons her in an abusive relationship thinking that this is what God wants, or believing that this is what she deserves.

That is why man has always used the words in the traditional wedding service to his liking. The words, are claiming to be what God said, such as "that the woman was to 'love, honor and obey,'" and "for better or worse," and "I now pronounce you 'man' and 'wife'."

Never did Jesus preach, or live his marriage, by the word 'obey.' Each would listen to the other, and together they would determine a choice; and most certainly abuse was never, and never would be, condoned by God.

Eeshans believe that what had taken place from before the Mosaic Law/Torah came into being, and continuing up to and including when patriarchal Christian religions came into being, originating from God with no exception, seemed to give or imply that men have an innate knowledge of being identified as gods on earth by virtue of the fact that this belief stood uncontested, since there were no laws, or doctrines 'from God' that protected the rights of women.

LESSON 36

AND THE WOMAN ASKED MAN

HOW COME YOUR JESUS IS NOT THE JESUS I KNOW, LOVE, AND SERVE?

The fact that Jesus was made to look as though he supported man's thinking, Eeshans present that there is only one reason the traditional version of Adam and Eve was used and taught. It was for the same reason Mary Magdalen, as wife of Jesus, was dismissed, suppressed, and abandoned. The true stories would have threatened man's justification of their dominance over women.

It is this theme which has plagued women in every aspect of life, that is, until they realized that because of man's linear thinking they neglected to see that one of Christ's most notable teachings openly addressed his feelings, and played out in his actions and teachings, actually favoring no gender, no class, etc:

> "They came to him and said, 'Teacher, we know you are a man of integrity. You aren't swayed by others, because **you pay no attention to who they are, and do not care what anyone thinks for you do not look on the appearance of 'men' [should have been person]**, but you teach the way of God in accordance with the truth.'" (Mark 12:14).

What does Jesus think about religious, judgmental people who claim they speak for God regarding gender, sexual orientation, color etc. who want to love God? It is very clearly spelled out in Matthew 23:13:

> *"How terrible it will be for you, scribes and Pharisees, you hypocrites! You shut the door to the kingdom of heaven in people's faces. You don't go in yourselves, and you don't allow those who are trying to enter in either."*

What had drawn everyone to Jesus was that they knew he, indeed, welcomed everyone, and he recognized each one as a child of God; and, yes, he didn't care what others thought because he came to correct the errors made by man and restore the truth to the law without personal and material gain that he was God!

Eeshans believe as we are all God's children, as told to us by Jesus, and treated as such by him, that it could be possible that the male ego, through a consciousness formed around what men believed to be God's law, *was merely human law defined by self-preserving religious authorities*; therefore, in an effort to love God with his whole heart, soul, and mind, we find that perhaps men can only see equality defined as both being created male and female but in a condescending bow to a 'lesser gender,' who though made in the image and likeness of God, also still needs the male to access God. This thinking follows the pattern of how the traditional story was worded in such a way that the religious authorities actually believed the wording of the story would suffice for male and females alike. Then add the fact that what they say comes from God, puts a kind of imprimatur, i.e., an official license, on their words, or writings, that would cause people to believe they have the authority of God. This notion was widely promulgated and never questioned.

If the story read as it was intended, in truth it certainly would have to involve the first androgynous being which was separated into two, and, in marriage, becoming 'One' again. So, both would have to agree as one. However, it was worded in such a way as to get lost in the translation. The definition via translation of man's interpretation similarly acknowledges equality in definition, but it doesn't in actual practice.

The truth is most women were not ever consciously aware that they were different, weaker, or subordinate, even to God, until men told them they were. The citing of the differences not in defining the gender, but in comparison to male attributes, such as saying the reason a square and a circle are not equal is because they look different.[61] Women needed little to know, love and serve God, and were content until made to feel foolish, and that suddenly they were being robbed of their place with Jesus.

Women had always silently accepted discrimination and oppression, as did others who were different, offering up their sadness to Jesus out of love for him. One must be reminded, however, of the good men, the balanced men who treated women with love, care, gentleness and equality, despite accusations and persecutions made against them. These are the true representatives of Christ's love and example, and are most open to Jesus being married, with accompanying admiration and a sense of camaraderie. Eeshans are not saying that "ALL" men are discriminators, just like not all Catholics/Christians are responsible for what was done with regards to Jesus.

One will find that usually the members who try to keep alive their personal relationship with Jesus feel this sustains them and still retains them as a member in good standing of their church and denomination. This assuages their culpability for not addressing and acknowledging its errors. This also eases their conscience, for to these, He is the friend who walked in when everyone else walked out on them.

We are also saying that the discrimination label is not just on men; since we have, to a great degree, and witness daily, *reverse discrimination from women*,[62] other genders, and races of people, and even political parties. What we are addressing and pointing out, are what we find to be the origins and effects behind what was always considered and taught as rational, though not always logical, teachings given to Christ's followers. These mindsets, however, are also attributed to enabling a godless people who lack spiritual guidance and the knowledge of the transcendental to

---

[61] Both are shapes and equal as such, but a circle is not a square; the circle is not, however, superior to the square, or vice versa. – Ed.

[62] Anyone can be an oppressor.

become victimized, or so easily wreak havoc on each other. Bringing the truth is of the utmost importance to us even though it means having to illustrate what has affected everything, which includes: a) how changing the teachings of God; b) how changing the teachings of Jesus; c) how showing the truth as to why Jesus came to us; and d) how he lived and taught, became significant.

Most assuredly, the Jesus that women know, love, and serve[63] gives them strength to carry on despite what the church, or anyone else, claims. The Jesus they know was, and is, amazingly attuned to their connection with God.

Jesus' Teachings on Women[64]

- "It is not meant that a son should set aside his mother, taking her place. Whosoever respects not his mother, the most sacred being after his God, is unworthy of the name son.
- "Listen, then, to what I say unto you: Respect woman, for she is the mother of the universe, and all the truth of divine creation lies in her.
- "She is that basis of all that is good and beautiful, as she is also the germ of life and death. On her depends the whole existence of man, for she is his natural and moral support.
- "She gives birth to you in the midst of suffering. By the sweat of her brow she rears you, and until her death you cause her the gravest anxieties. Bless her and worship her on earth.
- "Respect her, uphold her. In acting thus, you will win her love and her heart. You will find favor in the sight of God and many sins will be forgiven you.

---

[63] This draws distinction between the Jesus described above who sees women as equals and the 'Jesus' the church taught through the ages who appeared to sanction the belief that women were, and should be because of their nature, subservient to men. – Ed.

[64] Drawn from Elizabeth Clare Prophet, *The Lost Years of Jesus*, p.239. – Ed.

- "In the same way, love your wives and respect them; for they will be mothers tomorrow, and each later on the ancestress of a race.
- "Be lenient towards woman. Her love ennobles man, softens his hardened heart, tames the brute in him, and makes him a lamb.
- "The wife and mother are the inappreciable treasures given unto you by God. They are the fairest ornaments of existence, and of them shall be born all the inhabitants of the world.
- "Even as the God of armies separated of old, the light from the darkness and the land from the waters, woman possess the divine faculty of separating in a man good intentions from evil thoughts.
- "Wherefore I say unto you, after God your best thoughts should belong to the women and the wives, woman being for you the temple wherein you will obtain the most easily perfect happiness.

LESSON 37

What's Happened to Marriage

The need and meaning of marriage has been debated heavily and its importance lessened over the years, mostly due to the increased number of divorces. Why? Because as the number of divorces increase the solemnity of the sacrament diminishes, and so, too, the reasons and needs to be married. How did this happen? There are a few reasons. When the need to be married is lowered to the basic sexual drive, marriage loses its meaning. There is also abuse. Women live in abusive marriages because their mothers did, and so did their mothers.

Other causes for the decision for couples not wanting to get married include when one, or both, are not interested in keeping the love interest alive. There are those whose focus is the children and *their* lives, or lack thereof, and of course there are those whose aches and pains (not serious ones), are just enough for constant attention. Any one of these are most or all of what happens with age, or the fear of getting older. When these things happen, a marriage becomes as meaningless as the paper the license is printed on.

It is acceptable these days to have committed relationships over marriage, especially where if dissatisfied, one or the other, can call it quits. There were also laws that gave certain states reasons to prohibit marriage certificates to certain individuals: same sex, interracial, marrying outside one's religion or creed etc. Where it was once simply obeyed, or accepted, today's generation does not feel the same. Their decision is not just rebellion against an establishment, but they think God is behind it. If you lived under the old Law before Jesus came, you would be following the Mosaic Law with the book of Leviticus as your commandments. Yet one would think this old law is still in effect, since the church under Peter still dictates it as such, and has formed doctrines and uses a system of laws and legal principles made and enforced by the hierarchical authorities called Canon Law to govern itself and its members, as an institution.

Over the years, marriage as taught by the church was primarily meant for the purpose of procreation. It was also only available for a man and woman. However, the number one reason for bringing children into the world was, and still remains, to bring more souls into the world, with which to adore God. With that said, it makes God look as though marriage is a license for women to breed for the sole purpose of bringing worshipers for him, and not love. That is primarily why contraception was taboo, even at the risk of the marriage and family relationships being threatened, since contraception was not acceptable. It was said that it would incite promiscuity among the coming of age. If you recall, the church felt that by denying contraception they were protecting women from losing control over their bodies.

Let's take a look at what actually happened. Religion's way of thinking again made women objects for man in God's image and likeness, while making men 'gods.' Just as we said in the previous text, it's as though women don't know what's good for themselves and need men to guide them and keep them under control. Who keeps men's bodies under control?

By this we mean, that along with pregnancy, whether wanted or unwanted, came the mindset that it was always the woman's fault, especially if the pregnancy fell under the 'unwanted 'category. Often, stress entered the picture when it was a financial strain on the income, and it put men under pressure to provide for extra children. Either way, it was the woman's fault, though she could never say no, since this would be deemed against God's law to deprive her husband sexual relations, and as failing to uphold her duties as a wife. What is amazing is how when another man showed admiration for three or more children, the husband took the credit for it all. Children witnessing negative, or dysfunctional, family life forms a bad opinion of marriage, adding to the list of why marriage may not be seen as a positive option, or worse, that 'this' is what marriage is.

Even in situations where a man would abuse, or beat, the wife, it was seen as alright and acceptable for just cause, even by many priests. Again, there was only the criteria set by man, in his image and likeness, and authority over woman, this became the template made to look as though it was from God.

Because the truth about Jesus' marriage was expunged by the patriarchal church of Peter, the person of Jesus could now be 'viewed' as powerful and iconic for having women surround him, but he was 'free.' Though he might be tempted, He rose above the act of sex, which in the masculine gender was superhuman.

As God, who was seen by church authorities as giving rights to husbands to lord over their wives, and for the wives to be subject to their husbands, made it very difficult for a woman to get an annulment in the past; but it was much easier for the man. Things have evolved 'a bit' over the years.

All of the above not just hurt women, their desire for marriage and desire for a family, but also relieved the man of his sense of responsibility. Though they were/are told they were to honor their wives, to cheat on them due to the women's negligence, and/or irresponsibility for getting pregnant. or at times to include illness, and of course desire, it was an unwritten law that God would understand this 'offense.' These are what made marriage nothing more than a license and vehicle to satisfy sexual desires.

Once a few women began to stand up for themselves and take the blows from the church who denied them Jesus in the Sacraments. Others came along, hoping and trusting in Jesus' love.

What happened as a result was that Marriage, and all it was meant to be, was no longer anything but a means to almost forcibly hang on to the person you wanted for mostly selfish reasons. We are not saying that this is true for all, but we are merely giving an overview of how things deteriorated. These sins and offenses find their origin in being subject to only a human consciousness. They cry out to God for vengeance, and women aren't afraid to go to God for help.

LESSON 38

PROOF THAT UNCONDITIONAL LOVE FOR GOD EXISTS

What is unconditional love? Unconditional love is defined in the dictionary as affection without any limitations, or love without conditions. It is also known as true altruism or complete love. It is the type of love which has no bounds and is unchanging.

This is Metta- the love of God. How closely related is a woman's love in comparison to God's love? A woman's love is resilient. A woman can love without receiving love in return. She will work hard for less than a man. She will do anything for the love of God, her loved ones, her children—for humanity.

With the Pope being the 'Vicar of Christ, 'women had always felt that he would hear and understand their plight. What they found was that he was not the Vicar of Christ, but merely the successor of Peter, or perhaps by the Pope's own words, that he is just the "Bishop of Rome."

There is no hope of equality within established patriarchal religions, nor was there ever. Without the acknowledgement of Jesus' marriage, women have little chance of hope in changing these rules/laws, with regards to the priesthood, or equality, at this point, since the future looks bleak in regard to this.

Addressing inequality is not a single issue; but it effects every level of a woman's life. The bottom line is that we find by the Pope's own words that it is because women's bodies are not like Jesus' that they are restricted from becoming priests. That's like saying such outlandish things as that a priest is one whose physiology, and physicality, of the male gender must compare to Jesus; and more preposterous is the argument that without men there can be no priests, and, thus, would be the end of the Eucharist. Did anyone ever explain to these men that *without women there would be no men*? True, a woman's body is made for birthing; however, this is because it could withstand more pain, and endure more punishment, and does so at the risk of her own life, which is to bring life into the world. One would think that all of these things would cause women to measure the degree of hardship, or injustice daily, but rather they will display grace and kindness: for pregnancy and birth are not the result of a 'curse' but are a result of love; and despite what many may be inclined to think, love is what dispels the hardship and daily injustices. That is why healing of the greatest hurts can take place with one act of kindness. "Love covers a multitude of sins."

Despite the odds being against them, despite any efforts that end with little change or difference, women have trust in God. They rarely blame God for the wrongful treatment inflicted on them; rather they thank God for their resilience!

They don't focus on the labor and pains of child birth, but see the wonderment of having the capability of growing another human being inside their own body. When she becomes a mother, she becomes a mother to all children.

Women are not perfect and they know it, but they will not be defined by their imperfections and will rise to their abilities and potential. A woman's heart always goes to the aid of those who have been beaten down, even if only in prayer, because she knows "Jesus loves her."

Eeshans wonder how the church attests that in order to become a priest only the male gender body is acceptable, as if commanded by Jesus Himself. This in itself would nullify all that was said of the character of Jesus.

The faith and endurance of women always came through their faith and many today feel and believe that God has had just about enough.

Just by the virtue of the knowledge of an all-loving God, women know that there is One, who is like Jesus, and when She comes, She will claim and profess She is the one who has stewardship over "all others." What is amazing is that any religion with hope of salvation knows that it will take the strength of a 'good man' and the unconditional love of women to accomplish what God desires for humankind. Who has the right to say this? His wife does.

If Jesus' marriage was eliminated from *all official written records*, one would think that no one would be the wiser. This is not true, since you will find, as you continue to read. All one needs to do is watch the trend of increasing women's rights and privileges over the years as proof that the Holy Spirit and his Divine Feminine consort have been moving and changing what was always meant to be but ignored.

LESSON 39

WHY YET A NEW PRIESTHOOD

Why could the Levitical priesthood not satisfy the debt of humanity? Could it have been because it could not be by a mere man that God could be satisfied, but rather only by a *Divine Priesthood that was Sacredly Balanced*? God was not in need of men; yet, God desired a Priesthood and laws that would end corruption and allow God's love to permeate from the priests to the people, like a window through which sunshine passes into a room. There was no way a perfect and spotless sacrifice could come from this Levitical priesthood, since it did not have a liaison who necessarily would have to also be *divine*. It was, indeed, not balanced.

The priesthood necessary needed to be likened to what is seen in God's eyes: God and humans as One who became Two, and the Two became One. The result should resemble the fruit of the 'love' in Marriage, i.e., one brings life with God's word, the other gives life, like the leaven; and, as the 'Logos' impregnates the heart, the other gives birth to love. This is symbolic of the first fruits to be given to God. In no way does it 'take for itself what is only due God." Nor does it prohibit any gender, because of physiology/physicality, from worshiping or loving God. It would help bring the joy and witnessing of a living word testifying to "as above-so below," and "making the inside like the outside," etc. The Priesthood would reflect under God, the one [the High Priest] being humankind, separated into two genders (the two Natures of Jesus Christ/and Divine Consort) sharing in a specific love of God, presenting as a whole, as a sacrifice by completing in each what the other does not have, while entering into the union of the transcendental/human sacrifice. This was the Priesthood necessary, and this Priesthood would bring glory to God. As this would not come through the Old Law, a New Law would have to come into existence: a Law that destroyed corruption that could only come into existence by way of God. Furthermore, it would have to be God made human in order that the translation would not be lost.

With the Order of Priesthood in the line of Melchizedek, this should have happened. The Plan was laid out, many were called, but the few of the few that were chosen refused to turn away from the old to the new. This sadly went on to spread the reaction, which because of the right circumstances accelerated dramatically. With the imbalance continuing, and God's directives being compromised to gain success, truth and salvation were altered to meet the challenges Christ's modified spirituality posed.

So once again the real teachings of Jesus were hidden away amongst omissions and dissolutions of writings, paving the way to what some may argue as probable good intentions of some, but, Eeshans feel, it was power and greed to others.

Even though the ramifications of these lies and alterations regarding Jesus' teachings, the Divine Feminine's time was at hand. It began with our Foundress' directive to go to Rome and see the Pope. What she was met with began a series of events that accomplished all that Jesus wanted. In the room of heads of State/diplomats, in front of witnesses the prophecy of Padre Pio came to pass. As blood flowed from the wounds of our Eesha, in response to the presence of "Peter," after an awkward moment and quick approval of her work, everyone was asked to leave. Blood had flowed over the ring of the Pope, as Jesus commented, "Behold Ecce Homo."[65] As she and her Priest were quickly ushered out through the residence, the large ominous doors were closed fast and bolted. Outside the door to the hallway, she was greeted with the Swiss Guards and

---

[65] While the literal translation of this seems to say, "Behold behold the man", it is important to understand that when Jesus said this he was deliberate in saying 'behold' twice. He was fulfilling his words to Peter, "Then I will make her a man," I have made her a man. When you see her you see me, for the Woman in your presence encompasses the Man. On the human level, this event paralleled and completed the image of Jesus before Pilate, in this context, his wife in his place before the modern 'Pilate,' Pope John Paul II. – Ed.

with men who were like Vatican Secret Service officials. As they told the Swiss Guard that they would handle the situation, they escorted Eesha to a very lavish restroom, where they handed her towels and held plastic bags in which she could place the bloodied towels, praising God that she was there. "Padre Pio!" they exclaimed, and thanked God for her coming into "this evil place."

Later she was contacted about her story, and asked that she would write it down and that a special courier would come to her house to pick it up. It would be not too long afterwards where the Cardinal of Baltimore would try to intimidate her. Then not much longer after that, was the founding of the "Place" and the birth of the One, who is like the Son of Man. The Child was whisked off to heaven in fulfillment of scriptures. What happened next was full disclosure of who she is. From there came a sequence of events to include the forming of two orders, the Sisters and the Brothers; next the resurgence of her Kallahs marking the Eternal Priesthood of the Eternal Consorts. and then the Marriage Feast of the King and Queen's Son and his Consort, was now in the world. Having fulfilled the necessary scriptures, with Eesha's identity revealed, the Kallahs brought back, and the Marriage Feast providing the return of the Sacred Food by the woman who encompasses the Man, it is now time to reveal, and provide, what is necessary for Salvation, to those who believe and want it.

Meaning "there are more ways to kill (skin) a cat (in this case a Christ!);" "If at first you don't succeed ..." is another allegory pertaining to killing Christ. If by his Crucifixion he does not die, then kill his teachings, or better, 'kill his wife.'

Living a lie for 2000-plus years does not make it true (but the gravity of the wrong will exponentially increase). Killing Jesus was a good plan, which, carefully thought out, would seem to jeopardize any attempts for a 'religious' insurrection, and which would be the end of the Jewish religion of the day, since it would also squelch the belief that Jesus was the Messiah and life could go on, status quo. However, looking back now, even though Peter's plan to take the coveted role as 'leader, 'it eventually led to the apostolic priesthood proving to be the equivalent to the parable of the wheat and the tares: God's directives being the wheat, and the church of Peter the tares (weeds).

Jesus told this story[66]:

> *The Kingdom of heaven is likened unto a man which sowed good seed in his field.*
>
> *But while men slept, his enemy came and sowed tares among the wheat, and went on his way.*
>
> *But when the bade was sprung up, and brought forth wheat, the tares (weeds) appeared too.*
>
> *So, the servants of the landowner, came and they asked, "Sir, did you not sow good seed in your field? Where did the tares [weeds] come from?*
>
> *He told them, "an enemy has done this. The servants asked, "Do you want us to go out and gather them up?*
>
> *But the Landowner said, "No. If you do that, while pulling out the weeds, you may uproot the wheat with them. Let them both grow up together until harvest. Then I will tell the reapers to gather together first the weeds, bind them in bundles to burn them; but gather the wheat into my barn.*

Jesus allowed the church to continue in its ways, until the fullness of time, before reintroducing his wife and the Eeshan Religion. If this was too soon the weeds would have overtaken the wheat. The church would've tried to stop it. You see, it is better that both grew along side by side, for even though the weeds look clearly different from the wheat, it's easier to see the ugliness of the weeds, and much easier to pull them out and separate the wheat from them. The weeds will be gathered and burned. The wheat will be protected. The church's priesthood and deceit severely clashes with the Truth.

With the return of the Divine Feminine, God's people have eternal security.

Even though those from Peter on in the church thought it could kill Christ's directive, and the Truth by killing his Mary, they stand now in stark contrast to the wheat.

---

[66] Matthew 13:24-30.

LESSON 40

THE LOVE BETWEEN A HUSBAND AND WIFE

How is this a way to "kill Christ?" Love has always been the center of Christ's teachings, especially the love between a Husband and Wife, as in his marriage, but also the true love of soulmates, and in this case, Twin Flames. Being attracted and united in God's love, this is the love of a male and female that brings about the desire to adore and glorify God by adoring and loving your spouse.

Children are the fruit of the love of the husband and the wife but not the purpose for marriage. It was this old way of thinking that brought stress into the marriages. There almost appeared to be an unspoken 'code' among men, that years ago if a woman did not get pregnant the man felt emasculated. In biblical times that was turned around by calling the woman barren, as if God was punishing *her*.

It is no wonder why Jesus' choice to enter into a marriage without conjugal relations, a choice for him and his wife to not bear children, that raised this marriage to a higher level. Aside from the restoring what was lost by Adam and Eve, Jesus and Mary wanted to show that their love was not Root Chakra-based, meaning just an earthly marriage, but was founded on true and genuine love.

During this time too, Jesus used their choice to raise his wife, mother, and all women to equality among men, and their transcendental choice allowed for the eradication of the stigma that marriage was for procreation, first and foremost.

Even though we know only of Jesus' part in the salvific mission, in the revealing of his marriage 'we now know' by the definition of marriage, that each share in the other's love, pain, and death, equally.

Mary was Jesus' whole world. That someone would hurt her, then or now, would figuratively kill him. That is why we can say that there are more ways to kill a Christ. That is why we can say that Mary, being the Female Christ, experienced death at Jesus' crucifixion. Each of these examples show how they shared everything, from life to death.

As we said, it was all about the eradication of corruption. This is what the Eeshan Religion is all about.

Our goal is to identify, point out to the world, and destroy that which is at the foundation of chaos and war. We want the world to be a better place. We believe that the Divine Feminine is here to end the falsities from the beginning of the control of the human consciousness, due to entropy, and which has continued on, weaving between humankind's prayer for peace all the untruths that have been successful in bringing about the loss of Jesus' identity.

LESSON 41

JESUS IS GOD—NOT A RELIGION

In searching for a religion or spirituality to practice, it seems likely that one would look for something that fits the mindset and changing lifestyle of today. In most countries, both religion and culture were one, and this played an important role in the perception of God and Jesus over the centuries.

This perception, especially under the sole guidance of the human consciousness, affects how we image God, and view our relationship with the Divine. Everything that we believe to be right of wrong affects, what we are looking for in a spirituality, such as how the deliberate use of masculine pronouns was a battle between the 'faithful' that sought to keep the image and likeness of God masculine, without thinking or wanting to believe that it gave way to the way men addressed this issue. It was not the same as how women saw this issue and for good reason. With a long patriarchal history, males could lord over females,[67] and men over women, by using this simple tactic, including the fighting between women, that it seems plausible that the repetitive comments actually enabled the Catholic church's stance to remain steadfast in its refusal to ordain women. Simple and trivial complaints like this did actually play into women's fear, resulting in the Popes declaring that it was because a woman's body was not male, as was Jesus.' Because of the grip of the church's authority over the minds of all, women naturally wouldn't go against the 'Holy Spirit' either; nor would they go against the Holy Spirit because the duality of God was never revealed. Therefore, they couldn't consider that the Divine

---

[67] As may also be the case in same-sex relationships.

Feminine, the Holy Spirit's consort, that was bringing on these urgings. Now it seems that the Pope's words are coming back on him and past popes, as there is a shortage of priests to epidemic proportions, and they can't use women, as women don't have a body like Jesus.' In fact, with the Pope's words, this discussion is over and women can't ever be considered for the priesthood again.

Could it be that because of the hierarchy's brazenness women have stopped going to church? That explains all the empty pews.

Jesus is not a religion. He is not owned by the Catholic and Christian faiths. He is God. Being God, he is not subject to what humans say is his "job description," nor is he subject to our laws, philosophies, politics, and opinions.

Everyone has a right to discover, know, love. and serve God; and we are all called to do so by God. Vocations to God are always found from a calling through the heart.

One can only imagine the stir it caused when Jesus, as God, included not just his wife, but other women, and had little children help, too.

Why? Because for someone like Peter who witnessed those things about Jesus that made Peter exclaim that Jesus was the Messiah now finds himself in a quandary. Peter's lip service is so blatantly obvious that it is easy to see how shallow the man was. Declaring Jesus 'Son of God,' and even witnessing the miracles, yet, despite all of this, he disagrees and refuses to conform to the transcendental consciousness, and he'd rather deny Jesus to save his life.

Now, that comes with the fact that Jesus, being the Son of God, has actual witnesses. The Divine Masculine of God could not come in and attempt to change what was the structured hierarchy and mindset put into place by men, since the men chose to listen to the 'God' their Fathers taught about, and stayed with what was considered the natural order for genders.

Jesus as God saw the fulfillment of scriptures regarding being met with a 'rebellious people.' The God/Man saw how women's involvement induced in men the fear that women's analytical minds and intuitive minds began to rise up, thus, initiating the return of equality, which was something that increasingly became more than Peter could accept.

To bring about such a change not just in the religion but in the culture, surely was another solid reason why Jesus was not ever going to be seen, or accepted, as God and Messiah! God could never have a Son, and would never send a Messiah to uproot what the religious leaders interpreted and used as God's own laws, especially regarding women's place and rights!

In recent times, attitudes and attempts to end racial tensions and gender discrimination etc., to no avail, sees God's people searching more and more for the 'real' God in places and religions where one would least expect. God's people want God, not a God re-imaged by humans, but one who lives up to the description of a higher, Supreme Being who knows all things, sees all things, and is everywhere present—one God who can end this mess and bring faith, hope and love to all of us. A God who understands transgender, gay or lesbian lifestyles, and can explain why these are wrong, or if they are truly created and loved as they feel they are. People don't need a religion, *they need God.* They need to hear God, and not be jolted into more confusion as to the identity of a human being by other human beings.

Another example of understanding the identity of a person is to realize that God wants us to strive to become the best we can be. This is also what is meant by 'conversion.' This means that God gives us opportunity to change. Perhaps when we were younger we did things that were not good, or which by today's standards can be considered hurtful. One must remember that conversion is when a person recognizes this and changes their ways so they no longer fall victim to those things they were involved with previously, and have since grown and have learned from their mistakes. If a person displayed prejudice, or discrimination, in their words, or actions, and hurt someone, or offended against someone's race and/or culture, but have since changed as they better understand how wrong or immature they were. we should accept this change in good faith, unless they prove otherwise. None of us are born perfect, or have never made mistakes. Suppose we never let a former drug addict forget what they were, or kept an alcoholic forever bound to their past addictions, by reminding them of their past constantly, thus, never giving them the confidence they need to move on? What good then is rehabilitation?[68] We have commonly seen how many people growing up and being socialized in certain families and social circumstances, and associated with negative elements in their elementary, high school, and college days, they were raised as not to see these prejudicial, or racist, things for what they truly were. People were not as sensitive to these things as later generations, especially due to lack of guidance through Jesus' true teachings.

When efforts were made to correct these issues the generations that came before were given an opportunity to change, this set in place the need to right the wrongs of peer pressure, and even religious conditioning, which overlooked these glaring problems. They overlooked these things because they were guilty of the same things for lack of seeing all people through the eyes of Jesus.

Conversion has its foundation in Christ's teaching regarding new life, and when one has authentically changed for the better, society should not continue to punish them, especially when good works and true conversion are evident. Devotees of the Blessed Mother were told during Marian apparitions that Our Lady spoke of conversion and the need for conversion of sinners. We know that Jesus sat and ate with sinners, and, as a result, they changed their lives. This is conversion. To love Jesus is to be converted. Eeshans teach that conversion is an ongoing process, a daily choice. Thank goodness God gives us a chance to do better. Thank goodness God doesn't judge as we do.

God's word is needed more today than ever. God's 'word' must be clear and precise so that there is no ambiguity. The mere use of the wrong word in the past, or that word which carries more than one definition, can be the cause of an even greater or lesser meaning. Remember when President Clinton said: "It depends upon what your definition of 'is,' is."[69] The explanation that was given was, "If 'is' meant 'never has been' that is

---

[68] On the other handsome groups naively protest the loss of rights of proven hardened criminals and they feel that these criminals should be rehabilitated and brought back into society.

[69] Paraphrased. – Ed.

one thing; but if 'is' meant 'there is none currently,' then the statement was correct."

Yes, we have become a society of words. Perhaps because we are seeking the one who is said to be "the Word" of God. Maybe because there's so much we are finding out about Jesus that we desperately are seeking 'his' word now. What did he really say?

For if he is God, his word should not only mean something, but reach those hearts who have ears to hear, and really want to hear.

That is why, Eeshans study to find where things went wrong. Eesha showed us how just looking up the definition of the 'word' helper gives great insight into how two or more people can hear a word and not hear the same thing.

Most men, then and now, believed women were there to serve man. When looking up a word one finds sometimes more than one meaning. Which one in particular is chosen to substantiate the reasoning behind the translation that reflected the goal imparted to Eve by God? This has everything to do with all that has contributed to root problems that allowed for double meanings.

For example: "God created woman to be a helper." Scrupulous? Maybe if there weren't centuries upon centuries of consequences and discrimination. Eeshans looked closely and the word helper means *partner*: "the one used to be the one who gives assistance to someone; make it easier for someone to do something." That sounds fine but this is the definition on which we again show how words can confuse, since a helper is "one who takes part in an undertaking with another with shared risks and profits."

'Helper,' under this definition would then be equal to Adam, as was intended from the moment they were one, then separated, and then one again through marriage, even after the fall and into present times.

If you look at 'helper' as just someone to serve another in whatever capacity they chose, the meaning is changed. The fact is, upon recognizing the true meaning of helper, and how both together, according to the 'true' story could have accomplished even the consequences of the fall, men still preferred the second definition; whereas, women were there not to serve God (as Jesus made perfectly clear when he talked about love of

God), but to serve man, in 'accordance with 'God's' Law, or the Law they were told came from God.

Eeshans attest that the lesson to be learned here is that there is no reason that one cannot go to Jesus as God, or be guided by God, no matter the situation, no matter what their birth religion is, no matter what the church says, 'BECAUSE JESUS IS NOT ANY OF THESE—JESUS IS GOD'.

If Jesus is God (which believe it or not was quite the issue in the Catholic church), and he became human, he would, indeed, take on all that being a human consists of, which is not what man wants Him to experience. That is why man could not conceive God having a duality as a soulmate/twin flame, because it would have to be reflected below.

To keep this truth, the Catholic Christian church reimaged Jesus so that there could be no female involvement aside from the Virgin Mary, whose title and involvement varies with Christian beliefs.

Whereas most religions have female counterparts, it has been said any religion who has no goddess(es) is halfway to atheism.

If Jesus was a religion then who could believe that he could understand human love if he did not experience it or share true love?

For all that is good comes from above. This love then filtering down to us and all that goes with Jesus' love for all other genders, if passed on, should bring peace. Not as we always hear it, i.e., the peace which is the 'absence of conflict' (i.e. freedom from war), but the peace and harmony of both divine and human, the male and female, energies, in Sacred Balance.

What we are saying is that if Jesus was a religion, then all that he 'is,' is what the church teaches. If that religion has no Sacred Balance, then there is something wrong with what the foundations of that religion and that church perpetuates this error.

If what Jesus' birth, life, death, and resurrection were all about God's love for us, because he was married, it wouldn't make him less than God, but would prove that he was truly God as God is the Creator of all creation perfectly balanced. God can never be subject to a religion or bound or subject to man's laws, God just "is."

LESSON 42

SECTION III: WHY WE ARE PLAGUED WITH SUCH THINGS AS ILLNESS, SUFFERING, AND SADNESS? BECAUSE WE HAVE A GROSS PHYSICAL BODY

How many times has this question come up within your mind, or at a tragic time, or even just in discussions with others?

Perhaps we can shed some light on this. The choice Adam and Eve made resulted in *entropy*. This means that our body is made from matter, and this is the disordered and flawed state of being human. It is said we live to die; often it is said, from the moment we are born, we, indeed, begin to die. A transcendental body is made up of light. There is nothing there subject to decay or disease.

Once the choice for physicality was made by Adam and Eve, and after they took their first steps towards physicality, there was no turning back to being immortal and keeping the human body. Even Christ's body was not impervious to hunger, thirst, and pain etc.

What this means is that once they left their transcendental world, they were subject to time and a gross physical body. This body, as you are aware, is made up of, everything within you, which, because it is matter, began to break down immediately; and though a little different than for us, time was stretched out a little longer—by several hundred years.

The physical aspect of Adam and Eve's life together began with a choice, and the final step to becoming a physical/human being, was in the eating of the apple. This part of the story is really intriguing; however, it will be discussed later.

Because the transcendental consciousness was replaced with the human Consciousness, we see how imperfect we are, meaning that we have flaws, and except for the soul, the body does not live on forever, even though some have this feeling of immortality in their minds! The feeling of mortality does resonate through our minds and that comes from the feeling of 'self,' which we call the biological clock.

With the choosing of a material body Adam and Eve didn't count on the very things God forewarned them about. This very first choice/sin, altered everything about their life for it became a path to death in different ways, and not just the loss of life of this body. The mark of original sin is the collateral damage for us as descendants, and as a result this forfeited our ability to see God in his entirety, and live forever free from disease, suffering, loneliness, sadness, and poverty etc. Yet, even though we lost these abilities, God "compensated" us by first bringing the Divine Presence to us in Human and Sacramental forms, and merit to the side effects of entropy, because the only begotten child experienced these things, and made them ways for us to see the works of God within us, and to be glorified by them.

This 'mark' however, is very interesting. Once the soul is placed within the body, this 'identifiable mark' of original sin, which is placed upon the soul, shows that the soul has entered into 'time' via a 'physical' vehicle, and not through a transcendental, or begetting process. It is now subject to mortality. Thus begins the process of entropy, which causes the consequences that lead to death of the body; but it is very clear that original sin means death to the soul.

Once the body contains within it a soul marked with the Original sin/choice, like a kind of weed, the mark of entropy will begin to release the seed, and fructification of many continually unfolding consequences of heath of spirituality, mind, and body of both suffering and death.

You need not fear; however, since God is watching, He has placed a guardian over you, and is still present here in this world, and is really the cause for human joy for those who believe.

Like good parents, God knows that unless we experience, and are accountable for our choices, we learn nothing; and knowing that our choices can cause future problems, or issues, for our children to help us to realize the importance of heeding God's word. This, too, was paramount in Adam and Eve's post-transcendental life.

We do the same with our children. There is no difference here, since God continued to guide Adam and Eve, and taught them about sacrificial love. He showed them that the things once given freely, are appreciated more if they are worked for. Thus, we try to teach our children by experience and knowledge ... though our advice often goes unheeded.

It is often said that entropy basically means that at birth we begin our journey to death, but with God involved in our lives, even though the death of the physical body occurs, the death of the light body and soul can be conquered.

All those issues of the mind, body, and soul that we are subject to are because of entropy; yet God continues to provide human assistance through doctors and medicine, for science and technology are all instruments of his love. With faith, we evidence God's help more clearly, and often through one's faith we find healing, including even miracles, which connects us all to the divine. Sadly, however, entropy is what allows for sickness and illnesses of all kinds to enter all of our body's systems and vital organs before birth, and after. God uses this to test our faith, hope and love, and not in a negative way, but in a positive way.

Realizing this may help us to understand the different infirmities that plagued people in biblical times. That is why Jesus often used miracles to heal people from terminal, or chronic, illnesses deemed incurable. The miracles were used to establish that through 'him,' the person had contact with God. Secondly, through miracles he performed, he used them as an example for hope, and proof, of an afterlife, dispelling doubt and teachings contrary to physical death being the end of everything in a person's life; but Jesus also used miracles involving elements and food.

Another reason miracles were important was so that Jesus could successfully get the people to see *him* as God, and how he was their way, truth, and life. He worked towards convincing them that what he was telling them was from God, even though it came from one who seemed to contradict the Law. This made him one who was apart—from the warning from God. What Jesus was teaching about God, along with His miracles, did not conform with what was taught before.

Isn't it amazing that Adam and Eve were told by God NOT to eat of the Tree of Knowledge of Good and Evil, and placed a guard so that they could not go to the Tree of Life?[70] Because of Jesus, we profess that this same God is now telling us to eat of the fruit of the Tree of Knowledge of Good and Evil, and to run to the Tree of Life, who is Jesus, who is human, who is also the Divine Masculine of God.

Jesus had a lot to accomplish in order to bring the people to accept who he was and why he did what he did. Yet, he was/is adamant about this as being the only way. With limited time, he was purposely steadfast in telling everyone that only those who choose to believe in this salvific Christ will once again have access to the transcendental everlasting life.

We know that entropy did allow for the body to be the physical encasing of the soul, if only temporarily. Original sin/choice would mean death to the body, but would also be death to the soul if not for Jesus' death. For those who believe, but in the event are not baptized and nourished during the lifetime of the person, where death would be the result, if there is at least one who could speak on their behalf and to make the mysteries to available to that person, they will be righted. This very well can be the acceptance of the Divine Feminine. If by chance this can't take place, their love and faith in Jesus/God will, indeed, be determined by God.

Due to the fullness of time, and God's love for us, when Jesus came, by all that His sacrificial life entailed, the indelible "mark" of original sin remains to show that we were born and not begotten. The curse is destroyed by Jesus' death on the cross; the consequences of the sin remain, and the way to the transcendental is secured in the Eucharist of the Marriage Feast of the Lamb and His Wife.

We are freed through Baptism by way of Jesus' death, where as his side was pierced, and both blood and water gushed forth, there is the witnessing to his marriage. It is written 'the spirit (the Holy Spirit), the water (Mary Magdalen), and the blood (Jesus)—bear witness on earth as prefigured at the Marriage Feast at Cana. Eeshans profess that the same

---

[70] If the couple ate of this Tree of Life in their 'fallen' condition, they would have been locked in that state forever by eating its ratifying fruit. – Ed.

would have made a difference in world affairs if one had known through the years that Mary Magdalen had shared in this lifeline. Unfortunately, the side effects of the original choice to seek physicality, would and do remain serving as a reminder of the importance of God's guidance, as well as the reason we are earthbound. It also serves to show us the need for a 'Way' back to the transcendental by using our free will to follow, and enhance, the desire within us to find our way back to where we belong, which is with God.

As Baptism is one of the Mysteries of God that Jesus gave to us, there are a total of seven which are necessary in order that we stay on track with Christ and his Wife.

LESSON 43

SACRAMENTS OF GOD

Jesus essentially taught, and gave us, seven Mysteries, which we need to ensure us success with connecting our humanity to this beautiful transcendental life. These are typically called 'the Sacraments.' Eeshans offer seven Mysteries that are the seven Sacraments, only in their entirety. Each mystery reveals such deep allegoric and symbolic truths, and each in and of itself transcends human understanding; Eeshans require a rite of passage from one sacrament to the other before God. That is why we feel, that as an entirely separate belief system is carried through our religion, to become Eeshan, one would be required to receive all seven sacraments.[71]

For example, Jesus showed us the first step: baptism; but baptism alone does not guarantee Salvation, but is rather an initiation/induction into God's salvific plan. All new inductees will require reception of all the Eeshan Sacraments, as our beliefs regarding these Mysteries are different than what one originally was taught under the church and by previous Christian denominations. Baptism is a most powerful tool for it inducts members into the faith. Because it uses the powerful words, "in baptism you die with Christ and at death you Resurrect with Him," it still brings about a different sense of alpha/omega, which at one's death causes one to be fearful and guilty for leaving the church. And it should not. It has been witnessed, time and again, that it is actually powerful enough to lockdown one's spirituality ... despite what the heart tells them. It is, indeed, a false sense of guilt.

---

[71] Priesthood, if this is the path a person takes. – Ed.

Only salvation through Jesus and his wife, and by way of the spiritual food of the Marriage Feast, known as the Eeshan Eucharist, does the ultimate union of human beings with God take place, however. At death, Eeshans believe that to be more focused on the love and trust one has with Jesus covers a multitude of sins placed before Him.[72] Matrimony is at the heart of the Eucharist, especially for those entering into the ultimate union of human beings. Confirmation at the time of Baptism when an infant is presented, vs. baptism and Holy Chrism as an annual renewal by choice, carry two different meanings. With the first one, the infant has no choice; whereas, in the second, which is presented later to a Confirmed adult, one is supposedly renewing these vows and promises of free will. This should not be taken lightly.[73] These, along with the Mystery of the Anointing, are by far the unfathomable mysteries, which are preparing the individual for strength through any illness of mind, body, and spirit; and at the onset of death, one may be given all of the Christs' Mysteries, at once, in preparation for the soul's release to go before God. One obtains all that is necessary for God's Salvific plan for the everlasting life, as Jesus commanded.

Since acknowledgment and contrition of sins is key, and another mystery required to attain the fullness of our transcendental state, this is the Mystery of Forgiveness, and it is by far a different experience, which always encompasses love of God and love of neighbor to include good works.

The statement, "to have Jesus," means more than just 'knowing, loving, and serving' God, it means just what he said, *to eat and consume God*, in order that we awaken the light body within us and have union

---

[72] At death, if a person can honestly speak from their heart that they love and trust Jesus, the love covers a multitude of sins. That's how powerful love is. They may not believe in 'any' teachings, but that resonates with him.

[73] To be clear, if in good faith a person does these things they are not in any kind of sin or bound to something they can't get out of. The church's sacraments are not complete in themselves and you will see why as you keep reading. However, if you are going to make these vows, be sure that they are between you and God, not 'you to the church, to God'. Any vow to Jesus through love does not fall under evil; at the same time, it's important to remember that the fullness of the sacrament is not there. The innocence of the person's love for Jesus makes up for that.

with the Light of the world himself. What does it mean to transcend via the Eucharist? The ingestion of the Eucharist was meant to be the spiritual food necessary for our souls and light bodies. It's the antidote to the fall to the human consciousness, since it counters the ingestion of the fruit which brought the need for a Savior—One who can only be God, and One who is *Sacredly Balanced*.

So, you see, as a mystery unfolds, the soul is sealed, and is guided to the next mystery. Each of these mysteries are so vital to reaching the transcendental consciousness that the Eeshan Religion will not accept solely the sacraments received by a previous religion, and, in fact, will re-do the mysteries upon initiation into the Eeshan faith, but only after the individual is totally aware of, and understands, the true essence of the mystery. This does not exclude people coming to Eeshan rituals and ceremonies with the intention to participate; all people of all faiths are welcome. Rather what it means is that people formally seeking initiation into the Eeshan faith would be expected to live by the more informed, and respectful, appreciation for the uniqueness of the Eeshan sacraments.

LESSON 44

WHAT DO YOU KNOW ABOUT GOD'S LOVE?

Early on, we shared some facts about the 'What' of God. Here we would like to share the Eeshans beliefs on the 'Who' of God. It is the 'Who' of God that most feel they are familiar with. Eeshans, on the other hand, feel we have a more complete understanding of the 'Who' of God. It is from the 'Who' of God that we find a love Eeshans refer to as *Metta*.

God is *Metta*. *Metta* is perfect love, a love so perfect, that it can only originate in God. It is an extension of God. It is so powerful that we are begotten since we are extensions of God when we enter into this love. It is sown when found and reaped only in the consuming of God, if you follow Jesus, and believe he is the Divine Masculine of God, and Mary, His Wife is the divine Feminine of the Second Person of the Holy Trinity.

To understand the love God had for Adam and Eve, and, as Jesus taught, is now necessary for all of God's children, it is good to follow the Plan of Salvation from its inception to Jesus, Divine Masculine of the only begotten child of God, and His reason for becoming human, living, marrying, and dying on this earth.

What better way for God to prove their love than to allow the only-begotten Child of God to become human and guide us back to the transcendental life we were destined for! Yes, we say 'they're', not in the sense that there is more than one God, but in the following way.

God as Male and Female, so loved us that as one Being, three Persons, each sacredly balanced, shared in the separation of each by gender, in order to reverse the consequences due to Adam and Eve's choice for the physical and apart from the transcendental.

God, the first Person of the Holy Trinity, Divine Masculine and his Female Consort "separated" into two beings, to allow them both to become human. The Divine Male would become known as Melchizedek. The Divine Feminine of the first Person of the holy trinity, would become human, and would come to be known as the Blessed Virgin Mary, in order to provide a spotless body, which was necessary for the birth of the Divine Male gender of their only-begotten Child. As their only-begotten Child, both would become human, by way of incarnation, The Divine Masculine, along with his Divine Feminine consort, would sacrifice all to break the bonds of the Original Choice, and bring us back to immortality by awakening the light body and nourishing it with a new Spiritual food, which by virtue of their sacrifice, suffering, and Jesus' death on the Cross, and Mary's sharing of his death, makes up our spiritual food, which is the only antidote for mortality.

Emitting the Light of His Divinity attracts the suspended light body within us back to the Light of the World, Himself, who is known as the Son of God.

Reflecting the Father in heaven, and identifying himself at the perfect opportunities, the Divine Masculine through mastery of words, since this is who He is, He even moved Pontius Pilate to identify him, by his words: "I demand by the 'living God,' that you tell us if you are the Christ, the Son of God;" and, thus, by these next words Jesus was identified and acknowledged Himself before witness: "You have said so. And in the future, you will see the Son of Man seated at the right of power, and coming on the clouds of heaven."[74] He was the Divine Masculine of the Only-Begotten Child. A truth they would never understand. He is who is also rightfully titled, "the New Adam," which, under the belief system of the Eeshan religion, would make his wife Mary the new Eve, his other half, as they were separated from one being.

Jesus claimed that when we see him we see the Father. As Jesus taught us that his Father is our Father, we have proof of God as a Father with

---

[74] Matthew 26:63-64.

a Father's love. Being the Masculine part of the only-begotten Child, it could only be Jesus that could stand with the authority of God to speak for his Father, and as a new Adam. Being the divine male consort called Adam would then bring into play a divine female consort to represent the new Eve; and they would have to be one via God's image and likeness, through marriage as Adam and Eve were, before and after the transcendental life. The difference here is that here they would be humanly joined together in a marriage reflecting the transcendental, thus reversing the choice (made by Adam and Eve) before the sacrifice and necessary for the reconciliation between us and God. In no way could his Mother occupy this place; however, being that Jesus' Mother identified her as wife of the Father, who was her eternal consort, came to earth as part of the Salvific plan.

That perfect 'love' of God was lived by Jesus, as Man, with all the characteristics of a human man. The restoration of God's original plan for us after the Original Choice/Fall, most certainly would have to have been reflected in his life, in every way, and it was.

This is the love the Divine Masculine Father intended, and provided with the Divine Masculine gender of the only-begotten Child. The Male gender of the Child would experience all that a human Man would experience, including obedience to God and poverty sans material wealth. He would not rely on his Divinity, except in rare instances, which would identify His role as (active) Redeemer, Messiah, etc., who was to fulfill the criteria of being the perfect victim, altar, and sacrifice, as stated in the aforementioned text, the liaison between humanity and God. By example, he would turn to continual prayer and meditation for strength against temptation and experience sacrifice. In order to reconcile humanity with God, the begotten descendants of Jesus and Mary Magdalen would have to be able to relate to both consorts as one being, which is in and of itself what chiefly defines marriage. Life here isn't perfect; thus, both Jesus and Mary would have had to experience everything that human beings go through. Jesus would be a husband and teacher as the active component in the plan of salvation, since this time period would not only complete his salvific mission, but would also raise him up among humans as the perfect priest, altar, and victim with a gross physical body that dies, since also on a more personal level, He not only offered himself at his Father's will, but indeed sacrificed the love of his life, his wife, and the children they could've had together for the whole world. His Wife offered back to God her Husband for love of God and of God's children.

Jesus would not only talk, but would lead the way. Starting with his teachings on love and forgiveness, He would then lead them along the path in preparation for their salvation. By his own baptism, He showed them they must choose to be baptized to become children of God; thus, with His Father's voice witnessing to God's authority that of Jesus' authority as God's Son would, therefore, be an indication to the people to do as Jesus did. Having his followers do the same, the baptized people were prepared for the next step. By setting up a template of what others must do, Jesus had them follow Him and set His wife next to him as an example of one who shared his body, which in effect was necessary to follow in order to return to the transcendental, immortal life He promised those who followed and would follow him. This example would be the template He laid out for them. By these steps of choosing to do as He did and his ways of enlightenment and initiation they learned. He showed how forgiveness of sins meant contrition for one's own sins and offenses against God. As living a good life outlined in and by Jesus' teachings and example, along with his voluntary sacrificing of all He loved, via his passion and death, for us, the indelible mark placed on every soul was removed—Jesus and his wife would once again provide the sacred "Bread" necessary for life everlasting.

During his short life here, Jesus showed and gave all that would be necessary for humanity for a lifetime. He, along with his wife, would provide for His presence to remain with his people, so that they may share in what Adam and Eve shared, which is in the opportunity to reserve any, time day or night, or perhaps for just an hour, to spend with God the Divine Masculine and Feminine. Yes, whether with an hour taken to worship God, or observing God's real presence in the Sacramental state, or a minimum of a daily or nighttime prayer to know, love, and serve God, the Son, and His eternal consort, one would be strengthened for whatever hand life dealt.

Next, He made it possible for all His priests and priestesses, both men and women, who by their love for God and all of God's children, would (by their vows), be given the right to become the special vessels, by ordination and consecration of themselves to the Divine Consorts, by whom the sacred and mysterious alchemical words of the Christs could be spoken.

By the authority of the co-Saviors, Jesus and His Wife, who was, is, and always will be his Eternal Consort, restored the mystery of the lost transcendental marriage in their Mystical Eucharist, only found through, with, and in the Sacred and Divine Marriage Feast of the Lamb and His Bride. This eternal, transcendental life, as God, wholly Divine, wholly Human, wholly sacramental was once again available to us, even as it was before, but as it had been in the beginning, because it is God's gift to us, and, by right of free will, we must choose it.

In His Resurrection, Jesus takes on His glorified transcendental body, and gives us a glimpse of the life that Adam and Eve experienced, where they were no longer subject to the effects of entropy, especially death; but will be freed once again from physical, mental, emotional, and psychological suffering of life in this world.

Thus, we have at our fingertips, and by God's love as parents, the opportunity in this world, the privilege to eat the sacred and spiritual food, and to transcend at that moment into God, the Light of the world. With the strength from this holy, and sacred bread, who is the Light of the world, and the real physical presence of Jesus and His Wife, we have the opportunity of being the leaven, enabling us to touch, and be touched by the Holy Spirit, by whom we are able to stay connected with God from whom we draw happiness. We are filled with God's spirit, and it is from this spirit we have the ability to persevere with steady persistence, and purpose, despite all difficulties, obstacles, or discouragement we find facing ourselves.

We are the leaven each time we talk and laugh with friends, in wholesome and loving, uplifting, encouraging, and, of course, materially and financial ways, just, to mention a few.

LESSON 45

UNDERSTANDING JESUS' SACRIFICE

When we think of the love that compelled Jesus to do his Father's ('only' his Father's as taught in Christian religions) and Mother's will, we have to remember that in order to offer a salvific sacrifice, Jesus too, had to experience a very deep *personal* sacrifice, not just that of doing His Father's/Mother's will. Think of how great a sacrifice it was for both Jesus and his parents and Jesus and His Wife. They had to give up the person they so deeply loved, who was their whole world; and on a very deeply personal level, the thought of Jesus and Mary's never having a human life and family together was devastating to them; and Jesus' arrest, scourging, and death on the Cross ripped through Mary's heart, as well. God, as human beings, was not sheltered from the heartbreaks, heartaches, and endless difficulties we all face. Their life was from the beginning the ultimate sacrifice.

> *Ask me not to leave you, or to return from following you.*
> *For where you go, I will go.*
> *Where you lodge, I will lodge.*
> *Your people shall be my people and your God, my God.*
> *Where you die, I will die and there will I be buried.*
> *May the Lord do so to me, and even more.*
> *If anything, but death, part you from me.*[75]

---

[75] Ruth 1: 16-17.

Even following his passion, and death, at that time, there still came the unthinkable separation of the two—Jesus' return to heaven. Mary couldn't comprehend his leaving, as she thought they would never be separated again. Even as their Divinity made this true, Mary would remain, thinking she would continue his work. As it would happen, as the with the Cornerstone, so be it to the Keystone. Mary's life was always in jeopardy, until which time she died. Following the life of Twin Flames and Soulmates, their relationship would remain as such, until which time it would entail suspension of Mary's consciousness, in order for it to enter into supramentalization. (Then once again Jesus would be united with His 'human' consort in these end times, in order to prepare her for the continuation of their salvific mission to fruition.) Yes, this certainly was a sample of a transcendental life, and proof that it was real, and possible, living the way of true love.

Only by their continued love for God's people, through, with, and by this way, can we obtain this rich and full life resulting in the absence of emptiness and fullness of God's love.

LESSON 46

PARENTING LESSONS MEANT FOR ALL ADULTS, AND FOR REARING OF ALL CHILDREN

Jesus 'life here was spent witnessing to us that, contrary to what we were told, God is not an angry vengeful God/Creator but a loving Father and Mother God. Examining Jesus' parable of the Luke 15:11:32, the story of the Prodigal Son, and in Luke 11:11, "which of you fathers if your son asks for a fish will give him a snake," shows this to be true.

It was also why it was extremely important for Jesus to share with us, and establish that not only did He share in a human life with his mother and heavenly father, but that there was an 'eternal' relationship that existed between his Mother and Father. He did this by calling God His Father in heaven, and Mary His Mother, making them Divine Feminine/Masculine. With his reference to the crowd telling him, "Your mother and brothers are here," Jesus replied, "anyone who hears the will of God and does it;" He was referring to his Divine feminine Mother as God.[76] He knew that His sacrifice in conjunction, which the sacrificial love and life offered by their Only-Begotten Child would bring salvation to all

---

[76] In the sense familiar to most Christians, this parable would reflect anyone doing the will of God being related to him as the Son. In the transcendental sense this passage links the below with the above, as in 'As above so below.' Thus, those who on earth who do the will of God reflects the relationship 'Above' where God is his mother and those who do the will of God are related to him as the Divine Masculine Son in an eternal sense. – Ed.

of humankind, which is why He used every opportunity to speak of 'his Father 'in heaven, and his Mother here with Him on earth.

It was so important to reveal his human Mother to all. In this way, it identified her as Spouse to the Divine Masculine part of God, whom he called Father; and it was they who brought him into this world in such a way that revealed his Mother's love for her husband: "For whoever does the will of God, [identifying his Mother and Father] is Mother, sister and brother to me." In doing so, He identified Joseph as a foster father, but if you noticed, He also kindly waited until Joseph died, out of respect.

His identification of His Mother, is not *only* linked to all those who hear God's will, and do it, but to Mary Magdalen's love for God that *she too gave her yes and would give her yes again if necessary*, leaving her place in heaven to become human to God's will.

The first Person, as our first Parents of the Holy Trinity, gave Adam and Eve their original form and life, but their begotten child enabled the restored life to play out as God intended, in the truest sense. This Child[77] witnesses to the true love of God, as soulmates, in order to bring us back to God. That is why it had to be the Second Person of the Holy Trinity: this Child again had to be the Sacred and Balanced, eternal (not created) Consorts, who by being the 'only begotten 'Child of God, as a deity, could be the only transcendental one who could represent "the created Adam and Eve," as the first "children" of the First Person of the Holy Trinity.

As one can see, to have not related to God as Masculine/Feminine, or Father/Mother, eternally, and in their Divine and Human forms, created a downward spiral and has done so historically, since the onset of the story of Adam and Eve.

In the whole of the Christian world this has affected the development of our consciousness. Jesus gave us the right to call God our Father and His Mother our mother, yet what went wrong? How is it today, knowing this, that Christians communicate their disapproval of God, as Divine Masculine and Divine Feminine, and speak as if the Divine Masculine alone represents creation? Most apparent is the disregard by those who claim to follow Jesus, and to know these truths by His own words, yet,

---

[77] Who became Jesus and Mary.

agree to accept that everything had been created in the image and likeness of a Masculine God?

That is why the familiar story of Adam and Eve is condescending and disrespectful to the first beings created by God because that is NOT how their life began, nor how it continued.

Life as we have come to know it, *is because* of a tailor-made story, one whose flaws and errors have continually altered the course of human history.

Pre-Jesus, the God described in the Old Testament scriptural accounts is portrayed as being angry, punishing, and almost vengeful, which is very contrary to how Jesus described God, and this is juxtaposed against the background of there being no clear sense of any afterlife for souls. Over time, even Marriage appeared to not be based on love, but scriptures made God concerned only with being worshipped and wherein men (not husbands) are allowed to offer worship and have 'wives' by design for providing future adorers for worship of God, since women were not 'worthy,' even of 'life.'

This is not consistent with the teachings of the God of love and mercy that Jesus spoke of with such fatherly familiarity; and again evidencing that what is written can not necessarily be considered the truth, since ten percent truth and ninety percent lies do not make a teaching *true*.

Jesus 'parable of the father who rejoiced at the return of the prodigal son is certainly opposite of a father who punishes him for a disappointing choice. Though his choice was disobedient, and made by free will, Jesus tells how we find not a father that the son was afraid to come to when he sinned but a father who is seen bestowing a welcoming kindness towards a son, who hopefully realized, that he went against his father's wishes, and yet his father rejoiced and celebrated his return. If this father was one of mercy, how much more loving is God?

Yet, Old Testament scriptures, as far back as Adam and Eve, portrays a God who appears to invoke fear, not love, and guilt, rather than seeing innocence. This and other parables show a definite distinction between the Old and New Testaments; and, thus, what was believed in the Old Covenant, therefore, cannot be correct, after Jesus. So, if Jesus taught the contrary, then whatever had been taught contrary to that was wrong. If there was nothing wrong with the way things were in the Old Testament, there would not have been a need for Christ, his teachings, or his passion, and death. Knowing this provides the reason why so many people ask, 'Why would God send his own Son to die?'

LESSON 47

God's Timing

If the religion of the Old Testament time was not doing what God desired, then why did it take so long for Jesus to come?

Things of heaven don't play out in time as one would expect. First of all, *there is no time in eternity.* These are contrary to each other. That is why there is no measure of time with creation, or the length of time from when Adam and Eve came into being or fell from grace. All happened outside of time. Time came into existence as a consequence of our first parent's choice. To be sure, it certainly wasn't the result of a few days, weeks, months etc. of 'our' linear time.

In this earthly existence, when time came into existence, God allowed for other factors to play out first to get the best possible results. This is what is called the *fullness of time*. It's very difficult to comprehend the fullness of time because we live in time; and God's ways are not our ways, but God's way is the best way. The fullness of time can come into fruition when people get to the point where they are so desperate that God must intervene. The time has come now where people are once again desperate for intervention, since they realize they have no chance of survival if left any longer on their own; or, they have the realization that they *"aren't" God,* after all. Just maybe there is enough of God's people, who realize that they really do love their lives, and that there has to be someone greater than them that loved them enough to create them, and wants them to be happy! There are many reasons, and perhaps all of these, and more, are why we find ourselves not knowing what to do anymore.

We have become a people of instant gratification and have very little patience. This connotes the cause as being due to living only by the human consciousness. We don't know what to do next! Our flawed reasoning, and corrupt outlook, of life have created mayhem. Every day we hear of crimes in which defenseless victims are maliciously injured.

We demand answers, where, if balanced with a transcendental awareness, we would realize that we were given the know-how, the reasoning, and intelligence to figure out that our priorities have not been, but still are, way off base. This is where God and humans differ. God decides when the time is right to get the best possible results. We, on the other hand, work on emotion.

Living balanced with both the human and transcendental consciousness, we see how God works with a perfect love. By trust and faith, the desired plan will change and alter all lives, having the best possible outcome, in order to bring about a greater good, and to help correct matters in ways that will bring out the best in a person. This will come about not by infringing on free will as humans do, but by guidance, the way Jesus intended.

In order, however to get back this balance, it is necessary, these days, to learn about the transcendental, since it is this consciousness that has been missing. It is only with this Consciousness that one can begin to understand God's mysteries and all the unfathomable truths which are necessary for our Salvation.

PART I

GETTING BACK TO THE TRANSCENDENTAL

LESSON 48

THE REASON FOR GOD'S DIRECTIVE TO OUR FOUNDRESS

Once the realization occurred of what has been taught, and happening, as a result for the last 2000-plus years, our foundress realized that she knew from a very early age what Jesus revealed to her, more precisely, over the past 30-plus years, regarding humankind, that there was a stark contrast. How could this be? What had been the teachings by which we lived didn't coincide at all!

Gaps in scriptures, the 'whys' and the 'whats' that Jesus followers have still, and what had been happening over the centuries, were almost instantaneously revealed as *wrong*. Questions to which we were told to believe in faith were finally answered, and what's more the answers made sense.

Once the pertinent facts were brought to light, along with modern source material, the Paschal Mystery made perfect sense. It was obvious that what we were hearing was truly from an entirely higher plane of spirituality, unlike we had ever before experienced.

Without a doubt, the whole truth had to be revealed to ensure that God's people had a choice, which was not one to be made under duress, or fear of loss of salvation for questioning one's faith or religion, and which was not a choice that was already made and handed down to them, but was ultimately a choice which required one to think and pray in order that one finds that personal relationship that reorders one's life and resets priorities.

Coupled with what our Foundress taught, and with the help of the advancement of technology, and the resurfacing of the many of the gospels and other writings, once on the Index of Forbidden Books, we were now able to fill in the gaps and find satisfaction. Not only did we find the information backed up evidence of what we had been taught, and doubted, since the onset of the pre-Eeshan Religion, but we also continued to find truth and answers to more and more questions. Along with our foundress' teachings, what we discovered showed us that what we were now hearing was absolutely more in line with what seemed to be at the heart of today's issues with God and God's people.

How could this be? With every new discovery, and Eesha's teachings and explanations, we continued to ask ourselves, how and why, if all of what we were told over the years about Jesus was true, were we so blind that we couldn't see why the reason occurred for the continued departure from God and from any spirituality today? We concluded that we were not just innocent, but we were in an actual spiritual lockdown, which would not enable us to freely look beyond what we were told. More frightening, in the wake of a chaotic world, the onset of evil staring us in the eyes, such as scandals, and dwindling faith, and the lack of desire to comply with Jesus' directives, lies that one question that everyone is afraid of being asked: why did *Jesus* fail? Since wouldn't things have gotten better, not worse?

As Eesha explained with an infused knowledge, and from what flowed from the consciousness of an eye witness, it became ever more apparent how much more about Jesus' life was omitted, and countless numbers of his teachings were altered, especially more than what we first surmised? With that said, we were able to see, and finally had many explanations for, why nothing had changed in the world for the better, and furthermore, how the Christian church's history truly evidenced how deep the corruption was, since human influence on the origin of and the cause of pain and suffering, some of which is even identified as works of evil in Jesus' name!

It was always known that when Jesus came, it was the beginning of the "New Law;" one must ask why; then, were/are the Catholic/Christian religions still teaching part of the Old Law, and does anyone see how combining the two Covenants affects and even *alters* what Jesus brought to God's people? The foundation that was built and given by Jesus is clearly opposite of those leaders and self-proclaimed authorities within the church at large. Actually, it is just like those Pharisees, Sadducees, and other religious leaders whom He rebuked when He walked the earth! What a surprise and dismay!

If he came to show us the truth, and is it not obvious that what Jesus addressed, and corrected, has, by far, been lost in what has been taught for over 2000 years by those who were responsible for leading God's people? If one remembers, at every opportunity Jesus corrected those religious leaders for their claims to be mouthpieces of God, not only because of their behavior but by putting too great a burden upon the people with their man-made Laws and their keeping the people away from God.

To have eyes and not see, and ears and not hear, points to lack of all Jesus gave to us in and from a transcendental nature. For the human consciousness will not lead us to enlightenment, rather, it will lead us to more human guidance.

LESSON 49

WHY DOES GOD USE ORDINARY PEOPLE TO BRING ABOUT VITAL DIRECTIVES?

First of all, despite efforts to stop the prophecies from being fulfilled, Jesus came as an unknown to God's people. Another answer was so that during His time, as the leaders and teachers had become irretrievably corrupt, and the spirit and letter of God's law was blurred, Jesus, having little status, could work directly with the people outside the authority and leaders of the time.

It is said whenever God's message cannot get through to the people, or the conditions become hopelessly degraded, God will intervene. Sometimes ordinary people are used to make people think, and bring about change, because they are in a position to see things a heavily conditioned person cannot. Because those leaders were authorities who had ears to hear and did not, and eyes to see but did not see; therefore God's message came via prophets, mystics, apparitions, and revelations, etc. Though most were used by God, NOT ALL were "chosen by God."

Without a doubt, however, these methods of divine to human communication have always been a controversial subject matter throughout history, but even more so in recent times. We find many predictions, or prophecies, that have inundated humankind usually center around natural catastrophes, or warnings, about impending man-made conflicts and war.

Then there are apocalyptic books and writings that have misled people making the above even less credible. This does not mean that God would no longer use those means, but better to move people by the words of those chosen that would reach a person's *heart* rather than using words of fear and intimidation. Ordinary people often fall suspect by a church that claims to wield the authority of Christ, let alone one who claims God's intervention has come through them.

We find the church, at large, though appearing to have Christ's best interests at heart, has in fact found ways to limit, and, even destroy, the transcendental way of Christ, as God intended for humanity. How? First by confining and restricting interpretations of scriptures to align with its own narrative by discouraging certain reading materials, as well as prefacing that the danger of exploring any reading would be outside of the established boundaries of orthodoxy.

One such noteworthy reference is the Book of Revelation. It is generally considered common Christian doctrine used by those evangelists and preachers of the gospel.

According to the church, this Book contains Christ's teachings and there are to be no further additions to 'revelation,' because, with Jesus, all prophecy and revelation is complete, closed. What the church is saying, however, is that the Book of Revelation is purported to contain God's plan for human beings played out from beginning to end.

Eeshans believe that a very particular understanding of this position is taken out by the Catholic church, and some Christian denominations that followed in their wake, in order to prevent any later adverse additions, or amendments, to the doctrines they created.

Because the church has become so powerful, any 'authentic mystic' coming forward with a genuine mandate from God to teach and heal would be suppressed, or would be vigorously invalidated, or discredited. Nevertheless, God would even in this case, employs another avenue to accomplish the divine purpose of the mission. But why has such caution been employed? Eeshans feel that the above reasons were merely a cover story so that the true purpose, or in this case, "truth," would have no chance of being revealed.

We, as Eeshans, see this as not only another effort to serve the church's claim to protect the sacred image and person of Christ, but also to rather serve its own interests of self-preservation, as in 'the case is closed.' Eeshans feel, however, that it was, and continues to be, a means to prevent any discussion or dialogue regarding Mary Magdalen's original place alongside Jesus, especially in a *co-redemptive* role which would usurp the church's authority and doctrines.

It is important that we make clear the church's stance as we're describing it here is not intended to mean that Jesus did not speak through the book of Revelation, but that they are referring to the Person of Jesus as being complete through the totality of Christian Revelation, as a whole. What Eeshans are saying is that the church's official position with regards to Christian identity and beliefs not only prohibits its members to accept that there can be a correction of consciousness with regards to central doctrines, and the *origins* of those doctrines,[78] but also prohibits the development of a transcendental consciousness, regarding the fullness of salvation through the medium of Divine Masculine and the Divine Feminine of the Second Person of the Trinity.

People in these modern times are more and more coming to sense the rising tide of change brought on by the Divine Feminine in these eschatological days, and yet the church historically withheld the means by which a human consciousness could adequately develop to understand and evolve towards the transcendental. More so, however, Eeshans see how all these things can affect the mindset of people towards the introduction of Eeshan beliefs adversely, especially if presumed to be contrary to Revelation. How?

To the 'average' catholic anything that is written, or spoken, outside the sanction of church authority, or mainstream, Christianity is not accurate, nor can any public mystical phenomena be witnessed, or apparitions or private revelations be included, for real since they are conditioned to believe only within certain parameters, and all 'phenomena' outside that can be explained, or is derided, as trickery.

In summary, while the doctrine that God has spoken definitively, and finally, through the revelation of Jesus, and there can be no further revelation, this doctrine is also at the same time, incomplete because a central component, and that is Mary's true and actual role alongside Jesus which was purposely omitted and hidden away. In conjunction with this

---

[78] Consider how some basic doctrines about Jesus' identity would expand or be altered if Mary's position and role alongside Jesus were in place from beginning and maintained.

confusion, the average believer has been conditioned so that any reference to Jesus' marriage must immediately be condemned, without further thought.

Therefore, even while the doctrine being 'closed' is 'technically' correct, it is *incomplete because this central component of that doctrine was purposely omitted and buried*. Thus, the arguments of the church, or all those who follow suit regarding there being 'no more revelation,' would not apply to the what the Eeshan Religion is based on, i.e., existence of Mary Magdalen as the Wife of Christ; the point is that it is precisely *that* part of the original revelation that was buried.

To be clear then, the Eeshan claim is not something invented in modern times, which would fall outside the church's concept of Revelation; rather, *it was always there* from the beginning of Jesus' own life and ministry. It was just hidden away and buried over time.

It appears that if a biblical reference supported the church's view with regards to Jesus then this reference quite possibly was altered; then, any reference to Mary, his wife, can be made to look as though its origin comes from outside rather than inside.

Any "prophet" after Jesus can be suppressed by the church's authority, as the church holds Jesus as the Prophet and the Law. However, what about an ordinary person who by supramentalization who is one with Jesus? This changes everything.

God is not bound by human beings whether in authoritative and leadership positions, or in what they believe or don't believe. People actually have been conditioned to believe that if they think that they know better and they don't believe, then it's not true. So why does God use 'ordinary' people to bring important directives directly to the people?

Catholics are told that they must believe the teaching authority of the church (the Magisterium) regarding the Deposit of Faith, since it is Divine; it is also said that anything else determined by human faith in the credibility of assertions of truth of one kind or another must submit to the church's authority. The church allows the faithful to believe that God did promise to teach his people, but if any public or private revelations are conflicting with the Deposit of Faith they are said to be to not be credible. It also states that no private revelation can ever be necessary for salvation, or, against what the church deems, against traditional or Sacred Scriptures.[79]

To go outside the church's teachings makes one no longer in union with the Pope. God, however, can avoid the red tape, debating anything for the Salvation of Humanity. In End Times God may use a mystic 'in ordinary clothes' simply to bring about 'truth' that the 'over-intellectually dressed' just cannot see.[80]

However inconceivable, it's true. God always used ordinary people to bring to light what God desired. It's been proven time and again, even within the Catholic church, that God has often worked "outside" what was always considered 'his church.' It is written, "And God will teach his people." Using Old Testament scriptures that had been interpreted, and one that appears to have little alterations, we Isaiah 28:26 is pertinent here, " ... God instructs him/her and teaches him/her the right way."

The answer is simple. If one is not satisfied with the way things are going, and wants change, *God will not go to those who do not desire to change what they are doing*, but a prophet will be used to convey the changes necessary to please God. One working within the organized religion would most likely be persecuted, shunned, etc.; thus, instead, one will be used who can promote change by messages, or actions, which otherwise would be stifled.

In light of this, we find how both Jesus and Blessed Mother apparitions were most often given to ordinary people, often children, to present truths that, to this day, are still not all accepted even within the church at large, and to include some of her more popular apparitions where she identified herself as the Immaculate Conception.

We find in Deuteronomy 18:18, where God said, "and I will put My words in His mouth, and He shall speak unto them, all that I shall command Him."

---

[79] So Eeshans conclude that predictably the institutional church, i.e., the 'Holy See,' considers itself as beyond the possibility of error. – Ed.

[80] Consider the quandary of God speaking to an ordinary person versus a "divinely sanctioned authority;" this was the role of the Old Testament prophet, or a prophet like John the Baptist. – Ed.

It was once believed that in order to be able to speak God's words, one must be a 'navi,' one who is empty of oneself, or has complete openness to God. These have been part of all Abrahamic religions.

Prophets have existed in many religions, and cultures, throughout history, such as Judaism, Christianity, Islam, and in Ancient Greece, etc. Is it only due to the lack of faith that people have been made to feel that there can be no real prophets; or, perhaps, it's because we are a modern people who feel that education and knowledge lends no necessity for prophets; or, that anyone who claimed to be a prophet is either mentally ill, and has the attention of the uneducated, superstitious, or those looking for doomsday/apocalyptic predictions in which to believe.

Within the church are those who bound by laws of the church, and do not allow for any actions or messages outside what the Magisterium approves;[81] thus, they feel nothing is going to happen, and tomorrow will be much like today, with no fire falling to the earth, no judgment day, etc. These people never allow for anything that which defies the testimony of their senses, and reasoning and logic, especially *their* reasoning and logic, that is.

There is, however, within each of us, a trigger which does surface when there are great fears upon us. It's an innate warning that occurs when there is some form of a prophecy or warning, even if the patterns perceived are decades in the making, and that is triggered with catastrophic events. An example is when Nostradamus predicted the end of the world with signs that will occur in nature. So that throughout the decades, whenever there is the onset of catastrophic hurricanes, erratic weather patterns, etc., people go back and begin to look at his quatrains and prophecies as possibilities; whereas, for the most part, under normal circumstances, these prophecies are ignored.

Fearful prophecies appeal to all kinds of people, be they religious, secular, and well-adjusted, or sometimes causing the person to become a 'survivalist,' in storing food and water, buying bomb shelters stocked with

---

[81] i.e., If God is going to 'speak,' and catholic tradition says he has, it is going to be through his own chosen mouthpiece, the Pope, and Magisterium, etc. – Ed.

everything one would possibly need to live through a nuclear war, or a cosmic correction where all life can be exterminated.

These things, as recognized, as the consequences of seeing problems too great to solve, or that the bible said so, are often simply discounted as being wishful thinking.

When "signs" seem to grab attention such as when the number 11 is seen everywhere, for example, or when the animals are acting differently, an antichrist seems to appear among us, this "root" doomsday alarm sounds, and economic and solar flares, and the switch of magnetic poles begin to become possibilities in one's mind. One becomes surrounded with stories, videos, YouTube stories of UFO's, and sea monsters. These are not laughing matters, but they definitely point to the human consciousness and it's both rational and irrational concepts and plans.

To reiterate, there is a marked difference between prophets of the Old Testament and what people consider 'prophets' of today. In the Old Testament, the prophet's duty was to bring God's word, and Jesus was the last of these because of who He is. Ordinary or noted people such as Nostradamus or Edgar Cayce, and visionaries like Tesla, did not bring religious messages, but to most people they are seen in that category. So, they become "approved" prophets, especially when certain "signs" are thought to appear. On an ordinary day, when people are doing ordinary things, you have a greater chance of avoiding persecution by those people who are called "trolls" if you predict weather changes, world events, etc., even if the predictions fall short, but there is an even greater chance of people attacking you if you say you talk with God.

When predictions prove to be drawn from an infused knowledge not found in textbooks, that makes the heart listen, and one's faith suddenly becomes clearer and clearer, it is then that one can find that God is teaching and guiding us (in these times in the form of the Divine Feminine). Maybe it's because there are no fear tactics employed, but rather a transcendental spirituality is being taught. She has been rejected, as was her husband, but she continues to teach about a loving God, not a punishing God.

For 30-plus years she has gone out, and continues to go out to the byways and highways, to bring in those travelers to the Marriage Feast: "for those invited refused and were not worthy."

LESSON 50

GOD IS GREATER THAN HUMAN ERROR

What exactly is it that we have been witnessing with regards to religion? Is it something that Jesus always intended but was suppressed? Is it a gift that God knew would be most effective in these times? Whatever the case, we do know that God's timing allows for free will to be enabled; and, at the same time. our right to choose should bring solutions, not more problems. So, when we reach a point where the human consciousness has our souls crying out to God (for they recognize that something they are hearing is efficacious in producing a desire to change our ways and/or promote a change in the Consciousness of the world). Today we have become a people:

- of haughty eyes
- of lying tongues
- shedding innocent blood
- who have hearts that devise wicked schemes
- whose feet are quick to rush into evil
- who have become false witnesses that pour out lies
- in desperate need of spiritual help.

Perhaps, in God's plan, it had to take 2000 years, because we are slow learners, or maybe it would take that long so that we would better see the end result of a flawed human consciousness leading us. God's ways are not our ways, and letting the patriarchy's plans play out may just be that catalyst intended that was meant to open our eyes to see what and who Jesus really was and is, more clearly.

What we have to show God is that our love and faith is stronger than our stubbornness, and not just in times of personal tragedy or catastrophic weather etc.

In any event, it is without a doubt time to change the consciousness of the world, as we are in the fullness of time, where the need for God is imperative. We are witnessing the need for salvation from God, which will deliver us from ourselves. Following the example of the Divine Parents, where the only-begotten Child was first, One as eternal Consorts, then, secondly, as Jesus and Mary, followed with Jesus' return to heaven, allowing for his eternal consort to carry out the much-needed conclusion of God's plan for our salvation, in these end times.

We have seen enough to believe that there are prophecies and scriptures now being fulfilled. We are witnessing one such prophecy of 'the Woman encompassing the Man,' made possible by an unfamiliar process recognized by those outside of certain established, and socially acceptable, religions and spiritualities.

We believe Jesus is now saying in these revelatory times, "come I will show you my wife, the wife of the Lamb" (Revelation 21:9).

LESSON 51

HERESY OR ENLIGHTENMENT?

When one finds that they are at odds with what is generally accepted, especially in Catholic/Christian faiths, they are said to be in heresy. When one attains spiritual knowledge, or insight, in particular as having a more informed sense of spirituality and the things of God and the Divine, they are said to be *enlightened*.

Once we as Eeshans opened our mind to the things of God and Christ's teachings, we found enlightenment; and despite some that may be labeling us as heretics (it is usually those who don't practice their own religion, but a revised version of it), we don't fear answering questions, since truth brought us to the Eeshan Religion, and since we were never satisfied with what we had settled for in our birth religions.

In fact, we feel freer and more knowledgeable, and were truly drawn to glorify and love God. With what we practice spiritually, there's a sense of contentment in knowing that God is there and understands human beings better than other human beings do.

We no longer feel that Jesus left us to our own devices, as we were guided by the Holy Spirit to question and *seek truth*, and it was to his Divine Feminine that we were led. She, too, has been ignored and reimaged to conform to man's own agendas for himself.

We no longer are faced with trying to make a case for 'blindly' accepting those "truths" that we were told came from God (but to Eeshans, they didn't). How could the things of God be contradicted with the very things Jesus taught, unless the things of God were not heeded in the first place? However, that's what happened when Jesus lived on earth, and obviously it is clearly what happened again, when one changes the transcendental to reflect a human desire, and we try and understand God through the lenses of human logic. The outcome is that nothing makes sense.

Through our Eesha's teachings, and by attending her mystery school, we found what happened. What we found was exactly what we included in the beginning teachings of this book, and they adequately proved to be more than a hunch or suspicion. What we found pointed to a myriad of hidden and concealed evidence, which sadly seemed to have been covertly communicated to God's people by passages that *were* changed, omitted, or destroyed with the intention to redirect, or present a somewhat similar path to God. The results showed a splintering off of teachings into many versions and paths, each one different from the other, with not one evidencing the 'Way' back to those things God intended for us.

Even within the UNIVERSAL church itself, there is evidence of conflicting versions of what Jesus taught and meant. When these gaps were filled with information from Eesha, and along with other sources completing the puzzle, the once vague teachings of Christ became virtually transcendental and satisfying, to include topics such as:

1) Could the use of these altered stories suggest this was a way and means of controlling the faithful?
2) Were these involved with other measures specifically used for the retention of power and authority in the name of Jesus?
3) Why does history reveal a repetitious fear as a tool used in an effort to prevent the loss of followers from the very beginning of so many patriarchal religions, especially in the entire Christian world?
4) Could and did which serve as a means to accomplish the paralyzing of any effort used to expose this sin was so great, and the threat of losing or dying without the church's blessing was so frightening—that the sin or offense against God became so great in minds of the faithful that we became likened to sheep before the slaughter?

It's no secret that the sense of guilt in religion, without a doubt, has always been handed down and repackaged in various ways over the centuries; but what remains consistent is the sense of inhibition, blindness, and deafness on the part of the soul towards God as a result of all this, since the mind has been essentially imprisoned in darkness. God is Light. Without God, there is only darkness.

Where's the harm when a story or teaching is changed? Well, take for example in the story of Adam and Eve, where the central axiom has always been their "sin," defined solely as the 'transgression of a law,' and this caused the need for salvation.

We believe the real story found that the couple fell victim to *delusion* that there was a better way of mirroring[82] the love of God. We see it as 'the embracing of an illusion,' while exercising free will under duress, which resulted in consequences testing the true love of the male and female beings and the power and strength of marriage, and the need for loving God with our whole heart, whole soul, and whole being, especially within marriage; thus, showing what happens to humans if they don't stay connected with this beautifully, Sacredly Balanced God, and when they are not being spiritually nourished. Finally, our view takes into account what emerged because of the only-begotten child[83] being God's parental mercy, forgiveness, and love, which is certainly not at all defined in the traditional story.

What is found instead, is that while reference is made to the "Fall," or "Original Sin," focused only on disobedience of God's law, these elements self-locate the reader's attention in what mankind has overlaid as a word play that became a means used as a foundational tool to keep in place a failed gender equality today.

Today God is not defined as by Jesus, but by the same human consciousness that defined God in the Old Testament; there is too much similarity between the Old Law and New Law that contradicts Jesus as Messiah, Savior and Redeemer. Finally, what has been taught through

---

[82] 'Mirroring' is important in this context over and above the term 'expressing' because mirroring denotes the advice they were given by the serpent to *imitate* God's love ... not channel it, not express it. A mirror image is not the actual thing; also, it is in reverse. – Ed.

[83] We believe that as God is Divine Masculine and Divine Feminine, they begot an only begotten Child, one who is like them—infinitely and sacredly balanced and undivided in unity.

the centuries, in no way gives the reason for, or completes the mission and purpose of Jesus' life, death, and resurrection, nor does it restore what was lost by the fall to physicality. It shows no acknowledgement, or need, for the transcendental element in spirituality, or the purpose of life here, or the need for God in this world.

It has been said that over great periods of time, when the actual event is recast, and promulgated through the troubled conscience of humanity, it is bemired in illusion to reflect more and more not the true God who is love, but a projection of any given group's, or nations, dominating gender. Again, this is not the God that Jesus revealed, and 'this spirit' had no part in his mission.

With an enlightened *purusha*[84] (consciousness), we truly learn, and are enlightened, and change for the better. We've all heard that "God works in mysterious ways," and as a result should in effect apply this to things and events in our life. Eeshans believe that the failed human consciousness must now bow to the Age of Enlightenment, the Final Testament, and follow the True 'Way' that Jesus planned for us, or to otherwise continue down the path of indignation, as was the path of those who walked away from Jesus at his 'Bread of Life' discourse, which was due to more reasons than just what has been taught. These reasons will continue to be unpacked from many perspectives throughout this book.

---

[84] Sanskrit term meaning "pure Spirit," "Self," or "power of Awareness." – Ed.

LESSON 52

Is Anyone Out There?

Even though Eeshans believe that the mistakes humans make are more of an offensive nature, there is still sin. Sin is more than just an offense, since an offense in and of itself is compared to human weaknesses; whereas, a sin is a deliberate act against God or neighbor. Offense, on the other hand, often is followed by remorse, and one eagerly sets out to try and make up for the hurt. There are different forms of sin.

We've heard of venial sin. We've heard of mortal sin. Mortal sin condemns one to hell if not forgiven, since it separates a person from God's plan; and, thus, the person has no means of salvation. Few, however, understand the sin of which Jesus' spoke, and yet there is no greater sin than the 'eternal sin.' This is the sin that Satan committed, and is eternally unforgivable and not understood, since when one attacks God by saying what he desires is evil, or at the source of evil. So why wouldn't an all-loving God forgive someone in this state, such as Lucifer? The answer to this question is found in the fact that Lucifer places himself in this state precisely by the refusal to seek forgiveness, due to the fact that the narcissism he possesses doesn't allow him to see himself as less than perfect, i.e., God, and so the position he enters is 'unforgivable' and it stays that way. We must remember that first, Lucifer was a *created* entity, but he believes he came into existence on his own, and that is why he sees himself equal to, or greater than God. And from this place, he challenged God: "I will put your throne under my throne, and destroy you." So because he was *created*, Lucifer cannot see that an infinite God cannot be destroyed.

Something very similar happens too often today when one chooses to "hold God responsible" for evil, or tragic things, in his or her life.

Like Lucifer, a person who blames God for all the evil in their lives, or in the world, cannot see God for who God is: limitless love and infinite mercy, using the appearances of joys and tragedies for a higher end. Human beings start out perceiving with a fallen nature, which means they cannot help but be subject to illusion from the start; they cannot see the grand scheme, or the big picture of God; nor are they easily able to see Lucifer's plan either, which very subtly led to entropy: Adam and Eve allowed themselves to be guided by a created being whose intellect, reasoning, and will was already corrupt, instead of turning to God for their guidance.

When a mind becomes corrupted, the illusions they entered into become their 'truths,' their 'realities' *for them*. As it has been said in the world of professional stage actors, playing a good villain depends on seeing the villain as "the hero of his or her own story." For human beings limited to only the human consciousness, this delusion spreads from a root sin like envy, jealousy, covetousness, lust, etc. From these an entire perception of 'reality' ensues. As what happened with Lucifer, we see the same pattern with human beings.

Simply, this also is the sin that one commits when we say that someone "won't forgive God" for what has happened to them, since "that's not what a loving God would allow." It is the sin that blames God even though the consequences are the result of *humans'* actions; since God knows our weaknesses and yet won't stop us from harming ourselves. One the other hand, when we do good, we don't acknowledge God's intervention. It is also the sin that kills innocents in the name of God, whether it is actual physical death, or that which, in the case of pedophiles, or similar wrongdoers, causes the death of innocents through perverse immoral acts of the perpetrators, giving the impression that the spirit of Jesus desires such things. It is calling God a liar by ignoring, walking away, or downplaying, as did most of the disciples and followers after his "Bread of Life discourse." It is deliberately disconnecting the Bread of Life discourse from what Jesus said, and did at the last supper, as though we have a choice in whether or not to follow Jesus' "directives."

When the Spirit of God is compromised, life takes leave. This was the state of the world in biblical times when Jesus came on the scene.

Isn't the spirit of God being attacked daily? Have we so lost that healthy fear of God that we actually dare to think we can judge and ignore God's directives?

Well, in countless ways we have, and just as those faithful people of biblical times prayed and pleaded for God to send a Messiah, their own image of what the Messiah would be like prevented them from recognizing not just him, but his wife. Eeshans believe the same goes for today. God-loving, God-fearing (respecting) people are crying out for vengeance from God, and guess what? They, too, are waiting for a Messiah they have formed in their own image. To change this mindset that was derived from years of being told what to believe, we now find, all it takes for God to respond is to have faith; since faith is born of truth.

We feel as a people we have reached that point in time where our prayers have been answered, but as before we cannot see because we are blinded with fallacies, which will not allow us to see beyond what we have been told, and see the Messiah is back, only not in the same way we may have imagined. Remember those times when you watched the movie "Passion of Christ," and said to yourself, "How could these people not recognize that he truly was the Messiah?" You most likely said that *you* would have known and believed. Can you say that now?

God sent the promised Messiah to free the enslaved people, but due to blindness what they couldn't see was the bigger picture. The enslavement that God was freeing the people from far surpassed the bondage of any government, and due to the altering of scriptures, there is only the record of the Divine Masculine avatar Jesus. We know little, except that He was and is to be the Way, the Truth, the Light, and the Life.

If an Avatar(s) is (are) ignored, or re-imaged, by the human consciousness, the final result is the same as before his/her presence, or worse than the condition before the previous Avatar. It doesn't end there, however, as the loving God will send another, or bring to light the one disgraced by the ignorance of humans. This will continue up until which time, God calls an end to all things.

Jesus was the active Messiah, the Savior and Redeemer, who by altered scriptures, was shown to have come in response to the pleas of the people. These pleas were not seen by all, since Jesus did not come to change what most of the people of that day expected. Jesus was coming for a much greater reason, which causes one to wonder if anyone knew for sure what the bondage of sin meant. We are taught that he came to free all Adam and Eve's descendants from original sin/choice. Yes, we said the active Messiah.

What was actually accomplished by God, and missed, was that God, as a Man, came to us showing us how God didn't desert us after Adam and Eve, but was guiding us back on the path of righteousness to where we belong, *with* God. This means, it was God coming out of God who came forth.

> "Whenever righteousness wanes and unrighteousness increases
> I send myself forth
> For the protection of the good and for destruction of evil,
> And for the establishment of righteousness,
> I come into being age after age."[85]

Though the above is not a Christian verse, Eeshans nevertheless see in it how the presence and Word of God has permeated human experience, and made appearances to human beings, long before even Judaism appeared on the scene. If God is omnipotent, omniscient, omnificent, and omnipresent then there is no way that we wouldn't find God's presence, especially under other names, such as Jesus being known in India as St. Ish, and also known as *Issa* (who was renowned), thereby bringing all people together; however, we would also have to find Jesus' teachings within these to include the life-giving sacred bread, in one way or another. We are not claiming that Jesus is just one of 'many,' we *are* claiming, however, that the many are of the one God (Jesus) in likening him to a diamond with many facets. Yet, the line of truth, that links all to Jesus in the above verse, is that Jesus comes out of himself[86] throughout the ages.

---

[85] Bhagavad Gita 4:7-8.

[86] In the Vedic conception, God 'expands' himself according to time and circumstance, to share in relationship and to enact pastimes, called the divine 'Lila' (play). – Ed.

Throughout recent times, however, people seem more conditioned to believe that the living presence in the Eucharist is more symbol, or myth than truth, more memorial than the reality of Jesus, with the option of believing it is a memorial rather than his directive becoming more 'acceptable.' One must remember that God is not bound by human law, but is the author of "Law," and that man is bound by God's law.[87]

It is the Eeshan perspective, that what we have been taught via the Christian faith is not only imbalanced, but by what's been omitted, has forfeited the life exchange and transcendental entrance of which Jesus spoke and gave us. Most of all, we are cheated out of knowing God's greatest love story. Once again, we have fallen victim to the same fears and doubts about God, linking us to biblical times when those who didn't recognize the Messiah eventually doubted the reality of his coming.

Even though one may live in a religion with expunged truths, and teachings, and important events, still, through faith and love, one can receive the benefit of God's gifts, although without the fullness of those gifts. As those of other religions do not fall under the same criteria, or belief system, as the Catholic/Christian religions, the onus of this tragedy would fall on whatever religion claims to be the true faith founded on Jesus; since their strategy was supposedly based on a forthright responsibility to go out and teach all nations.

---

[87] But God's Law is not properly understood by man. – Ed.

LESSON 53

How God, as Jesus, Began the Age of Enlightenment, but Allowed for Man's Free Will to Disrupt God's Plan of Salvation

Eshans believe that it is clearly the fullness of time. It is always in 'the fullness of time' that God causes a major change to take place. One major onset began with Jesus' birth. This marked the beginning of change as humanity knew, even if it was not aware, a climactic event took place. God became human. The details surrounding the incarnation of God in the birth of Jesus from scriptures are few. The fact is, as God is all-powerful and all-present, everything God knew no boundaries except those He chose as a Child. Growing up, the Divine family experienced major obstacles, and as we do, attempted to make the best possible decisions, sans using their divinity. Joseph would strike the human balance for this divine human intervention, facing the most unusual set of circumstances that no mere mortal man ever did. Everything God is, and does, however, penetrates and permeates all ages, since the past, present, and future are all actively present in God's eternity.

Jesus' incarnation, as was his eternal consort's incarnation, about which there is nothing written in biblical times, continued to play out simultaneously.

We spoke of the only-begotten child whose Divine Masculine side was incarnate, as Jesus (whose birth was from an *Immaculate Conception*), and born of the Virgin Mary. That does not say that Jesus' conception was not. It just makes one aware that the Mother of Jesus had to be more than human and sinless.

Jesus' part in the Salvific plan was to be the *active* consort of the only-begotten Child, insomuch as he would be the most visible, and being the outward aspect of the Divine Masculine of God; and for that time, would fit into the way things were. Deemed by religious leaders to not ever mention (or put any attention on or acceptance of) His marriage, would allow for all the focus to be on Jesus as the teacher, as this was the mode of lifestyle chosen to identify Him.

It was deemed that His marriage, to this 'type' of woman Magdalen was considered, would take away from His being God, and because of His attitude towards women, would be the end of the 'new religion' before it got started. Though it was so not acceptable, little could be done about keeping away His wife and the women who worked with and were taught by Him. He taught primarily outside the temple; and, therefore, worked outside the 'human religious structure,' even though it is written that the synagogue/temple "was His Father's house." Yes, the age of enlightenment had begun!

Jesus, however, proved to be the greatest Temple within Himself, since He with his wife carried within them the perfect knowledge and perfect plan of salvation of humans (from which they could teach).

Jesus began as a teacher of Jewish values and customs, and worked his way to the spirituality necessary to implement his plan. Those considered teachers at the time were also considered arbiters and authoritative judges.

Jesus on the other hand did not desire to be an arbitrator; rather, he wanted to probe the attitudes motivating His questioner, while implicitly rejecting His request. In this way, He almost immediately began incorporating those characteristics which triggered an onslaught of enemies, of which equality of women was first and foremost. He was different from the other teachers who roamed along from place to place with their disciples.

Aside from being a teacher, He was considered a healer and prophet who displayed powers from God. That is why when questioned about His *s'mikhah*,[88] He replied that all his authority came from God. One must be clear, however, that there were also sorcerers and magicians who performed tricks and wonders. Jesus had many obstacles to His work.

Even upon returning to Nazareth, his home town, He met with obstacles; He went to the synagogue to read. It was here that He read from the scroll of the prophet Isaiah that was handed to him. Scanning the scroll Jesus found where it was written:

"The Spirit of the Lord is on me, because he has anointed me to preach good news to the poor." Eeshans believe what was meant by "to the poor" takes in a lot of ground here. The poor were in many cases those who barely got by, and therefore did not have the means to be educated, thus accepting whatever the "religious leaders" told them. He also could have meant poor in spirit who were humble and can be likened to baby birds who await food with open mouths! The poor in spirit are empty of themselves and await the living word as eagerly as the baby bird, since the poor in spirit are humble, and look for nothing for themselves.

He also knew that the rich were preoccupied with other matters; and, without a crushing reason, truly did not feel a need for a savior, but understood why the poor did.

Jesus also meant that those who were living in sin, and didn't know it, needed a strong faith to overcome all they were going through, and by far needed the Messiah, since theirs was a life where all they had was God.

"Having read the scroll, He handed it back to the attendant and sat down. All eyes were on Him; and He began by saying to them, 'Today this scripture is fulfilled in your hearing.'" (Luke 4:16). This was Jesus' public proclamation for making corrections of the laws and the recognition of women's equality, while attesting to His intention to open the eyes to see, the ears to hear. His words implied that, as the Son of God, He had a deliberate intention to lead God's people to the "Lighted 'way' of truth and life;" and for those who followed Him and abided by His

---

[88] A specific type of recognized bestowed authority/credential by which a teacher could interpret and explain the law. – Ed.

directives. The rest of that passage acknowledges, and was not necessary for Him to repeat:

"Because the Lord has anointed me, to bring good new to the afflicted..."

Here Jesus gave the reason why He came, while also identifying that he was the Christ, the anointed one who came to all of us who were afflicted by Adam and Eve's choice for physicality.

"He has sent me to bind up the brokenhearted..."

Here Jesus gave meaning to our lives, that, despite how the world has treated you, He, as God knows you, loves you, and for that reason, your life has meaning.

"He has sent Me to proclaim freedom for the prisoners and recovery of sight for the blind, to release the oppressed..."

Here, as in all of the above, Jesus was teaching a transcendental Consciousness, not a human consciousness; therefore, one must not read these words literally but to understand what has happened to the soul when for whatever reason it is separated from God, and how He addresses how people have eyes to see Him: and yet do not see, and ears to hear but do not hear. Because of Jesus, if one believes, they *will* see and hear, as He, who is the Bread of Life, will not just nourish, but united with the light body within them, and as Light of the world, to also escort them into the transcendental everlasting life.

"To proclaim the year of the Lord's favor..."

This passage along with all of the following verses made it known to those who were blessed to know, that He was the Messiah, who came to change the consciousness of the world!

There was no reason why Jesus, who by His love for humankind, and whose mission of salvation (along with his wife's), would bring the restoration and reversal of the original sin/choice, if He taught the story that had been dictated. He also wouldn't have caused issues for Himself with religious teachers. Instead, by His teachings and actions, which were contrary to what the religious teachers upheld during those times, He would bring merit to the consequences of listening to these Pharisees, Sadducees, and chief priests, since He knew the people were innocent, doing as they did only what they were told; and as Truth, He taught Truth.

As a result of man's ego, closely mirroring an oppositional defiant disorder, along with free will, God's directives were once again altered even within Jesus' own immediate group and almost immediately after Jesus ascended back to heaven. Why? It was apparent that already at least half of his apostles were afraid that they may be arrested and put to death, as Jesus was, even after the Holy Spirit gave them strength.

You will find later on how the apostles, under Peter strategized a plan that would (at least temporarily) ward off persecution. The plan was to utilize those directives of Jesus that paralleled similar practices of their birth religion, and in a generic way, sans Jesus' wife. The women who followed Him would be returned to their status before Christ, and would no longer pose a threat to the known religion of the time.

As time went on, we find that, when aligned with man's desperation to be successful in obtaining security and success, and without compromising their original agenda to continue on, there was still an unrelinquishing of the origins in the Jewish faith. To succeed in their plan, the leadership of those in the early beginnings of the church, i.e., Peter, would have to find a way to stop anything that could disrupt the status quo, one way which was the prohibition of women from leadership positions, and by destroying any, and all, evidence of this that might be discovered afterwards. Later this problem would find its solution in a convert whom we would come to know as St. Paul. He would ease the differences, and as Peter split the two cultures (Peter taking the Jews and Paul the Gentiles), Peter's freedom to exercise his own beliefs would come to pass; thus, maintaining a very similar structure to what he had been born into, sans Jesus.

Then afterwards, as time went on, even these 'changes' would have to be modified further by Constantine, in order to guarantee a unified body; thus, establishing the institutional, formal organization of the church which would continue all the way up into present times. As the church became more established, it adopted and developed new doctrines and outlined new traditions. Throughout the years there was always a need for changing and modifying what eventually became known as Canon Law. (This is primarily what was used against the cry for female representation as apostles and as such making them worthy to be priests).

What happened next, due to the failing of the church leadership in following the path of the transcendental, once again for fear of persecution, and concern over losing and retaining followers, a problem which persists even today, the leadership centered on spirituality focused *human*-based directives, rather than on the transcendental, which was something they could not comprehend could begin to happen. Their reluctance caused the people to fall victim to a deeper, more humanly centered rational consciousness that was the same as the consciousness that Jesus was met with in the guise of religious authorities of the time. Who would have known? We have only this to discover if one was strong enough, and courageous enough, to peruse through and present their opinions. But who can stand against a two-thousand-year-old established church that had taken down anyone that was considered dangerous to its survival, or having a different point of view, or a heretic, as in the past? You would not be alone. In fact, you would be in the best of company.

Jesus' way almost always provoked opposing arguments, which He had to constantly deal with; and those who tried to trick him would eventually provide enough 'evidence' which would bring about His arrest. He was labeled a rebel, a lawbreaker, as were all those who followed Him, and amid the rumors of His getting arrested His still continuing to teach, certainly frightened some of his apostles. If only they, to include those in opposition, 'all' would've seen Jesus for who and what He really was, and had gone beyond the 'rational, logical' consciousness, they would have seen the true God, and understood better what Jesus meant, when He said, "Where I go you cannot follow;" yet, the time had come, and it would take his death and resurrection to open the gates of heaven. During the time, Jesus taught publicly, and despite the growing threats against him, knowing his own future, Jesus made it clear that he was not afraid. That is the reason he faced His enemies and lived according to what He taught. That is why he said, "Fear not the one who can kill your body and can do no more, but fear the One who can kill both your body and soul …" He did so that others would see the importance of what He taught, and what may be necessary for salvation, while loving God, above all things, and our neighbor as oneself.

Jesus spoke to the women saying things such as, "it is better that you would starve your children of food than to starve them of me." If listening with a balanced consciousness of both transcendental and human, one would know that He meant to show the seriousness of a parent's decision to keep children apart from Him, who was indeed God; and not intended for good parents to take this analogy literally, as in corrupt sciences of the human consciousness.

Moving on after Jesus' ascension, the apostles now separated, not just to spread his teachings, but also for those closely aligned with Jesus, to get away from Peter. Trust was weakened, and there were those who were frightened, but still remained steadfast to what Jesus had continued to teach through Mary Magdalen. There were those who felt compelled to make compromises by combining the Old Law with a 'New Law,' as you will see later.

Those who tried to do Jesus' will, and stood by Mary, his wife, eventually had to move on to do as Jesus asked, and to go and teach those who wanted to hear, until which time things became so violent that it was impossible to stay together. By this time John had taken Mary, the Mother of Jesus, to Ephesus.

There were searches organized to find and get rid of Mary Magdalen. These became relentless. More stories circulated about her, but one in particular was the story of Mary being put on a boat without oars by Peter and a group of men that surrounded him from his Jewish connections (not apostles), in hopes she would meet with her demise. What we are witnessing today are the results of those choices and changes from earliest times.

Remember when we mentioned that Jesus had the *active* role in the "Plan?" This is where we begin to show why, and how, we believe God is reintroducing the truth about the role of the Divine Child today. As the Eucharist has been previously taught to be Jesus solely, with the understanding that he was the Divine Masculine of the only begotten Divine Child, it is now revealed that the Eucharist, as the church understood and presented it was incomplete, since it was meant to be both Jesus and Mary in Sacred Balance. As Jesus is understood as the Son of God, it would only make sense that Mary would be the divine Feminine and counterpart in that Second Person. It is now in these end times that she would also be introduced in the *active* role (whereas, during Jesus' earthly life she was in the passive role).[89] It is important to remember that the fullness of this unfathomable mystery is contained only in the Eucharist found within the Marriage Feast. Since as this mystery plays out through the Eucharist, it brings with it Jesus' counterpart and Eternal Consort, and fills in the gaps, bringing about the completion of the true Salvific Plan, as only it can.

His Divine Female counterpart, in the person of Mary Magdalen, is she who was always His inseparable Eternal Consort; and like him, became human in order to complete Christ's salvific mission. During the time they both lived on earth, she was seen as the passive consort who stood alongside with him as his equal, teaching the Kallahs and ministering alongside of her husband as soulmate and partner.

Who better to send to us in these end times, but His consort, his twin flame, his Divine Feminine counterpart to the Divine Masculine of God. No one knew him better, since she shared his Divinity first in eternity, and then here on earth marriage, and in the Eucharist prefigured in Cana on their wedding night, as they shared in a tantric,[90] transubstantiated way, their bodies, blood, souls, and divinity in this world, as no one else could.

---

[89] At the time of Jesus, Mary could not be brought to the forefront because of the social structures in place regarding women, many of which are still in place to this day in the Middle East. – Ed.

[90] The deepest expression of love to be unpacked as the book continues to unfold ...

However, as you know, eventually Mary Magdalen died ... or rather, was it time to let her human body go and prepare for the next phase of God's interrupted plan? One thing is for sure, after her life as she knew it, she left her body, her remains were buried, and, as stories have it, it was dismembered and used for relics of power; but as her spirit returned to God, her consciousness was laid in a state of suspension, awaiting the fullness of time, at which point it would return and find its place through the process of supramentalization, which some may describe as an imperfect kind of resurrection, because the body chosen is not in its glorified state, but in a purely human state, once again.

LESSON 54

WHAT WE KNOW ABOUT THE ONLY BEGOTTEN CHILD OF GOD

THE FRUIT OF THE SACRED BALANCE OF DIVINE MALE/ FEMALE AND WHO JESUS AND MARY MAGDALEN ARE

Jesus is familiarly known to people by what Catholics and Christians called the Only-begotten Son of God, Savior, and Redeemer, who suffered, died for the sins of the whole world, and who Resurrected.

Eeshans hold a *deeper understanding* of this remarkable Man. We know that actually there was an only-begotten Child-and the Divine Masculine, as well as the Divine Feminine of this Child, who was separated, and became a human male and female; and each, though Sacredly Balanced, needed to become One again.

When the only-begotten Child was separated, the incarnation of the Divine Masculine, who has come to be known as Jesus, and his counterpart Mary (Divine Feminine), imaged and complemented the first created transcendental being, who when separated became Adam and Eve. The Divine Masculine of the only-begotten Child is eternal, as he is human; and together he, with his wife, are sacramental.

The first Person of the Holy Trinity, being Masculine and Feminine, would become the first Divine/Human marriage witnessed on earth. We are told that the Father, the Most High God—the Divine

Masculine—announced through an angel, His favor on Mary, and His desire to have a Child.[91]

His desire was not just to have a Child, with just any woman, nor was it to have a Child outside of marriage. The Blessed Mother, who unbeknown to her, was already the human incarnation of the Divine Feminine/Eternal consort of the first person of the Blessed Trinity. What was necessary, because she was now the human representation of the Divine Feminine, was for her to *exercise her free will*:

> *The Angel said, "Do not be afraid Mary, for you have found favor with God. You will conceive and give birth to a son, and you shall call him Jesus. He will be very great and will be called the Son of the Most High. The Lord God will give him the throne of His father David and will reign over the house of Jacob forever, and of His kingdom there will be no end." And Mary asked the angel, "But how can this be [happen] seeing that I know not a man [or in other words," since I am a virgin]. The angel's reply was, "the Holy Spirit will come upon you, and the power of the Most High will overshadow you; and the Child to be born will be called holy—the Son of God." With that said, the Virgin Mary replied, "Let it be done unto me, according to your word."*[92]

With that she was placed in a euphoric state, and because of her *Yes*, the Most High awakened her to who she was, and impregnated her through a kind of begetting process, using a transcendental womb in which to carry the Child, while maintaining her virginity. She was special in her own right. With all that is known, and believed about Mary by Catholics, via Sacred Tradition and Sacred Scriptures, she really was, and still is made to be less than who she is!

---

[91] If God came himself and asked her, there would be no choice; so by the angel being the messenger, she was provided the room to make a completely free choice. – Ed.

[92] Luke 1:30-36.

The fact remained that the Divine Feminine spirit was, and, has been, ignored in the person of the Blessed Virgin Mary, despite the fact she brought the Eucharist into the world!

Even as Christ's Mother, she was/is a woman that the church had/has concerns about. So much so, she was defined *only* as bringing Christ into the world, even though Jesus made the point to call to witnesses' attention that she did God's will. This omission, and the deliberate exclusion of her being the Wife of God, in and of itself, lessened the person of the Blessed Virgin Mary. What damage was done? The defamation of her character is one example. The attack on her virginity, then, and, in present times, is another. The church obviously thought that it was better that Mary's person be attacked than to risk these truths that could lead to Mary being worshipped as a Goddess. The repercussions of these truths, becoming known, and her marriage to the Divine Masculine, first Person of the Holy Trinity, would bring back the notion that God was behind the equality of genders.

Regarding the outrageous attacks on her virginity, it is well demonic to say the least that she would lower herself to partake in a sexual relationship for pleasure, knowing she was actively married to God the Father. That, too, is the reason that Joseph was not involved with God's plan.

Her purpose for coming to earth, and her key role in the participation in the plan of salvation, was to bring the Divine Masculine gender, their Son, delivered into the world to begin the Salvific plan.

The Husband of the Blessed Virgin Mary is known to Eeshans as God the Father. In this account, we understand that Jesus was raised by his mother, and God had chosen Joseph as the foster father, or male figure, to offset rumors of an illegitimate pregnancy.

The Mother and Child were placed in the protective care of Joseph, who also provided a basically sufficient patriarchal family structure under Mosaic law. The family was human in every way, as God the Father's and the angels' care, was not obvious, or visible, in any way to anyone.

As rumors about a prophecy of a King being born circulated, it was necessary that the Holy Family often moved for safety reasons. As the Child grew, it became necessary to observe some of the "rites" of their religion; however, it also required that they take Jesus away, so as not to be chosen for and drawn into an arranged marriage. Having him travel with his great uncle, who was a metal merchant, allowed him to spend a lot of time in what is now Avalon, England.

As a pre-teen and teenager, He was taught and studied lessons at the hand of His mother, and had His presentation in the temple where He exceeded the priests' expectations. There were times, when He was not traveling, that He worked as a carpenter with Joseph.

At the age of 17, He left his homeland and traveled to the Himalayas to further His studies in spirituality, and, being so very brilliant, it wasn't long before He became a Master of Spirituality. While there, He took the name 'Ish,' and became known for His teachings, especially regarding women. Those who taught him knew He fulfilled all the prophecies and qualifications of the Messiah, and that He would one day return to his land to fulfill his duty to marry, suffer, and die.

LESSON 55

THE DIVINE BECOMES HUMAN

Though human, Jesus' body was not affected by the fall from the transcendental/Divine life to physicality; being God, His body was the result of impregnation by the Divine Masculine, Husband, and formed in the spotless, immaculate womb of the Divine Feminine, who became Mary in order to bring to pass God's will and promise to humanity.

Mary (the Divine Feminine and counterpart of God, first Person of the Holy Trinity and Mother of Jesus Christ), became human via a transcendentally/divine impregnation into the person of Anne (Hannah), who was the elderly and childless wife of Joachim. She was chosen to bring into being the first Divine Feminine by Divine means.

To find anything out about Anne, one would have to check mention of her in, an apocryphal tradition, in the Gospel of James. Accounts of her birth had been condemned as an error, in 1677.

According to Eesha, the conception of the Virgin Mary took place under the Golden Gate, where Jewish tradition holds this as where the place where the Divine Presence enters. It is also known as the Gate of Eternal Life and the Mercy Gate; it is also the Gate through which Jesus passed on Palm Sunday.

Being God the Father's eternal Consort, Mary could not be subject to sin, and her conception could not be created by human means; therefore, her soul was free from original sin as it was protected within the womb of Ann (Hannah) into whom the Divine Presence of Mary was placed by the very hand of God, without ever having contact with Ann's body. Her very essence was encapsulated in a special womb designed by God, the Divine Masculine of the first person of the holy trinity, her husband. She was nourished and grew, and at the fullness of time was removed the very same way, in a kind of 'divine cesarean birth,' meaning the birth was achieved by a begetting process, and not in the same way as a human birth, since there was the absence of the need for the use of the birth canal, just as what would take place with the *birth of Jesus*. This truth later became known, as being initiated by the Virgin Mary herself, in an apparition to St. Bernadette Soubirous, in 1858, as the 'Immaculate Conception.'

Jesus received his humanity through Mary's sinless body. His body was formed within her womb, and she gave birth to Him by extraordinary means. His body was subject only to entropy of time, meaning the flesh that formed His body was pure, just as was Adam and Eve's was before the fall, but similar to ours, since it was not impervious to hunger, tiredness, pain, suffering, etc., since this was as the plan of salvation dictated. Contained within Him was a singular grace, which caused His body a preordained life expectancy of a little more than 33 years. So, everything he had to accomplish in a human body, to include His passion and death on the cross, had to occur in these 33 years.

As we mentioned earlier, we have been taught that the only-begotten Child of God, did the Will of His Father, but we were never told that the Father's Eternal Feminine consort was identified by Jesus as the Virgin Mary in her human form. Of course, as the Three Persons of God share in all things equally as one God, each has a Divine Feminine consort-whom we were never taught about.

When the Divine Feminine of the First Person became human, it only stands to reason that the Second Person of the Blessed Trinity's consort would also become human. However, it does not stop there. As Melchizedek was the embodiment of the First Person of the Trinity and carried the royal line, so must his wife, the Virgin Mary-who came through the line of David. Thus, as the Second Person of the holy Trinity became human in the Person of Jesus, He carried the royal bloodline of David, and founded the beginnings of "their Priesthood as Male and Female" under the Order of Melchizedek. It was made known that no male would be allowed to offer a sacrifice at the King's Altar because the altar was intended for woman to celebrate the Marriage Feast of the King's Son at Cana.

Few know how God's plan for the Divine Feminine of the only-begotten Child. Mary Magdalen's line came through Her father, who was of the Tribe of Benjamin. Furthermore, God's plan always included the astrological signs in the creation of human beings. Mary Magdalen's father, Cyrus, said to have been a direct descendant of the royal bloodline of the Benjaminite Tribe, was a Sagittarius; a most fitting detail with regards to Mary Magdalene's role due to the fact that Sagittarius is the sign connected to the Divine Feminine and Wisdom.

Providing proof of His Bride and prophesying what was to happen, Jesus used the following to clarify His Wife:

In Matthew 21:43 Jesus states, "Therefore I say to you, the kingdom of God will be taken from you and given to a nation bearing the fruits of it." This is referencing Jesus being apart of the Tribe of Judah bloodline, and passing His blessings from the Tribe of Judah onto the annexed Tribe of Benjamin, of which Mary Magdalen was from. From there, he tells the parable of the King's Son. Legend has it, that the parable included the Bride.

Condensed Parable of the Wedding of the King's Son[93]

There once was a King, who was a powerful King over a great and mighty kingdom. One day, the King began to plan for the wedding of His Son. So the King made public His intent for His Son to be married and promised great blessings and favor toward the one who would become the new Bride. The King sent messengers to announce the search for a Bride to be chosen from among all the virgins in the Land. The King devised a plan to find out which of the virgins would truly love the King's Son. He produced a "Book of Wisdom" with hidden messages throughout the book. The virgin who found these hidden messages and understood them would properly prepare and practice for what would delight the King.

---

[93] Adapted by: Brother Bill of Notes from the Wilderness Blog.

Late one night, the King sent out His messengers to announce the coming of the Bridegroom for His Bride. All the virgins began to awaken and get dressed to go out to be chosen, but they had no oil in their lamps to light the way. While the unprepared virgins went out to find oil, the true Bride was chosen, for She understood the hidden messages of the King, to Love from a pure heart and keep His decrees. However, the virgins who were not chosen were given the opportunity to apply to be followers of the Bride and take part in the Wedding Feast of the King's Son and His Wife.

These women, the virgins who followed the Bride, would come to be known as Kallahs. "And in that day seven women shall take hold of one man, saying, 'We will eat our own food and wear our own apparel; Only let us be called by your name, To take away our reproach.'" (Isaiah 4:1) Eeshans believe that this passage from Isaiah was meant to deter women from pulling away from the patriarchal religion of the time by instilling fear of the consequences of disobeying what they were told was God's law. However, if that was true, then God would be subject to the interpretation and consequences of the human consciousness of man's law and not the Author of the Law. We see this many times when man's interpretation is quoted in the bible, yet one example, is the Virgin's yes to bring the birth of the Divine Masculine of the Only-Begotten Child, showing God working outside of the Mosaic Law

The Divine Feminine of the Only Begotten Child's role would be to become human just like the Eternal Divine Feminine, the Virgin Mary, who is consort to Jesus' Father. Mary Magdalen and the Virgin Mary were to find their soulmates in order that they fulfill their destiny, which would be sealed with their "yes."

Eeshans believe that every attempt was made by Jesus to not only redeem His Wife and further Her role, but to instill in all the need to stop discrimination and prejudice. Jesus' parable of the Good Samaritan was used to point out that all are God's children, which in that case meant all those cultures and people who were shunned by the religious authority at the time.

The Samaritan woman at the well, was one in particular with whom he "shared" all of who he was. Not only was this person a Samaritan, a despised religious people at that time-but also a woman. His conversation with her in front of His apostles and His Wife proved that He supported this woman who went out in public and before male forums. She would not be silenced. This was a precursor to how Jesus' knowledge of the rejection of His Wife would take place because of the religious leaders and Peter but how His Wife's future role, we find like the Samaritan woman, shows how She will overcome and complete His Mission and will not be held back or stopped despite the apostles rudeness or hostility- or because of Her gender or nationality. The Samaritan woman was the herald to Mary Magdalen as John the Baptist was to Jesus.

They mirrored true love, and as soulmates, spent every moment of their life and in their marriage doing God's will, and together did all that was necessary to restore humankind back to a life with God. After Jesus' ascent back to heaven, and upon Mary's death, her spirit returned into the arms of her husband, but her consciousness would be suspended, until which time another body would be chosen as a vehicle for the return of the Divine Feminine.

LESSON 56

THE WOMAN WHO WAS THE ETERNAL CONSORT OF JESUS

Though she, too, was born human, little is known about her divine side except that she took on the human form of Mary Magdalen, as her 'Yes' to participating in God's salvific plan. Her Yes came in her desire, out of love of God, to exercise her will to accomplish God's plan for us. Where the Virgin Mary gave her Yes to having Jesus, Mary Magdalen gave her 'Yes,' to first accepting God's desire to become human, and, again, when, not knowing who she was, and that she was already Jesus' eternal Consort, and under such unusual circumstances, she accepted His proposal for marriage.

In both cases, both female counterparts became fully human, while being fully divine, but with one qualification, since Mary Magdalen, as the human consort, there would be the necessity to relate and experience the effects of the original choice in her flesh in yet a third Yes, beginning with the receiving the 'apparent crucifixion marks' of Her Husband, who died on the Cross, to remove original sin and show their Oneness of Body, Blood, Soul, and Divinity.

This is so because her life would have to mirror her Consort's; and, therefore, her sacrifice would be necessary until which time the Salvation Plan played out.

Both were needed to bring about the Bread come down from Heaven in the Eucharist of the Marriage Feast, thus marking the fullness of 'eschatological time.'

Since there is no other woman who was ordained to carry the title 'Immaculate Conception' in traditional religions other than the Mother of Jesus, the question now arises about the conception and birth of Mary Magdalen. In traditional circles, the thought that Mary Magdalen was of virgin birth would be absurd and blasphemous; but what is the truth? Some say, she, like John the Baptist, was conceived, but not born with the mark of original sin. Or that was she born with original sin but freed upon her first glance of her 'human/divine consort'? Perhaps it's too early to answer this question. Perhaps it should be the reader who determines this answer for himself or herself.

It's a deep mystery wondering how this woman, so loved by Jesus, whose life was altered because she offered herself as victim, became known as a 'harlot.' No one was guiltier than those who took this horrendous story and used it to ruin her life. Mary, violated by seven thugs at the age of fourteen, in an effort to save her sister from them, never blamed God for what happened. Where did her strength come from?

Her reputation as being a prostitute, at the hands of human beings, was as ridiculous as Jesus' reputation for being a criminal!

It is also interesting to note that the name of Mary Magdalen's mother was Eucharis, without the "T," almost as though she was awaiting the arrival of Jesus to complete her name, which would then become the legacy of her daughter.

LESSON 57

HIDDEN QUEEN

Some of God's most beautiful mysteries are often revealed through the suffering and sacrifice of those who love beyond purely human, especially through *Metta* (Divinely originated Love). As human beings are guided only by the human consciousness miss the most spectacular signs, Mary was one that was missed.

We've heard, 'when others saw a shepherd boy, God saw a king,' which makes reference to King David. When others saw a carpenter's son, they missed the Messiah; and when everyone saw a 'prostitute,' Jesus saw his Eternal Consort. God had sent "their only-begotten child" to save the world,; however, the world rejected them.

Until recent times, Mary has still been hidden away, and that is until her husband came back for her, as He promised he would; so that the whole world would know and hear the truth.

There's a little flower which describes the life of another beautiful flower, and this hidden flower is Queen Mary Magdalen. The flower is called *Eucharis*, and is a small genus in the Amaryllidaceous family, whose true bulb is found underground with above ground petiolate leaves. The species of this genus can be grown in situations without much light, which is called the understory rainforest habit. There are photos of this plant that went through major stress, including root disturbance and defoliation. It, indeed, responded by flowering. The plant was then starved of water for a couple of months, and then watered again. During dormancy, it did not lose its leaves. The flower is small, white, and star-like (6 points). It is distinctive from any other species.

Disgraced and falsely labeled a prostitute, Mary Magdalen's marriage to Jesus was deliberately 'hidden for centuries,' or in other words, the knowledge of it laid dormant, but survived the prevention of its knowledge of the love they shared. This starving of Mary to the right to her titles, does respond in a similar way as the small, pure white, star-like (6 points) flower, *Eucharis*, and is, indeed, truly distinctive from any other species.

Eeshans feel that if Mary Magdalen was not conceived, but was born in original sin, it may have been a necessary component for the sake of all those souls who are in need in this world and who would be restored to purity with each encounter she had with them, and, then, restored permanently, through the reception of the Eucharist from within their Marriage Feast. Jesus, by virtue of his marriage to Mary, created a cleared pathway for the redemption of all souls, and especially for this faith-deprived time.

LESSON 58

JESUS LOVES MARY, OR JESUS AND MARY SITTING IN A TREE K-I-S-S-I-N-G

Oh, yes, we have heard all the stories. How sad it is that we cannot accept Jesus as truly man. Even though we were told he was human in very way. Some can't imagine him dancing when he was raised Jewish in the Middle-Eastern part of the world. Others cannot accept that followers of Jesus, as well as Jesus himself, drank wine, and often didn't fast, since we forget that wine was not just used at religious ceremonies but at weddings and other happy events. Those who were not in his company were shocked and pointed out how the one they followed, who was John the Baptist and his disciples, didn't drink and always fasted. Jesus never criticized John for his fasting but rather gave the reason for why Jesus and his disciples did not. [Luke 5:33, Luke 18:12]

Bread and Wine-Psalm 103–105:16

"You cause grass to grow for the livestock
and plants for people to use
You allow them to produce food from the earth—
and wine to make them glad,
Olive oil to soothe their skin,
And bread to give them strength."

Is it so surprising that Jesus would use all of the above, including salt, to bring about the recipe for the very food that would be used as key ingredients for the Marriage Feast to strengthen and gladden not just the body, but, via transubstantiation, the soul?

We find how very significant wine actually was, and would become, to Jesus and His disciples. It identified him as Messiah, as Bridegroom, and other more cryptic mysteries which He would eventually reveal.

One cannot think of wine and not think of Jesus, including the very controversial Marriage Feast in Cana. The Marriage of Jesus and Mary Magdalen in and of itself was vital to God's plan of salvation.

Let's begin with the love that Jesus and Mary Magdalen, as the Bridegroom and the Bride, and as husband and wife, shared on earth. Their love for each other was perfect and true but not without its challenges and problems. It is said that light is emitted from our finger tips and lips. Remember the first time the one you loved held your hand? Do you remember the ecstatic feeling that filled your whole body? It was the same with Jesus and Mary. It happened when they saw each other for the first time at Mary's family home.

MARY REMEMBERS:
[her recollection from the Greatest Love Story Forever Told]

It was the first time in eleven years that they saw each other. As Mary turned the corner to see who the "special guest" was that Lazarus was welcoming back into town with a party—her heart nearly stopped when she saw Him. Those eyes! Those eyes were the eyes she looked into that day He rescued her. It really was He! There he was—the one she dreamed and fantasized about since that day. As she walked towards him, He smiled. Eleven years and He was every bit as handsome as she knew he would be. Mary was not one to show weakness especially in the presence of a man—even this man.

It was rather upsetting actually. Her mind quickened to all those dreams of her hero coming into town and whisking her off her feet in front of the whole town vindicating her from the jeers, hecklers, and gossip she lived with.

Every fantasy she had, every romantic notion of His return boiled down to finding that He came back to town to look for 'a wife'—not looking for her exclusively. Rumor had it that he had no money, no job, and that He was staying with his recently widowed mother—to care for her. Perhaps those qualities that she emulated[94] *about him when He was seventeen, were no longer there—or, worse, were never there.*

Pretending she did not totally recognize him, Mary greeted Jesus graciously trying to not be so harsh in her judgment that it carried into unkindness—after all He did rescue her. Perhaps she was being insensitive in her thinking, not giving any consideration as to possible consequences that He encountered. After all, eleven years had passed.

Mary could sense that Jesus, seeing her approach, was immediately taken by her. Exchanging courtesies, Mary found it difficult not to exercise candor regarding Jesus' return—in hopes of finding a bride. Jesus did not seem to be uneasy with the topic and shared how He felt it was time.

Mary simply couldn't get past the letdown from her own thoughts of how she imagined her life would be with her hero, only to discover she couldn't have been more wrong. Graciously excusing herself she sought out her brother. Upon finding Lazarus near the kitchen, she unloaded on him in a harsh whispered voice. "How could you, brother? How could you bring Him to this house! He is the last person I ever wanted to see! I spent years trying to forget, trying to move on and now—it's all back, every hurtful memory, every moment of pain-every ..." her words trailed off when she noticed a shadow to her right. As she turned, there He stood. "You, Mary, were the first person I wanted to see," He said calmly, gently taking her hand. Apologizing to her, that He heard what she said, He interrupted once more saying, Mary, I was not one of those who hurt you."

---

[94] He was everything she looked up to and admired, everything she wanted to embody.

> Getting past her uneasiness, it wasn't long before they both realized there was a genuine attraction that existed between them; but things were certainly different for her. He was human, and though she could no longer escape into her fantasies about His being larger than life—she could now come face to face with the reality she spent so many years running from.
>
> With that, Mary felt it was better that she left. As she gathered her wrap, she couldn't help but look one more time into those 'eyes.' Without thinking, she found herself giving into an unexpected impulse and kissed Jesus.

This kiss was not the '*sacred kiss*,' but there was no escaping it; however, this energy, indeed, did pass between them. This kiss led to Jesus' responding in a precautionary way. Any kisses Jesus would share *before marriage* would amount to a kiss once in a while on the forehead. As powerful and exciting as one would think his kisses would be, to Mary it was disappointing for her, since, once again, she had imagined for years the kisses she might share with her beloved. They would be most beautiful and filled with passion. However, once married, it would be their kisses that witnessed their divine connection. That is why Eeshans stress that though their kisses were, and still are, a very controversial issue they were more than just public displays of affection.

These kisses they shared were without a doubt very disturbing to those who witnessed them, even though they were far from sensual kisses in a public forum, but to those who couldn't love, they caused tremendous intrigue, indignation, and anxiety. The reason it aroused this was, more than likely, because it was the sacred 'catalyst' responsible for accelerating Adam and Eve's transcendental euphoric union. For one who cannot love, who is evil, as in the case of Satan, this would be a reminder of what is at the core of the bitterness, which is the envious, jealous, and murderous outlook of which he was composed.

The Sacred Kiss that would be shared between Jesus and Mary, would be the 'key' to their entire love story. Their marriage would begin with it, and would be repeated throughout their human marriage, and it would bring life to each other. Their kisses contained *the most extraordinary*, transcendental component, and the only way we can experience this kind of love is to have our *human marriage in union with theirs.*

These sacred kisses were Jesus' way of giving life to his wife and awakening her self-awareness as his eternal counterpart, since Mary's kisses brought the fullness of her love and *ignited* Jesus' most sacred heart, since love is life.

> *"Love is like a friendship caught on fire. In the beginning, a flame, very pretty, often hot and fierce, but still only light and flickering. As love grows older, our hearts mature and our love becomes as coals, deep-burning and unquenchable."*
> —Bruce Lee

Can you only imagine how powerful an "eternal love" burns. However, as powerful as the light is that passes from fingertips and lips, there is yet another very powerful connection that human beings are capable of sharing.

With their kisses was the exchange of breath. Their breath was an anomaly. Breath is what we need in order to live; it is what we give to bring back life to others in emergency situations. We don't think about breath until we can't breathe. Breath carries light, life, and love.

Both Jesus and Mary sustained each other with a divine breath, and it emerged as does a sun yielding their life together as one.

Divine breath is the same as the Word of God. When it leaves God's mouth, it never returns empty, or without accomplishing what God desires, nor without succeeding in the matter for which it was sent. In the kisses exchanged between Jesus and Mary, along with light, the very breath itself is exchanged and inhaled by each.

Once again, we must reiterate that there were no physical marital relations shared between Jesus and Mary. Their kisses were the primary, profound, and transcendental mode of their love, that rendered unto them a totally exalted, transcendental consummation. This sublime vibratory experience was not only shared throughout their bodies, climaxing and strengthening through the infusion of true love, but within His Light

Body and that of his wife, that also sent vibrations outwardly into the world. This is how Jesus and Mary communed on the highest, most intimate level, even unto the conquering of death and Christ's Resurrection.

This is the love that Jesus uses to continue to commune with his eternal consort with profound receptivity then and still, efficaciously, since she lives among us in this material world.

> 'SO THIS IS LOVE ... HMM,
> SO THIS IS WHAT MAKES LIFE DIVINE
> THE KEY TO ALL HEAVEN IS MINE'
>
> (FROM WALT DISNEY'S *CINDERELLA*)

How can this be, in this world today? Eternal love does not end, thus, we use the word, "eternal," The process by which Jesus and Mary Magdalen can continue to share the eternal components of light, breath, and love is called supramentalization, which is the thread that connects the physical world to the transcendental world and vice versa.

LESSON 59

SUPRAMENTALIZATION

Supramentalization is a concept/process, which appears throughout Eeshan texts, and is essentially a reference to how Jesus' eternal consort, who lived back in biblical times, can live in these present times, and how that same person of Mary Magdalen, in the time of Jesus could be in present times, without drawing, or relying on the common conception of reincarnation.

While the concept of reincarnation has its own root possibilities and merits within other religions, as Resurrection has within Catholic/Christian faiths, it is not to be confused with the manner in which supramentalization is used in this document. In summary, it is said, "supramentalization refers to a physical divinization, the rising of a human being through the various layers of existence to the transcendental realm to the Source of Being; while simultaneously the Divine Source of being is drawn down into the physicality of the person." In other words, it is how the Divine Consciousness has been, and is, established upon Earth. This process brings the Divine Feminine aspect of God (again by Ishvara) and localizes it in a person (here being Mary's consciousness into Eesha), which, having descended in fullness, was filtered through into human form.[95]

This also is not to be construed as channeling, for this is not just a form of communication from Jesus, or Mary Magdalen, to a human being through mystical means, or an interpretation of non-verbal communication into words; nor is it the fullness of realization of the Divine

---

[95] Explanation adapted from some of the writings of Sri Aurobindo. – Ed.

Absolute in the heart-mind field, as with yogic meditation. It is also not locution, which has been accepted by the church as the Divine talking to a person through the 'mind's eye.'

We find that variations of the supramentalization process have been found, and continue to appear, in various cultures and in various time periods, as well as in different philosophies.[96] These approaches to spiritual life are found among ancient Persian dualists, Jewish and Christian spiritualists, Gnostic groups, New Age groups, and, to a degree, theologians such as Teilhard de Chardin; however, it was Sri Aurobindo (a mystic/sage from India) who most closely approximates the sense of supramentalization used here in this text.

Here, the understanding of the substance of Ishvara is vital to understanding its role in attaining enlightenment and understanding the transcendental consciousness; but most importantly, it's *the combination of the two* that not just differs from the human definition, or rationalization, since when logic and reasoning are applied to supramentalization of Mary, it greatly pales in comparison to the fullness of the supramentalization process with Mary, and this is because of who she is. This is so, because Ishvara and all of what you have been reading, most assuredly shows a more complete picture of why God gave his directive to our Foundress. Here's how.

Ishvara, which is the very essence of God in the world, is transcendental to the physical universe of time and space, and so is not subject to time; and, whereas, Ishvara is eternally present and complete. Jesus would be the male manifestation of this descent (Second Person of the Holy Trinity), thus, his name/title '*Ish*' would fit the definition of Highest

---

[96] When the pure energy of the Divine enters into the world in this way, there are reverberations of this action which result, and that spread out, with a variety of effects and in varying degrees. They might be called 'physical reactions' to transcendental actions. For example, when Jesus was born into the world, the earth was changed, and there were reactions among the people of all kinds; even the physical universe itself was substantially altered; when Jesus died on the cross, there was a tremendous earthquake. When Mary Magdalen died, the community and spirit of believers under Peter's direction and control were 'cemented,' and made permanent in quality, since once Mary was gone there would be no possibility it could be changed as that window had been closed (until these present times). – Ed.

Reality, ruler, king, and husband; and the definition would also fit, first the Virgin Mary, and then Mary Magdalen, and presently *Eesha* respectively. We began first with explaining how the Virgin, who was the human form of the Divine Feminine, came to give birth to the Divine Male gender of the only-begotten Child of God her husband, thus transitioning from the Old Law into the New Law of God; next, the Divine Female of the only-begotten child of God, took on the form of Jesus' wife Mary Magdalen, during their years on earth; and, now, lastly, as we find ourselves transitioning from the New Testament to the "Final Testament." We find Mary Magdalen's consciousness via the process of supramentalization complete with the very essence of God, beginning from the person of Mary Magdalen into the person of Eesha for this, the Final Testament in these end times. That is why her name would be encrypted until her awakening and reception of her title *Isha* (pronounced 'Eesha') came about. Thus, the title Eesha carries these meanings or translations: God, Supreme Being, queen, or special self.

LESSON 60

A Brief Description of the Eeshan Salvific Plan (Eeshan Transcendentalism) and the Return of Ishvara

Because we call ourselves a 'Religion' for purely structural purposes, we don't want Eeshan Spirituality to be confused with how 'others have defined *religion*.' We feel it is better defined a as transcendental, "ancient," mystical, beyond Merkabahalic and Kabbahlic[97] way of being, brought back into consciousness, not as one defined before, but by God's directive, by and for love of God, in order to meet the spiritual needs of the people in these modern times. Our attempt to represent the true teachings of Christ and the real reason for the Messiah(s) is unlike any other.

We want to reorder feelings, imaginings, actions, and beliefs about God that have arisen in response to the direct and mandatory directive of the sacred and spiritual. As this attempt expands in its formulation and elaboration, it became a process in which it created meaning for itself in an effort to deflect what we as God's people have become accustomed to in defining religion.

We want the Eeshan way to become a sustaining basis by people originating in and representing the transcendental experience, thus continuing to sustain a faith that will continue to grow, so that when Jesus returns-he will find FAITH.

---

[97] These are an integral set of esoteric teachings from Judaism to its later Christian, New Age adaptations. – Ed.

TRULY we can be identified then as the continued salvific mission of Jesus Christ and his Wife—returning once again, only this time as being carried on as was originally intended; and at the fulfillment of God's promise, to finally represent to the world, the woman who would crush the head of the serpent.[98]

To those who desperately want to know more about Jesus' purpose for being born and living among us, and why it seems God has forsaken us, while showing the world that Christ's mission did not fail, you are welcome to peruse our sacred texts. Indisputably, as disbelief in God and persecution reigned over Christians throughout history, we find this spirit of history repeating itself in these present times. If you believe there is more to God/Jesus than what you have been taught, you may be interested in our spirituality and practice.

God's plan for salvation (though halted by, and, under appearances, precluded by the false impressions surrounding Mary Magdalen), seen through the urgings and calls of persistent memory, we find in these present times that the lack of the transcendental spirituality (a spirituality which Jesus shared fully with his wife) in biblical times has not only been extended, but has blossomed in this present time period.

If we look at the suppression of Mary's role as Jesus' wife, and look at it as seeing *God in charge, and as Eeshans prefer to view it* with a more positive train of thought, we could surmise that what had taken place was destined to re-emerge approximately 2000-plus years later, again by the will of Ishvara. Eeshans believe Ishvara was suspended at the demise of Mary Magdalen's life and memory to allow for the choice of the patriarchal mindset of Peter's religion to play itself out. It was safely secured during the suspension of her consciousness, and then, as promised, the hand of her husband reached into the world of time and space as human consciousness understands it, and resumed the continuation of his original mission to see it through to its completion.

---

[98] Adapted from "WHAT IS RELIGION," DARC.ORG, COPYRIGHT 1996 by Paul Connelly.

The gap in time was part of the plan of God to allow for the gospel to spread, since the free will/choice within man's world advanced to a point in time where all the developments under human direction (with the exclusions of God), whether a cause for joy or a cause for sorrow, reached a crescendo. This casts an intriguing, as well as a greater and more fascinating, light on Jesus' telling the disciples that *it is better to refrain from pulling up the weeds sown among the wheat, to allow everything to grow together for a time out of risk for pulling up the wheat as well, because God will intervene and will sift the wheat from the chaff at the proper time (Matthew 13:24-30)*. In other words, let human beings run the course they create for themselves until the time comes for the plan of God regarding Jesus/Mary or Ish/Eesha to be completed and to be fulfilled.

Time, while being a hurdle to humans, is not a hurdle for God, and the importance of properly understanding supramentalization, especially when talking about Ishvara is central and essential in order to understand the mystical underpinnings of this book. To dismiss this mystery as a nothingness, or a fiction, is the nature and error of logic and reasoning deduced by the human consciousness. It robs one of unfathomable mysteries of the Divine.

LESSON 61

REPITITION, REPITITION, REPITITION

As we said, you will find that all we discussed in the foregoing text will be further unpacked as you continue on in this book.

It is said that the purpose of repetition is to increase the depth of understanding: as in the Latin expression, *"Repetitio est mater studiorum"* (Repetition is the mother of all learning).

Let us 'repeat' once again why it's important to repeat. By repeating, we learn. It is often the case that when people feel that they have learned a new point, that it later fades; and they return to their usual course of thinking amidst various backdrops of past methods of learning.

This writing is organic. It is alive and is meant to continue to speak whenever one begins reading and even after it has all been read, just as if as it was spoken it was absorbed, as though it had always been in your heart consciousness, and your mind just realized it. Think of it as the heart consciousness being cyclical, or female, and the brain being linear, or male.[99]

It can be reread without one feeling that it has been 'finished' in one's heart. It is an ongoing event taking place in the heart, which is why it is referred to continuously as a 'transcendental' piece of writing. Moreover, it will no longer appear to be "new," or "newly introduced," because it already became 'part' of your subconscious memory. For example, without thinking, when you are asked, "Who made you?" the response is more

---

[99]This book is written from the standpoint of heart consciousness; that is why it reads so differently than most all other books which are written from a certain agreed-to current standard of logical flow, logical structure, vocabulary, and so on. – Ed.

often than not, "God made me." Question: "Why did God make you?" Response: "God made me to know, love, and serve him in this world …"

These questions and answers are "engrained" in you.[100] They are a part of you from your earliest years. That is why repetition is so important here. Most of all that you have been taught over the years is engrained in you, your thinking, your beliefs, etc. Anything outside of what you know, or have learned, over the years is "new" and somewhat entertaining, *but not absorbed*, as those two little questions regarding who created you and why. We don't wish for you to be entertained. We wish to break through the barriers of that which you 'learned' so that you can be enlightened from a fresh, transcendental perspective.

Therefore, if your intention in reading this book is to be entertained, or if you are coming from a place of skepticism, then this book will not benefit you.[101] It will somewhat upset your spiritual fabric, since what you have come to absorb by the human rational consciousness, will do battle with your desire to 'want more.' Why? Because you have also been conditioned through worldly learning not to seek answers, and not to read *anything* that will cause you to have doubts about what you have been taught to believe.

Reading should open doors and not only expand all boundaries but also push the limitations of an individual. Transcendentalism prevents one's mind and conditioning from becoming a 'stumbling block' to God and the Divine. Life has meaning and purpose; and books, especially transcendental reading, can help you to explore and to learn the blessings and greatness of this life; whereas, life by itself, without a positive guide, cannot reach such limits.

To read this book, and to understand it, must be approached as you would spirituality, because it IS a spirituality in itself. You must detach from former habits of reading. Some, if not most of the knowledge you have obtained with Christian guidance, as well as any theological education received, may not allow you to fairly process the information found

---

[100] Spelled 'engrained' purposefully, as the qualities from this lesser used spelling evokes a connection to the 'fallen nature' and the effects of entropy. – Ed.

[101] It may do the very opposite! – Ed.

in this writing. We are not saying that what you read was negative, but it may be wise to just try and abstain from thinking from the standpoint of your root religion. It may prove to be incomplete, or even too rigid a template, to seeing another version of God's Salvation Plan.

It is sometimes necessary to break this common habitual form of thinking and learning, even though it may serve one well for other pursuits. In this case, breaking that former pattern, and, allowing oneself to absorb divine energy in the form of repetition and spiritual guidance, will be helpful in creating the conditions for the budding of transcendental modes of thinking, feeling, and perception. That is why we try to impress upon you the need *to meditate or pray daily*. It is also the one way you can send positive energy and God's grace to anyone, anywhere, in the world, and even beyond it (i.e., purgatory).

We cannot impress upon you more strongly that repetition is the mechanism behind the operation of the *mantra* in the heart. By way of the organic transcendental voice which supersedes the best of writings, the disciplining of the mind by repetitive forms of imagery, and by good transcendental reading, will direct it continuously back to where it needs to be. Likewise, the repetition that occurs in this text is essential to the budding of a new way of thinking and perceiving one's own sense of history and time.

The mind is thus trained to continually return to an *eternal event*—one that is outside the limitations of time and space, or the confines of what human beings have taught themselves to believe about history and the 'truth' of events. Thus, what appears to be repetitious is in fact a deliberate mechanism for awakening the capacity for a transcendental awareness.

LESSON 62

CHOICE AND RESPONSIBILITY

Though we are sharing all our opinions and core beliefs, these, indeed, are ours. As Eeshans, we believe that so long as a person finds faith, hope, and unconditional love in the spirituality they practice then they should feel free to remain where their heart lies.

We tell everyone we meet, and it is important for the reader to realize that whatever you do in life, a wholesome, God-centered RELIGION and/or SPIRITUALITY, which knows no unjustified, or incorrect attitude, and does not teach and spread negative behavior towards an individual, or group of people and view, and which tolerates no discrimination, are the true guides to happiness and understanding.

There is only one thing that you can take with you when you die, and it is the one and only thing that God judges you on. **It is how you loved, and how you accepted love.** Nothing else matters. Nothing that can be attained here on earth, be it wealth, power, or fame, goes with you when you die, nor does it impress, or sway, God's judgment of you and upon you.

The principles of exercising full, personal responsibility relative to a religion, or to spirituality's belief system, are for the reader to consider. Eeshan books, articles, etc., are written to help you make the best possible decisions for whatever personal situations you encounter. The fact is, when one is trying to determine whether something is right or wrong, it goes without saying that moral law is of the uppermost importance. Moral law was always known to reflect a general rule of right living which was universal and unchanging in that inherit in it was the sanction of God's will, of conscience, and of man's moral nature, and of natural justice as revealed to the human reason.[102] Today, with the ever-lessening of God's importance to human life, and as the human consciousness continues to evolve with reason, logic, and expand without spirituality to guide it, we find ourselves confused and empty. We have been watching the pillars of faith, which we felt were unshakeable, be proven to be hollow and defective. Universal laws have not changed; however, mans' interpretation and translations make them appear to have be susceptible to change—so, now what?

We are teaching from the transcendental consciousness, that is one, and that is supernatural and beyond the ordinary, or common experience, as Jesus had taught in His earthly life, and He now continues to teach through his wife. *Your decisions* must reflect these laws, and the right thing to do must be applied, depending upon what moral law was violated in any given case, or scenario. Jesus is NOT responsible for pain or suffering in this world, and He explains this when He says (regarding a lame child), "Neither this man nor his parents sinned," said Jesus, "but this happened so that the works of God might be displayed in him."(Jn. 9:3). This passage, if not taught correctly, does not allow for saying that it is because the human body is flawed in its conception, but just because it is, indeed, human. Today we know more about genetics, and DNA, to explain congenital and hereditary health issues, but people did not know in prior times. They were taught that these things were God's punishment due to sin of their parents, grandparents, etc. This is a perfect opportunity to clarify that God didn't strike these people ill just for some personal glory. This one line written is not the fullness of what Jesus taught; and is a perfect example of errors that were handed down through the centuries. Sadly, it was this kind of mentality that so called modern day "mystics" caused groups of people to believe their 'bloodlines had to be cleansed.'

In other words, we must be careful what we do to each other as human beings. It is not our right to play God based on what *we* like or dislike so that it becomes an excuse to impose harm upon on anyone in the name

---

[102] "Moral Law." Merriam-Webster, Merriam-Webster, www.merriam-webster.com/dictionary/moral%20law.

of God. There is a moral code for this. This code should be practiced in conjunction with *what Jesus taught*, and not outside of it; *and certainly not before it (as in the Old Testament)*.

Our books are intended to serve as a guide and path to God, to holiness, to decency, and to the equality of every person; however, a person must exercise *full responsibility* for the choices they make, and to base those choices in the light and foundation of Metta, or God's Love. If your choices are selfless versus selfish, humanity-centered versus self-centered, the end result is you have to live with the consequences of your choices. Choosing selfishly, and thinking without responsibility, is not only foolish and unrealistic, it is also chaotic. Every ripple grows into a wave.

Not all situations are black and white. This book shows that the one constant that can be relied upon for locating one's self, and where to base the mind to make good decisions, is Love. If God is in your life, then you must make choices of your own free will, and not the free will of someone else. Choices must be made for the good; and each person must make those choices knowing that accountability belongs to oneself; and, therefore, you cannot blame anyone else for the outcome. This applies to all decisions that are made.

Good decisions should be centered on proactive spirituality. You know your decisions are good when they are made in the knowledge of, and in the light of, morals, values, and ethics. Morals refer to one's inherited belief systems, values refer to what comes from *within* the person himself/herself, and ethics refer to what actions a person exhibits themselves, without coercion from exterior 'laws,' for their own good and the good of all. We also have the responsibility to choose leaders that do the same. We must also get away from backing those leaders who cannot move beyond sour grapes, and, in turn, deliberately stifle solutions, or obstruct justice, out of spite.

In conclusion, the path to true enlightenment—the enlightenment Jesus taught—is in remembering that Spirituality is necessary for all of us, and that the concept of a life comprised *only* of math, science, logic, or philosophy, as some believe, is wrong and is and always will be disproven by love.

Living in believing that one needs no guidance, or understanding, except that from within their own human consciousness, is flawed, and wrongly excuses an individual from accountability.

> *Cheap grace is grace without discipleship, grace without the cross, grace without Jesus Christ, living and incarnate. Cheap grace means living as though God ignores or condones our sins. But forgiveness means that sin is real and must be dealt with. The denial of sin is not grace: it is a lie.*
> —Dietrich Bonhoeffer

NAMASTE:
MAY THE DIVINE LIGHT WITHIN ME
BOW TO THE DIVINE LIGHT WITHIN YOU

PART II

BEGINNING YOUR JOURNEY

LESSON 63

Attaining Enlightenment

THE EESHAN GOAL IS TO BRING TO YOU WHAT EESHANS BELIEVE HAS BEEN MISSING FOR CENTURIES. THIS CAN BE DESCRIBED AS THE SACRED, HOLY, AND MYSTERIOUS MANIFESTATION OF POWER AND PRESENCE THAT IS EXPERIENCED AS BOTH PRIMORDIAL AND TRANSFORMATIVE, INSPIRING AWE AND RAPT ATTENTION.

WE BELIEVE THAT WE PROVIDE FOR THE NECESSARY BREAK AND DISCONTINUITY FROM THE ORDINARY, BRINGING, OR FORCING A RE-ESTABLISHMENT, OR RECALIBRATION, OF PERSPECTIVE BY OUR EXPERIENCES, AND YET WE BELIEVE IT IS TO BE SO UNFATHOMABLE IT IS SEEMINGLY ORDINARY AND NATURAL, AS THOUGH YOUR SOUL IMMEDIATELY RECOGNIZES THE "TRUTH." WE BELIEVE BY REPEATED EXPOSURES TO OUR PERSPECTIVE THAT YOU WILL EXPERIENCE GRADUAL PERCEPTIONS OF MYSTERIOUSLY CUMULATIVE SIGNIFICANCES OUT OF PROPORTION TO THE SIGNIFICANCES YOU HAD ORIGINALLY INVESTED.[103]

In other terms, when one finds a key, it is inevitable that one would begin thinking in unlocking a door, or object, revealing something valuable, mysterious, or mystical. The ineffable truths presented, herein, to the

---

[103] Adapted from "What Are the Sacred and the Spiritual," DARC.ORG, Copyright 1996, By Paul Connelly.

reader rank highest among any memory, record, or traditional facts any human has been given, and which unlocks more truths, so deep within our core, we feel that one without guidance we could reach only *fathomable* realizations about God; whereas, with guidance, one could enter into the *unfathomable*, as though they were ordinary.

To do this, Eeshans believe that revealing our unique point of view, and what we consider to be "our" Sacred Writings, require such a key to understanding, and to unlocking the wonderment of the mystical in what you are about to read. Let's begin with examining what you are looking for.

How Do 'You' View Religion and Spirituality?

You will find that our beliefs pose a very different approach to the more familiar Catholic/Christian doctrines that are most familiar to you; therefore, you should sincerely approach them with a sense that religion/spirituality is, indeed, a personal choice, whether with a personal God, or a different understanding of Supreme Being. Without a true connection, you will not experience the fullness of that belief system. In other words, you can't claim to be Catholic in the real sense unless you actually practice all of the beliefs inherent in Catholicism. To do otherwise is to just award yourself a title of your own accord.

Too often people do *just* that. They stay in a religion where they do not have any connection, do not really believe in, or practice what it teaches, or they recast it according to a personal preference, or claim of a spiritual experience. Few people see anything more than obligation sans any transcendental, or spiritual, connection, regardless of the impromptu 'arguments or preaching' of grandparents and family members who claim they believe, or to have 'found Jesus.' Studies show that people often live and stay with a belief system not by choice but via pragmatic reasoning. Most of the time it's only religion to them, as interpreted and translated through the human consciousness, and just handed down to them. Forty to fifty years ago this kind of belief had been instilled through one's birth religion as something you do to show people you are not a communist or a pagan. A friend of mine said she felt forced to return to church to look like a good parent.

Others, too, in a way, feel forced into a religion from outside sources, and not by agreeing with its teachings, but due to issues regarding finances. such as lowering tuition for a school, or belonging to a church in order that the cost of tuition goes down, which is a small price in exchange for safety of their children. Some cannot let go of what they believe as their parents, grandparents, or someone they love lived by it. They, therefore, go along with it, but do not really believe in the religion itself. The list of scenarios is, indeed, endless.

There are those instances where people just stray away because they didn't get anything else out of it, save a sense of being judged. Some leave their birth religion thinking that living free of a religion, or spirituality, gives them freedom. Most will find that a particular religion, or spirituality, is the basis, or foundation, for a strong and emotional connection on which they can rely, especially in times of distress. Their faith lends them strength and closure that helps when there is no rhyme, or reason, for personal tragedy. For others, God gives merit and a positive outlook for one to continue on. That is why spirituality must come from within a person in order that he or she will live by it, since actions speak louder than words.

Religion or spirituality should never be based solely on the experience of a particular person whom you like or love; otherwise, you are only sharing in that person's belief system, and you will ultimately become disillusioned and disappointed (because it's not *your* experience). However, this is precisely how the human consciousness dictates and defines religion, which is to include how Jesus is perceived.

For example, if you are an atheist, and feel that the only difference in what you desire. or want in life, is from those with a religion of spirituality, and that to them God does not exist, you should think carefully about this, since to have believed and received the same result of an atheist is to have lost nothing, but to be right you have gained everything. Whereas, an atheist without belief in God, discovers they have lost in both instances, since if they were right they lived only for the moment, and in fate, without ever seeing the beauty of destiny and hope. Without God, there is no change possible, and, therefore, there is no hope.

Though non-believers feel that to have a strong spirituality lends to a brainwashed, emotional, and dangerous thought process, which overrides a free will, Eeshans view their religion and spirituality as the immortal soul's mission to make its way back to its Creator. In searching for the 'more' of what you feel you need, remember that religion must come through your own soul's desire to do what is natural to it, and that is love. An internal, rational decision towards finding what you need will always be consistent in soothing your soul, and building strength through love and not hate, relying on faith and not fear, and finding strength discovered in the face of your own weaknesses.

Today's advancements in technology and science have also made an impact on people. For many people, science, especially math, is a constant, and cancels out theology. There has been somewhat of a more positive outlook, since science (metaphysical science included) searches for answers, and these topics include God and Jesus.

Even before the time of Jesus, religions set the criteria for sin, contrition, absolution, and penance. Depending upon the priest, your spirituality grew or lessened. Have you ever wondered how it would feel to go to confession to Jesus, back two thousand plus years ago? Eeshans feel that if people had that opportunity, even atheists would go.

Everyone needs a way to detox their soul just as they need to detox their body.

But today, confession, as in years past, has failed to do this. Barring the scandals over the centuries, from the fear tactic up to today's failure to see sin, where does a soul go?

WHAT DO YOU WANT?
WHAT WILL SATISFY YOU?

Beginning a spiritual journey requires a desire to be pure of heart, soul, and mind. Purity can be defined in the sense that one must rid oneself of all those things that come between a loving God and yourself. It means you want to access your soul. You want more than those things that are material, and are searching for those things which satisfy from within. It means you want to better understand who God is and who you are. You want answers to your questions:

Why did God make me? Why must I know, love, and serve God? Why is God in heaven and why are we on earth? What happened? Why did Jesus have to come, suffer, and die? What's behind his resurrection? Let's take a look at the soul.

LESSON 64

WHAT DID JESUS FOCUS ON?

Jesus always focused on eternity. Where we should be focusing on this, instead, is that we should choose to focus on time, and all that goes with it. That is why transcendental spirituality and/or religion has become foreign to us. We always have too much to do. We have missed out on so much, and time has quickly gone by, and guess what? After all we worked so hard for, we didn't get to enjoy any of it. Well, when someone says, "stop and smell the roses," what this means is that God is certainly lacking in your life. You have so many things to busy yourself, you never took the time to see God's greatness, love, and beauty. All of which is always present; whereas, your 'stuff' is going to fade away, or someone is going to come along and change it to what they prefer, or so on and so forth.

It seems the more we are told to focus on God the less time we have. Without a doubt, we are driven by time. From the moment we wake up, to the moment we go to sleep, we concern ourselves with time. We even concern ourselves with the concept of controlling time when we sleep. If we can't sleep, we drive ourselves crazy by calculating how much time we should've been asleep, how much time we have lost trying to fall asleep, and how much time we are going to have when it's time to get up. We constantly check our phones for the time, to schedule our time, and to compare time with others, and the time it takes for them to do something versus how long it takes us to do the same.

Therefore, when someone says you have to take time and spend it with God there is a disruption, because you feel God should understand how little time you have. Surely, God knows that with that little free time you have, you want to do something important that you have been putting off, such as spending time with your kids or getting to do those chores at home you never have time to do, or by just taking some time for yourself. All day long you are doing things for someone else. The last thing you need is to feel guilty for taking a little time for yourself.

We bargain on the fact that we "know" that God understands. How attentive are you with even those things that you want to do that are much more important than an hour with God? Realistically, an hour with friends seems to be more refreshing and relaxing than going, and listening, to a homily, or sitting in front of the Blessed Sacrament, or praying before a tabernacle. Even when we are relaxing, we are working, and never think to just sit quietly and to consider all God has given us and just how blessed we are. That is until we have an emergency, or what we now feel is that important that God should take the time to listen to us.

Thank God, God is God and we aren't. The truth is, God does know and understand daily life, but what God doesn't understand is the missed opportunity to be there. Alright, then if you have such time restraints, why do you? Did you know, that if you take time to visit with God, you will be rewarded with more time, and that you will accomplish more that if you did not visit with God? Things do work out much better when God is part of your life.

God speaks to our hearts and often even to us directly if only we chose to listen. What Jesus taught was very interesting, because it was interesting enough for people to set aside being busy to not just go to listen to him, but to also spend hours and days being with Him wherever he was.

Clutter makes us miserable and stressed. Cluttered cars, homes, offices, and desks are outward manifestations of the condition of our minds, hearts, and souls. Peace[104] is not only the absence of conflict but the

---

[104] Ananda Coomaraswamy, in his intriguing essay "Shaker Furniture," writes: "Just as we desire peace but not the things that make for peace, so we desire art but not things that make for art. We put the cart before the horse. *Il pittore pinge se stesso*; we have the art that we deserve. If the sight of it puts us to shame, ***it is with ourselves that the re-formation must begin***. A drastic transvaluation of accepted values is required. With the re-formation of man, the arts of peace will take care of themselves." – emphasis mine, Ed.

absence of clutter. However, if you feel that it is a quick peace you want, Feng Shui may help; or, perhaps, more likely something like Ayurveda may be for you. Sometimes it is an interior anxiety created by systems in the body being out of balance that may be unfamiliar to the mainstream populous, and these include knowing what your *dosha* is. Did you know your blood type has a lot to do with your eating habits and personality? Did you know that your zodiac sign does, too? There are other factors, that once you become aware of them, and what they really are, they are no longer 'weird' or 'pagan.' Top of the list, however, is spirituality. Everyone, no matter who you are, needs spirituality.

There are wonderful doctors that 'you should seek out,' and if you have one, 'Go to him/her.' Seriously, most clutter is an outward sign of how one feels interiorly. When people have healthy minds, uncluttered and focused, they can clean up clutter, and begin to organize their cars, houses, offices, etc.

Perhaps we need to understand of what *we humans are made up*. Let's just take a moment and glance through a few facts to help you awaken to a new you, one in which you are, indeed, alive and thinking.

First, you must clear your mind. You must stop thinking and over thinking and obsessing. You must make a positive decision to do this. Next, there are many ways in which to calm your mind. There are wonderful oils, tones, exercises, vitamins, and supplements, all available to help you feel your best. Once you "do" something as simple as taking a multivitamin, or changing, or rearranging the furniture in your room, your mind becomes alert and active. Then your attitude will change, and your confidence will grow because you are coming out of an induced spiritual coma caused by the illusion arising from the spirit of the world, into which you have willfully chosen to escape; and because of that your reality has been altered and it has helplessness has engulfed you. What happens next is that you make a conscious effort to get your focus back to living, and not just existing; thus, becoming a better person.

LESSON 65

THE SOUL

It is said that the soul is comprised of three things:
A mind to think, a heart to feel, and a will to decide.
(Anonymous)

The soul is such a fascinating and mystical part of us because it is immortal. It is that part of us that belongs to God, and thus is where it gets its immortality. This is what separates human beings from all other life forms. It is for this reason that we come to know, love, and serve God, but we can only be free to choose what God, as our Creator, has imparted to us. Why? Because we have the freedom and peace that comes from being created with free will. The soul, you see, is, in a way *trapped* in the body. The body is part of the earth, and is physically encompassing, or rather imprisoning, a divine entity. The soul's only hope to avoid evil, and not face eternal death (the one sentence that does exist), is for us to make 'good' choices.

What we seek cannot come from us, but from One who became like us. Our soul is the God particle found within each of us, that though immortal, needs to be nourished in order that it sustains life.

That very special "immortal/divine" quality is only possessed by humans, though all living things have souls. This is because our soul links us to the mystical and divine; next is our consciousness. It appears that our consciousness lies somewhat dormant these days for the most part, but we do, indeed, have one.

As the soul is that incorporeal essence of a living being, or, for humans, it is the way of one's existence and the reason for one's life, our 'human' soul sets us apart from other souls, since it acts through the body as will, desire, commitment, faith, and love... because it is our nature.[105]

Because of God, we are the only beings/creatures that can transcend beyond our physical nature. That is the what made up the persons of Adam and Eve. After their choice to physicality, it is only by Jesus as the Divine Masculine and active consort who died on the Cross, who together with his life-giving wife, were the Second Person of the Holy Trinity, God, and Human, that gave us back the ability to transcend through the vital Sacred Food.

The soul has a mission. The Chabad[106] exhibits this by the saying, "Everyday the soul is challenged by the conflicting needs and desires of the animal soul; here the divine reality is obscured by the dense selfhood of the body and physical world around us." It continues to say, however, "that it is here in the arena of hidden truth and perpetual challenge, the soul can fully express and actualize its divine power."

This is what Jesus came for. It is because of Jesus that we can once again gain access to WHAT this wonderment of the soul is. It is in the soul's ascent back to its origin that we gain true wonderment.

The soul, however, can either rise above the challenges, and realize the hidden truth, or it can fall into sin.[107] Because the soul is the divine component in our corporal body, it makes sense that there must be a light body within this gross physical body we have, to house the soul; therefore, as the physical body will die off and decay, the light body will travel to its final destination.

---

[105] The capacity of mind in animals and other forms of life limits the intelligence to function only in a way controlled by nature. – Ed.

[106] Chabad is one of the largest Orthodox Jewish movements within mainstream Jewish tradition today. – Ed.

[107] It's noteworthy that in Christian Orthodoxy, sin is often understood more in terms of falling into illusion, as opposed to transgressing laws. – Ed.

Lesson 65A

Sin

There is, however, something that can affect the soul, such as illness to the body, whether limiting or deadly. It is called sin. Sin is said to cause 'entropy' of the soul. If you had the opportunity to ask Jesus how he would describe sin, He would probably say, "Sin is compared to both malnutrition and cancer." It is compared to malnutrition because the degree of sin starves the soul of a much needed spirituality, which provides for the presence of God; and it is compared to cancer since if the soul is grace-starved, it does not allow, or rather it actually even *terminates* any means of obtaining the sacred food necessary for everlasting life. Each time we commit a sin, we accept, or choose, a path away from the transcendental, since it is by the human consciousness that we begin to 'serve our humanity' better. It is when we choose self-gratification over spiritual gratification that the soul misses out on the presence of God for strength and the sacred food for life.

The seriousness of sin makes a difference in our behavior and judgments.

When we sin, we weaken the subtle body. The more serious the sin, the weaker we get. It doesn't have to be a mortal sin; it can be a habitual or 'venial' sin (known as the lesser sin) that eventually causes confusion, and we find we can't make sense of things and lack clarity. The more entrenched we become in sin, there is less and less attraction to grace.

We feel disconnected, restless, and insecure. Often when there is a lack of subtle awareness, we become clumsy in our physical bodies. Emotional drama, unhealed conflict, suspicion, and paranoia are also present to some degree, along with being scatter-brained, uncontrollably reactive, and being a magnet for negativity. Without an awareness that sin affects the mind, body and soul, we become unaware of nearby opportunities to help ourselves by getting rid of our sins, because we are unaware of what our subtle energies are doing.

Take all the above and apply that to 'mortal' sin, which is a sin that so rapidly terminates spirituality. Here, we are looking at a spiritually terminal cancer, since it leads to death of the soul. Here we have total loss of immortality *by one's choice*.

When we commit a mortal sin, the soul is totally separated from God. Yes, one mortal sin cuts us off from God. The soul is literally cut off from life. It has no ties to the transcendental. It becomes mortal.

It does have ties to eternal death. As we said, without ties to God, the soul is at the mercy of the human consciousness, which in and of itself is flawed. Enter now the consciousness. The consciousness here is the human, rational one; it relies solely on human reasoning with all that is caused through a fallen nature. God, and anything good, are marred by thoughts of selfishness, jealousy, and envy. Covetous feelings are aroused, and the person can no longer see anything positive, or good, in anything, or anyone. The person becomes obsessed with finding fault, and reasons to hurt someone, rather than make peace, even with someone they do not know. The person become enthralled with bitterness and is captivated in and with anything dark. Sometimes they appear to be happy, but this happiness is in their enjoyment of bad things that happen somewhere, or to someone. They are slow to forgive, but quick to judge and hold a grudge. It is not because the target of their hate has proven to be worthy of unyielding rage because the hater cannot see beyond themselves and their anger.

Why does this happen? This happens because the soul is so closely related to the subtle body. The subtle body is so closely linked to the light body, with the difference being that it is a very thin kind of membrane, similar in form to the physical body, but is not *attached* to it. It keeps its form, which protects the soul and its light just as it did the bodies of Adam and Eve. It's transparent, etheric, and wise. The subtle body is affected by the state of the soul.

According to the school of Kundalini Yoga, we have ten 'bodies' within us.[108] They are:

---

[108] While there are a number of different perspectives in each religious persuasion from which to view the relationship of the body, mind, spirit, and soul, Eeshans feel that

1. Soul Body
2. Negative/Protective Mind
3. Positive/Expansive Mind
4. Neutral/Wisdom Mind
5. Physical Body
6. Arc line
7. Aura
8. Pranic Body
9. Subtle Body
10. Radiant Body

While each of the bodies are interconnected and interrelated, it is the "subtle body" (which we form throughout life) whose purpose it is to take the soul and light body where they need to go upon death. It connects us to the unknown, both personal and impersonal. It is through the subtle body that we are able to tune into the subtle energies of the nonphysical dimensions of reality, or the infinite unknown. We 'refine' our connection to our soul and subconscious within the subtle body.

When the soul leaves the body, it leaves thorough the vehicle of the subtle body, and takes with it the history of all the soul's experiences, as recorded. Unresolved subconscious emotional imprints are all taken with us in the subtle body to be worked out. Some say these things get worked out in the next lifetime, but in the case of determining if you will go to Heaven or Hell, this acts as the recorded history of your life at the end of your life, or as you are dying (as when someone says their "whole life passed before their eyes"), or upon committing the mortal sin, as in the case of receiving the Holy Eucharist without absolution.

Whenever the soul is in sin, the subtle body becomes weakened and crude; and when this happens, one knows that all the other layers have already been affected. By grace the subtle body stays strong and communicates with the soul to help one feel calm and intuitively strong.

---

the breakdown according to authentic Yoga systems are often the most useful, detailed, and true to experience. The system being used here is drawn from the teachings of Kundalini Yoga. – Ed.

It appreciates beauty and feels compelled to stay healthy of mind and body, along with a desire to help others. God's light permeates to all the layers of our being and God rests in our hearts.

When the soul is affected by sin, this is communicated to the subtle body, and unless we take action, the sin will continue to not only grow, but metaphorically starts to eat away at the subtle body. therefore, making it weak, and creating more hate, and has no ability to see good. This can, and usually does, manifest in our physical, mental, and emotional states. The more we sin, the less connection we have with God, until there is no carrier of the soul to God.

Serious sin also "shorts out" the soul's memories, identity, and history in the material world. In other words, to enter into an act that brings on instant judgment, and condemnation, and should we die, the soul and light body experiences UNIMAGINABLE, INCOMPREHENSIBLE PAIN, AND EXTENDS THIS PAIN TO ALL THE OTHER LAYERS OF THE BODY, forever, and without ever having any lessening degree and with no one able to stop it.

Lesson 65B

Why Won't the Holy Eucharist Absolve Mortal Sin

The sacred and divine will not tolerate evil. It is against the 'All' of who and what God is. When the Light of God permeates through us, especially in the Holy Eucharist, it gives illumination, knowledge and life to all the layers of our being; therefore, the penalty for receiving the Sacred Eucharist in mortal sin is set in place by God, so that immediately God's light and presence leaves the soul, since it detects darkness. If darkness is detected, the soul is immediately judged, and one's whole being is condemned to hell.

As many times as the person had received the Sacred Food and Drink, is as many times as the sin is 'compounded,' and as many depths in Hell that the soul shall be driven down. Does this seem odd?

You would think the Eucharist would void the sin because nothing is impossible for God. Right? Nothing is impossible with God; however, deluding oneself into thinking that God absolves this kind of sin, is as foolish as thinking that one has the right to defame the Body, Blood, Soul, and Divinity of the Person and spirit of the Savior, as though God is on the same level as a human being and will just allow it. Human beings are 'created beings' of a fallen nature. They are mortal beings, meaning that their only life is that which God 'allows' for the opportunity to have everlasting life. We have no 'right' to this life; it is a 'gift' to us from God, the Creator, Redeemer, and Sanctifier.

There are different reasons why people delude themselves into thinking they can receive the Eucharist in the state of mortal sin. First, someone who commits a mortal sin is already deluded, and can't see beyond himself or herself, let alone see the truth. The longer they are in this sin (even if regret sets in), unless they come back to God with true contrition and the promise to not do this anymore, *they can't, or won't* be able to stop.

Because of this, not taking action can, and will, result in remorse. It's almost as though they force themselves to commit this sin. Some people who are in mortal sin, can delude themselves into thinking that God understands why they do what they do, and that God is alright with this. This, too, is dangerously naïve, and upon receiving the Eucharist, their sin is compounded. Some joke about going to hell for what they do. They joke that hell is not so bad. These are deluded into thinking that they prefer hell, since it will satisfy their desires, and they will be with people just like themselves. There are also those people who think they can't go back to God, and those who believe that their sin should be allowed despite God's law. Mortal sin blasphemes God. But good people forced to do evil acts can be forgiven so long as they have contrition and come back to God, in grace.

Hell exists, and is a place of incomprehensible pain, agony, and rage; and it is not a joking or laughing matter. It is a place which houses those people who are considered pure evil, and is defined as doing divine purging, which is brought on by a purpose, a will, an intent, time, and a counsel, so that it produces a desired effect for those who purposely did an immoral and cruel act, without any feelings of guilt, or remorse, and who acquired satisfaction doing it. You may say because a person received the Eucharist in the state of mortal sin does not make them 'evil' like murderers, sadists, etc. Well, let's just let you figure this one out.

Without a doubt, lastly, there are also really evil people who were born evil and who cannot be helped or rehabilitated. A pure evil person gets joy out of wickedness and by being depraved. This is a person who seems to have been born with no conscience. Hell is a place for those who have deep-seeded (and deep-seated) hate down to the core of their being, for themselves, for others, and mostly for all things good, especially God. There *is nothing in hell* to 'satisfy' a soul, even souls like these. Hell is not a reward for souls like these; it is a punishment. Once sentenced to hell by God, or by one of God's laws that is set up to automatically send the sinner to hell, everything good they did in life is forfeited; and there is absolutely no mediation by saints or angels on behalf of this soul, as God's judgment is final. And, if anyone is wondering if there is a chance that God will have a change of heart for those in hell whose sin(s) are/were compounded, and held against them, the sentence remains the same even in the final judgment, again with zero recourse before God.

So where is God's mercy? If any of these people feel remorse, or contrition, while alive *they have until their last breath* to beg God's mercy.

Your attitude towards mortal sin is important. It can mean the difference between life everlasting and eternal death. It can be a very slippery slope towards eternal sin for those who have no contrition, love, or respect for God. Belief in God is absolutely paramount, and beyond what is written above, where you go after this lifetime: this is, indeed, God's choice.

Eternal sin curses the very Spirit of God; this is an unforgivable sin, deemed so by Jesus. This is the sin He said was the unforgiveable sin against the Holy Spirit, meaning it will never be absolved.

Lesson 65C

How Jesus Changed the Way We Look at God's Laws

Sin is as misunderstood today as it was in previous eras. Back in biblical times, much of how sin was viewed was outlined according to both oral law and written law of the Judaism/or Hebrew religion, but often in a very scrupulous way, i.e. the book of Leviticus.

Surprisingly, Jesus stayed mostly focused on how much God loves us, how we are to love God, and how to live according to the directives given to God's people.

The letter of the law was so feared back then, that loving God had nowhere near the focus Jesus placed on it, especially in one's daily life. One did not love God, but more or less feared a Spirit who was genderless. Understanding God's (in the sense of 'His') ways was expressed in the form of burning sacrifices, and asking for absolution for sins.

Living scrupulously under God's Law was what was mandatory for that time, which accounts for why Jesus' approach to God was so well received by the common people. Before Jesus started teaching, it is wise to say that people lived with the feeling of oppression and enslavement. They lived more from the perspective of obeying what they were told were God's Laws for fear of being punished, and their yoke was hard, and their burden was heavy. That is why Jesus told them that what God desires is 'love.' God's yoke is easy, and the burden God gives you is light.

Jesus eased the fears people had of a punishing God by not only telling them that they were children of God, but also by telling them that God was their Father.[109] He used stories and parables *to change* what had been handed down by man for centuries, and to emphasize God's love and forgiveness for sins in a similar way that the father did in the parable of the Prodigal Son.

---

[109] While Jesus crossed many lines by drawing the intimate and familiar connection between the soul and God using the term 'Father, 'and while His mother, the Blessed Virgin, was the Divine Feminine First Person in human form, He did not elaborate extensively on God as Mother because, given the impacted foundations of the patriarchal mindset current in His time, the gradient of acceptance for such a notion was as yet still far too steep. 'Father' was already controversial enough. – Ed.

Lesson 65D

How Sin Has Been Viewed Before Jesus, During Jesus' Time, and in Present Times

What was a sin and what was not a sin, was blurred by the interpretation of God's law so that God's love was only that which did not offend him, essentially meaning that God's love in the way Jesus taught was nonexistent.

Today, people are still disillusioned by what Jesus taught and what he meant when he said of the authorities, "Do as they say, not as they do." What this meant was not to preach the word of God, and then not live it; or not to say one thing and do another, as though God is not aware.

That is why a spiritual teacher must, and should, always imitate Christ's life and teachings. A bad spiritual leader will deem everything and anything scrupulous if that teacher is also in the state of sin. For they do not want to judge for fear that they will be judged.

The trend toward thinking and defining sin independently of God is often done for precisely the same reasons. Humans often tread where angels fear to go, especially when it comes to God.

There were instances, too, when faith and love of Jesus may be at a high, but a person will still be hesitant, or reluctant, to do something that is right before the eyes of God because it is contrary to man's. Why? Because usually if it implied spirituality of any kind or a religious undertone, it was because of fear of some kind of punishment, or being ridiculed and made to look crazy.

Jesus is God incarnate, and his purpose was to restore us back to the life God intended for us, using what pain, suffering, and the consequences of entropy, of all kinds, to bring us to the reality that this world was not all there is, but that the heaven of which we all dream, existed. He addressed those things necessary to attain this goal. He taught how to identify sin, and He explained sin, and its consequences, and He also told us that if we had contrition, God would not only forgive our sins, but also that all of heaven would rejoice. Jesus also taught what we as God's children must do in order to attain that transcendental life, and that would be to eat the "Bread come down from heaven," which was greater than any riches a man could possess.

Today we choose not to see sin. We want to define what we think God should accept as our standard for living. Sin, therefore, has becomes what *we* define it is, not as what we described above. What *Jesus* taught and what we have been given by ordinary 'men' differs greatly. A good guide of course, are always the Ten Commandments; but as Jesus said in John 9:39, "For judgment I have come into this world, to give sight to the blind and to show those who think they see that they are blind." Though the Ten Commandments outline how we are to live, we find that even with these, rather than 'Though shalt not', Jesus condensed them into "Thou shall 'love God' above all else, and with our whole mind, our whole heart, and our whole being, and love our neighbor as our self!" He took the Old Law and made it New. This was to emphasize love. Who better to teach love than Love Himself?

Many atheists believe that *'sin is a platform, a special organization existing for moral propaganda, materially interested in the maintaining of popular ignorance and religious enslavement, and not to bring about a closer relationship with God its Creator, Redeemer and Sanctifier, let alone a more wholesome and decent development of the mind, body, spirit.'* In other words, like fear, sin drives the masses.

The fact is, sin, even a little one, is in reality, a direct act that not only offends but violates God's law and makes the soul sick or weak. In other words, as we mentioned above, being in sin skews our outlook on what is important, and what is not important as Jesus taught, causing a gap that always, in some way, separates us from God. After your first lie, haven't you noticed how it became easier to lie time and again?

The sin that Jesus focused most on was the rejection of Him. This continues today. So, what is essential for us to gain everlasting life is, indeed, getting to know, love, and serve Him as God, and witness to, as well as believe in, his salvific mission. Once you are introduced to the truth, those who do not accept what Jesus' Way connotes will be held accountable for this sin because as he said, implicitly, and as a matter of fact, that He is God. If he was just a man, the consequences would change. This is something that should never have been debated within the church of Peter.

Our conscience is there to guide us, but as sin becomes easier and easier as we believe we are not accountable to anyone, and eventually we can no longer hear its urgings to stop. When the general consensus regarding the state of your soul is less important than anything else in your life, something is terribly wrong somewhere. Accordingly, sin is not just linked with any particular religion. It is wrong inside, and out, of a religion.

Jesus taught in John 8:34 that sin is a master to whom we become enslaved and only truth will set us free [John 8:32]. Jesus' works and miracles were performed to show His divinity and to prove his power over sin, and that He was who He said he was. This is why the debates regarding Christ as God, Man, or both are contrary to this teaching and, thus, leaves way to human self-interpretation and/or reimaging of the person of Jesus.

In John 15:22, Jesus teaches that with Him we have a choice to have everlasting life, or to live in a temporary state here. Those who rejected Him in the face of indisputable evidence by His teaching and His works, as people so often do today, are lost. Eeshans believe this, but what if the truth was never really taught? What if what was given as truth, and drove God's people *backwards*, instead of forward?

You can only witness exactly how prevalent sin is, if you *know* what sin is.

We are told the confusion comes due to the struggle with the widely diffused and deeply engrained prejudices of human beings. Couple this thought with being united under a particular belief system, which is said to be mind control, which stifles individuality, along with those who compound the problem by their prejudices, and there you will find sin. Sin begins in the heart. The heart pulls away from God. Next the mind takes over and begins to supply reason. Then the act is committed.

Jesus' calling card was love. Yes, those who reject him, are blind, since to love forgives a multitude of sins; so to love much, then much is forgiven. To love little, then little is forgiven.

LESSON 66

THE HEART

Jesus spent a lot of time talking about the heart, and this was for good reason. What happens in the heart truly affects the soul. It is the vehicle for the transcendental. Once it is darkened, it can no longer see the light, or, in this case 'the' Light, the Way. It is said that the heart (and solar plexus) region is our "second brain."

Neurocardiologists say the heart's intimate connection to the brain shows it is an information processing center that can actually act on its own, without the cranial brain being involved. The heart can connect, and send signals, to key brain areas known for regulating emotions and perceptions. Thus, the heart brain can receive, and respond, to stimuli before the cranial brain processes it, and as the scientists call it, split-second 'body premonition.'

Another fascinating finding was how the heart's electromagnetism, the largest in the body, 'can affect and even synchronize with another person's brain waves,[110] since it seems to be sensitive, and receptive, to the heart energy of others, making empathy paramount.'[111] This is what Jesus was talking about when he taught, "where two or more are gathered." (Matthew 18:20). That is behind the success of Jesus' ministry. That is why the heart is the center point of prayer and meditation.

In the Eeshan Religion, the heart is taught how to be deeply entrenched in the transcendental and mystical. The light mind is necessary for the Divine to be fully expressed;, so, therefore the heart consciousness

---

[110] Willitts, Chris. "The Heart Has a 'Brain.'" SELFFA, 19 Sept. 2019, selffa.com/heart-has-consciousness-knows-before-brain/.

[111] Cf. mindfulmuscle.com

must be engaged in order for the fullness of the Divine to reach through the physical to free us, as we journey to the transcendental life brought to us by the only-begotten Child of God. That is why a darkened heart is responsible for the greatest separation between a person and God. The heart consciousness carries the memories and emotions that could be found to go along to a new heart transplant recipient. This is important to remember, especially in the process of supramentalization, as you will see, in which we unfold the mystery behind the sacred and divine union of Jesus and Mary Magdalen. There was such a powerful connection between the two that there is no doubt that both would carry with them the love of the other from eternity and back. Jesus spoke of the darkness of sin within the heart many times. Why? Because no one knew the human heart better than Jesus, and none expressed more concern regarding the heart than his own male apostles. Eeshans feel the negativity and pettiness he faced along with their inability to completely transcend is a perfect example of why it's important for the heart to stay close to God through a strengthened spirituality.

Did you know, that having a close relationship with God and being positive, as well as communicating positivity with those around you can ease stress? Studies have been done to show that high ratios of heart coherence are able to alter DNA conformation according to a person's intention. Intending to unwind, or rewind, the DNA had corresponding effects on the UV spectra. As human beings learn to sustain heart focused positive feeling states, the brain can be brought into entrainment with the heart.[112] The conclusion is the need of addressing the *heart* as the center of consciousness.

The universal law says that negative energies attract negative energies and positive energies attract positive energies. The heart is light when we are positive. A light heart serves both the individual and those it encounters. Spirituality guides the heart to positive energies and acts like a lamp.

---

[112] W., Charles. "Heart Consciousness—the Next Frontier in Brain and Neuroscience." NLP Coaching & Time Line TherapyR—The Tad James Co, 27 Dec. 2017, www.nlpcoaching.com/nlp-coaching/heart-consciousness-the-next-frontier-in-brain-and-neuroscience/?no_mobi=1.

Jesus says we should be the light in the world for all those to see your good deeds and praise the Father in heaven. Love should grow out of spirituality. That is why we need spirituality. Spirituality brings love into the heart, and sets the guidelines for love of God and neighbor. A heart-filled spirituality is always in the spirit of giving and sharing and not in the taking without contribution. Fear not, however, since God needs only the tiniest spark to come to the rescue should you need help!

It is spirituality that keeps the heart on the path, and Jesus is the spiritual food desired by the heart that the soul needs. In other words, it is a pure heart that rises above human rationality and strongly urges you to nourish your soul, which will determine if "you" will go on to live with God in eternity, or, due to your choices, deign you to be forgotten in eternal death.

That is why strong spiritual guidance is important. That, too, is the reason Jesus drew so many people. The people were starving spiritually; that is why the crowds came and soaked in all He told them. Their souls were like sponges in an oasis.

LESSON 67

SPIRITUAL GUIDANCE AND THE NEED FOR RENEWED TRUST IN GOD

A strong spirituality focuses on God first and foremost in SUPPOSEDLY grounding one in truth. That is what Jesus brought to those who followed him. We give to God what is God's. That is, we know, love and, serve him with *total* love. Spirituality, and all that goes with it, must have its origin in goodness. Eeshans believe that "all" are accountable to the God who created us, and ransomed our lives, because God is almighty, omnipotent, omnipresent, omniscient, and omnificent, BUT God will not help if we don't ask and believe, since God *does not infringe on free will.*

As it is necessary with all living things, there must be a system in place to protect, defend, and preserve freedom and life for all, especially for those who cannot defend themselves, or are of an innocent and impressionable age. We believe God had a system in place which, by man's hand, fell short; and, thus we lost a lot with regards to spirituality. Now in this fullness of time, God continues to reveal another system that will work so long as we do our part.

Seeing the need for a renewed trust in God, we have witnessed the innocents cry out once again for help. These are those who believe Jesus is the Messiah, but feel they need him now more than ever.

Jesus had promised a helper for those days He lived on earth, one who would work in conjunction with his wife and James the Righteous to continue Christ's work, as only they could. In keeping with his promise, we find Jesus takes the lead once again returning for the Bride He adores. She is the Divine Feminine, teaching and guiding us, as a people under

God, on a path towards our original state, and once again, God's plan for our salvation is continued.

Once again, we can be at ease knowing that we have not been abandoned, despite ourselves, and that we are in the hand of one who is like Jesus, but this time, we aren't under the reimaged God, one who is resembling the 'golden calf.'

We trust that God, as Divine Feminine, will fill the earth with the truth of Christ, giving all the ability to let go of what is 'comfortable' and embrace the truth.

It has always been said, especially by converts, that too much grey area, and unanswered questions in traditional Christian religion, have led people to wonder if God really exists. So many questions have arisen, since the truth has been so blurred.

At what point does life begin? When do we receive a soul? Does the soul determine when life starts, or does it start at conception within the body? So many questions in such a diverse world of human beings who want answers, or rather, maybe they just want the truth.

Eeshans believe that humanity became even more confused when the spirituality that the Christ taught was altered to portray a similarity with the Old Testament religion, consequently anything supernatural has become to most figments of one's imagination. Where God once used phenomena to move the hearts of people, answers seem to head the list today.

There are those who need answers to questions, such as: Is Jesus truly the Messiah for all people, because we are told now it is ok to think that He is Messiah for us, but others are still awaiting the true Messiah to come to them? In other words, is the Second Coming only for those who believe that Jesus is the Messiah? If it will be the second coming for us, then for those who never believed he was the Messiah, what will be the First Coming to them? Who will come for these people? Will there be others like Jesus? Will there be a Messiah from within each religion, and who then will be the greatest of them? Will it be Jesus? Or will it be One in whom all see their Messiah? Other questions also include: can anyone justify a Jesus, who has been reimaged by religious leaders so much that no one has any fear? In fact, who will those religious and priests fear, when they have masked the serious crimes, and continue to allow the horrendous acts of so many more priests and parochial nuns, not just presently but over the centuries? They certainly don't fear Jesus, but they justify the use of barbaric methods to get anyone to repent of acts they deemed sinful, especially against a child.

This is where spiritual guidance is vital, and that is, true spiritual guidance by which one can only get God's answers from GOD! Those who were supposedly called by God to a religious vocation to propagate his message turn around and abuse children, use women, and perpetrate severe punishment, and were not equipped to guide, as they themselves were misguided.

Along with true spiritual guidance, education is vital. Education, however, should never be a tool used to bring about a loss of innocence by making any person feel unworthy to approach God. Nor can the killing of a person, the killing of innocence, or the killing of a belief that is God-fearing to the point of depriving one of a wholesome, kind, loving personal relationship with God or others, be justified.

Love, not fear, always leads one back to the One who loved so deeply. the One from whom they received life, and that would be God. Then that love would trickle down, as God intended to parents/guardians and to a good government. All of these give life in their own way.

Eeshans believe the omission of Jesus' spirituality and teachings on the transcendental level left the weak, hungry, homeless, and innocent vulnerable to those teachers and leaders who sought to form imbalanced minds in the young and led their hearts further away from the transcendental life God designed for us through Jesus. Teaching our young people is very important.

Today where the children find it difficult to accept any religion, where they feel they will be forced into the thralls of religious superstition, or worse, abuse, we fear that without proper spiritual guidance, they can unfortunately be seduced by religions of persecution and violence.[113]

---

[113] While accounting for why people turn to violent/extremist positions in religion, this also sheds light on why many women who have been abused all their lives easily could turn to such things, due to effect on bruised minds by the powerful psychological force of persuasion. Many women stay in abused relationships as well because of this phenomenon. – Ed.

Though many of our young people seem to be fascinated by social, scientific, or given in some way just a theorist's impression, we find it somewhat refreshing that there is evidence out there that may be conveying to young minds some integral outlook regarding God, the Divine, and supernatural element in the creation of universes. This may not be the phenomena the baby boomers experienced, but actually it may be a start of an even fuller and more mature understanding that God is much more vast a mystery, and subject, than what was originally imagined.

Without spirituality and/or spiritual guidance, the splendor of God, as well as the much needed belief in the supernatural and Divine, is forfeited. When this happens, the human consciousness takes over. and logic without the balance of reason comes into play. One consequence of this is the redefining of sin.

Without a God or Supreme Being in human life, sin becomes obscured. If there is no greater Being in our consciousness than ourselves, then there is no one to be accountable to, leaving nothing for us, except this very temporary life. More people are living in mortal sin today than ever, even before Jesus, since before Jesus people had no concept of God's plan of salvation, and since there was no common belief in an afterlife, only just a notion of liberation from a political oppression. More people are less interested in the mysteries of God, and parents neglect teaching their children about God because they do not believe themselves.

We have become a people more involved in social and political realms. This all filters down to social justice, humanitarian issues, and those authorities who have deliberately been giving conflicting answers on so many mainstream issues plaguing people today, such as whether women's representation is, or ever was, validated adequately, thereby, excluding women from being accepted in leadership, or liturgical positions; the exposure of the proliferation of pedophilia and the constant deliberate creation of confusion surrounding doctrine and practice, along with the obvious deliberate Vatican doubletalk fostering confusion used to sidestep issues, and hide behind created controversies, resulting in a kind of spiritual apoplexy, and setting further precedence for the way our world has been so far shaped.

The greatest cause for today's global issues is this: the ignoring of the first commandment of Jesus to love God with one's whole heart, whole soul, and whole mind, while loving one's neighbor as oneself. He did not say, "love God by focusing ONLY on your neighbor as yourself." Time after time, Jesus used these words and lived these words to the fullest from birth, via his private life and marriage and pubic life with Mary Magdalen. Should these things have been part of his story for the last 2000-plus years, well, many of today's issues would not even have come into being.

The 'Time of Enlightenment' is upon us, and one must understand now more than ever that a liberal approach to sin is far from right; however, how can anyone argue about what is happening without the guidance of God as a center point? If God came in the Person of Jesus, why is there still confusion about so many issues? Not knowing the love of God discourages love of neighbor. We know nothing about the ways of God; yet we act as though we do.

We need to change hearts. We need to dispel the darkness and let in the Light, so we may find the peace and love Jesus actually taught.

LESSON 68

MERCY

Traditional scriptures talk about mercy in terms of what the human consciousness dictates as mercy. As a result, we no longer ask God for it, but have come to expect, or even demand mercy. We have come to feel that we are entitled by our own right to obtain mercy.

Though God is all-*merciful*, divine forgiveness requires contrition and the resolve to change and not commit that sin again; but with little to define what is right and wrong, what do we have to compare, as God has been reimaged by whatever any particular group needs, or wants, God to be. Let's look back and see how the one sin of so many basically is not to believe in Him.

One thing is for sure with regards to the things of God, human beings cannot judge on their own. They haven't the knowledge, the capacity, nor the impeccable omnipotent quality that only God has. As such, God does not just accept your wrongs as your weaknesses, nor does God accept with mercy that this is 'just who you are,' especially when you deliberately go against God and the commandments regarding loving our neighbor.

Ignorance is no excuse for ignoring God's law, or even human laws. Without law there is chaos. To think that you don't need God's forgiveness and mercy, or that you know better what is right and wrong by your own imperfect standard, is to set yourself up to being judged by your standard and not God's. Therefore, you are not only deceiving your own heart, and rationalizing love of pleasure, but you are essentially indicating that you have perfect intelligence and knowledge that far exceeds God's. One of the greatest errors of humans is to say, admit, or be accountable for the comment, "I don't believe in anything," which makes them susceptible to everything wrong, resulting in a misinformed conscience. Remember, the easiest person to lie to is yourself. Though God is all-merciful, His forgiveness requires contrition and the resolve to change and not commit that sin again. God does not just accept your wrongs as your weakness and accept with mercy that this is "just who you are," especially when you go against God's law and the law regarding your neighbor. To think so is to deceive your own heart, and you are only rationalizing love of pleasure more than love of God.

Though mercy is what we seek, love of God is what is *necessary*. One's pathway to God is actually known and best understood by the soul of each person; in other words, this is from within, or interiorly. It's when one understands that the fruit of any religion, or spirituality, is the transformation and conversion from those things that hurt God and oneself, which affects all those around them negatively, and to an individual who respects himself or herself, and others. Mercy is, thus, defined as compassion shown toward an offender, an enemy, or other person in one's power. Mercy is the fruit of love. Loving God enables us to see the use of mercy towards one another. Without love (the transcendental love Jesus taught and teaches today through his wife), real mercy does not exist. Confusion exists.

Boasting a system of beliefs, and not living it is likened to one who appears religious, yet continues to hurt others with an unbridled tongue.

You must enter into a spirituality with a clear sense of peace and desire knowing the difference between right and wrong, decent and indecent, knowledge and ignorance. One should also remember that whatever deity you worship should be the source of good-not evil.

Once you realize these things, we encourage you to find the path to God, or that Supreme Deity that fills your heart with joy, and leads you to become the best version of yourself, and it is there that you will find mercy.

PART III

LESSON 69

AN EXERCISE IN PREPARING TO WALK THE PATH OF TRUTH, ENIGHTENMENT

*W*e put together this little exercise to help give yourself something of a break before continuing on. A lot of information came your way, and, like ingesting food, the mind too must take a break to digest what has been presented to it. When we say the 'mind,' we mean the enlightened mind, and this always means to include your consciousness. So, if you're ready: close your eyes and let your body relax in a kind of mini Shavasana [the quieting of the mind beginning with stilling the body]. Though Shavasana (the "corpse pose") is a yoga practice done usually in a supine position, what we are asking is rather to relax your anxious state of being. What enlightenment requires is the getting away from the "thought" that a busy mind means a productive mind, and promising that you will allow more intuition-minded activity. It has always been taught by yogis that those who follow intuition have the right answers, and that unbridled thought limits our choice; this is usually wrong for us and hampers our intuition. Learning what type of personality you are can help with this exercise. Quieting the mind may be very difficult, if, for example, you are a "type A personality" and when in shavasana (especially as a beginner) you are subject to the human consciousness alone: you can't wait for it to be over to get back to the three dozen things you have to get done on your to- do list. There are some people who when trying to still the mind, but instead fall asleep, and this is not shavasana, but, rather, this most likely is exhaustion. The fact is, quieting the mind is very difficult. So, remember that shavasana is not allowing your mind to control you, but rather you are taking better control of *your mind. Now, close your eyes, relax your body. and still*[114] *your mind. If you cannot lie in a "corpse" position, relaxing the body [as people may get alarmed if they find you doing this at your work place], practice in a sitting position, on a park bench, on a chair, or in a quiet place, etc., becoming comfortable, and focus on relaxing whatever part of the body that is tensed, and to avoid focusing your attention on that discomfort. Try not to think about anything except becoming relaxed. (about 3–5 minutes), then take a few very deep breaths, and imagine your journey beginning (about 2 minutes). Now WE SHALL BEGIN.*

---

[114] Not to be confused with 'stopping' the mind or thought altogether. – Ed.

LESSON 70

FINDING THE KEY TO UNLOCK AN ENLIGHTENED MIND

We all have heard that the ultimate, and most elusive door, is that of our consciousness; this is where we 'store' our wisdom and peace; so, to unlock this door allows one to access and enter into the transcendental realm found deep within each of us. The subtle body is where wisdom is.

A master key makes it possible to unlock many doors. Jesus, the Divine Masculine of the Second Person of the Holy Trinity is this Master Key, and, when He condescended into this world, He lived and taught in such a way that it became impossible to keep the heart and mind locked up.

BRINGING HEART AND MIND INTO CONFORMITY

It is by far essential, even pivotal, to bring your heart and mind into conformity within the Eeshan spirituality. That is why we decided to take your consciousness on an Eeshan spiritual journey, using the legend of truths, mapping out a guide, and utilizing what we already provided for you, which contains all the central ideas and expressions that you will need, weaving through these pages like a lighted pathway.

Your consciousness will follow this light, which guides you as a kind of muse, taking your consciousness from an exoteric literal meaning and raising it to an esoteric inner meaning. The final destination is The Light of the world, and, of course. Jesus Christ. Although you may think you know all there is to know about Him, we think you will be rather surprised at what we are going to share with you, or, rather use, to awaken your Light Body.

You may at times find yourself going back to the stimuli you have been previously exposed to all your life, trying to compare what you are learning with what you have learned in the past, how you have, or have tried to live by that mindset. That's normal. For the sake of enlightenment, however, try to set aside those thoughts until you finish the book. At that time, you are free to agree or disagree, but you will have already begun to become enlightened, and by then you may have determined your dissatisfaction or satisfaction of your own religion or spirituality.

We have set up passages that we call doors. These will serve to show that a particular belief is presented and should you find you have strayed back from the path of enlightenment, the Key (Jesus through the teachings of his Eternal Consort) will serve to remind you that these are repeating Eeshan beliefs.

You will find, that though repeated several times, more information was added to present another perspective, or to deepen the knowledge you have already been privy to. These bits of added information will assist you in opening that once mysterious and elusive door to enlightenment. Think of these reminders as forms of your consciousness checks. These doors should help guard against the deeply probing skepticism of the human consciousness; and should ultimately prevent you from entertaining remnants of what may be coming from a former superficial spiritual life of which you may not be aware, or even be accustomed to.

Reviewing these passages will help you to be better prepared to unlock each sequential door, indicating a point, or juncture, with which the mind and heart is illuminated. If used correctly, they will lead you, each time, to a more richer and fuller understanding of Jesus' true mission and life that Eeshans believe has been locked away from the earliest times.

On the other hand, these doors are also intended to show the human mind's limited capacity to comprehend a *transcendental* consciousness, and will provide insight into how it truly differs from everyday, earthly, and common consciousness; and in some way help to "continue to remind" one how the rational human consciousness has been formed through upbringing, schooling, social conditioning, etc., and how this greatly differs from the transcendental. In a way, these little repetitive insights will help you to identify which consciousness you are in, at the moment you are reading about it. For example, if you begin reading and begin drawing from information you had been exposed to previously that causes you to question if what you are reading is unrealistic, or heresy, you will then know you are reading wholly in the human consciousness; so, take a deep breath and allow yourself to change your consciousness and approach what you are reading by asking yourself, "what if this is true?"

As we said, the doors we are talking about are identified with the "lock symbol."

Each of these locks will give you a 'heads up' about the next transcendental point. In doing so, before you continue reading, you have the option to go back and determine if you have begun to deviate from the path towards enlightenment, and have already dropped back to the earthly, or natural, mindset we so commonly rely on.

This is a reminder/warning that to continue via human consciousness is to fall off the path of enlightenment, and, thus, you will be limiting your spiritual growth by refusing to learn, or read, a particular Eeshan teaching/belief using a different perspective, which simply means you should read the writing with an open mind so that you may, in the very least, see what serves to solidify what *you* find is the fullness of your own faith.

Our beliefs need not be yours, but Eeshans feel that one basic step to **finding the fullness of enlightenment, regardless of your religion of choice, means you must be open to listening and understanding all views presented to you, and not just your own.** To attain this requires that you unequivocally need to return to that same quiet space through meditation, and focus through prayer before exploring the subject matter, especially if you truly want to understand the Eeshan perspective.

Try not to read ahead. Doing so shows your consciousness as belonging to the everyday human consciousness ... and this will bring with it consequences, which will result in you convincing yourself that any particular door is not necessary, causing you to tell yourself that you need only to get to the 'meat' of this religion. The 'meat' of our religion is Jesus Christ, true God, true Man. The only-begotten Child of God, born human to restore us back to the life that God, with unconditional love for us, which is the love intended for us.

Just one such consequence causes you to miss out on creating for yourself the ambiance experienced by it, and surrounding those sitting in the presence of Jesus. We believe that though it is impossible to recreate the physical moment in time, which would enable you to hear firsthand Jesus' teachings, and that by following the light, you may be able to transcend back and capture a deeper realization of His words by raising your consciousness to the level He intended for all those who followed Him. In this way, we may be able to provide for you the advantage his crowds did *not* have. Consequentially, if you start out seeking 'the meat,' and not the means by which the meat is obtained, that's exactly how you will view everything from that point on. You won't appreciate what went into preparing this transcendental life, and, thus, miss out on the spiritual food, that transcendental meal who is Jesus Christ, united solely as one to His eternal consort, being the victim, the sacrifice, the love.

Approaching enlightenment "your way" is exactly how the human consciousness dictates and works. So, if tempted, and you start to think all you want is to 'get to the meat of the teaching,' or belief without reading, or seeking enlightenment, will only result in desiring entertainment; whereas, in actuality it presented to you a chance to expand your knowledge. To skip everything else that seems 'boring' seems to be how we are wired in these times. To think of the meat of the topic at hand, deprives you of all the special spices you can add to basic food to enrich the taste. So, before you begin to skip through a transcendental document, thinking of 'getting to the meat,' instead think first, 'Do I wish to only imagine the animal body from which this nourishment came, serving only to give temporary satisfaction?' However, if you dare to allow us to prepare you a *spiritual meal*, you may end up saying, "I didn't think I would like it, but now I'm glad I tried it."

If you were sitting with Jesus you probably would first have been part of the greater teaching of Jesus that began with, 'Man cannot live on bread alone,' subsequently setting the stage for His most profound revelations and mysteries. You would have stayed to hear this new concept because, for some reason, you could relate to it.

Taking advantage of using the analogy of 'getting to the meat' is a perfect way to show you how when opening each of the doors will keep you on the path of enlightenment, and provide insights through, and beyond, the obvious. Meat weighs one down, and if eaten too late in the day, it makes one feel lethargic. Think of a transcendental reading as vegetables, especially greens, which are not only light-infused, but become light through digestion, which ultimately *feeds your cells' light*. This being a tremendous cancer preventative to the body, and can do the same for your soul.

Enrich your mind, body, and soul, by feeding them some spirituality, even if at first you don't like the taste.

LESSON 71

THE MASTER KEY JESUS, GOD, MAN, SPIRITUAL MASTER

DOOR #1 UNDERSTANDING JESUS' METHOD OF TEACHING HOW HE RAISED THE HUMAN CONSCIOUSNESS TO THE TRANSCENDENTAL LEVEL

Jesus had a very unique way of teaching. His teaching would always be adapted from things most familiar to the people. For example, He would often use a particular food to distinguish the difference between temporary satisfaction and true sustenance, or the difference between good and bad. Being God, and long before he came on the scene in the familiar areas of Galilee and Jerusalem, Jesus was known as *Issa* ('Ish'), Master of Spirituality in the Himalayas.

As with any teacher, He wanted His followers to be able to relate to what He was teaching in order that they would understand the difference between the human rational consciousness and the transcendental. Fruit, such as the fig, was intended to show good and bad spirituality in the eyes of God. Bread was, perhaps, the simplest and most identifiable earthly food people could identify with as it was necessary for life. Water was easy to see as sustaining life, while wine was seen as a drink which celebrates life. Jesus, by his word, would take His followers from eating the bread, made by human hands, to nourish their bodies, and use it to show how He could turn it into the Bread that has come down from heaven to nourish their souls.

Knowing that bread has a special social and emotional significance that goes beyond its importance as physical nourishment, Jesus took advantage of bread's importance and the common bond it had with His people, and He began to deviate from the human perspective of bread that makes sense, and raise its purpose to a transcendental meaning, predicting what will happen in the future.

In other words, he started with connecting bread's identification with being something his people could relate to as nourishment, and then simply began leading them into how it would become the foundation for the restoration and salvific mission for which He came. By taking people's common experience of bread, He divulged the most emotional, heavy, broad, and intense teaching about *spiritual sustenance*, as God to His children.

In order to teach the people about God's divine immanence, in conjunction with His teaching about bread sustaining human life, Jesus used instances of miracles to show that He also possessed this other nature, since He wanted to bring them around to the concept that He was God made man. Thus, He began to employ these concepts together as He spoke of the familiar bread, and *himself* as the bread come down from heaven. However, He began with simple teachings, which coincided with the planting of the wheat, which would lead to the processes involved up to the harvesting, or reaping, of the wheat. These, in turn, were introducing to their minds an early preparation and foundations for the Eucharist of the Marriage Feast and what we might today call 'the real Presence.'

These parables and analogies, along with his miracles, presented, in childlike terms, a teaching to the people of an otherwise overly complex, unfathomable mystery regarding God's 'real presence' (the understanding of God, as a person, again the Sanskrit term *Ishvara* which will unpacked as we go on), in order to illustrate to His people the difference between the bread used for the nourishment of their bodies, and a Bread that is necessary to feed the soul. It was mandatory for them to begin to realize that though being immortal, the soul still needed a spiritual 'bread' to sustain its lifeline to God, and thus insure its life even beyond death.

Because of their limited understanding of the mysteries of God, Jesus would always use common experiences, and moments, from 'their' daily lives so that people may relate to what He was teaching on a human level. More importantly, these would help people connect to Him, especially when He would speak on a subject, or difficulty, on a personal level, relating to an issue someone had, or was having. This would immediately result in the discovery that they were not alone, and proof that God was there for you!

This made them feel that this very holy man, who stood in their presence, didn't just listen, but understood their burdens, fears, plights, and better—He reassured them of the existence of a God who knew them *personally*. They would be enriched with each word and each moment they spent listening to him. The people connected with him, and this enabled him to continue to lead them back to the transcendental consciousness and a relationship with God they had never before known.

Jesus would also make use of things, or events, from his personal life, as well. If you examine his stories, or directives, they were often about those things that his apostles would be murmuring about behind his back. Issues such as whether one's place with Him, something they feared would get him, or them, arrested, changed what He was making with regards to a person's relationship with God in the Old (Mosaic) Law versus His perspective on this, etc.; and, of course, these teachings were nondescript, and he spoke to non-segregated crowds daily.

Jesus was known for his parables and His knowledge of God, and while emanating kindness from deep within his soul, He enjoyed laughter, and had a sincere interest in each person he encountered, all while making the very deepest doctrines understandable and applicable to their daily lives. He spoke on every level of understanding. He could speak to Royals, Pharisees, Sadducees, doctors, soldiers, thieves, as well as the greatest learned men, but, most of all, to the common uneducated people. Surprisingly, because of their inept ability to leave behind the human consciousness, Jesus would find that his parables would cause the minds of those closest to Him to become disturbed to the point where the purpose behind what He was saying became confusing to them. The reason that He would continue to use parables was to shake up their consciousness. It was amazing, however, how it was those who loved Him that understood these great teachings, and were able to apply them in their daily lives, but not His own apostles, since God has always revealed His highest and greatest mysteries to the most lowly and those most humble of heart.

A perfect example of this was when teaching His disciples, or those who followed Him, the purpose for which He came. Jesus used the people's understanding of how a grain of wheat dies, and how it is, once again, reborn as a spike, which then becomes capable of providing human sustenance. This was not just a one-time teaching. He mentioned bread many times.

That is why He also would invite himself to dinner at the homes of different people. Not only did He do this in an effort to bridge the gap between God and man by His presence, but by his breaking of the bread. He would always raise a glass of wine with the host, and after a while it became common knowledge that this is what to expect should He dine with you. That is how He would be identified after his Resurrection—by his breaking of the bread and sharing of wine. Present would always be oil, water, salt, and honey, as well.

Jesus would eventually use these gifts, along with this simple act of breaking bread and sharing wine, as well as using parables and related topics as opportunities to prophetically bring to light the Mystery of salvation and restoration of God's intended plan. He did this always with his wife close to him, linking the two as one. Little did anyone suspect that this simple food and drink would become God's greatest gift and the key to eternal life; nor did they suspect that this would be the outward sign of His love and devotion towards his wife, with whom He would always share the bread and wine first. This mirrored the love between Adam and Eve, and how his relationship with Mary was not just necessary for salvation but was also the template for marriage and true love.

This unfathomable mystery would have to reveal that the Messiah (as Jesus and Mary) was (were) here to save souls, and not merely achieve liberation from an oppressive government. Even the warnings of Peter, regarding the rumors of Jesus' arrest, should not have been the reasons the apostles[115] and the people should be afraid; rather, they should be afraid of the one who kept them from a spiritual food. This could only come about if those who followed Him knew and understood that 'He would be the wheat' that would die in order that this Bread from heaven would resurrect, and become the *Bread come down* from heaven, of which is the sustenance of the transcendental or Light Body.

Yes, this would become his most powerful teaching. This teaching regarding the wheat was one He would use in a prayer-like fashion, especially before the breaking of the Bread and sharing of the wine. He would initiate this little ritual before partaking of any meal.

Then, Jesus took this Ritual further. As time was of the essence, Jesus gave the Bread of life discourse, a Mystery so intense, that because of the opposing laws of God dictated by their birth religion, many had to walk away and leave Him. Dictated by what they had lived from birth, this was against everything that their religion taught them to believe.

What Jesus wanted them to understand was that what He was telling them was much more than just a teaching, and that, specifically, it was the Presence of God He was instilling within them, being that the Sacred Food, which was once lost was also soon to be available again.

It did not end here, and to further complicate matters, He involved his wife Mary as a key component in fulfilling his Father's plan to reverse what had happened and why, which will be revealed more thoroughly later in the book. Mary would share in the pre-meal ritual often repeating after Him, in an almost echoed manner, the resounding words.

The starting point to His salvific mission was bringing people away from the notion that everything of this world is temporary, and that everything will die. He was going to prove that there is an afterlife, and that He alone was the only One who could accomplish this and provide the means to enter/travel upon this lighted path.

---

[115] It's important to keep in mind that not all the apostles at all times were in agreement with what Jesus was teaching or talking about. Even at the time where the rumors began flying, some felt it was necessary to 're-explain' what Jesus meant, and others tried to interpret what Jesus was saying through the lens of their birth religion. In any case, by this time, they were seen and known as fully invested as formal disciples of Jesus.

As we said before, in the religion, at the time Jesus came, there was no real definite understanding, or hope, of an afterlife. Not only did the religion of the time teach this, but the human consciousness and logical reasoning discounted it, as well.

Surprisingly, early on, the Egyptians always prepared their Pharaohs and royalty for their journey to the afterlife; how ironic that under the 'one true God' imaged after Moses, this belief was lost until Jesus. Perhaps it was because the Israelites, around the time of Moses, wanted a clean break from Egyptian beliefs, or had the same problem under the human consciousness, as did Peter and some of the other apostles?

Lesson 71A

The Bread

Bread became the mainstay of Jesus' teachings, and He would continue to use references specific to bread. He referenced the manna God provided in the desert that was the nourishment for the Israelites as their bodies hungered. He used simple analogies, such as when He questioned what father would hand a son a stone when he asked for bread, or a snake if he asked for a fish, as another way of showing the love of God as the Divine Masculine in a parental role, as a Father, and they as His children. Here He was leading them to developing a mindset that a Father would not deprive his children of what they needed to live, AND that they could trust the Divine Masculine of God as they would trust their own fathers.

He divided the few loaves of bread with some fish to feed the huge crowd that came to hear Him speak, and, when, on another day the Pharisees attacked the disciples for picking corn on the Sabbath, Jesus retorted to deflate the importance they put on 'corn,' and used yet another opportunity to raise the bar about bread by re-telling the story of when David and his men ate the showbread after they had gone without food for some time. Also, the showbread, as it is also known, was consecrated and forbidden to be eaten by anyone other than the priests.

He wanted them to see, that when David ate the bread to save their lives, it was prefiguring the Bread Jesus was now describing, which many would walk away from, even though it would feed their starving souls, which once again 'was rejected for it went against the Law.' Jesus reminds the Pharisees that the Torah states, "All the commandments I command you these days, shall you observe and do, that you may live …" If you note, He did not give this as a 'teaching.' It was a commandment and not an option.

Deuteronomy 8:1 reads, "God's rules are to live by—not die by." Thus, the ancient Rabbis taught that virtually all of the 613 commandments are lawfully suspended to save life. Thus, David (as High Priest) and his men ate the showbread to sustain the body; and Jesus, using his authority 'as' High Priest, will be the Bread come down from heaven, will become the consecrated Bread that will sustain the soul, and it should be noted that as the sacrificing of goats, calves, or bulls was used to cleanse the earthy sanctuary to receive forgiveness from sins, Jesus' blood would cleanse the heavenly sanctuary and that this was necessary for the forgiveness of sins. Hence, it was necessary to keep providing food regularly to keep the body alive; and because of sin, He commanded that it would be necessary to eat the bread come down from heaven regularly to keep the soul alive.

This Mystery Bread was in keeping with the kind of food the soul needs in order to live. As a matter of fact, it was a transcendental light food that needed to be 'ingested.'

To reiterate, Jesus, just as the wheat, would have to die so that like the spike of His body would become the bread that God commanded His people to eat to nourish the soul housed within the light body, which was created and formed by God; but due to Adam and Eve's ingestion of the apple, their light bodies were imprisoned within the gross physical bodies *necessary for them to live in the material world.*

Jesus knew that most who called themselves disciples would not understand this concept, let alone accept any other 'concept' that required the eating of any food containing animal blood, let along *human*. You must remember that the notion of Jesus being God, and God commanding them to eat His body and drink His blood, since Life was immediately rejected for so many reasons outlined in the Judaic religion. However, what you probably didn't know, was that among these, Peter, too, would be the first to be guilty of not following Jesus' command to no longer be identified by the food they ate, since that which was once unclean, is now clean.' Why would He tell them this? Of course it was so that the food did not identify their religion and/culture, and more importantly it was in preparation for the acceptance of eating His body, blood, soul, and divinity, which caused those others to walk away and, prophetically, that they would never come back.

At the surprise of His apostles, after his Bread of Life discourse, as the crowds began to disperse, and walk away scandalized, Jesus was unaffected by this act of insolence.

When He questioned those who were His apostles, if they too were to leave, it was a means by which He was testing their faith. The reason He was not bothered by those who walked away, it only prefigured those who would always lack faith in Him and His words. What affected him, however, were those who followed Him, and were taught by him daily that were led by their fear. That is why when He asked them if they, too, would leave, they then asked where else would they were to go, since He offered the words of eternal life. Yes, those few of his own apostles, who should already have had faith, remained; however, not all believed in what he said. But they really did have nowhere else to go at the moment. For them to leave Jesus at this time would make them fools, and they were to be looked upon as rebels, without a powerful leader, and if He was arrested they would be arrested, too. A few however did believe, oddly enough, Thomas was one; Philip was another.

As we said, Jesus' teachings centered on bread began early on in His ministry. He taught in parables, He taught metaphorically, and He taught metaphysically, but He never catered to the human consciousness, and always illustrated his teachings with examples of all kinds to exhibit that, as the body is temporary, earthly bread is not enough to keep you from dying. No matter how He addressed it, one thing was clear, for everlasting life, and that is we need the Bread come down from heaven, and that is necessary to conquer death, and restore us to our original transcendental form, and to insure everlasting life, and once we are on this path, it is the only means of being saved. This Bread would come to be known as the Eucharist; and without this Eucharist, this bread of life, all that one does has no sustenance,[116] even to include good works done in His name.

---

[116] Eternal life won't come solely from performing good works and preaching Jesus' word. Something more is required. Jesus said so himself.

One must understand, that Jesus knew it was not essential for anyone to completely grasp (intellectually) what He was saying, since teaching in the transcendental bypasses the mind, and goes straight to the heart; but for those who lacked faith, and refused to transcend, they would be blind and not see, that without the Eucharist, salvation is no longer an option.

Unfortunately, even those closest to him lacked faith. That is why He did not feel he had to justify His discourse.

The apostles themselves continued to struggle with Jesus' command to do so, however, it was different for them. Again, they spent day and night with Jesus; and yet few of His own would fully accept the changes Jesus was instituting. They failed to see that what Jesus was teaching was based on God's love for everyone, and just as with the miracle of the loaves and fishes, this bread was not only 'meant' for 'everyone,' it was necessary for all who sought salvation, or, rather, for all who wanted what Jesus promised.

It was also difficult for them to understand, since they lived only in the human rational consciousness and since their birth religion did not put faith in an afterlife.[117] To not believe in an afterlife would not allow for one to think, or understand, beyond this world; and to not enter into Jesus, as He intended would not allow for the acknowledgement and acceptance beyond what a human rational consciousness could understand and interpret.

Eeshans believe Jesus' Bread of Life discourse was a real problem for many, especially for Peter; and one will see how this was the beginning of the end.

As Jesus had made efforts to get Peter on the same page, Peter became more and more the stumbling block not just to Jesus, but also to himself and all others seeking the transcendental. He would perceive Jesus only through the faulty human consciousness.

---

[117] Egyptians did have a concept of 'everlasting life,' but the Jews at the time of Jesus did not share such definite views of the soul continuing to live on after the body's demise, even while there was discrepancy between Pharisees and Sadducees about 'resurrection.' – Ed.

To better help you understand the difficulty of accepting Jesus' teachings and directives, we present a before, during, and after moment taken from an eyewitness account referencing Peter.

Jesus foretells how a future incident showing Peter's resistance to the new covenant and his rigid attachment to the old covenant will be revealed, as in John 21:15-18:

> When they had finished *'eating,'* Jesus said to Simon Peter, 'Simon son of John', do you love me more than these?' 'Yes, Lord," he said, "you know that I love you." Jesus said, "Feed my lambs." Again, Jesus said, "Simon son of John, do you love me?" He answered, "Yes, Lord, you know that I love you." Jesus said, "Feed my sheep." The third time he said to him, "Simon son of John, do you love me?" Peter was not 'hurt,' but was embarrassed and annoyed because Jesus asked him the third time, "Do you love me?" He said, "Lord, you know all things; you now that I love you." Jesus said, "feed my sheep."

We find proof of the above in Acts 10 how little Peter understood with regards to the transcendental.

It is there we see Peter just 'beginning' to realize just how different this new religion, begun by Jesus, was from his birth religion, and how limited Peter's ability was, due to conditioning of human consciousness, to accept Jesus' teachings on a transcendental level. This caused him to continually be the 'stumbling block' Jesus prophesied about.

It was during Paul's confrontation with Peter, where Paul addressed all that Peter was failing to do, that is significant. Peter had not been having, nor attending, worship services where the Eucharist was distributed. This caused unrest among Peter's followers, since they, too, began to dwindle in numbers at worship services, and thinking that if Peter didn't go, then they didn't have to go. This shows that the Bread of Life discourse made little impression on Peter all along.

Another time, when Peter was on the rooftop waiting to eat, and he had a vision. In the vision, a sheet was lowered from heaven, containing many different animals. A voice encouraged him to eat. Peter balked, realizing that some of the animals in the sheet were forbidden under Jewish law. Three times the sheet lowered, and three times Peter refused. This vision had two purposes.[118] Jesus had given a new law where the once forbidden food was lifted, meaning that the rules about dietary restrictions no longer applied, since those who follow Jesus are to be recognized by their love for God and neighbor and not dietary laws. Since Peter was told what God has cleansed, he did not call the food unclean. After the third time, the food was taken back up to heaven.

Secondly, and most importantly, it signified that this was a spirituality that welcomed everyone. Salvation was open to the Gentiles as much as it was for the Jews.[119]

It was then that Peter received several messages from a 'Gentile' centurion, (someone deemed unclean and who ate unclean food according to the Jewish religious standards) who was looking to accept and follow Jesus' way. This was a real conundrum for Peter, as we see that his birth religion was still very much alive in him. In a vision, Cornelius, a very prayerful man, was called by God to go see Peter that he may witness his desire and find out what he would need to do to follow Jesus.

Though Peter told them that he perceived that God is no respecter of persons and in every nation, there are those who were righteous, and who are accepted by God, which we find later that he chose to work only with the Jews, and told Paul to work with the Gentiles. Thus, once again, Peter may have spoken the words of Christ, but his actions were still those of his birth faith. That is why the influence of Peter's teachings, and his example regarding what was given to Jesus' followers was limited, if not totally stifled, the fruits and gifts of the Spirit which intended to free us from oppression and discrimination, and to make possible the freedom to change. Today, we see even fewer conversions from other religions, even fewer from the Jewish faith.

---

[118] Acts 10:11.
[119] Acts 28:28.

LESSON 72

DOOR #2 THE RISE AND FALL OF THE TRANSCENDENTAL LIFE EXPERIENCING PHYICALITY IN A PHYSICAL WORLD

The following is presented to help you as you journey towards enlightenment. When approached with an open mind and faith, AND used properly, this will continue to unlock the consciousness, thus opening doors to truth and enlightenment; but if you insist on only seeing those things presented to you strictly through the earthly fallen nature, one that will only permit you to view what you read with the consciousness that Jesus was met with, you will not.

This human consciousness is affected by a mind corrupted by subsequent ignorance, since Adam and Eve, due to the onset of entropy, and you, will fail to see how God's plan for salvation began with the restoration of what was lost to us by the choice of physicality and who we truly are before God.

It goes without saying that once Adam and Eve developed gross physical bodies things would have to change, such as the way in which they lived and reproduced, as well as their relationship with God. Aside from the obvious, one may wonder if there are any physical remnants of the once transcendental bodies they had; and would those markers follow down the line of descendants?

Lesson 72A

Tracing the Physical Back to the Transcendental

When Did Confusion Begin?
How the Template to the Transcendental Inprint is Still in Our Body; and What Changes had to be Made in the Physical Body to Compensate for the Loss?

The human mind, because of entropy/time, is automatically drawn to a darkened and finite reasoning; it is darkened in the sense that it is not open to enlightenment. This is due to the original choice of Adam and Eve to take on a physical form, which brought them out of the transcendental nature, which before boasted of a timeless form absent of time and gravity into a physical form made of material energy, vibration, and the earth/gross physical body, which was subject to decay.

Eeshans believe that Adam and Eve's mind, as well as the minds of all their offspring who were begotten before the fall, and transcendental-minded people, were/are respectively, governed by the third eye.

If what is being said is true, after the 'fall,' where once the gross physical body began forming, there would still have to be evidence of the transcendental light body somewhere within. Since it would only make sense that God would allow proof to compare what was before and what came after the choice to physicality, especially if Jesus, as Divine Masculine, came with a salvific plan for us.

It is necessary however, that you leave behind your fears of what you were taught was 'evil,' and let us introduce, and explain, to you to some of the things you feared over the years as being a means to take you away from Jesus, and to explore those teachings He taught privately, and which have been backed up, scientifically, medically, etc., today.

What was once referred to as the third eye, is also referred to now as the pineal gland. This small endocrine gland resembles a pine cone; hence, the name. It is considered to be the seed from the tree of knowledge. It is located in the epithalamiums, near the center of the brain, tucked in a groove between the two hemispheres. It is often called the "principal seat of the soul" where all our thoughts are formed. Throughout history it was believed to be and regarded as a 'mystery gland.' Eeshans believe, that when Adam and Eve chose a physical existence, the pineal gland was 'encapsulated.' If you take a look at the pineal gland, you will see that it actually hangs down, as though in a falling position.

Though it is thought that it is responsible for various limited aspects of sexual development, we believe that there continued to be limited activity in early years of development once the human being descended to total physicality. and its secretion of hormones became restricted. There remained some ability to function, enabling God's plan of salvation, but in order to reproduce, as we know it, the pituitary gland replaced the transcendental functions, such as the begetting process.

One way the pineal gland is restricted is that it secretes its hormone, in sync with circadian rhythms, releasing more in the dark and less in the light, and the opposite of its original function where it functioned transcendentally, or always in the light. As it secretes less melatonin in adults than in children, it is said to inhibit sexual development, which is a natural result of a human condition versus the heavenly.

Spiritually speaking, Eeshans believe that after puberty, the pineal gland shrinks, and releases less melatonin, then the pituitary gland takes over.[120]

We come to see how important our journey is through different phases of our life. mad that the need for spirituality from the closing of the fontanelle (until it reopens at our death) is known in many spiritual traditions. One such book is *Following our Bliss*, by Don Lattin. Here, the author tells how participants often seek the help of a Shaman, to find

---

[120] Anissimov, Michael, and Niki Foster. "What Does the Pineal Gland Do?" WiseGEEK, Conjecture Corporation, 3 Nov. 2019, www.wisegeek.com/what-does-the-pineal-gland-do.htm.

guidance and spirituals answers, which help guide a child from adolescence to adulthood.

In our understanding and use of metaphysics, we know that as the pituitary gland takes over in puberty, due to the loss of the pineal gland's function, and because entropy sets in, you will find that the pituitary gland is in a dropped or fallen position. That is why the position of the pituitary gland, the size of a pea, weighing 0.5 grams, protruding off the bottom of the hypothalamus, at the base of the brain, is depicted like a fallen entity, deficient of light; whereas, the pineal gland is one whole gland representing the transcendental being, which was created, and sacredly balanced, before God separated its complimentary components into two, which were still functioning as a whole until the Original Choice.

Due to the absence now of the begetting process, along with the pituitary gland, hormones must set in order for sex to be introduced. As this was new to Adam and Eve, God explained the changes that would now take place within the physical body, as well as in their daily life. This is where God explained what Adam and Eve would now experience in Gen. 3:16. This is not to ever have been represented as in a punishing way, but in God's effort to instruct them as to how these new bodies are different from what they had before.

This next section is not only proof of this, but carries a very pretty, and spiritual, attachment, or as Eeshans believe, a direct line to God. The relationship of the pineal gland, the third eye, as it is called, to the fontanelle, is as follows. The fontanelle is surrounded by sutures in the skull, which are located on the top, back, and sides of the head. The fontanelle is located at the center of the top of the head, where the sutures intersect; it is often called the 'soft spot' at the top a baby's head, which allows the head to collapse slightly to get the head through the birth canal. The growth of the skull is associated with religious ecstasy and the baby's one-on-one link to God. This means that there is a constant flow of grace, etc. from God to the baby. Thus, we often say the angels are playing with the baby when we see a smile etc. It is this open spot that channels to the pineal gland. Eeshans believe that this is why a child should be baptized before the fountain closes. Associated with the pineal gland is the path to higher consciousness, clairvoyance, and enlightenment. Is it no wonder that it would be another facet indicating that there is so much more to the human child. In fact, it shows the divine contact until which time the fountain closes, and the child loses the direct contact it had with God, as it matures and must now 'choose' to seek God? Some feel this is also where the light, soul, and spirit enters the embryo. It is said that as the child approaches the age of two years, this age coincides with the closing of the veil, or cutting off of light, and direct contact with God, with the closure of the fontanelle, and, perhaps, the soul, light, and spirit of the child recognize that it is now imprisoned within a physical body, and cannot escape the flesh.

Once the fontanelle closes, and that divine contact is gone, this is when parents, godparents, etc. serve as guides to keep the child on God's path and the way back to the transcendental, by teaching them Sacraments and the mysteries of God.

Light fascinates babies, and they often stare at incandescent light for long periods of time. It is amazing how their eyes will turn in any direction light is shining. Could it be that the light they see is so familiar that it calms them? That little familiarity that comforts them during the transition from the transcendental to the material, or physical, world reappears again in near-death experiences.

We are told that as the biological eyes begin to focus, and that is around the time the pineal gland closes, which is within a few months after birth. In the Balinese culture, there is a ceremony when a child reaches six months of age. Prior to that time, a baby is never allowed to touch the ground, because the child is still considered to be a heavenly being. In her book, *Eat, Pray, Love*, Elizabeth Gilbert tells us that only at this ceremony does he, or she, become a child of the earth by lowering the child for the first time to touch the earth with their feet. At this time, the pineal gland is closed off in order to prevent the transcendental begetting process of reproduction.

It is now that the pituitary gland becomes necessary to govern the rational consciousness and human sexuality/reproduction. It is also significant to mention, at this time, that pre-pubescent girls go through an enlightenment period before the pineal gland shuts down entirely. That is why so many girls between the ages of 9–12, seem to suddenly fall in love with Jesus. This is a very important time, since this surge is at the brink of the encapsulation of the pineal gland, which will prevent the return to the transcendental-like the gates of Eden prevented Adam and Eve access to Eden, unless one chooses to follow Christ's directives to follow the 'Way' back.

As this truth has been made 'optional' by man, the fulfillment of God's promise to send a woman to crush the head of the serpent is now upon us. It will now be by she who can, and will be, the one needed for our return to our origin and to live transcendentally with God.

As human sexuality is found in time and outside spirituality, the opposite was true of the pineal gland, which at one time moved one towards God, and, thus, the love of soulmates begot children transcendentally. That is why one who loves God totally, and does not have earthly children, are thought to carry life within them, and to beget children for God. You will find how important this fact is as you continue to learn about Jesus and Mary Magdalen. Without this transcendental connection, and the continued darkening of the mind and heart, via the awakening and functioning of the pituitary gland, human sexuality has, over time, become selfish and self-gratifying. With each generation, there is less and less need for commitment, or a need for a soulmate; yet, because of the void that comes from this mindset, in recent times, there seems to be a growing, almost innate desire for one.

As previously mentioned, Eeshans believe that even with the 'curse' (the original choice which caused mortality), at the onset of death, one experiences, once again, a taste of the transcendental because the body is dying, and one's light body is being drawn forward from it. The awakening and decalcification of the pineal gland prepares to release the soul at death which had been safely tucked away within the light body, where it been imprisoned within the 'gross physical body.' When the pineal gland opens this time, the soul is called to acknowledge the mysteries of God, Life, and Salvation; which upon professing said mysteries, the path is cleared for the soul to leave the body. It is during this time of decalcification that the person's life passes before them, while Satan uses this opportunity to discourage and torment the soul. That is why it is necessary to know the Mysteries of God, so that the pathway is free of obstacles, as quickly as possible.

Eeshans believe that in cases where someone is dying who may not know the mysteries of God, that someone be there speaking the mysteries, and, thus, easing the spiritual distress and pain of the loved one, or any other person. This is the reason the line, "Pray for us sinners, now and at the hour of our death," was so wisely included in the Hail Mary.

Another sign of our transcendental origin that is found within each of us is how the pineal gland/brain resembles the uterus, which takes us back to Jesus' teaching of 'as above, so below,' and how the pituitary gland resembles the male reproductive (testes), and how the male/female bodies seem to take on the other characteristics towards their later years, as the male body produces more estrogen and the female body more testosterone. This gives witness to the male/female union, imperfectly, of course, but the two-gender identification of God, who contains within the Male/Female genders found within each of us according to God's image and likeness.

As the human brain has been the subject of tremendous study, there has been so many accounts of near-death experiences.

With the flawed mind, in the state of the human consciousness, one is guided by the mind; whereas, in the transcendental, 'you' would be 'guiding' your mind, as on a lighted path. The disconnect caused by the rational mind will cause the information your mind receives to remain limited to what you know and/or have learned, and, thus, the transcendental element will be processed incorrectly. This again is where sin originates, since a flawed consciousness is a flawed conscience, and the end result equals only flawed negative thought processes. We could go on and on with examples of God's love and guidance towards Adam and Eve after the fact, but what's fascinating is that peoples and cultures all over the world share in God's goodness through their own traditions and belief exhibiting the goodness and vastness of God, or a Supreme Being.

That is why it's important, for one who desires enlightenment, to understand all of what Jesus was teaching. From those teachings on loving God above all else and loving our neighbor as our self, forward to the source of Light and light food necessary for the nourishment of the transcendental consciousness, we find a deeper, more intrinsic, and essential meaning behind Jesus as Light of the world. Understanding that the Light is Jesus, one sees how it is necessary, while alive, to attain 'perfect' enlightenment and understanding of the things of God. He is the Light Himself, and those things that contain light and nourishment to our light body can only come from someone perfect. He (along with his Eternal Consort) is the only perfect one. As part of his mystical body, we are positive extensions of the 'Light of the World,' and, thus, we are light beings, or, as Jesus said, we are lights in the world, and should be witnesses of the fruits of the Spirit by spreading acts of kindness and patience.

Meditation and prayer illuminates our path. An enlightened mind does not see itself fearing the unknown, nor does it feel threatened to the point of anger. It is devoid of judgment, and is open-minded, and sees the world with great clarity, with no bias, or conclusions, based on limited, preconceived information. We promise you that regardless of whether you accept our sacred beliefs or not, this is the BEST approach to a more heightened, richer, and deepened spirituality.

LESSON 73

DOOR #3 JESUS, THE 'WAY' TO ENLIGHTENMENT, AND WHAT DO WE MEAN THAT JESUS IS THE 'WAY'

When we hear the word 'Way' we think of a method, style, or manner of doing something, or a road, or a path. Jesus is not only all of these, He is an actual human 3D material/transcendental gate we must consume, and go through, much like walking through a doorway, only in the form of a person, and light. Imagine walking through a person.

Let's begin with reviewing what we learned about transcendental versus every day, or earthly, rational consciousness. This lesson is important because, due to the lack of guidance, and despite Jesus' incarnation, teaching, suffering, dying, and resurrection, little has changed with regards to how humans interact, evidencing how little they have transcended.

Eeshans believe that in giving you a transcendental book about our spirituality. with no guide to follow, will only result in the same consequence, which is no change whatsoever. This is so, because the mind, being flawed, would unconsciously resort back to what you have been taught your whole life regarding Jesus' life, death, and resurrection, which includes hearing only the universal church's version of Jesus' mission, and you would entirely miss the "world's greatest love story" ever told.

Failing to understand, and, continuing on any 'path,' rather than following the Way, does not take you in the same direction, instead, you would find only the faulted human definition' of what is meant by Jesus being the Way.

Eeshans want you to learn, and have the same experience and connection, as those who lived at the time of Christ and came to hear Him. We want you to see the person of Jesus, how He loved, and, essentially, how He 'thought' what his mission actually was, and the reason why he died.

Lesson 73A

The Genius of His Parables

As we mentioned before, during His time on earth he taught everyone using the people's surroundings, lives etc., in *parables*. Today people still ask why Jesus used parables. One answer we were always given was that he preferred this way of teaching, since people could relate to what he was saying, using themes and things related to their daily lives, however, it doesn't stop there.

The most important reason, thought, was to divide the people into two groups. The first group would listen to the parables and stories like little children listen to shows, cartoons, and stories read to them, solely for entertainment; BUT, the second group were composed of those children who actually received more than just entertainment from his parables, a lesson on kindness and love, a sharing and caring to be learned, and good habits to follow, including manners. When Jesus' crowd grew, he chose parables to see who learned from them, and who sought God, and who just listened to the stories and became confused, afraid, and disinterested after a while; since those people wouldn't grow in love of God. These would be the people who eventually would desert Him.

As we said, Jesus knew and understood people, and the mentality He would be faced with since this was a fulfilled prophecy and a reoccurring theme, which began in *Ezekiel 12:2:*

> *"Son of man, you are living among a rebellious people. They have eyes to see but do not see and ears to hear but do not hear, for they are a rebellious people." And in Jeremiah 5:21, "Hear this you foolish and senseless people, who have eyes but do not see, who have ears but do not hear.*

Confused with Jesus using parables, we find proof of this even within His followers, since a few asked him why he didn't speak 'plainly.'

Knowing that most of who heard him were influenced by the human consciousness He spoke of, as Jesus says (Matthew 13:13-15),

> *"Though seeing they do not see; though hearing they do not hear or understand. In them is the fulfillment of the prophecy of Isaiah: 'You will be ever hearing but never understanding; you will be ever seeing but never perceiving; for this people's heart has become calloused; they hardly hear with their ears, and they have closed their eyes. Otherwise, they might see with their eyes, hear with their ears, understand with their hearts and turn, and I would heal them."*

You will find, in particular, how those who spent day and night with Jesus would prove how "many are called, few are chosen," as we continue to unpack Jesus' teachings and the stumbling blocks placed in His way.

As a result, we are faced today with the same rebellious people, and things are worse than what He encountered in that time. That's because of who He was and is, what He came to do, and what He did for us.

LESSON 73B
AND JESUS SAID, "..." ("WAIT, WHAT DID HE SAY?")

As Jesus' words are meant for all ages, we see how he effortlessly revealed the importance of foretelling and warning us that his words would be altered; however, what happens when his warnings are ignored and/or omitted? Or what occurs when His words are used for the purpose of protecting the changes which reflect another agenda?

Once Jesus' words lost that transcendental quality by not being taught and accepted according to the way He commanded, His divinity became scrutinized by the most surprising teaching body. The opinions over whether Jesus was God and Man, or just Man, abounded in none other than his own church, which claimed to be founded by Christ and holds his truths; yet, the church did not agree on these truths as dogma until approximately AD 325, as dictated under the authority of Emperor Constantine, who at the time was a non-Christian.

We believe that the Christian religion, under continued poor leadership from its inception to today, actually, in many ways not only erred, but resorted back to a non-competitive, safeguarded, and a watered-down version of social and secular issues, and was an entity which taught only earthly things and heard only earthly words, even while clothing itself in religious dress. That is to say, that the direction people are going in today is little different than what Jesus encountered when he began his public ministry with his wife. Eeshans believe this makes way for how, after his ascension, so much of what Jesus taught was not only omitted, lost, or misconceived, but so lacked in truth that today reverence and conversions are practically speaking, relatively few.

It's not hard to figure out why, if some of those closest to Jesus didn't convert, or teach according to the New Law; how, then, could they, and their successors, lead others to the transcendental when they had no experience of it themselves? That is why Eeshans believe it is time to show that when Jesus ascended, many people, including a couple of his apostles, resorted back to their previous ways of thinking according to the Old Law, living almost just the way Jesus first found them. Because they continued to define His teachings for all ages, on the lower human consciousness, and with no one to guide them to a higher level, we see the reasons for the breakdown and collapse of what eventually grew to become the Catholic church. (Most telling is that, truthfully, the Catholic church actually 'cannot' go back, and revise and correct its dogmas and doctrines, and various other positions that are drawn from these, because to do so would essentially mean to abandon what she claimed she had all along, which was an inerrancy that came from God, which they hold has been preserved them from error in faith and morals, and guides the interpretation of sacred tradition and holy scripture.)

Without anything more than what they were given, we can see that, as people did not have, and/or lost, the transcendental qualities of Jesus' "Bread of Life" discourse, over the years, confused Jesus' teachings, and applied purely human consciousness-centered practices in its place. Knowing nothing else, the people would feel complete as followers of Jesus. Doing the basics, such as worshiping on the Sabbath, acts of kindness under the guise of simply living decent, wholesome lives within their own way of life, was their own interpretation of 'Christ's way to salvation,' which became the foundation from which all the Christian-based religions today were built upon. Sadly, they never comprehended that though this is a 'path,' it is not the '*Way*,' or where one finds the fullness of Christ's love and salvation.

Excluding Jesus' command to eat the "'Bread' (Jesus) come down from heaven" is to not believe, wholly, in Jesus being more than just a man, or, to believe he was merely a man with whom God may be working, but who was most definitely not God. As humans, we feel only those things that are logical and rational commands could come from God. To view Jesus as being anyone but God, in the flesh, allows for our choice regarding His directives.

This, in and of itself, shows a lack of understanding and acceptance of who Jesus was/is and why he came. To know and understand the whole story would negate any 'debate' as to the necessity of the Eucharist, and would relegate Jesus' teachings to being optional.

It is no secret that what the church of Peter is today, with its own problems, mirrors what it was in its early days. Sadly, again, we see more of the same.

As the early church was struggling, divided, and on the brink of extinction, some declare that it was because there was no template such as the Torah to teach his people. Eeshans present that Jesus' teachings, the Beatitudes, the Two Commandments, and Bread of Life Discourse define, most accurately, His plan, and that He left explicit directives all of which many were later changed for a more 'acceptable,' and 'less controversial' goal. Peoples' feeling around such atrocities was to focus on Jesus and their love for him. This would be fine; however, they never really knew about what Jesus taught. Basically, they were told what to do, and believe what was given, and never read the bible (if/when they could read), since they would not understand it, or be drawn to misinterpret what they read, that suffering should be offered up, and so on and so on.

No one ever would suggest that there were changes made, or that these changes included the elimination of the writings of those apostles and followers, who thoroughly understood Jesus was the Son of God versus those who feared controversy and persecution; the people were conditioned to fear excommunication and eternal death.

To sum up what Eeshans believe in this connection includes:

1. Jesus was the Divine Masculine of the only-begotten Child of God who became known as the Son of God who came into the world to awaken the light body within;
2. Jesus intended that he and his wife would together give nourishment to this light body and strength to the soul and the subtle body; and by his life, death, and resurrection He showed the "Way" with "Truth" and by his marriage to Mary Magdalen, His eternal consort who was the Divine Feminine aspect and eternal consort of the only-begotten child of God,

3. They provided a template for a transcendental life, mirroring their marriage, and finding its origin in, the marriage of Adam and Eve.
4. Thus, this provides what the soul needs for its continued ascent back to God by, with, and in God through belief in the Eucharist and thereby achieving everlasting and eternal life.

LESSON 73C

"THEREFORE, SEE WITH YOUR EYES, HEAR WITH YOUR EARS; UNDERSTAND WITH YOUR HEARTS, AND TURN, AND I WILL HEAL YOU"

How much greater would be the meaning of His words if all were taught and lived fully the way Jesus intended.

With that in mind, when you meditate, or pray, remember to ask that "your eyes be opened to see and ears to hear by leaving behind this world and allow yourself to enter into an enlightened world."

It will be quite an experience for you to see just how deeply you have been conditioned to "not think," and to find yourself, perhaps, for the first time, awakened and able to see how deeply deprived of the highest love of God, neighbor, and life you could have had. Maybe for the first time, you can count yourself among those of whom he spoke in Matt. 13:16: "But blessed are your eyes because they see, and your ears because you hear. For truly I tell you, many prophets and righteous people longed to see what you see but did not see it, and to hear what you hear but did not hear it." Perhaps, you knew these things all along; yet, were forced in some way to suppress what you knew, interiorly, and intuitionally.

LESSON 74

DOOR #4 THE HUMAN CONSCIOUSNESS AND ITS 'FAR REACHING' EFFECTS ON RELIGION AND LOSS OF SPIRITUALITY TO ITS FOLLOWERS

What 'consciousness' was lacking that Jesus was teaching and talking about?

Without a doubt it was the transcendental consciousness. He knew that the people had been living with only the ability to perceive, think, and feel according to an everyday human consciousness, and witnessed first-hand how that the so familiar human consciousness conditioned their everyday lives and decisions. By today's standard, that is the world we live in, entirely framed around what human beings need, enjoy, and they think only according to what they perceive, or are led to believe ... "like lambs to the slaughter."

Religion, or spirituality, still in many cases, dictates our life, though often not true to its total belief system, it was different back in biblical times. Back in Jesus' time, the religion was also their culture, and was dictated by the higher authorities who claimed to rule by God's oral and written law.

Today, in many places, the culture and government still abide by their system of beliefs, but for our western culture, the media and social media seem to have replaced religion and spirituality around us, and is more apt to play a greater role, and it is often seen by many as responsible in forming the foundation for how we think, live, and make decisions. This is our conditioning.

Both 'ancient and present time consciousness' flawed and imperfect, is what Eeshans believe has brought about, once again, the fullness of time, and the need for a Messiah and change. When humanity's needs have been lowered to the very basic laws of humanity and are based only on the limited, five senses of taste, touch, smell, sight, and hearing (and are prone to error), with sight and hearing in the forefront, God responds with an unfathomable love.

Jesus knew, that in order to reach the people of his time, and in order for them and all who came after them to be saved, he had to draw them away from self and back towards the transcendental consciousness, which deals with God and the things of God.

As in today, the human consciousness at that time was also something that was conditioned not only by individuals in power, but also by those in charge of groups of people, whether it be interest groups, companies, societies, governments, nations, and so forth. Unanswered promises, scandal, death of innocents, and death of the innocents' trust in established religions are at the heart of, lack of, and unbelief in God.

Back in Jesus' time, Judaism guided its adherents in both practice and belief. As the Torah says nothing on the afterlife, no one was sure if the soul could exist without the body. Some believed that the righteous would ascend and enjoy a second life in Olam Ha Ba,[121] and the bad people will go to Gehenna, limited to twelve months. Some believed it was more important to live a good life here. In any event, it was the concept that the Messiah would be born poor, die, and then be resurrected that would stir controversy. This is written in 1 Corinthians 15:19-20: "If we hoped in a Messiah in this life only, we are of all men most to be pitied. But now the Messiah has been raised from the dead, and thus is the first fruit of those who are asleep." No matter what the belief of the group, without a doubt followers were affected and lived accordingly; and each of these shapes its members according to what it feels is best for the "survival of that group and its goals."

---

[121] In relation to Jewish eschatology, 'world to come'. – Ed.

LESSON 75

DOOR #5 CITING DISPARITIES BETWEEN THE HUMAN SPIRIT AND THE TRANSCENDENTAL TRUTH; THE THINGS OF GOD LABELED HERESY, TO WHOM BELONGS THE POWER AND THE GLORY?

Anytime a teaching goes beyond the material or rational human consciousness, especially that which involved miracles or the supernatural, either fear or denial, grips people. Jesus was not exempt from this, and His miracles were often deemed sorcery by the Pharisees, especially He was doing something which came from outside their priesthood. So, after witnessing his miracles, it was only natural that they accused Him of sorcery.

> "The chief priests, temple priests, Pharisees, Sadducees, and Sanhedrin, accused him of many things (Mark 15:3). "Then one possessed by a demon, blind and mute, was brought to him and he healed him, so that the blind and mute man both spoke and saw. And all the people were amazed and asked "is not this man the son of David? But the Pharisees, having heard it said, "This man does not cast out demons, but by Beelzebub the prince of the demons." And Jesus knew their thoughts and said to them, "Every kingdom divided against itself is brought

to desolation; and every city or house divided against itself will not subsist." (Matthew 12:22-25)

This darkness that surrounded Jesus was not just limited to outsiders; it also came from within those who would follow him and claimed they loved him. There were witnesses who were cured by Jesus who came forward at the "influence" of the chief priests and Pharisees, who then in turn gathered a council to set in addition to others' false testimony and charges of sorcery against Jesus. The way they manipulated it was by saying that he was doing extraordinary things that were inexplicable, and which can only come from evil. Eye witnesses to his walking on water and raising the dead increased his following greatly each day.

To let him go on, more and more people would start to believe He was truly the Son of God. This made the Pharisees and Jewish leaders very scared. They also feared that the Romans would rob them of their place and destroy the Jewish nation, making their autonomy impossible, and, therefore, He must be discredited and eliminated.

Without the transcendental consciousness, all of these things were seen as leading Israel astray and into apostasy.[122]

Eeshans feel that is why and how the transcendental truths (the divine substance) behind the teachings of Jesus were eliminated in order that a particular goal be reached and/or keep everything status quo.

---

[122] Taken from the Babylonian Talmud, which is a commentary on Jewish laws composed between A.D. 500–600 [Neusner/Green, p.69]. This is a text about Jesus and his death. The Tractate Sanhedrin [43A] and [Lenski, 225, Acts 10:39, Galatians 3:13, Geldenhuys 649–670, John 11:47–48, cf John 11:48 and many more describe all of the above to include Christ's Passover, His arrest, scourging, death on the cross, and more. – Ed.

LESSON 76

DOOR #6 NEW AGE OR NEW KNOWLEDGE

Things that Jesus was very much attuned to, things he talked and taught about (such as light, energy, vibrations, chakras) are still considered today by many as "pagan" ideas and practices, including the zodiac and stones and crystals, etc., which were, and are, still considered as belonging to the realm of magic, witchcraft, and sorcery, and are seen as somehow threatening. Yet, the Ark of the Covenant utilized many of these at the request of God. Would you believe essential oils and different mineral elixirs frighten Catholics/Christians; however, they are all part of the Ayurveda and holistic natural medicines used effectively today, and passed on from generation to generation, and these were also used in biblical times, since there was no medicine as we have today? Yes, still considered 'New Age,' it is redefined, and when put in a book listed "natural remedies or holistic medicine," so it does not pose a threat.

When you look to science and medicine today, you will find how the above have already been implemented into our lives. Who wouldn't rather use garlic instead of an antibiotic? Or who would use frankincense instead of an anti-inflammatory? What if just by your zodiac sign you can determine what illnesses you are prone to? Or what if you were told that the use and benefits of switching from regular white table salt to Himalayan, or sea salt, is against your religion, even though people travel to the Dead Sea and the Salt Lake in Utah for their benefits and that doctors agree? How about if there are people who are afraid of Yoga, or chakra cleansing, because they were told they are 'pagan,' or sins against God; however, Jesus Himself as a human, studied, learned, and taught these in the far east, in order to deepen meditation before he traveled back to his homeland? These practices helped bring to his followers from all regions not only the realities of those things transcendental, but also especially the *unfathomable* truths of the Eucharist, and his being the Light of the world. As people from all surrounding regions came to hear Him and be healed, Jesus used and shared his knowledge of these other cultures, which served to show that God is NOT confined, or restricted, to a particular religion, and that isolating God's light under a bushel basket does not promote growth, love, sharing talent, and skills with which to generate new ideas but causes phobia and the imagination to become darkened. Therefore, not only can we not hide our light, but we have no right to hide the "Light of the world."

Did you know the use of essential oils were used for illness and anointing back in biblical times? Stones, semi-precious and precious, were used on the Ark of the Covenant, as well as on the High Priest ephod (breastplate).[123] What if by studying your blood type and your name that your personality, diet, and health issues can be determined? Well, it's true.

Eeshans know that one way to protect a system of beliefs is to base everything on only part of the truth that works to your advantage, and to demand the elimination of anything, or anyone, that threatens the end result of a goal. There was no difference back when Jesus began teaching, in lieu with what we are facing today.

Eeshans present the following examples of such acts and deeds over the centuries with regards to Jesus and the methods He used to accomplish the goals of uniting people by the realization that we are all God's children.

---

[123] This was the garment used by the High Priest which contained the 12 stones and the Urim and Thummim—which were oracular means to question God and receive 'answers' about courses of action to be taken. These means were considered approved divine communication, compared to Jesus' own communication with God and the miracles he performed which were, by contrast, deemed 'sorcery' by the religious authorities. However, Jesus performed his miracles not from an outside source, but were from within because of who he was: he was *God*. – Ed.

LESSON 77

DOOR #7 WHO HAS THE RIGHT TO DECIDE WHO SHOULD RECEIVE CHRIST AND WHO SHOUDN'T, IF CHRIST WELCOMED EVERYONE, EVEN WOMEN WHO WERE FROM SHUNNED CULTURES, SUCH AS THE SAMARITAN WOMAN

Though the Eeshan Religion and Spirituality only cites the questions of error(s) as far back as the Old testament, i.e., the story of Adam and Eve, up to, and, including Peter, as Christ's stumbling block at the time of Christ, we decided to list a few examples of how a religion can continue to manifest 'truth' of a particular avatar, as defined by a particular religion, and still have its own political goals met, and still survive in the midst of undisputable error.

What if, in all that we were told, for example, "necessary steps were taken to protect the sacred," yet you found, or discovered, that there were a lot of missing references, with no explanation that filled the gaps of mystery, and better explained a teaching than without it? Would you feel the same, or would you want to examine all that was found along with what you were given?

There are many examples of the use of power of the church throughout history and this use of power was not necessarily used for the good. We know, for a fact, that there were many disagreements with regards to what was being taught and what the people thought and felt; thus, leading to the many protestant denominations, as well as the break of the

Orthodox from the papacy and western Christianity. In regards to some editions of the Talmud, from 1239–1775, the Roman Catholic church, at various times, either forced the censoring of parts of the Talmud that were theologically problematic for the church, or simply just ordered the destruction of copies of the Talmud. Could they have contained excerpts of Jesus and Mary Magdalen's marriage, or writings on the controversial leadership of Peter? Why would they have done this? It would serve two purposes: 1) The Jews could have put the details in there in order to discredit Jesus as the Messiah (So-called messiah married to a prostitute, etc.); while, 2) the church would seek its removal in order to erase any possible reference to Jesus being married. Opposite sides of an issue (in this case the identity of the Messiah and Savior), can, hereby, be seen as benefitting one another willingly, or unwillingly, and, yet, together serve the same goal.

Eeshans present that this is absolutely possible. Examples of how the church controlled not just those things within her own institution but also outside of it there are seen in these moments in time also such events as during the Middle ages in which a series of debates on Judaism were staged by the Roman church and by converts, including the Disputation of Paris (1240), Disputation of Barcelona (1263), and Disputation of Tortosa (1413–14), because it claimed that the Talmud contained insulting references to Jesus. Therefore, numerous times between 1239–1775, numerous copies were destroyed, or censored. Following the invention of the printing press, the Talmud was banned by the Pope. Other printed editions were censored. In 1559, it was placed on the Roman Index and banned. In 1592, the pope ordered all copies of the Talmud, and other heretical writing, destroyed, whether expunged or not. The total prohibition was in place until 1775, but the censorship remained in force. As a result, many references to Jesus were removed, or changed, and subsequent manuscripts sometimes omitted the passages in question entirely.[124,125]

---

[124] "Jesus in the Talmud." Wikipedia, Wikimedia Foundation, 16 Nov. 2019, en.wikipedia.org/wiki/Jesus_in_the_Talmud.

[125] It is not generally known that Jesus appears to be written about in the Talmud, but one can consult the existing research done by scholars and see the numerous references to a "Jesus" who is guilty of various improprieties and sins against God and Israel, ranging

Door #7 Who Has the Right to Decide Who Should Receive Christ / 313

Just in these instances alone, we feel our suspicions are justified in citing the case for the reasons we feel these are perfect examples of what is behind the expunging and destruction of any and all passages surrounding Jesus' marriage to Mary Magdalen, thus showing that the patriarchal religious authorities coveted and replaced Mary's role in the plan of salvation under Peter's name, which resulted in failing in its responsibility (due to the lack of attention) to safeguard the spiritual needs of God's people. This problem was essentially inherited from the presiding religious culture of that time and it still continues up to present times.

In the case as to why the decision was made to separate, and remove, the ending to the Lord's prayer (given by Jesus himself and honored by believers in reciprocal response in early centuries) from the Faithfull's liturgical practice, by those whose spirits were moved by the "Holy Spirit," we present it to you, the reader, to discern:

"For Thine is the Kingdom, the power and the glory, forever and ever! Amen."

How could this be taken out, especially when praying the Our Father? We are simply told that "there was no doxology," meaning that this wasn't part of the original prayer. How sad is it that when the people are moved by the Holy Spirit to use it, and it is rejected, even though it was evidently

---

from his coveting an innkeeper's wife and being a frivolous student under a prominent rabbi who practiced magic and turned to idolatry (Sanhedrin 107, Sot47a); He was sent away in his early years for misinterpreting a word which He should have understood and to the practice of sorcery and magic through which He led other Jews into apostasy (b Sanhedrin 43a-b); other references include Jesus' punishment in the afterlife being boiled in excrement (b Git56b, 57a), His execution (b Sanhedrin 43a-b), and so on. There are many other references too numerous to mention at this time, but suffice it to say for this context that Jesus was a problem for both the Jews, who had to show proof of his not being the messiah so as to eliminate the risk of further converts among those who hear about Him, and the church, who took drastic measures to ensure there were no possible references to women, especially his wife. Surprisingly, in lieu of all that was censored: beyond his not being the Messiah, but to include His being sent away for "misunderstanding a word"(yet he IS the 'Word'), His misconduct and sorcery charges, along with his being outside what the religion of the time was holding as 'common truths' (i.e., treatment of women, and/or his being the source of his power as God) the Catholic church still refers to the Jewish religion as "our elder brothers in faith". – Ed.

scripturally based, and inspired by the Holy Spirit, as well as intended to increase fervor and direct the intention of the *faithful*.

One should remember that over the centuries, many, many prayers came from ordinary people, as well as saints. and were readily accepted. What a shame that this little add-on was permanently left out, when, in fact, it gave such honor to God. It is the absence, or rejection, of these little efficacious prayers that we believe affects the personal faith of the people as a whole.

LESSON 78

DOOR #8 FAITH

Jesus' teaching revealed how the transcendental form of consciousness rises above the physical world, along with all that happens in it, with regards to human thinking and the way it is shaped. Interestingly enough, faith was key to attaining the fullness of what all those who followed him had who may NOT have understood but believed because He said so.

Transcendental consciousness is the path to enlightenment, but faith provides for the desire, and the fortitude necessary, in conjunction with meditation, prayer, and fasting, for this consciousness. Today, as back in Jesus' time, these were deemed weak, frivolous, and unrealistic, ineffective methods in comparison to the tools of fear, intimidation, oppression, force, and the power and violence of war. Living during a very volatile time, the one most powerful tool Jesus knew and used then, as well as what He looks for now, is to reach the people in ways that would restore their faith. Faith in Him with complete trust in who He is, is based on spiritual *apprehension*, rather than proof. That is why he said, 'Blessed are they who have not seen and yet believe.'

What Jesus did was to always use the most effective way to reach people, and the most effective method is by drawing on people's *experience*. Unless a person experiences what He was teaching, He could not show the power of faith, or the love of God. One such way to build faith in God is to reset priorities and to show that there is no limit to the power of faith, and how it touches the very heart of God. For example, He knew that limited encounters with one's own, or a beloved's mortality, makes the person realize the temporary nature of life and the passing of all things. He knew that how one thinks and feels at a funeral, or after a brush with death, suddenly opens their eyes as to how much they really love those around them, and what is most important in life; and to this day, when we are in this situation, we respond the same way. A brush with mortality causes us to rethink the way we are currently living. It causes us to see what a gift it is to be alive; and it compels us to reach out to people we haven't spoken to, forgive more easily, and to try to reconnect with family and old friends. This is sometimes thought of as a 'rude' awakening, but it is preferably known as *vairagya*, a point of view where one sees one's life in perspective against the backdrop of eternity, and what truly matters in life comes quickly and profoundly into perspective and focus.

Experiences such as these shake one out of the 'sleep' that human beings essentially live in during most of their waking hours where they do not consider the temporary nature of human life, or how important loved ones are, or tell themselves they have no real connection to, or sense a priority with regards to anyone but themselves. It literally lets us see how much time we have wasted obsessing over mundane practical tasks when we could be making better use of our time helping to better ourselves and/or properly care for others.

At one time or another, *vairagya*, at its peak in the moment, resonates through our hearts and 'makes a compelling case' for us to see clearly those priorities that should 'always' guide our lives. It should make us more determined to live life as though each day could be the beginning of a fresh start, or perhaps thinking how this day could be our last. The power of *vairagya* makes everything, quite clear. In this one moment, our priorities are realigned without conscious thought, but by intuition; but *vairagya* lasts only a short time, leaving us to forget, and go on with our life as we had before, in a kind of sheep-led existence.

Knowing this, the perfectly enlightened man, Jesus, used *vairagya*. Raising a child from the dead, the widow's young son who was brought back from the dead, and, of course raising his friend Lazarus after he had been dead for three days, restored faith in those who witnessed these events; but the acknowledgment of the faith of the Centurion with regard to his servant by Jesus (who told Jesus he believed he would be healed just by Jesus' word) shows us that the less faith we have the less we esteem Jesus, and the more faith we have the less we esteem ourselves.

The works and miracles Jesus performed showed the value of life as seen by those for whom He performed the miracles, but more than that, they also showed the lack of faith He was met with. as prophesied, and, at times, by His having to point it out. Faith helped to establish the power of God with regards to overcoming illness and death. This was a step towards showing people that all things can be, and are, restored through this faith in Him as God intended.

Reconnecting with our transcendental consciousness creates an awareness where *vairagya* becomes more a way of *steady thinking and lifestyle*, rather than just for a temporary time. What happens is *vairagya* is the detachment, or renunciation, of all we felt was so important, until life happens, or in this case, death. Why? Because it increases the richness of heart-felt love, while at the same time helps one to arrange priorities in life more wisely.

Jesus knew that with this faithless people He could use *vairagya* to instill in them faith in God. Subsequently He would follow up these with a teaching. perhaps, on light, or His existence before Abraham showing His divinity, or any number of things that could be used to lead his followers to 'enlightenment.'

Providing examples and miracles, and teaching one's responsibility before God is the direction Jesus was taking every man, woman, and child He taught. Love God with your whole heart, your whole soul, your whole mind, and your whole being; and love your neighbor as yourself, as God's love is the path of transcendental thinking, since it is the way of God who is the perfect transcendental Being.

LESSON 79

DOOR #9 JESUS AND MARY, LIGHT OF THE WORLD: THEN, NOW, ALWAYS

Consciousness arises from the soul, or that inner light of awareness, and this aspect is eternal, in contradistinction to the body and the senses connected with it, which are temporary. They arise and they disappear through the natural process of this world of birth and death, especially if one lacks a Spirituality with a system of morals that connects with one's inner values and God-centeredness.

That is why it is important to keep the transcendental alive, maintaining the *vairagya* in our consciousness, especially when we are raising children while properly setting their priorities for which you and all adults are obliged to do in this world. You want the child to learn decency, wholesomeness, and an understanding of your beliefs with good reasons for why you teach these things via your life and actions. There is constant change and flux with the material world, and the body changes right along with it; therefore, without spirituality, the *vairagya* coming into being, after a brief period, passes away.

One must remember that the mind and senses are not the person, but the soul, which radiates the inner light of awareness, 'is' the person. To further move his people, Jesus knew He had to deal with those who have lived their lives away, not just from the rational mind, but from the emotional mind also. This is why he was called the Divine Physician. Not only was He a doctor of the physical healing, but He was also one of mind, body, and spirit. Jesus identified Himself as the 'Light of the world' for many reasons. As He (and His wife, as One) is the Light from which *our light bodies will come* via the Eucharist of the Marriage Feast, all who heard, loved, and believed in Him, had to be led into the Mystery of this holy and sacred mystical Eucharist. In doing so, these would become the leaven or the extensions of them. Unlike the unleavened bread from which everyone ate, Jesus taught that the Eucharist of the Marriage Feast is the leaven from which we become the extensions of the 'Light of the world,' and are to radiate this Divine light throughout the world by becoming part of him and his wife—*and not just mystically.*

The light body is contained within the subtle body, which gives it its form. It is an actual grid work of light and sacred geometry that brings together your physical, emotional, mental, and spiritual being. It radiates light energy, and electromagnetically links your multidimensional self with the infinite universe, and when in union with Jesus and his Wife, operates at the highest frequency of spiritual light. Because of their body, blood, soul, and divinity, it no longer operates the way that it used to. It now operates as a vehicle for the properties of God's Light and radiates these properties at all levels. It incorporates energy fields, but it also consists of the cellular structure of each organ, the molecule of each physical cell, the atoms of each molecule, the electrons and subatomic particles of each atom. It becomes capable of influencing the genetic code and chromosomal structure, which gives rise to personal traits and characteristics of the person. Mental and emotional transformation by these higher frequencies of spiritually divine light and life is where a new and different consciousness arises.

It is also important to remember that this gross physical body, which we use each day, *is not solid*, but contains crystallized, or coagulated, energy that is held together by a level of vibration only to dissolve back into energy at the end of our life. That is why, as we tend to focus only on the physical aspects of our body, we should also understand the other systems unfamiliar to us. We know of the circulatory, the endocrine, and cardio-vascular systems, and the more recent chemical and electrical systems, or "communications systems" to name a few; however, one should, through spirituality, become familiar with the vibratory and chakra energy systems of the body, as well as the other levels to include the subtle body. These, of course, were labeled taboo teachings even though they are most important in understanding Jesus and the Plan of

Salvation. In other words, for a better understanding of how we return to our transcendental form, we must understand the light body. Once we understand the light body, it becomes easy to see how, when the new energy of Jesus being the divine masculine part of God, along with his divine consort, enters into us by virtue of the Eucharist containing the divine love, light, hope, and joy, most assuredly transforms us by, once again, restoring the sacred balance, which connects us wholly to our transcendental origin, spiritually free of the obstacles due to entropy, allowing faith to heal our mind, body, and soul. This is 'why 'one cannot be in mortal sin and receive the Marriage Feast Eucharist without first getting absolved.

LESSON 80

DOOR #10 THE ULTIMATE TRANSCENDENTAL EXPERIENCE

THE EUCHARIST OF THE MARRIAGE FEAST: WHAT DOES IT DO AND WHY IS IT NECESSARY?

The Eucharist of the Marriage Feast of the Lamb and His wife is the ultimate transcendental salvific experience. Because from the moment we consume this precious Sacred Food it causes us to be ushered immediately into God and God into us, simultaneously. When we consume this Spiritual Food (that contains within it all the Mysteries of the Marriage Feast as intended for our salvation), the energies of mind and emotion that we call thought and feeling,[126] through this introduction of spiritual Light, become a new energy pattern. This energy pattern resonates with, and increasingly conforms to, the Divine inner nature of each human being. This further emphasizes why mortal sin is contrary to divinity, and, thus, condemns the soul to hell.

This in turn, will be manifested differently, since it affects the physical, mental, and emotional being, and since it separates out light and darkness at each level of experience, amplifying, and merging with that which is already light-filled within the self, and releasing and dissolving what is not capable in its essence of joining with the higher frequencies of light. This enables the consciousness that we have held within us for x-amount

---

[126] Wonderfully explained in newlightbody.org.

of years, the ability to change and transform, and desire to become the Divine blueprint God intended for us all along. What this means is that this faith, hope, love, and desire for what Jesus has given us enables us to stay in the state of communion with the Divine Nature of and with God.[127] By living in the state of grace, or purification, we would be living in a sacred and self-aware life on all levels, within this physical realm and beyond.[128] That is why He taught about one's inner light being put on a lampstand, so that all may see by it. In this sense, He is guiding our light body, and in turn we guide others back to him. Only the Eucharist of the Marriage Feast can bring that immortal part of us that can rise above the material world, and its darkness, towards him, thus making us divinized. This is the means by which we may live transcendentally once again.

Identifying himself as the "Light of the world," Jesus revealed He was more than just an enlightened man, but that He truly is God; and He does, as does His eternal consort, continue to awaken our inner light bodies with his words the moment we acknowledge Him. Simply put, it is necessary for us to transform back into light to enter into heaven, and that is why there are just a few humans who have been allowed to enter heaven with gross physical bodies: Jesus, the Virgin Mary, and Mary Magdalen. Jesus used the gifts of healing the sick, bringing people back to life, and walking on water to quantify his being the Light par excellence. That is why the connection of our light body to his is vital for eternal life.

Comparing the earthly consciousness with the transcendental, and the need to nourish the souls and consciousness with light food, witnesses to the fullness of the person of Christ as was expressed in his words:

---

[127] Beyo, David Dogan. "(14)-1-31 August 2009—Love Peace and Harmony Journal." Scribd, Scribd, 2009, www.scribd.com/document/386167788/14-1-31-August-2009-Love-Peace-and-Harmony-Journal.

[128] The above passages were adapted from newlightbody.org to further help explain what the Eucharist does for us when consumed, adding to the explanation of supramentalization of the Wife of the Lamb. The hallmark of Perennial Wisdom is evidenced in many places. – Ed.

"Your fathers ate the manna in the wilderness, and are dead. This is the Bread which comes down from heaven, that one may eat of it and not die. I am the living bread which came down from heaven. If anyone eats this bread, he will live forever; and the bread that I shall give is the flesh, which [we] will give for the life of the world."

Thus, this Eucharist is revealed as our "Light Food for the Light Being" within us, which connects everyone with God just as Jesus divinized his wife Mary, and desired that through them, with them and in them, *we* are divinized, and we once again connect to God perfectly.

This is that Light Food which counters the ingestion of the apple which led Adam and Eve away from the transcendental into the physical human consciousness. This and only this perfect Light Food is what is required for salvation for within it is contained the mysteries of God necessary to restore life back to what God intended all the way back to the creation of His most treasured created being—the human being.

Sadly, Christ's command was 'not' obeyed, but, instead, Eeshans maintain that it was *altered*. It was altered to serve the desires of man, presenting the Eucharist as being only the person of Jesus Christ sans His marriage to Mary Magdalen, who, though being his *passive* consort of that time, was necessary as co-redeemer in God's plan. In doing so, it not only cost us the fullness of what Jesus wanted for us, but without the ingestion of the body, blood, soul, and divinity of Jesus and His wife Mary as One, we lost the opportunity first to see clearly the fullness of God's plan, and, second, the opportunity to be freed from the bondage of the slavery to iniquity, and inequality, with discrimination as the consequence for ignoring this truth. This made the power of the truth weak and without cause lost the power necessary for positive change in the world.

Without the belief in the power of Christ's life, marriage, death, and resurrection what people received only served to lock them down spiritually even more, since the world knew Jesus and His wife. This time, God's people were enslaved within the system of beliefs under Peter in what was supposed to be freedom to soar with the Christs. Often, Catholics are asked this question: "If it's true that the Eucharist is truly God, why then aren't you down on your knees before Him in the Blessed Sacrament?" Well, maybe they were moved by the spirit, and saw what they have witnessed was not the Truth, and *that* is why people do not respond as they should.

Eeshans question, "If what was/is taught as truth by the church regarding the Eucharist, meaning that we consume Jesus' body, blood, soul, and divinity, then why have His people made so little change for the better in the world?" Ironically, Jesus Christ's legacy is that of peace and love. Where is peace? Where is love? As God is the source of these, we may conclude that without God these moral qualities of mind, heart, and spirit cannot be found. What *is* true is that we need *God* to love God, and we need God to love our neighbor. We need the spiritual food Jesus promised, which has to be God and, in fact, *is* God, not just for our own sake, but for the sake of the world and all who are in it. For only with this Food can we be the leaven necessary to lead people back to Jesus and Mary Magdalen.

LESSON 81

DOOR #11 THE FAMINE

THE CAUSE AND FATE

The prophetic famine has always been a source of concern throughout the ages. Eeshans believe that the famine is already upon us, but not in the way the human consciousness connotes. We always attribute famine to those countries where millions of people are starving. Some attribute it to the crisis of food here in our own country. Few feel that the prophecy could be related to 'spiritual food.' There is no wonder that this is the furthest thought from humankind's mind, since religion and spirituality don't seem to solve these issues; but organized religion has often appeared to be the cause. Even with respect to Jesus, those religions which claim Jesus founded them, are usually at the center point of the problems we face today and result in the corresponding lack of belief.

By virtue of the fact that discrimination between genders, religions, cultures, or over beliefs, age, sexual orientation etc., it would appear that Christ's mission here on earth, by man's deduction, and the purpose for which He came into this world, to suffer and die-seems to have *failed*. Despite our differences, love should abound, and so should kindness. Eeshans believe that if the truth had continued to be taught after Christ ascended, this would have set us free; for Christ did exactly that.

Today's religious skeptics claim that what is taught is a myth, and is not the Truth. The stigma of organized religion is one of shame and guilt, causing one to become dysfunctional, which lowers our consciousness with false notions about living life with God.

The Eucharist, who/which is believed by some and doubted by others, is as debated as was the issue of Jesus being God and Man, or both, etc. Even though he Himself said he was God, the truth of this was debated long after He ascended back into heaven; and still today even within the church. Think of it, if we can't believe the Word himself as to who He is and says He is, and we can disagree and debate on what He commanded as necessary for our salvation, who is this Jesus we are following, or better: why follow Him? To debate the two most important truths regarding Him, how then is He the key to salvation? So Eeshans conclude that there are still those who don't believe Jesus is the Son of God, some think he was just a prophet, and others don't believe that the Real Presence of Christ is in the Eucharist. So, these people obviously also think that it is not a necessity to eat his body and drink his blood in real time for our salvation. All of these disbeliefs successfully make Jesus no more than a man, and no greater than a prophet.

The Truth is: in many ways, these 'misconceived facts' have some truth to them if you consider that not all that has been handed down since Peter is true. It was "dimidiated:" *and made to look like the whole.*[129] We say this because whenever any human being dares to alter that which is God's, and still expects the same results promised by God, they are not only sadly mistaken, but, in fact, have committed a most grievous transgression against the Divine Will because they have tampered with the plan of Salvation. One needs only to see how the world is in chaos to see the consequences of doing so.

The prophetic famine, mistakenly taken as lack of food for the impoverished, grows because of the lack of the 'food necessary for the life of souls;' and because the Eucharist, taught to only be Jesus, has not been the fullness of what was promised by God, or given to us by Jesus. However, God is gracious, and that is why being only part of the whole, it could only sustain God's people for a short time, which is barely over

---

[129] By carefully controlling information and perceptions of pivotal theological references like the story of Adam and Eve, the church was able for a very long time to leave out Mary Magdalen's role and focus exclusively on Jesus,' to the "Frog in the Well" effect: i.e., the frog that lived its whole life at the bottom of a well had no concept of a world that existed above the entrance. – Ed.

2000 years, before it fell from being a directive to being only an option. Today, due to the lack of faith, the scandals within the church, and the desire to guide oneself, even one's personal innate desire to seek Christ in the church's Eucharist is becoming less and less, and feared to become non-existent.

The true Eucharist was to bring with it the following:

1. The energies of mind and emotion that we call thought and feeling,[130] through this introduction of spiritual Light, forms a new energy pattern. This energy pattern resonates with, and increasingly conforms to, the Divine inner nature of each human being.
2. It is supposed to create physical, mental and emotional effects on each human being as Jesus intended, and it can separate out light and darkness at each level of experience, amplifying and merging with that which is already light-filled within the self, and releasing and dissolving what is not capable in its essence, of joining with the higher frequencies of light. This enables the consciousness that we have held within us for x amount of years, the ability to change and transform and desires to become the Divine blueprint God intended for us all along. What this means is that this faith, hope, love, and desire for what Jesus has given us is needed to enable us to stay in the state of Communion with the Divine Nature of and with God.
3. The outward manifestation of anything apart from the Marriage Feast Eucharist is likened to temporal food. What has been offered to God's people is not the transcendental Food for Life, which Jesus taught, lived, and died for, so that we may be saved but a poor imitation likened to giving watered down milk to infants and is only mandatory a couple times a year; which means there is enough to keep alive the soul alive for a while, but not enough nourishment to sustain life for a long period of time and certainly allows for life and eternal life-threatening deficiencies.

---

[130] As wonderfully explained in newlightbody.org.

As we profess, Eeshans conclude, that the Eucharist that has been offered over the past 2000-plus years, is absolutely *not* the fullness of Jesus' promise, which came out of His marriage to Mary Magdalen, because that Bread from Heaven never reached Christ's followers; the people only received what 'man 'felt was all that was necessary.

Even as it may be half of what God intended for us, it is not what Christ came to earth for, not what the purpose was for his marriage, and not what He taught about, and what was instituted for salvation through the ages until the end of time. In its 'watered down' version, though it is sought for love of Jesus, and strength to endure whatever life brings, the people may only be reaping the benefits, and not the *fullness or the nourishment for the soul*, as he commanded; and is being received mostly by the faithful elderly, and even then only out of a sense of obligation. Fewer and fewer young people seek Jesus in this form. Why? Simply put, sadly, they feel betrayed; and do not find faith nor have they witnessed what was promised.

Possessing the light food, the Bread from Heaven, that brings with it the mystery of and solutions for ending the so called 'curse' or consequences of a choice which prevented humans from returning to their rightful place with God through the Sacraments, has become an option. Again, this makes sense.

As it stands, when a part of the original is altered, it is no longer the original, and, therefore, the end result is changed. What happens to the faithful is the same as any member of the Catholic religion who believes what they have been told, and, that is the members will seek out "any kind of help from God' when they are dying, but not as a source of strength throughout their lifetime. What does this mean? It means they will have the benefits of God's mercy, since God's people are not at fault.

What will happen to those who disbelieve or need proof? That is why God brought into existence the Eeshan Religion. Jesus tells us that after all He has done, if you still won't believe, you will be judged accordingly, since, "If I had not come and spoken to them, they would not be guilty of sin; but now they have no excuse for their sin." (John 15:22). In other words, you can't say "I believe in Jesus and who he is," and then ignore His directives, especially since Christ is providing yet another opportunity through the Divine Feminine to come back.

This is serious. Despite what one wants to believe, without the reception of the true Eucharist, this may be the difference between eternal life and eternal death. This means that the inner Light of awareness, which was a necessary factor in the Plan of Salvation, is now available, but if it is rejected, this Light will be *removed*, along with its ability to transform us physically, mentally, and spiritually. One would, without a doubt, be no longer connected to the Divine. Once again, humanity would have lost the means to radiate the properties of God, at all levels, thereby, losing the ability to be the leaven and to affect the energy fields that surround individuals, transmitting positive currents corresponding to the qualities of thoughts, emotion, and higher consciousness that we all carry. What has certainly been absent before, and is the purpose of Jesus' coming into this world, would be lost, this time, forever.

Almost immediately from the moment Jesus was incarnate, up to and including His ascension to heaven, this is the gift that had already been put into effect. However, after Jesus returned to heaven, Peter would not/could not leave his human consciousness, as predicted by Jesus, and, thus, truly became the stumbling block to Jesus' work. Peter and his successors' refusal were proven by the 'altered bread' that was given in place of the Bread from Heaven, all out of covetousness of Mary's place with Jesus. This decision was made and carried out without remorse. and passed along from generation to generation. He was called Simon Peter, and by his example his name will be known from generation to generation. **Oh Peter, you failed to feed his lambs, feed his lambs, feed his sheep.**

LESSON 82

GENESIS 1:26-27, STATES THE ELOHIM WERE MASCULINE AND FEMININE

Being born human, God would then have to mirror the image presented in Genesis 1:26-27, which states that the *Elohim* 'were' (plural), masculine and feminine, and humans were made in their likeness. The likeness of His Father and Mother, Jesus as the Son of God, would mirror all of What and Who the Father is as the Divine Masculine. Being omnipotent and infinite, He would be totally God and totally human, not a demigod. After his death and resurrection, He would also become known solely for the dimidiated salvific mission for which the second person of the Trinity came.

As God, being male and female in an uncreated human form, Jesus would then have an Eternal Consort, to marry for the perfect representation of God on earth, just as the original first parents of Adam and Eve. Using the feminine noun occurs in a substratum manner, such as in references to man's being created with the use of the earth and by God, who would bring the end to eternal death by His conquering death by his resurrection. He and His wife were destined to becoming to humankind the transcendental food necessary for the light body housed within the gross physical body, and for the purposes of realizing eternal life, or in other words, for salvation. Because of their mission as co-Saviors and co-Redeemers, there is access once more to the transcendental world of heaven.

LESSON 83

IS THERE A HELL? A NEW REVELATION?

HEAVEN IS ABOVE, HELL IS BELOW

Contrary to what others want to believe, Hell is a physical place where everlasting death is found. This still rings true despite the Pope's opinion of recent memory.[131] One cannot dismiss what God has created, though over the years, it appears those in religious authority believe they can.

When Jesus spoke of hell, He did not do so in a metaphoric way, or even in a spiritual sense. He spoke of it as an actual "place."

Hell is in the earth's core. It is hotter than the core of the sun. It is not just a 'state of mind,' but, rather, 'it' torments the mind, spirit, soul, and body. Jesus referred to the *physical* state, and sensation of a person, feeling consumed by the 'worm' that works its way through a carcass. Hell is not a transcendental world. Therefore, the pain, torments, and suffering there are real and never-ending.

Each of the counterparts of God are of each part of that Person of God. Whether divine or human, in this way Christ's church would be obliged to show the feminine complement to the masculine and their unified body. Being such, it would be duly obliged to beget as well as bring about *eternal life* through the human flesh of Jesus and Mary, who were also Divine when God said, "Go forth and multiply."

---

[131] Pope John Paul II, for example, 'updated' the Catholic understanding of Hell as being more a 'state of mind,' much in the same spirit that evil was also now more 'correctly' being taught as the 'absence of good'. – Ed

The fruit of all the persons of the one omnipotent God would be the means by which humankind would conquer death in a transcendental way, and, thus, bring about a new heaven and a new earth.

This '*rock*,' which is not capable of bearing the weight of its sin, will eventually fall apart. Though it was successful in keeping every member blind who remains loyal to it, as it was grounded in the human consciousness, beginning with Peter and on down through his successors, they are all bound to earth because it is not the kind of *rock* upon which you *build*. Instead of their works being recognized by Jesus, He outlined what was in store for any of them who made a fool of God and sinned against the Spirit. Obviously, Peter and his disciples would continue in their ways, despite all of Christ's warnings. So, what happened to Peter when he died? Well let's just take a look at all those souls that he cost Jesus and pray that he had contrition for what he had done, and what he had failed to do; since if He did not, one would pray that he wasn't counted among all those religious leaders, and those in authority, who took this path, since they are destined for Hell.[132]

Both Isaiah and Christ refer to "the worm" of those who are destined to go to Hell as those who will not die. This 'worm' takes on the look of the one who duped Adam and Eve. His was the face of a worm, a reptile. That means, this horrifying, terrible, gruesome place, houses "living" carcasses, which are prey to unrelenting predators, eternally.

Those who choose to deny this actual place are in denial themselves. For if they believe that because *they* say it's so, then God will hold their words as bound. How foolish to think that the church authorities aren't trying to do this and anything else that eliminates even the 'concept' of Hell, since to do this provides a kind of recompense for their own terrible sins.

Eeshans find it amazing that even though Hell is mentioned fifty-three times in the bible, and Jesus himself identified it, and talked about it, on many occasions, the church of Peter can deny its existence.

---

[132] As the saying goes, "The road to Hell is paved with good intentions." Perhaps too few consider the gravity of this as a real possibility, and prefer, unwisely, to presume upon God's mercy. – Ed.

But if there is a Hell, where is it? Throughout the history of myth, literature, and private revelations, Hell is located in the core of the earth. Even before scientific geological studies could be undertaken, there were always descriptions of extreme heat and molten conditions at the core of the earth. This turns out to be accurate, since such conditions do, in fact, exist; however, who could have known this all during the previous periods without an understanding of geology? Despite how ridiculous, or primitive, the claim of a devil in a molten hell in the center of the earth sounds to the 'rational' scientific mind of today, the physical descriptions of the center of the earth held for so long do, in fact, line up with modern science; and what's more, in the present context, we understand that Satan was exiled to the earth and bound to it. We know this from Christ's description of Hell as being made of fire and brimstone.

In fact, there are vents in the oceans that scientists say run so deep into the earth that fire spews out of them. What is inside these vents is called 'brimstone' and a fire so unimaginably hot that it continues to burn even beneath the water. Could this be a spiritually-based 'reality check' for the modern, skeptical mind?

Jesus not only spoke about Hell but gave warnings about it using different terms and descriptions, ranging from a garbage dump (Gehenna) to the torture chamber of Hades where there 'wailing and gnashing of teeth,' Thus, he spoke in detail of the place we call Hell in our language, long before modern science describes for us the contents of the earth's core. It makes one wonder.

In Matthew 23:33, Jesus speaks to the Pharisees, and says, "Snakes! Sons of vipers! From those who do nothing, even what little they have will be taken away. Now throw this useless servant into outer darkness where there will be weeping and gnashing of teeth."

In Matthew: 46 Jesus also says, "And they will go into eternal punishment (Hell), but the righteous will go into Eternal Life."

In Mark 9:43-48, Jesus says, "If your hand cause you to sin, cut it off. It's better to enter Eternal Life with only one hand than to go into the unquenchable fires of Hell with two hands; and if your foot causes you to sin ...," etc.

In Luke 6:24-26, Jesus says, "What sorrows await you who are fat and prosperous now, for a time of awful hunger awaits you who laugh now, for your laughing will turn to mourning and sorrow. What sorrows awaits you who are praised by the crowds, for their Ancestors also praised FALSE PROPHETS."

In Matthew 13:49-50 Jesus also says, "That is the way it will be at the end of the world. The angels will come and separate the wicked people from the righteous, throwing the wicked people into the fiery furnace, where there will be weeping and gnashing of teeth." (This is a comment that is meant to describe how intense the pain will be. Jesus' description is meant to show how one will bite down in response to such pain, anguish, and anger felt due to the separation from God).

With so much emphasis put on Hell, Eeshans agree that it is most unlikely that the church can, or has the right to go against Christ's teachings regarding Hell, especially if it is to assuage their own guilty conscience. It is most likely that those who chose to listen to Satan, or anyone who was warned but allowed Satan to sift them like wheat, will remain in an earthly place, since they cannot enter the transcendental one.

In Matthew 7:21-23 when Jesus also warns, "Not everyone who says to Me, 'Lord! Lord!' will enter the Kingdom of Heaven. Only those who do the will of God in Heaven will enter. On Judgment Day, many will say to me 'Lord! Lord! We prophesied, cast out demons in your name and performed many miracles in your name.' But I will reply, I never knew you. Depart from me, you evildoers (you who break *God's* laws) …" Could this also be in reference to Peter's refusal to heed Christ's warning regarding being so grounded in his birth religion that he is blinded by his own interests even in the face of God? It's no secret that Jesus had been so frustrated with the fact that Satan had his sights on Peter that He had to stress the fact that if Peter persisted in the way he was thinking and feeling, and being so caught up in jealousy and revenge, he may well have been on the way to warranting Hell?

How about you, reader? Do you recognize Satan, and how he waits and desires to sift you, and cause you to be blinded by what you so covet, that Jesus can't get through to you? Have you become so blind to your faults and weaknesses that you, too can, dismiss how serious they are before God? Remember, this is the same one who told Adam and Eve they would not die if they ate the apple, which was contrary to what God instructed them. Is this same being who tempted Christ with human temptations?

Can you see how this could be another probable reason why suspicion surrounds the vague rendition of the Marriage feast of Cana? To focus on noting only the nameless bridegroom and Jesus, as a guest taking action to make wine at his mother's request, and the fact that it was the first miracle Jesus performed. Not only does this make no sense whatsoever, but also Eeshans believe this story was placed in the forefront, and was most persistently and aggressively canvassed for all to believe. This was written defiantly to discourage any possible way to eliminate any 'means' that could link this wedding to Jesus and Mary, and foil Peter's plan to offset the true Salvation Plan.

Just think for a minute. If what the Pharisees were doing to the people caused Jesus to react with such anger as to call them hypocrites, dens/sons of vipers and snakes, etc., you can only imagine what He thinks of those who interfered with God's directive for humanity's salvation, and that is starting with Peter and it still continuing today.

The omission of Mary Magdalen makes Jesus' wife appear to be that much more threatening than once thought. Could it be that the church of Peter deemed her the 'woman who would crush the serpent's head, 'and having starved God's people, and the church, as the mock-bride, now becomes the harlot?

Jesus and Mary clearly taught how their marriage is the link to all the greatest mysteries of God, which again, begins with the fruit of their love and ends with the only means of salvation, which is the Sacrament and the Mystery of the Eucharist of the Marriage Feast.

The only antidote for salvation and the outward sign of this unfathomable truth, is Metta, which is the Eucharist of Love. With its origins in the Marriage Feast, it does, indeed, make the Eucharist from that church be seen as only symbolic of one reckless event, and not the means of regaining heaven.

The Eucharist of the Marriage Feast, by virtue of the fact that the genders of each person of the trinity were involved in the salvific plan, and by that right is the reason behind the Gospel passages where Jesus feeds the five thousand in order to teach that God is a leaven; and though it seemed an impossible task, Jesus told the apostles, to feed them, and those who were fed will eat and be satisfied ... prefiguring the Eucharist nourishing the soul. People understood feeding the body, so that is why Jesus would use the analogy beginning with the manna in the desert, which is the showbread he fed his apostles, and the feeding of the thousands who followed him. He spoke about wheat and leaven, which led to his bread of life discourse in John 6:47-58.

He continued to teach this, despite the fact that so many walked away from him after telling them that what they had to do was eat his flesh and drink his blood, otherwise they "would have no life in them." He held nothing back, since this is what they needed to acquire everlasting life; to not do this would result in their eternal death.

Jesus was more or less saying, "You could stay here and die in this exile or you can do what I command and live forever!" Even His apostles did not understand this teaching. We know this to be true because when Jesus became aware that His apostles were complaining about this, Jesus impatiently asks, in John 6:61, "Does this offend you? Then what if you see the Son of Man ascend to where he was before!" [In other words He was saying, "I bet it would make a difference if you saw me ascend to heaven right now"]. Once again, even though he was frustrated that He had to address the questionable looks and murmurings of his apostles, what He felt they should've been able to understand, or at least trust what he was saying, Jesus still, despite man's loss of any beatific vision, made use of the moment to show his love for human beings, God's most treasured creation.

In John 6, He continues, "The Spirit gives life; the flesh counts for nothing. These words I have spoken to you—they are full of the Spirit and life." *Mary* teaches us that in looking at Him, to remember that this is the same Word who continued to speak to Adam and Eve after their exile from their transcendental state of being, and through his conception, birth, life, marriage, passion, death, resurrection, and revelation, the Word continued in the person of Jesus Christ, who witnessed by, and shared with His wife, and this shows that His words make the continued divine, human, and sacramental relationship possible, once again, without interruption. By receiving, and becoming the Eucharist, those who follow will continue to follow Him and they will act as the leaven to the transcendental. All who come in contact with these will see this.

That is why the Holy Spirit, whose counterpart is the Divine Feminine, is necessary for human contact with God, and why she has returned for us. Since together the Holy Spirit/Divine Feminine is as necessary today, as with the Virgin for conception of their son Jesus, for the marriage of Jesus and Mary Magdalen, for the transubstantiation of bread and wine into the body, blood, soul, and divinity of Jesus Christ and his Wife, for the conception and birth of the one who is born Emmanuel. That is why it takes the Fruit of the love of Jesus and his wife to bring back the sacred hidden bread and drink in end times.

Since in these days, it is the Divine Feminine who encompasses the Man/God Jesus; and those who hear her words, will hear Him teaching as He did then, and will have eyes to see and ears to hear, since these will NOT be a rebellious people, but are those who are found at the highways and byways and invited to the Marriage Feast. These are identified as the remnant of the remnant.

LESSON 84

DOOR #12 WHERE ARE YOU GOING?

THAT'S NOT THE WAY, JUST A RANDOM PATH

We will continue to reveal Peter's long history of cowardice in following what Jesus taught, and his failure to let go of his birth religion throughout this book. We hold these beliefs as fundamental proponents in our Eeshan belief system. What we are presenting is not only a 'necessary proof,' as seen by Eeshans, but also we feel it is contingent to helping you to better see how Peter's leadership is the 'supposed' appointment by a very patriarchal religion, one meant to maintain a future in what they wanted people to see as Christ's religion, but according to the human rational consciousness; yet, it was not the official appointment by Jesus' hand. You will see how despite Jesus' warnings, Peter remained attached to the human consciousness and, thereby, was not able to follow Jesus to the transcendental. As Jesus points out, Peter was very dull in his understanding of the transcendental, or perhaps he was just not interested.

Could it be that Peter also did not thoroughly understand what Jesus was talking about vis-à-vis, therefore, he could not believe the Eucharist could be more than a representation of Christ? We say this because the Eucharist is not the primary focus in Peter's 'apparent' handwritten letters. In these, the focus is on good works, which is far from the Salvific Mission of Christ's Sacred Food.

Not having the "true Eucharist," i.e., the Spiritual Food (who is Jesus and Mary) that is necessary for salvation, which also finds its ROOTS in what was lost by Adam and Eve, subjects us to unforeseen attacks.

and does not allow us to be the leaven that is necessary to connect with all those who desire eternal life. In reality, it leaves them guiding themselves.

Let's not forget that 'patriarchal,' in this context, refers to Jesus without Mary; so if taken from the "patriarchal" description of the Eucharist, which would be Jesus' body, blood, soul, and divinity, as the essence of the Eucharist, one would expect that Peter, or his successors, could never allow the truth of the "actuality," and the necessity of the fact that the Eucharist was, indeed, the bodies of Christ *and his Wife*; Peter certainly would fall into this group of who guided themselves. This is not to say that Peter did not 'love' Jesus. We are not saying this at all. What we are saying is that Peter believed he loved Jesus more than Mary, as a woman could, because he was a man. Being a man entitled him to be seated by Jesus' right hand, the side of authority and importance.

That is why a true believer cannot fathom how, if he/she believes Jesus is God, and He is the Word of God, can pick and choose what directives to accept and which ones to ignore. The Bread who comes down from heaven is NOT an option. It is a command. Perhaps, we no longer understand that a command is an authoritative order, and this one comes from God. If you do not believe in this as the key, the ONLY possible way back to God, then there is no way that you can believe, nor should you try and enter into the other Mysteries/Sacraments. Why? Because all the other six derive their life from the Eucharist, and if one is serious about enlightenment, and all are seen as necessary for the preparation and acceptance of salvation *via the Eucharist*. The command/directive from Jesus that, "unless you eat my body and drink my blood, you will have not life in you" is not to be regarded as equal to all the unfathomable mysteries of God instituted by the Christs, but is the one, veracious directive, upon which all the other mysteries are dependent.

> "Many will say to me on that day, 'Lord, Lord, did we not prophesy in your name and in your name, drive out demons and in your name, perform many miracles?
> Then I will reply, 'I never knew you. Get away from me, you who break God's laws.'

> Therefore, anyone who listens to my teaching and follows it is wise, like a person who builds a house on rock.
> The rain came down, the streams rose, and the winds blew and beat against that house. It will not fall, because it had its foundation on the rock.
> But everyone who hears these words of mine and does not put them into practice is like a foolish person who built his house on sand.
> The rain came down. The streams rose, and the winds blew and beat against that house, and it fell with great crash. [cf. Matthew 7:22-28]

A perfect gospel reading with regards to an insolent and cowardly Peter being chastised by Jesus is found in Matthew 16:21–26, and serves as a prophecy regarding Peter's intentions and plans.

> Jesus' concern for Peter's continued outbursts of rage (which was sending conflicting messages to the others) caused Jesus to find an opportunity to call him out. It was now important that the others see the difference between human weakness in the form of concern and fear for oneself. To distinguish the two, we find the following manner in which Jesus showed the character of the whole.
> From that time Jesus began to show His apostles that He had to go to Jerusalem. On this particular day, Jesus began talking about how He would be rejected and suffer many things from the elders, chief priests, and legal experts; and that He had to be killed and raised on the third day. Peter took hold of Jesus and, scolding Him, began to rebuke Him: "God forbid Lord! This won't happen to you." But Jesus, at the shock of the others, turned to Peter and said, "Get behind me Satan! For you are a stone that could make

me stumble, for you are not thinking God's thoughts but man's thoughts. (Peter was worried about saving his own life. He didn't want to suffer the consequences of being associated with Jesus should things go wrong. Many, especially Mary Magdalen, knew the reason Jesus got angry as it was not the first time they witnessed Peter's behavior. His continued fears and 'corrections' of Jesus' teachings were born out of anger, especially those that involved the equality of women.) Therefore, it is highly doubtful that the man Jesus identified as a stumbling block to Him, would later become the supposed 'rock" upon which Jesus would build his church. Eeshans profess Jesus built his church upon Himself as Cornerstone and Rock of salvation along with His wife; not upon a human stone/or rock, which would crumble.

LESSON 85

DOOR #12A PETER, DO YOU LOVE ME?

Or will you reveal My mysteries to My enemies?

Peter, being strongly attached to the teachings of his birth religion, continued to adhere to the teachings of the Old Law, especially with regards to women. This continued in Jesus' presence and up until His Ascension; it became drastically worse after Jesus returned to Heaven, when Mary was even more targeted by Peter, and since Peter no longer had to watch his step, because Jesus was no longer there to come to her defense.

One factor in how the major events of Jesus' life, and how Peter went astray is seen by carefully looking at how his authority has been portrayed, and compare it with Jesus' comments and teachings, which often reflected Jesus 'rebuttal to an action, or comment, of Peter's, which is not to miss the many ways Peter would go behind Jesus' back in an effort to change Jesus' mind.

What was also intimated many times was how people (especially men who seemed to target Jesus' wife) continued to haunt Mary wherever they would go by portraying her as a prostitute. How did such a lie take on a life of its own? Well one must first remember that back then any form of adultery was never the man's fault.

Few know the 'true story' of what had taken place in Mary Magdalen's early years, and how Jesus was her Savior first, and then how He later publicly redeemed His wife by setting the story straight when He drew in the sand. Therefore, how effective could the truth be if the people were only exposed to *Peter's version*, and he was purported to be, as the church says, the 'first among equals' destined to be the leader, and in time, seen as the first "Pope?"

Over time, if enough people heard the altered version, it would become 'truth,' and Peter would then become known as the one being the closest to the Teacher, and the 'fisher of men.' How fitting such a facetious title. Good is relative to what one wants to see, or as one perceives as what is 'good.' That's how the Catholic church was able to justify what it did for 2000 years, since people would ignore the bad through their denial to protect what they felt contained a sacred deposit.

HERE'S WHAT HAPPENED.

Door #12B Jesus the Young Savior

When Jesus was 17 years old there was a commotion where seven men were dragging this young girl through the streets. Following the racket of the crowd and the screams of the young girl, Jesus ran swiftly trying to catch up with the noise. The men were shouting that the young girl of 13 years propositioned them and she was to be punished—when in reality, the girl had broken in on these men attacking her sister Martha. The times were violent. The men were always protected. The girl being young and innocent gave herself to the men to save her sister and thus the men used this as their excuse to drag her through the streets. As the men shouted punishment to the 'adulteress,' the women watched on. Taking her outside the area and pretending that they were going to 'punish her,' they took her to a cave. There the men felt they had carte blanch and violated the girl. The young man Jesus, hearing the jeers of the crowd that gathered and the accusations of the men, ran after the men in an attempt to go to her assistance. He knew of the girl's family and had often seen her at different places growing up.

Arriving at the entrance to the cave, the men held the young Jesus back to witness their violent acts, and his heart was broken. After their dastardly deeds, the men left only to spread the news that mercy was bestowed on the girl since they did not kill her as the law called for, but in mercy and out of respect for her family name, deemed her to be shunned and not marriage material.

Jesus ran to help her. He washed the blood from her with a piece of his cloak. which he tore off, and wet it with the water running from the wall of the cave.

Keeping a piece of the bloodied cloth and placing it in his cloak, He then wrapped her up in His cloak and carried her home, where he was met by her grieving sister and brother. The next day, Jesus left for the Himalayas to study.

DOOR #12C SOMETIMES GOD ALLOW BAD THINGS FOR A GREATER PURPOSE

Hearing of Joseph's illness, Jesus, now a spiritual Master, left the Himalayas to return home; since He was Joseph's only son. Being away studying and teaching in the Himalayas for eleven years, he was now twenty-seven and a half years old. Knowing, too, that it was his time now to fulfill his destiny, Jesus decided to stay after Joseph's death, and to care for his mother. It wasn't long before he began the process necessary to be a rabbi and teacher under his birth religion.

As Providence would have it, He was reunited with Mary Magdalen, and soon after their betrothal, came their wedding. Their marriage took place in Cana, and it would be shortly after Jesus would begin his ministry. He took Mary everywhere with Him when He preached. Though Jesus' reputation was world renowned, so, too, was Mary's, but not in a good way; and there were many who did not like the fact that Jesus married "such" a woman. Among them was Peter, Peter's brother Andrew, and a of couple others.

Though they thought that Jesus had no idea of the kind of woman He married, now that they were chosen to become His students, they feared that Jesus would be seen as outwardly defying the law, thus making a sacrilege of Marriage. Being the case, there were always plans in the making to bring Jesus to his senses, or to outright address their disgust at her presence. Thinking it was because of a 'man' issue that Jesus kept her close, Peter still couldn't stand the sight of her.

One day, while Jesus was teaching, He was met with a crowd of people that included Scribes, who were like reporters of that day, as well as Pharisees and other teachers. and Jesus knew something was up, since only those who were close to Him knew that He would be in that area that day.

As always, when He was met with Pharisees etc., there would be an attempt to trip him up using the law. While He was speaking in front of the Temple, a group of these teachers of the religious law brought a woman who had been caught in the act of adultery and threw her in front of Him. Now since men were never guilty of adultery, and it was always the woman who caused him to sin, it was a perfect opportunity for those who claimed they knew Mary's 'caliber 'of life.

"Teacher," they said, "this woman was caught in the act of adultery. The law of Moses commands to stone her. What do you say?" Knowing that Peter did not like Mary, and spoke unkindly about her even in Jesus' presence, Jesus suspected that He, and some others who felt the same way, thought that by putting Jesus in this position, they could infer the same about his wife; and be done with her once and for all. Thinking that being away for so many years, surely if He learned about her reputation, He would put her away.

But Jesus, knowing their hearts, stooped down and began writing in the dirt with his finger. The teachers kept shouting for an answer. Finally, looking back at Mary, His wife, Jesus stood up. There in the crowd were the men who defiled her eleven years ago. They now were accusing and shouting to bring charges against another woman charged with adultery. Mary Magdalen looked at Jesus, and, there in a public setting, in front of her husband, were the seven demons who plagued her. Never knowing when they would show up again, always fearful they would embarrass her publicly, praying they would not ruin her wedding, they were now right in front of her.

As was Jesus' plan, they came closer. Looking first at Jesus, they looked down and read what he was writing in the dirt. Jesus wrote, "Mary of Magdala, my wife."

The crowd was still shouting for an answer regarding the adulterous woman who was struck to the ground in front of him. The men came closer. Jesus said, "Alright, I will answer." He stooped down a second time, since those who were involved with the violation of His wife watched him trying to see what He wrote. Standing up again, Jesus looked out at the crowd which was now becoming larger.

He said, "Let he who is without sin, cast the first stone." At this time, these same men looked to see what He was writing, and found that it said, "I was there." With that they realized that He was the young, seventeen-year-old who was witness to their horrendous acts and dropping the stones held in their hands immediately left, as did the rest. Jesus spoke to the woman kindly pointing out that the crowd had gone; and he had nothing against her either as well.

Then He turned to his wife and kissed her. Now she was free! Free of the seven demons who haunted her mind, day and night; since her greatest fear was that the fabricated story of the men involved, which became truth in the minds of those who willfully accepted it for their own reasons, would, in fact, be revised and retold in an effort to not only hurt Jesus, but be the cause His work to fail.

By Eesha

Even though records of this confrontation were brought to the forefront, her reputation as a prostitute remained, along with expunging Mary from the collective memory of being Christ's wife; this became, in time, what was successfully 'remembered.'

Later, the church continued to strengthen irrefutable stories by unjustly making her the face for all the repented, sinful, prostitute, adulteress, demon-possessed women in the bible, and focusing, especially, on the one from whom Christ cast out seven demons. God placed within the hearts of many the need to cry out for justice to vindicate this woman, and to return her rightful titles, most importantly the title "Wife of Jesus."

As the church continued under its namesake, its teachings mirrored Peter's reluctance to transcend. and this continually filtered through to become what was presented as *Jesus*' teachings. To this day, even via the human consciousness, and the discriminating minds of the those who continue to accept those erroneous beliefs, Eeshans offer that they still have another opportunity to disregard such horrendous tenets, and accept Mary as a victim, and understand how the charges against her were false. Jesus, being her husband, as well as God, publicly redeemed his wife's reputation. This is one of those instances where the entire event was altered and revised so as to rinse it of its true purpose and import, supplanting the story forever after as something with a very different meaning. As for a punishment for all those who refuse to accept her, their choice will result in loss of the Divine Feminine/Physical/Sacramental form.

Adding to the decline of faith, and disbelief, in God were these omissions and many other covered up internal sins, especially by those who only claimed to have the truth. The continued propagating of false doctrine has indeed brought about the many empty pews we witness today.

Without belief in the Divine Feminine, this Bread from heaven is not in its purest form, and is no more than bread without yeast, since, without yeast, the bread does not rise. Therefore, without Christ's wife there is no resurrection of the body.

There is no fullness of salvation with a reimaged Jesus. If there is anything we are told about what Jesus said, or did, that differs from the

Jesus who is the Divine Masculine of God, it is a lie. In the same vein, to continually receive 'altered' bread, and not 'altar' bread, under the most innocent of means, condemns those in charge, and those in authority are guilty as charged for creating the famine of God's Sacred Food and Drink.[133] Since without the truest form of the Eucharist, or the eating of the Sacred Bread sans the leaven, there is no transubstantiation of the light bodies to the transcendental. With regards to God's children, there is only blind faith, which in and of itself, is the extent of one's belief; whereas, with God, they have eyes to see and ears to hear.

The weak and blind faith provided today, when accepted with a mediocre confidence, does more damage than leaving a religion, or spirituality, because its doctrines are questioned. God gave us the ability to think and reason. Remember, at the core of logic and reason we should find truth, and this truth should lead us to Jesus every time. If your spirituality is based on shaky ground, or faulty reasoning, you will not live it, you will just exist in it, because, eventually, you will be left confused.

What about the faithful who believed, and lived, wholly the Eucharist as Jesus Christ's real Presence in the Catholic Church, or other denominations? That's where faith comes in. Faith is the umbrella that protects the innocent, and it always holds a special place in the heart of God; since it is only they that are innocent and live fully what they were taught was the truth. Just as the unborn who was/is subject to abortion, these innocents do not suffer the sin, but are martyrs, since they receive the baptism of blood. In the case of the Spiritual Bread, which Jesus gave us as the lifeline, those who are content will be martyrs, since their loss is not of their own doing.

Both of these and those who were ever brought to, or taught, about the mysteries of God, while being subject to famine and death, are unconditionally loved by God. Their beliefs will sustain them as they fully

---

[133] But we must remember that the Faithful are not at fault, and receive the benefits of what they believe, although they may not receive the substance; they believe in good faith their leaders and teachers who they otherwise consider to be honest, truthful and knowledgeable. – Ed.

live their lives for Jesus; however, the weight of responsibility and God's punishment falls upon those who were the perpetrators.

The same rule applies with regards to those priests, presbyters, and religious who followed the Way of Christ as they were taught. and may still believe. Innocent, they are all blessed, as well as those individuals who believed they had the truth and lived their lives according to what they believed.

LESSON 86

DOOR #13 GOD'S USE OF ORDINARY PEOPLE AS PROPHETS

We know that ordinary people have always been used for the splendor of God; and with that in mind, you must remember that a prophecy involves a process in which one or more messages are allegedly communicated to a prophet by a god, or spirit,[134] to be communicated to other people. A prophecy is not one that would affect material needs, since these are of the lower consciousness but typically involve inspiration and interpretation, which Eeshans believe our truths provide; but prophecies may also involve a revelation of events to come which reveal divine knowledge. These prophecies will not play out until God decides it's time.

True prophets would be used by God because God promised that he would teach his people. As God is not limited to the ways, or laws, of man, He would, indeed, work through His people, as others could relate to them; but as long as there have been prophets there have always been prophecies of famine and drought.

For whatever reason, people forget that there is a difference between prophecy and fact. For example, hunger and poverty have always existed, and are due to the hand of man and nature. This is not a prophecy. What then would make a prophecy real?

A prophecy would need to be from God and be about something regarding that which would affect the true nature of the human being's

---

[134] "Prophecy." Wikipedia, Wikimedia Foundation, 7 Dec. 2019, en.wikipedia.org/wiki/Prophecy.

relationship with God, not what humans believe is the true nature, which to them is that of physicality.

So, therefore, if Jesus commanded that we eat the bread for everlasting life, and that falls on deaf ears and a faithless people, along with total denial of God's word with evidence provided by God, or if this bread has been altered, would this not be then something worthy of the work of prophet? Would this not be one of the most important prophecies? For what greater famine is there than to not have the Spiritual Food, the gift of God, that God tells us is necessary for life everlasting; and, thereby, wouldn't a prophet be sent? Yes, God would send a prophet, since it is about the loss of a sustenance that is affecting the true nature of the human being's relationship with God.

This warning is so vital that this particular prophecy regarding the 'end time famine' we are talking about, causes Eeshans to shudder as we witness the continued human consciousness limiting this simply to running out of food on earth.

What is being ignored, or perhaps is happening without God's people being aware of it, is an actual divine catastrophism; whereupon, the light body is no longer being fed, and, thus, the soul, the Light body, and Subtle body are experiencing an insatiable hunger and thirst that is welling up from deep within the soul. It is causing an unidentifiable restlessness and void within each person. The worst case scenario is that it continues on and causes a hopelessness, or confusion, where more souls can lose faith, at which point the human consciousness, rather than the essential transcendental consciousness, continues to be its guide. What happens next, is the search for comfort and answers from only in the material world.

For these reasons, a prophet is chosen from among the people, one who possesses a transcendental knowledge, one who has ears to hear and eyes to see; and one who is chosen to correct the people's course and reboot their thinking accordingly.

When obstacles to God occur, that which is godless at the hands of man, it naturally carries with it only a human mind, human senses, and human body, all of which is not balanced; since we are imaged, and likened, to God who is our consort by, with, and through our immortal souls.

Eeshans ask, "Was Jesus actually predicting the fall of the established human church and the vindication of His wife, as co-redeemer, to take place in eschatological times?" Upon the return of the Divine Feminine, Mary has raised up the Kallahs (Jesus and Mary as co-redeemers) as their extensions. Was the famine of the real Eucharist, the consequence of the church of Peter, for denying his marriage and altering Christ's teachings to once again dominate over women? In Luke 18:8, Jesus says, "I tell you, He will see that they get justice, and quickly. However, when the Son of Man comes will He find faith on the earth?"

Eeshans say, yes, since by, with, and in the Marriage Feast of the Lamb, and his Wife, the Kallahs will invite all those "by the highways and byways" (Luke 14:23-24), and urge them to come in, so that the fruit of the Marriage Feast of the King's only begotten Child will be attested to." (Luke 14:13) "When you give a banquet, invite the poor, the crippled, the lame, the blind, and you will be blessed." One thing is for sure, Jesus did predict the return of the Marriage Feast, and those who refuse it here on earth will not partake of it in heaven. Since, as he taught, 'as above-so below,' When (Luke 14:15) one of those at the table with Him heard this, he said to Jesus, "Blessed is the one who will eat *at the feast in the kingdom of God." Jesus was telling the crowd of the many excuses that were made for not wanting to attend the wedding feast of the King's son, and Jesus said, (Luke 14:23) "I tell you, not one of those who were invited will get a taste of my banquet."*

LESSON 87

DOOR #14 GOD TO THE RESCUE

God's plan for our Salvation came with no hesitation (even though in time it seems to have taken forever), and it didn't end two thousand years ago; it is just now playing out fully in these end times. All we are taught is a short account of some of Christ's teachings and an even shorter account of the Last Supper, his Passion, his Death, and Resurrection. To use only highlights of such an important event in God's Salvation Plan for humanity, is inexcusable.

God in his unconditional love already had the plan for our salvation immediately following Adam and Eve's choice. God, like all good parents, felt that because Adam and Eve made the choice to live in a physical world with a human rational consciousness, they should experience it fully, along with the consequences of their choice. They were told what would happen if they ate the fruit, but decided to ignore all the warnings; therefore, they had to be held accountable for their choice.

Yes, we all learn from our mistakes. In God's wisdom, their choice had consequences that they had to face, and as a result this provided an opportunity for 'us' to learn, and note the consequences, of not heeding God's warnings. You see, *this* is the basis of real prophecies.

It was important to see how decisions were made apart from God bring accountability, just as decisions children make apart from the warnings of their parents have consequences. We may not like it, but being accountable for our mistakes helps us to make better decisions and hopefully we will not make the same mistakes again.

Time and entropy, and the effects of both, especially on a body made of lower vibrations resulting in gross physical matter, was unlike anything Adam and Eve had ever experienced. Yes, they achieved knowledge, but it was a fallen human knowledge in an unfamiliar consciousness of lower vibrations. They already had "knowledge in the form of wisdom," but now they were disconnected from the higher spiritual ecstasy where they had enjoyed a constant flow of grace, and the one-on-one link to God.

This is attributed to the encapsulation of the pineal gland, which caused them to immediately focus on their physicality. Once encapsulated, the pineal gland was replaced by what we call the pituitary gland. With the onset of activation of the pituitary gland their spirituality was no longer a certainty. The transcendental body was no longer operational; and this new physical body left them vulnerable, and their limited and flawed knowledge needed guidance.

The omnipotent God knew what they had done, and knowing the consequences, He came looking and calling for them. God already knew what was going on in their minds and hearts. Taking note that they were hiding themselves, it was obvious that their fear and confusion had overtaken them. They were now under a human consciousness. With wisdom, God asked why they were hiding and why they did what they did.

Seeing their shaken reaction, and listening with patience to their reasons, God comforted them by explaining what they were now feeling, and why. For the first time, they needed God in a different capacity, and to explain to them what happened and how they were going to live. They were experiencing new emotions. They felt fear, guilt, and shame, which confused them to the point where their first reaction was to hide and cover themselves. That is why God asked, 'How do you know you are naked?' The Divine Masculine was calling to their attention that their actions were not that of a transcendental being but a human being. They recognized they needed help and were sorry, but as God pointed out, it was impossible for them to go back since they were no longer transcendental. The garden was not created to sustain physical bodies, and it provided only for transcendental beings. So, the couple had to now adapt to a 'new body,' which required attention never before needed by their transcendental bodies. God promised to be there and help them in this new life, but they would have to ask for help, since this change was of their own doing.

Next, God explained the human body as compared to the transcendental body. The Divine Feminine explained the human reproductive system as compared to the begetting they previously knew. With this new experience, the couple immediately worried about the effects this would have on children. Would they be transcendental or human? How will the transcendental children be affected, and will the children born be able to stay in the garden? Sadly, God told them that because they were human so shall the children be human as they are. Seeing their sadness, God explained to them that though they were forgiven they still had to live out their choice, and, so, too, would their human children. When the children, from this point on, were born, they would not have the advantages the begotten children had.

At this time, the human body was now beginning to become just a vehicle for a dimming light body because the soul was now affected by what came to be known as "Original Sin." The moment they became human, a mark was placed on them, which identified their souls as in need of redemption. Being the very first sin ever committed (thus, the title *Original* Sin), this understanding became the template for sin in us. That is why though Original Sin is forgiven in Baptism, the certainty of a spirituality is now 'our' responsibility as the template for sin being a side effect is still within us.

The first sin we commit is the most devastating to our soul. Even if it is a venial sin, and what we call "a little sin," for a soul filled with grace it is unfamiliar with imprisonment, and, thus, this sin is as catastrophic as a mortal sin. Though *we* don't recognize this, the effect of our first sin continues to play out as in a ripple effect. From that moment on, it gets easier and easier to revert to logic and reason for our offensive actions before God.

LESSON 88

AWAY FROM THE TRANSCENDENTAL— GENDER IDENTIFIERS BECAME STRONGER

As the light body continued to dim, their minds became more and more darkened. Time, along with its mortality, coupled with a fallen nature, began to affect Adam and Eve as soulmates. Each gender identifier became stronger. The linear mind of the male became more logical and acted on reason; whereas, the cyclical attribute of the woman gave way to intuition and emotions. Each becoming more self-reliant, competitive, and less interdependent caused more and more the influence and bad judgment, which explains the birth of Cain. The selfless love they once shared towards each other that was grounded in God seemed to be a waning; and they lost sight of the mirrored love that God shared between consorts.

As the attributes of each became stronger, the physicality and anatomy of the male rose to the forefront in comparison to the softness of the woman; Eeshans believe that this was God's design to be able to not only identify gender but would also begin to manifest their weaknesses, and strengths, in ways that would benefit them in this new life. Before, both Adam and Eve 'were encompassed 'within each other. Now they had to learn how to work together, and for each other, and discover what sacrificial love was for each other.

As we follow the male, we find that as he went further into entropy, and the fallen nature led to male dominance and strength, and the female became his helper, but not in the sense that she was inferior, but in the sense that she was his equal partner who shared in everything, as he did with her. This should have continued even up into today.

As time would have it, and as humans were imperfect and responsible for their own spirituality, with Satan still around to drive a wedge between the humans and God, the male mind would continue to be influenced. Man learned the weaknesses of women, and as nature would have it, he would eventually fall victim to seeing his strength as superiority, and human nature would continue to advance in this way. Predisposed males would fall victim to a conception of a solely masculine God, as we find was the mindset of the male dominant religions, such as found with the Hebrews, the Israelites, and Jews where the woman was more of a possession than another human of equal dignity, as we find illustrated in Peter's comment that women were not "worthy of life."

This is why the *true* story wasn't the one that was filtered down through human history. Rather, it was the fallacy of composition by *male ego* that resulted in a continued misconceived, or perceived, inferior nature of women; whereas, the female gender would then become defined as '*needing* the male gender,' or worse, to become a servant to the needs of men.

According to the 'traditional' story of Adam and Eve, which became the template for life in this world, was that man was made in God's image and likeness and not woman, since she was an afterthought, here to help, assist, or serve man, and to not challenge, or to take the lead, when he is unable.

Through the years, women were told that they were included in the noun 'man;' however, we know that this is NOT how it was played out in life. From the first time a male translated, and interpreted, the story of Adam and Eve, it was deemed that no woman had the right to have a personal relationship with God, except through a man.

Eeshans see that as we are subject by right, to know, love, and serve God, the male gender has been victimized, also, since men were taught just as were women, that *this is what God wanted* by design. The confusion caused by the deliberate changing of the 'wording' from "Male and female, man and woman, were made in God's image and likeness" to "man being made in the image and likeness of God," which has been handed down, and became the directive that men, too, felt they were obliged to follow.

Eeshans believe that as history repeats itself, God's people were told it came from God, and by those who were the authorities of God's laws. Just as in biblical times, they were faced then with laws, and rules, regarding God that made no sense. The consequence of this is that man, too, had been used as a tool to continue with this agenda. even though there are a greater number of men who do not accept women as being inferior.

LESSON 89

MARRIAGE IS DEFINED BY THE LOVE BETWEEN SPOUSES; CHILDREN ARE THE FRUIT OF THEIR LOVE

In biblical times, marriage meant having children. It favored men over women. A husband could divorce his wife if he chose to, but a woman would have to get her husband's consent to divorce him; however, the Law was defined as such that the purpose of marriage was to bring forth children, especially boys.

Over the years, the church told women that they were to be obedient unto their husbands and that procreation is an expected duty. Despite the ongoing growing concerns of pregnancy, there was no room for a woman to deny God children. Despite financial concerns, health issues, etc., the church denied contraception at the risk of women not being able to control their bodies.

Yet, even Jesus' own Mother is a perfect case in reference to not wanting to be married to avoid being impregnated. Not knowing who she was, she by her own choice refused to 'have conjugal relations' with a man, since her heart belonged to God. That is why when Joseph was chosen to be her husband, and she told him, emphatically, that even though their marriage had to be under the Law, she did not want to have relations. Joseph, desiring to live for God, entered into an agreement that they would live as brother and sister.

That is why the Virgin Mary proclaimed to the angel regarding having a Child by the Most High, "how can this be as I know not a man?" By God's own words, the Virgin's decision was upheld, and upon her 'Yes,' he revealed to her that she was the Divine Feminine, his wife and eternal consort of the Divine Masculine of the first Person of the Blessed Trinity.

In conjunction with God's Salvific Plan for humans, it was the decision of the Second Person of the Holy Trinity that they two, as the only begotten child, would become the Christ, and *his consort* would also live a transcendental life. This not only satisfied God's plan to reverse the choice of Adam and Eve for a physical relationship, but it also witnessed to marriage being more than conjugal relations in order to bear children for God. Marriage was for love. In both these instances, it was their love of God, and true love for each other, that was first and foremost. Isn't that what Jesus always taught?

Metta Love is defined by the sacred union of God as the 'expression of oneness in the sharing of each other' in each of the Persons of God; and the fruit of this love will be manifested by God's design. For humans, this is true love, and causes the desire within each to serve the needs of the other with no explanation, or law, to tell them it's necessary.

Understanding these truths is to understand Jesus' real mission, God's extreme desire for soulmates to marry, and become one as God is one, united to God and in God, thus, experiencing true love. What has been taught is opposite of that, which surely reflects the Old Law, and which Jesus changed, because it was *based not on love*, but on a 'Law' defined by human consciousness.

From the onset of the fallen nature of the physical, many things were written and set in place regarding women, i.e., formal teachings and laws saying that women could not access God directly, but needed the mediation of a male. This was, and is, still used as the reason and template for gender inequality in religious, social, and political institutions, as well as with exploitation of cultural and racial differences. Again, this is not a directive by God; but according to one legend, God was angered that Eve wanted a separate relationship apart from Adam.

God promised a Savior to restore what was lost as a result of Adam and Eve's choice; however, with the 'altering' of Jesus' teachings and life events, we find ourselves facing unreasonable expectations and consequences.

Truly these man-made laws replaced what "the cornerstone," who is Jesus, brought to God's people, and because of what He taught and stood for He was rejected. Isn't He still being rejected by those who claim to speak on Jesus' behalf, and who refuse to go back and tell the truth about him and why He actually died?

Jesus became a victim to untruths even after He was crucified, and resurrected when what He taught and died for was hidden away to protect the survival of man's laws, just as He predicted. If the truth had been upheld, we could have had a better life as individuals, and in marriages, families, nations, and a better world.

Hence, rather than embracing the fulfillment of that timeless prophecy of the coming of a Messiah, once again, we choose man's desire for the slavery of women, and prejudice of whatever peoples, or individuals, don't meet man's standard for life.

The reasons we had been given for His passion, and death and resurrection, pales in comparison to the truth of Jesus' actual mission, and as a result, is a very unconvincing imitation of what man declares God's desire is.

As Jesus is love, and all he taught was love, the claim that 'he came and died to rid us of original sin' barely can be called *truth*. To raise human love, as shared between soulmates to the level where it mirrors the love of Divine Consorts, despite Adam and Eve's choice of physicality, over the transcendental, makes the love that two humans share between each other a love that can be truly envied by *angels*, as it is the case for some, as you will find.

LESSON 90

CHILDREN

"Jesus loves me this I know; cuz the bible tells me so! Little ones to Him belong; we are weak but He is strong!"[135] This is one of the first songs mothers and catechism teachers alike would teach their little ones. When a child came into the world, parents wanted them to know how important they were to Jesus. His name was probably among the first names little children learned. However, today, that's not so much. Unless the children attend a Parochial or bible school, and unless they have parents who still are counted among the faithful, it is safe to presume that the only time a child, or children, hear the name Jesus is when it is used in a cursing situation, be it adults they know, or songs they hear.

Children love to hear about what they were like when they were little. Every child wants to know how their mom and dad felt when they were born and what they did together. They look to see all the little things the child did to make the parent swoon, or laugh, over them. They loved hearing how they talked with the angels when they were small. As the children grow, however, unless they are enrolled in instruction classes for the Sacraments, there is little else they learn about Jesus. One little memory they come upon, either in religion class or by pictures, is the one where Jesus is seated and a little child is sitting on His lap, and other children are standing, or running, to Him. The caption under the picture reads, "Let the little children come to Me." Each time throughout life, whenever this picture is seen, the little child within gravitates to it. And, it is rightly so.

---

[135] Poem by Anna Bartlett Warner and hymn adapted by William Batchelder Bradbury.

The fruit of true love, as Jesus says, is either the birth of a child, or an angel: or the begetting of either. How is this? When we are blessed with a child, or children, we see them and hold them and take care of them. When a child is not born either by miscarriage, or still born, Jesus calls it an angel. When a couple love each other so dearly but could not have a child, Jesus says their love is begetting children all of the time.

As the Plan of Salvation called for Jesus and his Wife to refrain from physical love, but express it in a tantric *transcendental* love, Jesus and Mary conceived with their kisses. So in love were they, but this was a sacrifice that would beget by them "all of us" who love them.

We know this, and we believe that as powerful as God's love was, their only begotten Child came into existence. What is hard to imagine/comprehend was that this same God whose love was so intense for their begotten Child, also has the same desire and love for *us* as *created extensions of them*. This love was so reflected for Adam and Eve, and for their descendants, that it became the foundation for the sacrifice of their only-begotten Child for salvific reasons. This Child came to live out a human life, and as from a kind of adoptive parents, teaches us how nothing else can compare to love, and how love overpowers everything, and that through them, we, as their begotten children, may find our way back to heaven. In other words, *we truly have the means to be reborn back into the transcendental.*

As any young couple, the thought and desire to have a child filled the hearts of Jesus and Mary throughout their married life. They made themselves available for any and all events that presented an opportunity to be with and assist with children. Jesus would run and play, and teach games to the boys; and Mary would be involved with teaching "dress up," and make little beaded jewelry, and do the little girls' hair. She would also help with making bread and meals, and though not always welcomed among the other women, found joy in doing and teaching those things she enjoyed.

Jesus and Mary dreamed of what it would be like to have a 'normal' family and sometimes Mary would wonder if perhaps there would be another way or sacrifice that would appease the God she so loved. At that time, the reality of their mission would often remain pushed back in the most isolated recesses of their minds, at least hers. Fulfillment of scriptures, denoting the passion and death of the Messiah, did not seem as realistic as one thinks. In fact, it really wasn't a part of their daily discussion until close to the time when Jesus began talking to his apostles about what He was going to undergo. Yes, their private time was spent planning and dreaming, just like us. Yes, they were realistic, but they were also young and in love.

Yes, Jesus loved and loves children. His feeling for all children never diminished even after He returned to Heaven. That is why the birth of the Firstborn of the Firstborn was, and is, still filtering into this world, since He is the Spirit of God and is all loving. As God once again lives among us, He who is called Emmanuel, the One who is like the Son of Man, the Third King, awaits His time.

God, as Mother and Father, are also greatly blessed as they have an unconditional love of their only-begotten child we know as our only begotten Parents Jesus and Mary.

Abortion is against life, that's true. It is against Life. But not all abortions are black and white. It is not always done out of selfishness, but more often than not, it is done out of fear. Sometimes abortion is done out of pressure from others. What we are saying is that there are a lot more reasons why abortions are done. Blessed are we that we are not in that position, or in those circumstances, that this thought remains outrageous. Have pity that you are not one of those who are. Children aborted are martyrs, since their death is not of their own doing. No special Mass, or ritual, for their soul is necessary. Their tiny souls go right back to God. Those women who have had abortions usually suffer this memory all of their lives. To continue to punish them does not come from Jesus. Did you know how many women who had abortions have given up marriage, or their own lives, over the sorrow they held in their hearts? No one can imagine, just like one cannot know the pain of a headache of another, since only that person who has the pain/suffering knows their own tolerance. As with everything in life, there are those abortionists, and doctors, who do abortions for money. God have mercy on these for they alone know their guilt, and at their death what the consequences will be, and those who are even remotely connected to this sin, are destined for Hell, unless they make reparation for what they have done. Justice for predators, especially priests, who have and continue to use Jesus to abuse innocents, will find themselves in the same vein as murderers.

Today at least we find another way of bringing back the love Jesus has for children with movies and books on miracles and visits to heaven. Whether you believe it or not, these things are still a connection—and a good one at that.

Truth be told, all things that come before Him will be as He said, "For you will be treated as you have treated others. The standard by which you judge, is the standard by which you will be judged."

Jesus was never at a loss when attacked, or put to the test regarding his life, His teachings etc. Not only having to deal with comments regarding his wife, but having no children was among the issues that He and Mary had to endure. Even some of those within His group added to the stress put upon these two young people who tried to make every day together special in some way. From complaints about the way He handled situations, which infuriated the Pharisees, to those who tried to say that the Mosaic Law, which came before he was born was God's law, etc., it was at the basis of the murmuring of the crowd. Knowing this, Jesus responded, "Do not think I will accuse you before my Father. Your accuser will be Moses, in whom you put your hopes." (John 5:45)

Thinking that Jesus escaped everyday stress, or that the decisions he and his wife made were easy, and without incident, could be no further from the truth. They lived a human life with all that goes with it.

It would be during these moments when Jesus would look to his wife, and be thankful that He had her near. Not being able to give her children made Him sad, and often He would sit alone on the beach and meditate. He would pray to God, His Father, and His Mother, to bless His wife for her love and devotion to Him, as well as her hope and strength in the midst of trouble and adversity, and thank them just because she was Mary. The one thing He would never do was discourage her from expressing hope in having children one day, nor the excitement of talking about what their son or daughter would be like.

Jesus and Mary did not live their marriage out of servile fear of God but lived freely in God's Light. As there is an opposite to a positive, we find how a transcendental choice can become inverted and justified in a human consciousness addicted to a drive or desire, so that one sees a sin to be embraced under the guise of a 'truth': i.e., "I can do these sins because Jesus already died for them and cleared me."

The human consciousness claims, for example, in this instance, that where there is no fear of God, there is no guilt, and, in lieu of this, corrupt reasoning replaces wisdom. In other words, this same mindset can be played out negatively, and this is how religious authorities, having no fear of God, were able to expunge his marriage and essentially erase it from history.

It isn't the fact that Jesus was married that is the main objective of this issue, it was because it went against the grain of women having a say in all matters. Being the Son of God, and having witnessed the strength of his Mother, and now his wife, Jesus blessed God for the gift of women.

This is why Jesus spent so much time including women as the focus for most of His teachings, emphasizing their cyclical thinking, rather than the diminutive linear thinking which we were all were taught. We see this clearly in His visit with the woman at the well for example, where He chose to give her the unfathomable teaching. Why? Because he knew she would understand this teaching as she did not have to "unlearn" what was taught traditionally. Rather, Jesus knew she had the "eyes to see" and the "ears to hear" what he was teaching.

As the "Age of Enlightenment" has arrived, because of God, women are experiencing a newfound strength *in themselves and their love of God*. Through the grace and strength of the Divine Feminine, and the strength of Jesus' love for them as the Divine Masculine, women no longer feel like they are victims, but survivors.

Over the centuries, whenever women claimed equality with men, mankind judged them from flawed human interpretations which Eeshans identify as bearing false witness against other genders. Whenever females rise up against unfair laws, they are immediately viewed as sexist and feminists, even though they are asked for examples of their mistreatment, or despite any efforts to present their claims. The struggle for equality, or any path, to change must begin with presenting facts; yet, when women have done this, another punishment in the form of an ad hominem occurs. Since so many attempts have been automatically rejected as sexist, equality could not be assured, until now.

As there are so many sins that cry out for God's vengeance, the time for the Divine Feminine has come, and once again Jesus' mission will continue to fruition, especially for the sake of the children.

Eeshans believe that we are now in the fullness of time, and the need for the restoring of our connection to the cosmic divine Sophia is being brought about by the hand of God. The Divine Feminine, his divine consort, has been awakened and now upon her return, will restore the sacred balance, so needed in these times. Her means and directives to insure equality are in the desire to represent to all what the 'divine couple' brought to the world through the love of Jesus and his spouse, Mary.

God knows that though this will disrupt and cause anger to the very foundations of many, if not most of the Christian religions of this day; however, through counterintuitive propositions, one should come to see the truth and the extreme love of God. Through this restoration of the transcendental relationship, that God desires to complete in us, the chances of making God's plan happen will finally come to pass.

For She who completes God in every Person of the Blessed Trinity, is present now as the Divine Feminine, to bring balance. By her love, men, or males, who have never felt women were the weaker, or a lesser gender, and treated them as equals, as well as women who have worked without issues against men/males, will be blessed as they band together to bring about the right solution, which is to live and raise all children as equals. For it is God's plan that men realize that the children must be brought into this world seeing no superiority/inferiority amongst human beings, and that the children understand that it takes both male and female to bring balance into the world. Children are our future and the extensions of us, and the human race is our family. Family does right for family!

Jesus' eternal Consort is here to bring the truth, since it was said: truth is learning and knowing that we have the power to change everything. We, as God's children, have the capability to bring about miracles, and with God, we can do much more than we presently realize. In order to realize this power, we need God to reassure us that we are on the right path, and that we are following the "Way" given to us by the only-begotten Child. This way, and only this way, can we find of what we are truly capable, as well as the many miracles "we" perform 'each day' of our lives, with God's grace.

LESSON 91

DOOR #15 THE CONTROVERSIAL JESUS OF NAZARETH: TRUE GOD OR TRUE MAN?

IF GOD, WHY WAS HE-REIMAGED?

Could the controversy regarding equal rights for all genders be coming from the same kind of thinkers who could not/cannot determine if Jesus was God, both God and Man, or just a man through whom God worked? Couple these debates with gender inequality, and you find yourself faced with indecision, inconsistency, and error, and this is within His 'supposed' own catholic church.

If Jesus is the one upon whom all Christian religions and beliefs are founded, then why has He and what we know about Him, to include his teachings, been the center of such controversy and confusion?

It just points to the fact that with the truth being withheld from the beginning, the foundations will surely crack and crumble, thus, this was the reason Jesus changed Simon's name to 'Peter' to identify him as a pebble (as in stumbling block), so as not to be confused with the Rock (as in foundation) upon which Jesus would build his church. With Peter's constant self-aggrandizement, Jesus found himself continually having to rebuke him, and letting the others know that this mindset impeded Jesus' mission, as opposed to furthering it; due to this problem Peter had no understanding of Jesus' teachings, nor would any of those who followed Peter's example. In connection we might refer to Matthew 13:5, which includes a warning that the seed that falls on 'rocky places without much soil' will grow quickly because the soil is shallow; but when the sun comes up, the plants will be scorched and wither because they have no root.

So, case in point, had the truth been properly understood, and propagated from the beginning, Eeshans feel there would have been no need for councils (which indeed came later). However, we will find that regardless of man's interference in the Divine Plan, God's will prevails and rights the Plan's course in the appropriate time ... as we see today with the return of the Divine Feminine.

Eeshans hold that if you believe in Jesus, then believe what he says about Himself, what He teaches, and His directives. Since to change any one of these is to reimage Him, and, thus, no one really has the truth.

When asked over the years, when, from whom, how, and where would help come? The answer is the when: 2000-plus years ago. The who you undoubtedly call out to is "Jesus." How? By His birth, personal identification, passion, death, and resurrection. Where? His birthplace and surrounding areas. And for the most part you would be right, if that was the whole story; but just like the beginning story of Adam and Eve was not told, thus, only half the truth about Jesus was told.

Little is revealed traditionally about Jesus' life before his ministry except for what is known as the Infancy Narrative. It was always deemed his 'hidden' life. Even the New Testament regarding His coming, as Messiah and Savior barely summarizes the weeks prior to and post resurrection, let alone the gaps of early years. The little that was taught over the centuries, failed to satisfy his followers over the last 2000 years. Then came the "The Da Vinci Code."

Without a doubt, whenever a magazine, or television show, etc., is presented about Jesus, many want to see it hoping to find "anything" outside the poorly composed, or scanty scriptural accounts, about the man who was also God, either good or bad. We have no account of how he looked, his background, how he spent his time outside of teaching, if he had a wife, children, a family, etc. Traces of stories, parables, *a few incomplete teachings, and some miracles, became the whole story* of what should have and continued to be the greatest love story ever told. When the church was asked these questions, we were told the questions and answers were not necessary. We had all we needed.

We always wondered, and continue to wonder now, how human was Jesus? Did he get headaches? Did he get disgusted? Did he get hungry? Did he laugh? Enjoy sports of any kind? Did he fall in love? Oops! What?

We were always taught that Jesus was like us in every way, except they limited the details to what we read in scriptures, that he was obedient to his parents. Didn't he try their patience? Or was that just the one time when He was, and that about his Father's work?

Truth is, Jesus experienced life. The list goes on and on, and everyone's soul, with love in it, wants to hear about Him. What did He do after the resurrection? What does He do now? How about today? His life didn't end after he ascended back to heaven; yet, you would think so by the lack of faith and belief in God. Perhaps, His life means so little to so many, because we know so little about Him.

How we began this section is a subject of which not many are aware. Did you know that as far back as the early church that not everyone believed Jesus was fully God and fully Man? Some thought He might be God, some, just a man through whom God worked. Some believed He was both God and Man. Among His own apostles there was doubt. Not all believed he was God, especially those who knew Him all His life.

This doesn't even account for the lack of belief in His Sacramental state, and the mystery encompassing His body, blood, soul, and divinity, which still to this day, though what was taught about the Eucharist was flawed, is debatable in some Christian sects, i.e., whether it is a memorial of what took place, or is it truly the Real Presence. and does the Real Presence of Christ remain after Communion, or does it leave immediately after everyone receives?

Even in the Catholic church, there are still differences of opinion regarding fundamental 'dogma,' even among its priests, such as whether the Presence of Christ remains in the Eucharist after Communion (thus, the need for Perpetual Adoration and bowing, or genuflections, before the tabernacle), or, as some priests believe, that the Presence actually does leave after the community leaves Mass, a term similar to one called consubstantiation; or whether a sacrifice is present at all, or if the Mass is just a memorial to Christ's death, etc. The same debates go on within the various Christian sects.

Questions regarding the Pope, and past Popes, always arise, and with little to no satisfactory answers given. For example, if the Pope is sovereign over 'the whole 'Christian world,' then how, if there are differences in dogma between them, and if many and great truths about Christ differ tremendously among the Catholics and non-Catholics, how then can he speak infallibility on dogma: what gives?

The debates regarding Jesus as God and Man are recorded in early church history. Eeshans hold that theologians talk Jesus to 'death,' and are no longer capable of knowing, loving, and serving him completely because of this.

What did Jesus say about himself? Jesus said "I am who Am. When you see me, you see the Father. I have come not to do my will but the will of Him (God) who sent me. Before Abraham I Am. Whoever does the will of my Father in heaven …" are just a few of the ways Jesus identified himself publicly.

Eeshans find that all the discussions, and debates, of noted theologians and thinkers such as Origin and Plotinus, in many ways held a tremendous insight regarding God. Then there was Arius, who was just sadly mistaken about God in every way; Athanasius and Gregory of Nyssa were major thinkers and writers, and then there was the work of the councils of Nicaea and Chalcedon. The fact that there was so much discussion of whether Jesus was Divine and Human, Divine or Human with the divine working through him boggles the mind. One must ask: Why?

In the end, all this discussion, debating, and philosophizing failed. People want to know 'Jesus' just as he identified himself. Because of Jesus, people *are capable* of ending war, prejudice, discrimination, and bringing about the kingdom of heaven by, with, and through us, where a new heaven and a new earth will result as God intended for us.

Throughout the centuries, God continues to give to the ordinary and average person, whose faith and love for Jesus transcended facts and logic, the unfathomable truths and the faith and understanding that are still debated today by the learned, academia, and the elite. As one would ask, why would God appear to an ordinary person, and not go to the Pope, or the higher echelons of the church, where there are those who are educated in theology? Two translations of James 4:6 are useful in this connection: 1) *God sets himself in battle array against the arrogant and proud but gives grace to the humble and lowly.*; 2) *He gives us grace enough to meet this and every other evil spirit, if we are humble enough to receive it.* Also, we may consider Luke 1:53, *He has filled the hungry with good things and sent away the rich with empty hands.*

Well perhaps those 'rich in knowledge' lack what's necessary for God to work with them. The perfect example of truth manipulated by the gospel writers is deemed Jesus' first miracle. Not only is there just one gospel that speaks about it, but what is written is flawed and incomplete. We know it as the story of the Wedding Feast at Cana (John 2:1-11), and it is the event that changed the world: but no one would ever know.

LESSON 92

DOOR #16 WATER TO WINE; WINE TO BLOOD

"IT'S ALL ABOUT THE WINE"

"Whenever a timeless mystery enters into time, the most powerful positive vibrations of epic proportion brings a disruption of negative energies taunting these powers and causing change."

At the beginning of his mission, we find Jesus, described as a 'guest,' at a wedding feast at Cana. There is only the mention of a bridegroom, and a dilemma which caused Jesus' mother such concern, that she approached Jesus for help. So, being focused on the miracle of the water being changed into wine allowed the writer to move the focus away from the bridegroom. We are 'told' that Jesus had to be family because Jesus attended with his mother; whose concern for the wine in the first place puts her in the position of not just a guest at the wedding, but the matriarch. This is due to the fact that it was Jewish tradition at the time for the mother of the bridegroom to be in charge of overseeing the food and drinks for the wedding feast. There is absolutely no mention of the bride, of which both normally would be mentioned, but again, biblically speaking, perhaps, it wasn't unusual that the focus was on the 'man.' Suppose we take a closer look at this event.

This one event marks what is truly the beginning of the foundation of Eeshan Transcendentalism. As our teachings begin to unfold, you will find that there is not one detail of Jesus' life, death, and resurrection *that is not important*, or *that can be played down*, without a cosmic effect.

This Wedding Feast, or "Marriage Feast of Cana," does not meet with the standards of other stories.

Starting with the miracle of the water being changed to wine ... this is of the utmost importance to Eeshans. It is not the fact that it was seen as Jesus 'first public miracle, but it was his first act done through His divinity, and that was the priority. We believe it was far greater than this, since it was the first time he *acted as God*; it was here that He effected a change in the fundamental building blocks of the material world, to institute a permanent, irrevocable 'time released' change into the fabric of existence. As this had to embrace both genders of the Divine, it was time now to awaken Mary's divinity. This would be complete, and perfect through the words He spoke into the water, which he identified to Mary as being 'her.' This is actually the source, the beginning of the alchemical words of transubstantiation. Transubstantiation came in two parts: first, at Cana, secondly at the Cross; then both were repeated at the Last Supper, with the template of the ritual to be used. So, it should be understood that the Last Supper was not the *institution of the Eucharist*, but was rather the celebration of Christ's accomplishment in the form also of liturgical instruction, that is, 'how to do this from here on.' The key component in this connection, however, to be kept in mind is that Jesus did *not* say "do this in memory of me"; this is simply how it 'got' remembered, recorded, and passed down under the spirit of Peter as the women were being simultaneously suppressed. The actual words included Jesus and Mary's marriage vows, which were finalized at the Last Supper by Jesus saying "*Do this in time immemorial*," and what he would come to say as his Omega, or last, seven words to Mary on the cross: "Mary, we will never be separated again." Transubstantiation would not be 'activated' until Jesus spoke the Omega Words to Mary on the cross (and the official public commencing of the Marriage Feast in ritual form would take place in what came to be known as the breaking of the bread on the road to Emmaus).

Thus, what is usually professed to be Jesus' first 'public' miracle, and which marked the beginning of His salvific mission should actually be understood to be a private exchange between Jesus and Mary, and the occasion where Jesus was inspiring in Mary a sense of spiritual mystery and fascination. Since as Jesus spoke words into the water, Mary asked, "are you speaking to the water?" and to which Jesus responded, "No, I am speaking to you."

One must understand that 'water' here is important, since the water used was the cleansing water, and it was transformed into the living water, which Jesus foreshadowed when he spoke to the Samaritan woman.

Prefiguring the alchemical process known as transubstantiation, and authoring the beginning of a mystery that has its origins in 'God' alone, Jesus who was the Christ, the anointed one, was the only one capable of changing water into wine.

If in this context we were to employ the scientific language of the following,[136] we might draw further insight into the magnificence of what Jesus was doing as God:

> In a similar manner, is the idea of changing water (H_2O) into wine (ethanol, C_2H_5OH) by forming an alcohol normally accomplished through fermentation in which organisms derive energy from sugar. For Christ Jesus to accomplish this instantaneously, would require additional carbons (perhaps through breath) brought into the formula. This power of transformation would be so magnificent that three of the four elements of life—carbon, oxygen and hydrogen—are recombined into a new arrangement so that a conversion of the elements of life could take place. Yet if our carbon-based body as part of C-O-H-N system can be transformed into light, cell by cell, how much easier is it to transform water into wine during a marriage feast, symbolic of a higher union and transformation?

This is why the two natures of Christ were important, in order to effect the transformation of the water (signifying the Divine) into wine, and which shortly would become 'their' 3rd sacramental nature.

Thus the power and mystery of the Christs' marriage, where two human beings become one body in the eyes of God, living in union as

---

[136] J.J. Hurtak, Pistis Sophia, p. 827.

one body, blood, soul, and divinity, becomes the means necessary for our salvation.

This mystery will eventually play out as Christ's life leads to His command for us to partake of this Body and Blood, that we may become begotten children of Jesus and His Wife.

This mystery is two-fold. First, though it is impossible to measure the love between Jesus and Mary Magdalen, we do know that it had a cosmic effect that is going to be played out in these present times. Secondly, their marriage is incapable of being fully explored, or understood, because when he shared with His wife the fullness of his body, blood, soul, and divinity in God's way, it is incomprehensible the vortices that were opened within human bodies and consciousness.

As we must ingest the Eucharist which transforms and divinizes us, we, too, enter into a quickening of our natural inner light of awareness; and this is made possible ONLY if we enter into what we call the Marriage Feast, ourselves.

On their wedding night, Mary shared with her eternal consort a most sublime mystery. The reawakening of her divinity and being reunited with her eternal consort is a mystery in and of itself, though they both would not rely on their Divinity unless God deemed it so. This is because it would be by their human form that the plan of salvation could begin and play out, and by way of their divinity that the gates of heaven would be reopened once again, allowing our entry back to our transcendental origin before the 'Fall.' Please note that it was only after Mary Magdalen gave her 'Yes' that this mystery would be played out on their wedding night, revealing to her who she truly was. This mirrored Jesus' mother's experience; whereupon she had to voluntarily give her Yes before she too found out *what her true identity was.*

This mystery of God's love and how our salvation began through this Man who is the Divine Masculine, and his marriage to Mary the Divine Feminine, is unfolded throughout our teachings, not just in summary, but with all we know via the consciousness of Mary Magdalen.

The Marriage Feast of Cana is the ultimate first step in bringing about God's plan of salvation. It is not only a witnessing of true love, but the marriage of Jesus and Mary Magdalen is the manifestation of the unfathomable truth regarding the consuming love God shares between Consorts. By Jesus and Mary's transcendental union, all that was done and was lost with Adam and Even is reversed, and restored, that we may once again attain what God intended for us all. It is our responsibility to God to follow this "Way"[137] and, upon our death, leave this place of exile, and to return home.

Once that the truth is propagated, we will come to see the beauty and wisdom of God. Life will be better, and even though we are in exile, we will appreciate all that we have. We will no longer be victims of a weakened subtle body, but will experience strength, safety, courage, confidence, and self-assuredness, as well as courage to act and speak the truth. We will experience the "I Am, the Light of the soul". This is the light that Jesus said we cannot hide under a bushel basket; nor will we have any desire to hide it. We will not view life as:

Phase One: Birth
Phase Two: What the heck is this?
Phase Three: Death
Phase Four: Now what?

This Marriage brings with it the sublime realization of the eternal consorts finding each other in this world and consummating their vows, not in the physical way of the world, which always involved the blood covenant on the wedding night, but a consummation of their marriage in a divine form which reached a crescendo and fruition at the crucifixion.

The changing of water to wine represented the pure union, and celebration of the love Jesus shared with his wife and her divinization; there was no need for a blood covenant at this time.

---

[137] The connection between Jesus' "Way" and the Tao meaning 'way' is worth noting and studying further. In particular, one might research the writings relating to the Tao, and then return to a renewed and deepened appreciation of Jesus being the 'Way', the Truth, and the Life (and Light). – Ed.

Jesus changed the water into wine on their Wedding Day, but later on, the Wine will be changed into blood with a drop of water signifying their oneness in marriage and ultimately their oneness in the shedding of blood for us, necessary for the completion of God's salvific mission.

Without a doubt, the presence of Jesus' mother was presented to establish her as the most significant woman in his life. Beyond the shadow of a doubt, Mary was the First Divine Feminine to become human. Through her Yes to giving birth to the Divine Masculine Son of God, not only did she reveal to the world that she was the Spouse of the Most High God, but without her yes, there would also be no salvation plan. Her Yes was the first of three cosmic impacts that were experienced in the world that would affect the entire human race. This, however, was not the intention behind mentioning her presence in the manner in which she was attending the wedding.

The author's purpose was to exclude the possibility of this event being *Jesus'* wedding. Therefore, using what would be *basic alchemy* to Jesus, it was the only choice they had. There were witnesses to this miracle; so, therefore, they needed something to take away from his marriage. Emphasizing Jesus 'first miracle prevented any more focus being put on the wedding as Jesus and Mary's own, in an effort to dissuade any further questions. This is why and how the transcendental connection of His marriage and subsequent Sacred Balance contained in the Eucharist was negated and successfully obscured all this time, as were countless other mysteries.

LESSON 93

Door #17 Adam and Eve Knew About the Marriage Feast Eucharist

Perhaps this is a good time for the Eeshan interpretation of KJV Genesis 3:19, which proves that God had already revealed to Adam and Eve the means by which salvation will be brought about:

> "The ground will no longer produce every tree that you have eaten of before and every beast of the field, every fowl of the earth will no longer be as you have come to witness. Instead you will work the earth for your food which will be the work of human hands until by 'thorns and thistles' shall bring forth to thee; and thou shall eat the grains of the field (this will be wheat and grains for bread). In the sweat of your face you shall eat bread, until you return to the ground; for out of it you were taken, and unto it you shall return."

Eeshans believe the lines have been reversed, or poorly rendered, and should read:

> God told them, life as you knew it is gone. "The ground will no longer produce every tree that you have eaten of before and every beast of the field, every fowl of the earth will no longer be as you have come to witness. Because you cannot live in the Garden, the Sacred Bread

will no longer be available to you, for now you have different bodies. Instead you will work the earth for your food. And the grains you grow, which will be the work of human hands will be made by you into bread; however, unlike the one provided by God. This bread is for these bodies. It will not sustain you as the Sacred Bread did. Your transcendental bodies were provided with the Sacred Bread, which contained within, the Presence of God, in the form of Light and the Sacred Drink was our covenant of love. These bodies are of the earth. They need a different nourishment. You will use these grains to make the bread necessary to nourish these bodies. You will have to work all the days of your life to grow what you need for your food and drink. When death comes, these bodies will return to the ground from which they were created. Because you have chosen these bodies they will not live forever for they are not made from 'the light' like your transcendental bodies; they are made from a substance—dirt—that cannot provide for immortality. Once the body dies, you will remain in a suspended state until the One who, being uncreated, becomes 'human and still be divine.' Being human they will make up for your choice and by dying will provide once again the Sacred Bread and Sacred Wine. Made from the work of human hands, the Bread will be the Real Presence of the Second Person of God being the only begotten Child, and as Divine Masculine and Divine Feminine will bring forth eternal life for the remission of sin; and the Sacred Wine, will become the blood of the sacrifice that conquers death and brings back the everlasting covenant between God and humans. Until that time, you [Adam and Eve] will have returned to the ground for out of it you were taken, and unto it you shall return.

This is: "The Bread come down from heaven, necessary for eternal life, for bread made from man will not provide everlasting life but only temporal life."

It is good to include here that Eeshan Transcendentalism contains within it an understanding of the place of chakras and tones and all those things attributed to a higher consciousness. These are energy points, or issues, found in humans, and begin at the "root chakra,' which is related to survival, our body, and our identity. The basic issues associated with this chakra are survival, trust, safety, and family, and all those things affected when one is grounded in the physical rather than the spiritual.

The template is still there in its original form, though closed due to the Original Choice,[138] coinciding with the punishment of the Serpent. The transcendental Bread reopens the chakras from the base where these issues begin, and where the Kundalini life force energy is dormant ("sleeping"), and is awakened to rise to the crown chakra, where the gate to paradise is located. Thus the Bread of Life is accessed through the physical, leading the soul back to the spiritual.

That is why the seed of the transubstantiation for the transcendental Bread had to begin with the gifts obtained by the work of the human hands, used for the bread of Adam, that God told him he would eat. This bread from Adam, that would only temporarily sustain the gross physical body, would later be the same bread used by Jesus for life everlasting. This is the link from man, used by Jesus, as the liaison needed for the reconciliation of humanity to God, and with Jesus being the new Adam. You see, it was important that Adam experience the difference between this bread used for the body, in contrast to eating the "spiritual bread" given for their transcendental bodies.

---

[138] The term 'Choice' will, henceforth, be used more frequently in relation to the event at the heart of what readers most commonly were taught was the "fall" and "original sin." The reasons are made apparent in the author's words. – Ed.

LESSON 94

DOOR #18 THE FIRST ADAM AND EVE BEGOT CHILDREN: HUMAN LOVE AND NATURAL BIRTHING

THE NEW ADAM AND NEW EVE: PERFECT TRANSCENDENTAL LOVE AND BACK TO BEGETTING CHILDREN

With the woman being the other half of "one" through marriage, Eve would now experience human love and sexuality; and, thus, give birth to human children by natural birthing means, since no longer would she and Adam have children by the begetting process.

Mary, Jesus' wife and eternal consort, would not give birth to human children, but would beget Jesus' transcendental children, since as it was in the beginning, was now via a tantric love on earth, until the fullness of time returns, and will ever be.

Jesus' mission was to restore us to our original transcendental consciousness, and being, the transcendental link was prefigured by God's command to Adam upon Adam's participation in the original choice.

It is written in the traditional story, that for them to have children, Eve would have to go to her husband to procreate through her physical desire, since no longer could they experience the begetting process. Three different Bible translations for Genesis 3:16 illuminate the point from different language perspectives:

Unto the woman he said, "I will greatly multiply thy sorrow and thy conception; in sorrow, thou shalt bring forth children; and thy desire shall be to thy husband; and he shall rule over thee."

To the woman He said, "I will greatly multiply your pain in childbirth. In pain, you will bring forth children; Yet your desire will be for your husband. And he will rule over you.

Then he said to the woman, "I will sharpen the pain of your pregnancy, and in pain you will give birth. And you will desire to control your husband, but he will rule over you.

Eeshans looked at these and other translations and wondered.

We believe that a loving God most certainly would have told Eve what to expect now that she had a human body. This would include everything a woman naturally goes through. God would have placed a magnetism to attract both the man and woman to each other; and, thus, they would enjoy her pregnancy, and this unique birthing process, just as couples do today. We believe God would definitely tell her how when it is time, all about the labor and birth. To emphasize pain and suffering as a consequence of not being able to beget children, would sound like a punishment to humans, but with regards to making the baby the reason for the suffering, it does not sound like God. Giving birth is painful, women are pushing through their bodies another human being. But what woman remembers the labor and pain after the birth? This sounds like something a patriarchal religion would look to say to women simply because a man could not comprehend this pain. A woman sees it as being natural.

Our God, identified to us by Jesus, would not exclaim: "Now when you want children you will be punished!" Our God would emphasize joy and amazement.

To tell the woman that she would have a 'desire to control the man' sounds as though this was the version most appealing at the time when contraception was introduced. Was this translation the fail-safe used to ensure men's rights to keep women pregnant and in the kitchen? Remember, the church refused to agree to women wanting to use contraception not only because it "prevented life," but because "a woman wouldn't be able to control her body."

What God actually told them was that both male and female would now be drawn to each other, at one time, or at the same time as the other, perhaps, still initiated by a kiss. We believe that each complimented the other, and the fact that God would put Eve under Adam's rule is absurd. This takes us back to Mary Magdalen's heart prompting her to kiss Jesus in the kitchen at the "welcome back" party Lazarus had for Him.

Yes, this whole experience would be very different to Eve, but don't you think that even if she was not told, she would figure it out and would come to understand that it is all part of the human reproductive system?

It is a God-given love that compels a woman to give birth; so, if it was meant to be a punishment from God, why would a woman have not just one, but more children? If childbirth pain was meant to be seen only as an extreme punishment by God, well, humankind would be nonexistent since it this is a joy of which most women dream.

After the Fall/Original Choice, and as the mind, body, and spirit of Adam and Eve, became more and more subject to entropy and the human consciousness, the focus on the gross physical body took the humans further away from their transcendental and spiritual life. As time went on, it is easy to see how a gap between man and God could widen. But one must remember that God, as a Parent, would be there watching over them.

With this in mind, this undoubtedly would be probable cause for the male ego, which is vulnerable due to linear thinking, to change texts to preserve the patriarchal leadership they so enjoyed and felt was 'correctly ordered.' Couldn't this prompt the reasons to put into writing all those things that could be construed as God's punishment of woman for loss of a perfect life? Could patriarchal religions, who didn't fear God, but desired to use God's power through their religion/culture, find it easy to make God the scapegoat?

If the story of Adam and Eve was true, as we were told while growing up, naturally, the male ego would look at the story and take a step back. Next by reason and logic, perhaps, he was tired and disgusted with working and providing all the days of his life. Perhaps, he began to see in the story that Adam had every right to be angry. If the human mind allowed itself to be influenced by Satan rather than maintaining a relationship with God, it would inevitably sink into darkness. So, could Adam, by the urgings of Satan, begin to blame Eve because he lost the perfect life?

If the traditional story was true, it would appear that God would be forcing Adam and Eve together, not as equals, but by saying the man has a right to rule over, control, and force the weaker gender to do what he wants.

But the God that Jesus spoke of does not fit this description. Wouldn't it make more sense to believe that the two beings, that were subject to a human life, would experience human trials, but do so with the strength they gained through their marriage?

Would the God Jesus spoke of watch how separation from the Presence of God, the lacking the spiritual food necessary for life of the light body, losing a transcendental life, having no grace from which to strengthen them, bring about a salvific plan in order to restore the life intended between God and humans? Of course, it would. Why would God desert the extensions of a love meant to be shared?

Despite their weakened human state, God would remain with them, and guide them, but the effort to continue in a relationship with God would require effort on their part. In other words, they would have to seek him out. God was no longer visible as in the past. God's Presence was now hidden from them.

Could the lack of God's visible presence result in the couple's continued confusion, temptation, and tribulation? Again, of course, it would. With the lack of God's 'visible' Presence, they would begin to feel they were not being watched; therefore, they felt they wouldn't get caught. The more times one gets away with a sin, or an offence due to a weakness, the easier it is to repeat it, and so on and so forth. Once caught, however the dynamic changes, and either one stops doing it, or tries a different approach to stay connected to this action by setting up degrees or times. "'I only did that 'once', twice,'" etc. One more thing, the feeling of being caught in the act, you must understand, is NOT contrition; thus it does not follow that there will be forgiveness. You were caught, and not truly sorry, not contrite. To be forgiven it is necessary to be contrite with the intention to not do it again. This takes will power. To simply say you are sorry is not enough. A conscious vow, or attempt to not return to this particular thing, must be present in the forefront of your mind; and the choice to not do it again must be carried through your life, not just for a time, but for a time and yet further time, until you no longer do it. Fear of consequences is not contrition either. To confess only out of fear of consequences is not forgivable, since one must repent because one knows what was done was wrong, and there must be a conscious effort to not return to the wrong, offending, or harmful behavior.

Not being in the Presence of God allows us to fall victim to our weaknesses. That is why Adam and Eve could become confused, and the temptations became greater, even though they knew it could lead them even further away from God.

In the Garden, when Jesus asked, "Could you not spend an hour with me?" He was telling those with him, regarding what was to take place, "If you stayed awake and spent this time you will be stronger in the face of adversity and fear." They would have seen His face, and that would make it more difficult for Peter, and the rest, to deny him later. They would've understood more about the role Jesus had, and found strength in 'his' weakness and vulnerability. To have comforted him, also, was the ultimate gift they could've given Him. What if God was asleep in the midst of our tribulations?

In present times, if one is connected to their church, spirituality, and goes to Mass, Liturgy, the Marriage Feast, you would be less likely to sin, for your mind and heart would carry those precious moments with God each day of the week. That is why going to the Sacred and Divine Marriage Feast of the Lamb and His Wife, the Mass, the Sacraments, a Worship Service, Adoration, and hearing the Gospels, the readings etc. are so important to attend.

It was because of entropy that the masculine qualities of Adam, that once balanced Eve, were now becoming more linear; thus, causing dissention between them; and the lack of Eve's cyclical feminine qualities were now causing Adam to be out of balance. Rather than complementing one another, they were becoming more independent.

If true, and Eeshans believe it is true, then the lack of the masculine attributes, which maintain half the sacred balance necessary for what woman lacks in her person, as well as the female attributes that would make up half the man's being, their relationship would have taken a much different approach.

As the humans continued on, with no guidance and lack of the Spiritual Food intended for life of the light body and spiritual nutrition, they began to succumb more to the human rational consciousness and become more fixated on the physical and material world, and with the lack of spiritual guidance, brute strength was equated with power and control.

Further down through the ages, male dominance would be grounded in the biblical testimony in the traditional story of Adam and Eve: that "man," and not woman, was made in God's image and likeness, even if everything else in creation shows the masculine balanced by the feminine. It is also not enough to say the masculine pronoun "he" when used in connection with God 'included' the feminine. It's like saying one has depth perception with just one eye, when in fact two are required.

Though Marriage was supposed to be that which brought harmony back between man and woman, instead the Old Law based on the first five books of the bible, became the biblical foundation for defining woman. Woman was:

- the one who followed orders, and was there for man's betterment,
- to be dutiful, fruitful, subservient as man had rights over her as directed by God,
- to love, honor and obey her husband for as long as they both should live.

Woman did not just lose her identity to the man, but because of the flawed Creation Story she never had one. Her husband, for all intended purposes, was her identity. This is very wrong. Losing one's identity based on truth is very true since those identities become one in marriage. Each one is the other's 'better half.'

Jesus, by his relationship and love for Mary, made it obvious that a woman should be beside her man. Males and females were intended to walk together, work together, and love. Marriage was the Oneness that was the ultimate mirrored image of God. No matter how you look at it, it reflects the Divine Masculine and Divine Feminine. This love strengthens the bond of friendship and friendship the bond of marriage, and the oneness shared between the two, since love overpowers all.

LESSON 95

DOOR #19 FROM FAMINE TO FEAST

In those days prior to Jesus, there was no 'spiritual food' for life everlasting. There was only a 'hidden bread' and a Passover wine, which subsequently should have reflected the Sacred Bread and Drink hidden back in the Garden of Eden, and which remained there after the gates were closed; however, it is the events such as in the Exodus that lay the foundational groundwork for the Seder. Jesus' Eucharist, on the other hand, at the last supper, did not. In fact, Eeshans teach and believe that what took place at the last supper, hallmarked that there actually was a "Spiritual Bread and Drink" from which the tradition stemmed from.

Feast Of Passover

The Feast of the Passover is known for its connection to Moses and the Jewish redemption.

Though Christian history and the celebration of Christ's passion and death is for mankind's redemption by Jesus, we can clearly see even within these teachings and worship services how greatly they differ in doctrine.

THE FIRST MARRIAGE FEAST WAS AT THE LAST SUPPER

Once one enters into the Eeshan Marriage Feast of the Lamb and His Wife, it is clear to see how greatly it differs in comparison to the Mass and Liturgy with which most are familiar. The link is back to Adam and Eve outwardly in its prayers, and the only ties to the Old Law are the very striking errors that Jesus would draw critical attention to. In so many ways Jesus tried to right the wrongs of the Law of the time that the religious leaders so vehemently defended. The people of the time were weighing the Law of God, as they were told and lived for generations, not being aware of the Sacred Food and Drink but yet being aware of a 'hidden bread,' known as the "*aphikomen.*"

Their notion of the importance of the *aphikomen* could now be seen, and used by God, as prefiguring not just the Eucharist, but Eeshans' believe more importantly, the meaning behind the aphikomen that Jesus used, was to protect His Wife from harm under Peter and preserve Her for these end times. However, they saw that which Jesus was teaching only as being against their well-established beliefs. Though the people were filled with a mixture of fear and suspicion, they were intrigued, but the authorities were filled with dread. What Jesus was teaching was highly inappropriate to them, making them (the religious authorities) feel judged daily by the very people they were supposedly judging themselves.

It is said that through the Mass, the Eucharist is the Fruit of Jesus' sacrifice and death; however, He actually brought about the return of the spiritual bread once given to Adam and Eve, which was lost. In its fullness, it could only be by the Eucharist of the Marriage Feast that this Eucharist is back to restore once again the Sacred Balance of which this world has never really known. It is only in the Marriage Feast, and not the Mass, that the Eucharist is complete with all that God intended to include the true meaning of the aphikomen—the Hidden Bride revealed in these revelatory times.

The Seder, if compared to the Mass, is mirrored after the bread made from the wheat that Adam would have had to work the very earth for; and from this he formed and brought to God the first gifts to receive

His blessing. God's desire for Adam to bring the bread to receive the blessing was for just that—to receive God's blessing. This was not a salvific Bread. The drink from grapes was also not salvific.

In the Mass, the Bread and wine brought to God by only male priests would not only show Adam's separation from Eve, but would also exhibit a dimidiated sacrifice. Christ's role as the Bread come down from heaven, without his wife's participation, would not be complete; and, therefore, *is not according to Christ's life, marriage, and teachings. It also would not restore what was lost via Adam and Eve's fall from the transcendental to the material life.*

The Marriage Feast is complete, and finds its origins in Christ's marriage to Mary, offering to God 'their' oneness and return of the original perfectly and sacredly balanced 'beings,' which in the eyes of God, is One like the Original Being before separation, as was manifested by the separation into male and female of the original couple.

Adam and Eve's descendants would live on man's bread until Jesus, the new Adam, and Mary the new Eve, married. That is why, from the Eeshan perspective, the Old Law is not *salvific*.[139] Since as Adam and Eve were the first parents of humankind, whose choice brought about our humanity, it is Jesus and Mary who would become our first transcendental parents, who makes us begotten children by their marriage.

And, it all started with the marriage of Jesus and Mary, who by their divinity would now take the work of human hands, which is bread, and along with this bread used the miracle of the water and wine to represent their oneness. As the water becomes His wife, which manifests as his eternal consort, it is without form, showing her connection to creation; and Jesus with His alchemical eternal words would then turn the water into wine, and show how their bodies were transubstantially/alchemically united, and Mary would take on his identity. In End Times, an even more 'remarkable mystery' takes place as Jesus' identity would now be in Mary's human and sacramental form, fulfilling the prophecy of "the woman will encompass the man." That is why we said that understanding

---

[139] The Old Law was considered a 'babysitter' by Paul. The babysitter has charge only until the 'parents return.' – Ed.

the return of *Ishvara* is important, since it completes the understanding of how the title Eesha can carry the meanings or translations as God, Supreme Being, queen, or special self, and would be revealed via supramentalization (more about this later). It is how we explained the danger of dismissing this mystery as a 'nothingness' is the nature and error of logic and reasoning deduced by the human consciousness, and how it robs one of unfathomable mysteries of the Divine.

Since as it was written, in End Times, God will gather those who desire a spirituality and do not need to be convinced, but rather seek to come to the celebrated Marriage Feast, just like in the parable of the marriage feast of the King's son. It will be for all those on the highways and byways who were called and believe; but it will not be for those who were invited but who refused.

The Marriage Feast of the Lamb and His Wife is the non-bloody sacrifice of their body, blood, soul, and divinity together representing both the bloody sacrifice of the two on Calvary and the non-bloody sacrifice on their wedding night where there was no bloody consummation.

Their non-bloody sacrifice would find its fruition in the consummation and sacrifice of love since Christ died on the Cross, and as Mary was pierced through her heart and hemorrhaged at the foot of the Cross. As life drained from each of them, they simultaneously died together.

On their wedding night Jesus' breath awakened Mary's Divinity. The Marriage Feast came into existence to do what Peter's church refused and failed to do. The church of Peter maintains an incredulity mindset towards/ against anyone constituting a contradiction involving questioning the church's doctrines. Why? Because they say their doctrines are based on Sacred Scriptures and Sacred Tradition. The Eeshan Religion acknowledges scriptures to the contrary, where Christ and his wife are revealed as co-Saviors and co-Redeemers. By their bloody sacrifice and unbloody transcendental salvific union they fulfilled God's promise to:

1. Punish the serpent for what he did and in doing so show mercy to Adam and Eve.
2. Send one who will cause enmity between the serpent's seed and hers; and despite His suffering there will be one who will smite the power of evil and bruise the serpent's head.

These two Saviors will 'reverse the consequences' of Adam and Eve's choice for the physical. We witness this in the greatest of all unfathomable mysteries, the one that truly defies human comprehension, the return of the immortal transcendental/light body.

In order to accomplish salvation for their descendants/children, the transforming of the 'Cana water into wine' is key to identifying Jesus in his human nature, using His divine nature and using alchemical words, to awaken the divinity of His wife from her human nature upon the consummation of their marriage, and which would be forever witnessed to by adding water to the wine in bringing about *transubstantiation*. It showed how the 'two' became one and could never thereafter be separated, thus uniting heaven and earth. It truly plays out the mystery of how He and Mary could never be separated once they were married, thereby, explaining in the sacred words, and in an alchemical code, the identity of the true Eucharist. It would also serve as an eschatological reference to the End Times, when Eesha would return to complete the mission Jesus began here, prophetically exclaimed by the waiter who said, "You have saved the best wine for last." It also connects the two historical moments in time (the one at hand and the one in the distant future), the first conducted at the hand of the active gender (Jesus) while the passive gender's role in the present moment (Mary), in the second moment in history, becomes active.

Because the church never recognized Mary and Jesus as married, they are guilty of robbing the people of the fullness of the Eucharist by presenting Jesus in a dimidiated way. From Peter on, the choice was for a patriarchal lens through which to view the meaning of Jesus' life and mission, thus, completely altering the purpose and focus of God's entire salvific plan.

The Sacred and Divine Marriage Feast is the Sacred Bread and Drink come down from heaven, and Eeshans believe it provides the 'only' means by which to enter into the plan of salvation, so long as there is grace (i.e., no mortal sin), and faith in both Jesus and Mary as co-redeemers in these end times.

This is what will bring about the faith that Jesus asked if He would find when He returns with His Gift. This faith, however, warrants strong belief in God's Salvation Plan to a tee. The Eeshan doctrines are not only based on 'spiritual apprehension,' which means it provides complete trust and belief in God and reasonable proof to substantiate our perspective. This faith, however, requires the 'desire for the transcendental spirituality' that feeds our hearts, souls, and minds.

It actually brings the power of God within us by the reception of the Sacred and Divine Eucharist of the Marriage Feast, enabling us to be the leaven that Christ taught about … in other words, to bring God to others by being the best version of ourselves that we can be. We do this every time we put others before us. It's what we do. Because we are all connected, with the power of God behind us we can do anything. We can move mountains, end hate, restore balance, unite with love, since we are God's children; and, therefore, nothing is impossible for us.

LESSON 96

DOOR #20 LIVING FOREVER VERSUS ETERNITY

The problem with losing touch with the transcendental, and living a purely rational human existence since time immemorial, is that it prorogated skepticism of anyone, or anything, that presented, or presents, any evidence that conflicts with what is taught; and the church did this. What was, and is, supposed to be seamlessly accurate at best is mediocre, and hardly translates into the Person of Jesus, or His message of 'love' and mission of salvation. As we said it gives the appearance of Jesus but mocks truth. Under this consciousness, the church determined what books were 'true' and which Gospels, books, and writings regarding Christ's life were 'false.' This is specific to what is called "indefinitely ancient," or, rather, "ancient beyond memory or record." In other words, what they claim has become known as ancient sacred scriptures, and sacred tradition, and has been enjoyed for so long that the church (both established and universal) does not have to prove how they arrived at what they believed. This is then enjoyed as true in and of itself because their teachings go into such a distant past that they are secure and comfortable enough to make anyone who challenges the established catholic doctrines look foolish and stupid, especially without basis in 'fact' or without solid 'evidence'. This is so because the universal church believes there is no other memory, or record, that can be used, or considered legal, by anyone who challenges what is taught or written.

Without the transcendental, we are limited not just in our relationship with God, and the things of God, but also to only those things taught and passed along. We live in time, so it's difficult to comprehend eternity, since eternity to the human consciousness still seems to connote a future. Then there is the concept of infinity. Mathematician Peter Ashley explains:

> "Infinity is a procedure in time. The universe is infinite, because you can traverse it forever (cross over it); and a number line is transverse because you can count it forever. Eternity is outside of time. A clock 'has the experience' of eternity because there is no memory and perception to create time. The now is the eternal, because although the forms change constantly it's always just now. What does this mean in the scheme of things? God sees everything outside of time, therefore a second, or a minute, has no gauge. That is why the term fullness of time has no real 'time' component."

There are as many explanations of these words as one desires. We have no concept of eternity, and even given the definition our sense of eternity, it comes down to 'endless life with God.' Jesus also used the term, 'life everlasting.' God was not created and no destruction can come to God. God's love is ceaseless, endless, perpetual. Eeshans believe that when Jesus spoke, He talked about eternity in reference to the spirit and soul as bodies are matter and deteriorate and decay. He used the phrase, 'Life without end.' As Adam and Eve were created, they possessed immortality and could live without end; however, they did not always exist, but were given, indeed, everlasting life.

All these meanings are here to help you better understand the Story of Creation and of the life of Adam and Eve. It shows how using 'time', eternity, and other such words allowed for the 'prorogation,' or differences, in stories in bible verses; still it allows for the church to claim it has "the truth," as no one can claim otherwise. That is what enables the church to establish a 'spiritual' lockdown by verse, Law, Tradition, and repetition.

That is why what we learned about God came about by way of habitual repetition of something, such as being asked the question, "Who made you," and the 'almost mechanical' response of "God made me." Learning about Jesus, and how He taught falls under that 'rote' spirituality we have all experienced at one time or another.

We can prepare for all kinds of events here in life, and we are even capable of, and do perform miracles each day; we find the strength to accomplish these by a kind of interior drive. There are works set in place, that because of God, for example, a single mom is able to raise good children alone; or a teacher who teaches children for less pay than they can live on. There are those, who, despite their difficult life, spend time with the elderly, or sick, after a hard day's work, and give to others in need when they have little themselves. Still the concept of living forever, though most familiar to us, plays out in the mind as living forever in 'this world.'

Eternity is blurred and most difficult to comprehend. We read about those who believe they had 'other lifetimes,' of reincarnation, of resurrection, and, then, there is supramentalization; but the reality of eternity is still a conundrum for us because it goes beyond the natural and the known; and without warning, our minds step into the unknown.

Living forever nixes out the concept of eternity. It appears that our view of eternity is skewed based on how we live and think today. Some pray that they live with God in eternity, hoping that it is a reward for the trials and tribulations they had gone through here. Some view living with God in a totally different manner. We know things about life here, and the things we would love to do every day, but to some, eternal life with Jesus kind of connotes a life of prayer with 'hints of things' we heard, including things such as, "We will look like when we were thirty-three because everyone in heaven is thirty-three years old" … "The only music we will be listening to is angels singing and harp music" … or "We will be happy and never get sick." These notions are relative to things we pull from within ourselves, and from our imagination of what we may have imagined Paradise to be. So, living 'forever' seems to be the better option versus thinking about living with God, based on what we were taught.

When you are young and healthy, images of a religious life, based on going to church, and only knowing what has been taught by the church, seems to forfeit fun and relationships and the things we enjoy here.

Even as we read this book, we are not applying ourselves wholeheartedly because we would rather believe we can have the best of both worlds.

A significant reason for this is because without a strong connection via transcendentalism, spirituality beyond the reach of human logic is translated into only our perceptions. The consequence here is that one may think they can't apply transcendentalism to everyday life because they are not *religious*.

If you continue to equate the transcendental spirituality with only these kinds of things and perceptions, or what other people tell you, your definition of spirituality is only an allusion to someone else's words. It's not your own experience. What we want to give you is a reality of the kind of life that will cause you to desire a spirituality where you will find a treasure in the promises of God that causes a love and joy within you to your core ... so that when you apply it to your daily life you will not only see more beauty, and enjoy your life with others more, but you will be less likely to focus on the negative, the dark side of things, etc. This all gives one a taste of heaven. Human spirituality without the balance of a transcendental spirituality is governed by illusion *and* sometimes even delusion.

Today, by way of *illusion*, the soul, in terms of *human awareness*, confuses the body and mind with itself in thinking the body and mind ARE the self.

And in the midst of this illusion, one becomes fearful because *body and mind are both temporary*, and by way of simple observation can only see itself 'dying.' Today, with social media, we wake up with feelings that we are surrounded by death by cancer, clawing at the door of life, along with diabetes, heart failure, and other known diseases. Even if you try to take a positive attitude, and translate each of these into thinking in terms of prevention and wellness, you are met with what seems to be an 'ongoing flu season,' or 'contagion' that is wiping out large numbers of people. In any event we are being robbed of hope. The golden years of life, where one once looked forward to enjoying retirement, and the rewards of an often lifetime of work have now been replaced with television ads, news, and social networking, as well as awareness billboards of imposed physical, emotional and cognitive limitations, showing retirement communities stressing memory and palliative care with helpless elderly people unable to care for themselves. It almost looks as though we are right in the midst of a controlled euthanasia program, which allows life to continue until the person seems to be exhibiting the first stages of end-of-life symptoms. It's like we are trying to work around the constant perceived resistance geared to block and stall any progress to offset this perception. There doesn't seem to be any allowance for retirement past sixty-five years of age, but rather an effort to eliminate anyone considered 'elderly' by watching, and categorizing, 'acute' and chronic' patient care. By implementing this way of thinking, by age propaganda through media and advertising, older people begin to believe they are 'old.' What happens on a spiritual level? As the soul affects the subtle body, without transcending, the soul is held in the grips of the quicksand effect of the illusion; it also thinks it is 'dying,' and behaves accordingly, in a seemingly endless flow of dysfunctions and breakdowns in various forms and guises.

Earlier we mentioned Plotinus. He was a philosopher who believed, and taught, that there were three beings at the center of the universe. These beings were good and were at the center of the universal laws. He called them the One, the Mind, and the Soul. This view is often found in some other eastern teachings where as the One is the All, from the All is the Mind, which contains within itself the scientific and philosophical laws, and the third is the Soul, which is defined as the principle activity in all that exists. He says the One is why a hunk of clay exists. The mind gives the clay form, and, through the Soul, the clay is given Life, and that's how it becomes human. The three are totally spirit. Anything that involves matter, such as the world and what is physical in the world, are bodies that are not thought of highly. Humans are a mixture of matter, and spirit, and if they focus more on their spirits, and less on their bodies, they can come closer to the Soul, which means coming closer to the One.

Lesson 96A

We believe in the First Person of the Holy trinity as Father and Mother, who is the One, and in the Second Person of the Holy Trinity, who is Jesus the Divine Masculine of the only Begotten Child of God, with His eternal Consort who back in time was known as Mary Magdalen, but today is known as Eesha.

The Second person of the trinity agrees with, and is in every way equal to, the First Person of the Holy Trinity, but will be Judge; and in the Holy Spirit, who is guardian of the soul's disposition to each Person of God, there is a Consort of Masculine and Feminine, which equals Sacred Balance; and each of the Persons share equally in all things—divine, human, and sacramentally. This, too, will be discussed about in later texts.

Jesus knew that the human spirit is sorely affected by how the mind feels, and that the mind affects a person physically. So, as He embarked on his mission, He did so knowing how God's children had already been victims of a spiritual famine. As such, He used physical healings to make them appreciate life; then He brought them to the awareness of life after this life.

Back then, death was publicly mourned a little differently than today. While it is true that the various groups (Pharisees, Sadducees, Essenes, Temple authorities, etc.) had differing, and in some ways, competing beliefs about the afterlife, the common people of the time were 'caught in the middle,' in a kind of nebulous agnostic-like stance towards the subject, with no one being certain of what to believe or disbelieve. This could easily translate into not believing in an afterlife, since all that one could be certain of was what was happening in the 'here and now' and in day-to-day life concerns. This really is much the way people think and behave today, even though there is a profession of belief in an afterlife.

Nevertheless, people still believed in some kind of punishment where a soul may be in Gehenna for a short time, but still there was no way that they would have a concept of *eternal* life or death.

Because of Jesus, we know about eternal life and what we need to sustain us while we are here on earth in preparation for life everlasting; since He is the active consort of the only begotten child of God. This is why he is the new Adam, for He, His love, and sacrifice, cancels out the masculine part of the first human man's involvement in the fall to the physical. How? By bringing back the knowledge of life after death.

Eeshans believe as people at the time of Jesus had no concept of eternal death, and no knowledge of everlasting life by way of examples and/or proof, which would affect how they lived their lives and how life is a precious opportunity, since how it is lived determines salvation.

Today, we are almost as ignorant, except we 'believe' in an afterlife. 'Live for today,' 'have it your way,' and other mottos, or slogans, subliminally affect our decisions in everyday life. This is important, since without knowledge of an afterlife we are left with a whole different belief system, and one that is to believe that we should live for the moment and for ourselves, allowing for the belief that life, ultimately, has no value or worth.

What happens without the realization of an afterlife is multi-faceted:

1. First and foremost, there is no need for a Savior(s)—just look around and see that without God there is only the need for purging and punishing according to man's law,
2. There would be no need for religion or spirituality, for man's law now replaces God's,
3. We find anti-diversity—and sadly it seems as though it originated in Catholic/Christian religions due to how Jesus has been re-imaged by man—not how he actually was/is,
4. Unless you fit the standard dictated by the church, you may be judged as not being a follower of Christ or being in sin,
5. People, as a result, will become cynical and suspect, not welcoming and loving—thus we would become a nation governed by fear.

Because of Jesus, we know what we need to do to return to our transcendental state. Jesus himself gave us everything to include proof of an afterlife, identifying himself as the Son of God, the supreme Authority on how to love God and neighbor, as well as the Food needed to transform us, and the "Way" that to leads us back to where we came from. To ignore this, and say there is no need for these things, means we are weak, and, by human consciousness, will be drowned by the torrent. We easily find the answer in Luke 6:46-49, & 7:1.

> The Lord said, "Why do you call me 'Lord, Lord,' and not put into practice what I teach you? Any man who desires to come to me will hear my words and put them into practice. I will show you with whom he is to be compared. He may be likened to the man who, in building a house, dug deeply and laid the foundation on a rock. When the floods came, the torrent rushed in on that house, but failed to shake it because of its solid foundation. On the other hand, anyone who has heard my words but not put them into practice is like the man who built his house on the ground without any foundation. When the torrent rushed upon it, it immediately fell in and was completely destroyed.

In other words, *Jesus is teaching that by not heeding His words, one brings wrought upon oneself; for in this world one cannot love God by ignoring the fact that we belong to a family—the human race. If we can't love those who we can see, we can't love One whom we can't see.*
For those who aren't clear about what he is saying, we see in the words of John Lennon from his song, "Instant Karma:"

> Instant Karma is gonna get you
> Gonna knock you right in the head
> You better get yourself together
> Pretty soon you're gonna be dead.
> What in the world you thinkin' of
> Laughing in the face of love,
> What in the world you trying to do
> It's up to you.

Instant karma's gonna get you
Gonna look you right in the face
Better get yourself together darlin'
Join the human race ...

If one continues on, in the short time we have here, not doing what Jesus teaches, one will continue to have ears but will not hear, have eyes yet will not see. For it is only in developing a spirituality that you will understand what Jesus taught about eternity, eternal life, life everlasting, living forever; for all these will be rendered meaningless otherwise, because one hasn't grasped time, which is what one is most familiar.

LESSON 97

DOOR #21 GOD SENDS ANOTHER HELPER

Without a doubt, we need a helper. Just as Jesus had promised when he was returning to heaven, and to insure his mission, here on earth, this helper would come to maintain the Sacred Balance; however, Peter did not continue Jesus' mission, and as things began to revert back, many of Christ's teachings were not carried on. With this reversal of what Jesus taught, and exhibited, in his private life, it wasn't long before things returned to the way they were before he began teaching. Once again, that familiar imbalance raised its ugly head, and the feminine consort, Mary Magdalen, was once again under attack.

Back then we heard that "the power of the Holy Spirit came upon them and they were not afraid," the 'they' being the male disciples. What had taken place, however, was that they made a choice—yes, a choice—to receive the Holy Spirit, but, also, to *reject* the Divine Feminine Spirit. The Holy Spirit is the Divine Masculine of the Spirit of God. His counterpart is the Divine Feminine. The two *as one* comes to us, but what we do with the Spirit's gifts is our choice.

The few of the male apostles, who were still attached to their birth religion in many ways, felt that Jesus, sending this helper, finally had given them 'the power,' since the spirit couldn't possibly have been for the women.

Though many are called, few are chosen, so, too, is true of free will, when it comes to doing God's will. Even though the Spirit had come upon both male and female disciples, you witness how the male disciples ignored the calling of the divine feminine to make things right in their culture. It was the beginning of a dimidiated spirit.

As God's original plan had been altered, or neglected, men's desire to stand firm on the old teachings of keeping women submissive remained. Only men would have the roles of priests, just as before, under the old Law, since it was always understood that it was *man* who was made in the image and the likeness of God, and woman was his helper, as laid down for centuries before Christ. Dismissing and losing texts to back up Jesus' all-inclusive directives, we have discovered the many different ways things were changed, mostly for political and power reasons. Men could have been well worried that their efforts wouldn't be accepted, and respected, by the rest of the established religion and culture of the Jews otherwise.

Once again, we are witnessing the *Fullness of Time*. The need and fight for the Co-Messiah today to stop discrimination of women, and evoke equality among 'all' people, regardless of gender, culture, race, creed, age, etc., has now been identified as a cry for God to do something.

As it stands, the church will never allow women full participation in leadership/liturgical roles, no matter the arguments, and is certainly steadfast against the notion of a woman being God's Eternal Consort. It would mean the destruction of all "it" held as truth and sacred.

The time is now, and the world needs the One who shares as eternal consort to her Divine Male counterpart. Yes, we need Mary Magdalen, the hidden Bride, the Wife of the Lamb, whatever her title, today. How can that be, as she died many hundreds of years ago?

How can this situation be rectified? Well, as her body died. her consciousness lived on, and now, in these end times, she is brought back, and her work, which was stifled in biblical times, continues through supramentalization.

Just as God the heavenly Father assisted our first parents and promised help after their choice, Jesus and his Consort are here for us. Jesus being omnipotent, witnessed and made every attempt to change Peter's heart, knowing of his cowardly personality. But, despite his love for Jesus, Peter would remain the stumbling block, and would form a kind of religious coup and reject Jesus' wife, as well as any other woman who got out of line.

Being so dull, in the words of Jesus addressing Peter, Peter was so blind and deaf that he didn't even see God's help. Rejecting the Divine Feminine of the Spirit of God, the third Person of the Trinity, who is perfectly balanced Divine Masculine/Divine Feminine, would allow men to exercise their free will for a time and a time.

LESSON 98

DOOR #22 WHEN GOD HAS HAD ENOUGH

Why now? Why would God send forth His Divine Feminine in these end times? God hears the cries of his people. Being merciful, God has declared this time the age of enlightenment: when the omega woman, who like the Alpha Divine Feminine, the eternal consort of the Eschaton, would now be needed to bring about the sacred balance to fruition.

The promised helper, also Sacredly Balanced, would be sent to keep His followers on track with Christ's 'true teachings.'

As you can see, despite Jesus' warnings, the 'dissent' of humankind's consciousness began immediately following Christ's ascension. The male apostles became frightened and continued to hide. The women, nonetheless, were made to relent for fear of harsh intentions and cruel treatment, and, despite all efforts, were made to listen to and obey Peter's instructions to be subservient to the men, as implied by the Law of their birth religion, in order that the new religion may continue. The Divine Masculine watched how his followers used their free will not to do as He directed and lived, but to once again start treating the women with disdain.

This poor treatment of women resumed as it had been before, and was witnessed with Peter denying Mary's teachings after her visions of Jesus, following His ascension. Peter made it a point to treat the words of the wife of Christ, as though she made them up. Peter commented that surely Jesus would not give his words to a woman.

Mary's place of equality alongside Jesus, in her role as matrix among His male apostles and followers, which she enjoyed as a 'free' married woman, was taken from her as His male apostles and disciples (those who followed Peter) began to unearth rumors, lies, and threats from her past, which under the Old Law, gave them good reason to do so. All these produced a desired effect, which was enough to replace the redemption of her husband's word. This continued up and until the church was getting more culturally embedded, established, and ever stronger.

It was almost as though a state of confusion, or bewilderment, had immediately set in. Around 591 AD, the first documented mention of Mary Magdalen, as a prostitute, was circulated; and of course, what further discredited her reputation was a sermon performed by Pope Gregory, in which he fused the three sinful women named Mary of the New Testament as one person.

As Jesus pledged that all things will be revealed in the Light, Revelation 21:5 reads: "He who was seated on the throne said, 'Look, I am making all things new! Write this down, for what I tell you trustworthy and true.'" At this time, in this age of Enlightenment, once again, Jesus is not only His wife's redeemer, but He also presents her to the world as his Eternal Consort and co-redeemer to the world. As the Divine Masculine's Spirit's counterpart is called Divine Feminine, God is once again answering the call of the people for a Messiah; only this time, it will be she who is the matrix of God's possibilities.

See in Revelation 21:8:

"But the cowardly, the unbelieving, the vile, the murderers, the sexually immoral, and who practice sorcery, idol worshipping (money, power), and all liars, will be thrown in the lake that burns with fire and sulfur." All according to his 'word'.

What happens when God has had enough? The above is what happens. Joel 1:3 says, "Tell it to your children, and their children's children, to the next generation." Jesus says to the women of Jerusalem on his way to Calvary, Luke 23:28, "Daughters of Jerusalem, weep not for me, but for yourselves and your children." Jesus was already witnessing what was going to take place, since the men fled and the women stayed.

God's law has been perverted in many ways, and it is written that, "The wheels of God's judgment may grind slow; but they grind exceedingly fine." Still, his Divine Feminine comes back.

The price of a weakened faith, and lackluster spirituality is the price we are presently paying, and have been paying, since the refusal to recognize Jesus' wife, precipitating God's people to fall out of love and belief in God, which stems from the intuitive, rational mind, which is guiding us. Thus, it is necessary for the Holy Spirit's counterpart, The Divine Feminine, to assist and guide our Way and help to propagate our spirituality.

Wisdom has always been the Feminine aspect of God. With the return of Mary's actual presence in the world, we should see abounding strength in women and a kindness so powerful that it will bring a swift equality and gender appreciation that will turn the tides of iniquity and restore a Sacred Balance within the hearts of human beings, who will in turn bring back the natural balance within nature as it should be.

You need not look far to find evidence for lack of faith as witnessed through the mindset and the controlling human consciousness today. As we mentioned, people simply don't want to deal with personal responsibility; nor do they feel they can function without someone they feel is stronger than they are and in telling them what to do. They feel trapped, and seem to be looking for a great evil that will end the world as we know it. Their cry for deliverance by an apocalyptic means shows how emotional slavery has, indeed, oppressed God's people leaving them with validation of their fear. Rather than seek hope, people seek validation for bad things in the world as the fulfillment of prophecies from sources they determined to be true, such as the bible. Others want a sudden universal or cosmic disaster. All of these bring a kind of sad relaxation and peace, because it is at the hand of someone, or something greater than they, and makes the origins of their fear and prophecies credible. With negative thoughts or emotions, one can't think clearly, and it plunges them into depression, and, depending on how we feel each day, this affects how we function.

The mind has many levels of emotion to work through. When it reaches the level where it becomes desperately overwhelmed, the end result is the rational mind seeking help.

Though the above doesn't seem like rational thinking, it is all that is left if one is deprived of faith and hope, and in most cases, we find that, more often than not, the individual will 'not' ask for help. Without faith in Jesus, who fosters the transformation of the mind and spirit, as well as the physical body, the individual stays at lower level frequencies and 'loses' rather than 'gains' the properties of God's light, and not only loses the ability to be the vehicle for his light, but also cannot accept it either; for darkness cannot be separated from the light of self.

LESSON 99

DOOR #23 WISDOM! BE ATTENTIVE!

Jesus, having a "wise mind" understood that this is when the soul is at the point of starving for light, and begins to rely on the body's form of nourishment; thus, we find the avenue where a person, without the feeling of purpose, as well as having addictions and weaknesses, begins seeking some kind of release, escape etc., and since the individual is not happy, feels empty inside, and sees no happiness. Nothing in this world can fill the void, or satisfy the hunger, for the only thing that would satisfy it would be light. Without trust and faith in Jesus, however, to whom do we turn?

Wisdom is the ability to think, and act, using knowledge, understanding, common sense, and insight. Wisdom is the virtue which, as a habit, or disposition, performs an action with the highest degree of adequacy under any given circumstance. This involves an understanding of people, objects, events, situations, and the willingness as well as the ability to apply perception, judgment, and action in keeping with the understanding of the optimal course of action.[140] It means control of one's personal and emotional reactions, as well as one's passions, so that truth can be found. It is the core essence of the universe. For wisdom encompasses the wisdom of the all-encompassing space, mirror-like wisdom, wisdom of equality, wisdom of discernment, and the all-accomplishing wisdom.

All things Jesus taught, He taught through wisdom. Plato said, "the mind is willing but the body is not." Jesus said, "the spirit is willing but

---

[140] Rudin, Peter. "Going from Digital Transformation to AGI: Are We Really Ready?" SINGULARITY 2030, 2017, singularity2030.ch/going-from-digital-transformation-to-agi-are-we-really-ready/.

the body is not," meaning that both were teaching that the body is like a prison, except Plato believed the body is not good, for as it ages, one is more imprisoned; whereas, Jesus said one should focus less on the body and more on God, since one can leave the body through transcendence, which is the goal always intended by God for us.

There is only one who is capable of turning the tide of faith in the direction of Jesus, since too much damage has been done over the years, and, now, especially with the scandals that have destroyed people's respect and admiration of the apostolic priesthood. That would be the Divine Feminine. Sure, there will always be good priests, just as there were saints through the years where there were popes and anti-popes, showing that it was *the faith of the people and not the leadership that continued to propagate the faith*. But this time, it takes more than an ordinary human being.

The Divine Feminine speaks with eternal wisdom. Eeshans believe as she speaks, it is written, the jaws from which move mouths to speak ludicrous words will be transformed.

Just as in the biblical years when Jesus taught his wife (who was not only human but whose divinity was also revealed once they were married), He continues to share His whole being with her in these End Times. She knows His mind, heart, and will. Two thousand years ago, she was present not just for His public teachings, but also privately, when He addressed His apostles and followers. As eternal consort, she was with Him before, during, and after His lifetime here on earth, as He was, and is, and will be eternally with her. They were soulmates/twin flames.

Eeshans believe the divinity of Mary Magdalen, which sprang forth *proelato*,[141] was "unknown to her at the time," but that she was made aware of it on her wedding night. She experienced *epathe pathos*[142] completely at the crucifixion, without the embrace of her consort desired. This mystery would be played out similarly again in end times.

Yes, we all know what is written in Matthew 16:18, "the gates of hell will not prevail against it," but, as we said, the interpretation of this verse

---

[141] Meaning always existing; springing forth fully and completely via the begetting process.

[142] Meaning sharing extreme suffering.

was to back up Peter's role as leader and authority; this doesn't mean the text is referring to Peter, but it could be made to *appear* that way (i.e., as when Peter purportedly was named the 'Rock' and the church was named the 'bride of Christ'). As with anything else, one sees, in a text, what they want, or need, to see to validate their agenda, and what they consider to be reality. Again, if one chooses to believe this, that is one's own prerogative. Verses were put together, scriptures were not written down/copied verbatim, and certainly were not arranged in chronological order. It stands to reason that if there's been proof that even one scripture passage in the bible is wrong, or has been changed, who is to say that any other scripture passage is without error?

LESSON 100

Door #24 Genesis 4:1 Says: And Adam Knew His Wife and She Conceived and Gave Birth to Cain, "I Have Gotten a Man From the Lord"

Eshans believe that many scriptural passages were altered; and this is one that was written that was conflicting with and contrary to what Jesus said in 1 John 12:8-12:

> He who sins is of the devil, for the devil has sinned from the beginning. For this purpose, the Son of God was manifested, that he might destroy the works of the devil. Whoever has been born of God, does not sin, for His seed remains in him; and he [Jesus] cannot sin, because he has been born of God. In this the children of God and the children of the devil are manifest: Whoever does not practice righteousness is not of God [Satan], nor he who does not love his brother [Cain]. This is the message that you heard from the beginning, that we should love one another.

And in 1 John 3:12 Jesus says:

> Do not be like Cain, who belonged to the evil one and murdered his brother. And why did he murder him?

Because his own actions were evil and his brother's were righteous.

In the above, Jesus was talking about Cain. Cain wasn't Adam's child, and we are sure that many will wonder how this could happen. How can Adam and Eve's first son be evil—and of the evil one?

After the choice for physicality, entropy set in. Over time, the effects of entropy worsened, since there was no spiritual bread or the constant presence of God the couple was once so familiar.

As the human mind darkened, Adam's male weaknesses became more and more prominent. He began missing the life he had before, and began to see Eve in a different light. As time would have it, there grew a separation between him and Eve. Eve would continue to pray to God for guidance, whereas, Adam pulled away from her and became more celibate. Adam began to blame Eve for what had been both their decision—a choice.

Sadly, the lack of Adam's desire made Eve vulnerable, since it was always the love they shared that made them strong in each other.

And I will put enmity between you and the woman, and between your offspring and hers; she will crush your head, and you will strike her heel. (Genesis 3:15)

Satan, being the master of delusion, came to Eve as a 'Son of God.' He told her how highly favored she was; she conceived and Cain his son was born. She thought her 'yes' was to God, but it was not God who seduced her. Her pain was great.

In bearing the male child who she thought was God's child, Eve proclaimed, "God has taken away my reproach." (Genesis 30:23)

History would repeat itself, and this was the proclamation that was enjoyed and proclaimed by Mary Magdalen on their wedding night because of Jesus. No longer was she the reproach of men; she was highly favored by God.

God's favor would continue during her and Jesus' lifetime together on earth. This proclamation would offset Eve's comment regarding Cain when she said yes to whom she believed was God's son.

What about the Virgin Mary? It would appear that she reversed this act of Eve with her "Yes" to conceive and give birth to Jesus. But one must remember that she was not a redeemed woman by, with, and in whom Christ would save and redeem. It would be Jesus and Mary His wife who would restore transcendence by Mary, conceiving with a kiss the true Son of God. Remember, too, it had to be the Only-begotten Child who would reverse the actions and choices of the first created child. That is why there were no conjugal relations in Jesus and Mary's marriage, and their 'children' would be the offspring of the Perfect Man, children who do not die and are born each second.

We stand firm in the belief, that in order to hide Jesus' marriage, the religious leaders after Jesus would be inclined to make his *mother* the integral woman in his life.

By God's design, a son would be born as the fruit of Jesus, and his wife, but it would be fulfilled in End Times, as a result of man's departure from Christ's salvific directives. In other words, Revelation 12:6 regarding End Times would be fulfilled as written regarding "the woman" of the Apocalypse:

> **The woman gives birth to a Male Child that is attacked by the dragon identified as Satan. When the child is taken to heaven the woman flees into the wilderness leading to "war in heaven" fled into the wilderness to a place prepared by God, where she will be nourished for 1260 days. The angels cast out the dragon. The dragon attacks the woman, who is given wings to escape, and then attacks her again with a flood of water from his mouth, which is subsequently swallowed up by the earth. Frustrated, the dragon initiates war on 'the**

remnant of 'her seed' identified as the righteous followers of Christ [*correction: and his wife*[143]].

Showing that nothing is impossible with God, the first born of the firstborn, the Fruit of the love of the Lamb and his Wife would occur in these end times. Showing favor to the one who had been disgraced, He took away once again her reproach in these times, too, by giving her a son to ease her heart, knowing she too would be denied and ridiculed.

Her love for God her husband will manifest in her work and through, with, and in her Kallahs, as they will go and teach what has been hidden or lost, that Jesus' mission will come to completion with the union of the Divine Masculine and Divine Feminine. For the first time since Jesus, both male and female, will have the opportunity to be balanced and equal.

In the fullness of time, when all she was asked to do is accomplished, as Jesus' wife, their completely divine/human child—**the one who is like the Son of Man** (Revelation 1:13)—will be fulfilled.

The Wife of the Lamb's proclamation when Jesus returns with the "Gift," will mirror what was written in Luke 1:25, as Elizabeth said of her pregnancy, **"The Lord has done this for me. In these days, he has shown me favor and taken my disgrace among the people."**

The same type of reproach was endured by Job. Job suffered so many afflictions that when his friends tried to console him he said: **"These ten times you have cast reproach upon me; are you not ashamed to wrong me?"**

Today, we hear the echo of Mary Magdalen's unrequited love for souls which seems to arise from a melodic, and almost rhythmic tone, by those who suffered the same afflictions at the hands of those who refused to recognize her as Christ's wife. The world is empty and out of balance, and its song is one of pain, because it does not relate to Jesus' teachings.

---

[143] "Christ" embodies the Sacred Balance of masculine and feminine, Jesus *and* Mary. – Ed.

It was because men refused to recognize Christ's directives, and chose rather to stay in the human rational consciousness, which Christ came to free them from.

The philosophy, thereby, would not reflect what Jesus taught, but only that which a human being, without God, can rationalize as truth. Without Jesus, there is no link to truth nor is there a connection to the transcendental life and Salvation.

LESSON 101

DOOR #25 THE PHILOSOPHY OF AN UNGUIDED AND SPIRITUALLY DEPRIVED MIND REVEALING THE CAUSE AND ORIGIN OF A TROUBLED LIFE

Since the dawn of humankind, after the fall from the transcendental life, there are as many philosophies as there are people. The trouble is that any philosophy without spirituality causes the human mind to fill the gaps necessary for human development and survival, with solutions only from the human consciousness. So maybe this section should be called "the consequence of a philosophy of an unguided and spiritually deprived mind," since spirituality seeks to live in the present moment, and philosophy deals with the mind and intellect. That is what religion[144] has become. Religion on and of its own, since Jesus' ascension, *has*, by and large, dealt more with the human mind and intellect, and lacks a balance that mysticism centered in the heart would bring. Sadly, the church was less focused on the spiritual essence which, without the truth, prevents a transcending of the human consciousness in order to live by the Divine Consciousness. That is why so few people believe in God or a greater power or Being.

We all embrace a philosophy, especially as we venture through life finding everything wrong with the way things are done, or the values or mindset and all the problems we are faced with etc., on a daily basis. Confusing philosophy as a form of spirituality becomes a problem, as one cites

---

[144] Chinmoy, Sri. "Philosophy vs Religion vs Spirituality." Biography Online, www.biographyonline.net/spiritual/articles/philosophy-religion-spirituality.html.

mostly problems, where if balanced, the other helps to find the good in one's life. As we find, "philosophy leads to endless debates, and as we have noted that religion, too, is seen as an array of disputes regarding which is the best choice, your spirituality should be the guiding way to how to live your life, and though not complicated, but should be the vessel of peace.

There are those who don't see any merit to this life, and are entrenched with darkness. Sadly, they were never taught anything but instant gratification, and were left to themselves to find an escape from a life, which seemed only to be that of pain and suffering, all of which is a virtual dead end. What alternative do they have than to turn to those things that they need to fill the void—an artificial means of satisfaction—such as drugs, alcohol, cigarettes, and, yes, food, or, lack thereof, even though with these they are destroying their life. Examples: when warned of a pending danger to their lives the response of many is: "Well, we have to die from something, right? Why not die doing something we enjoy." This is a cry of a people who seek an escape from this world complete with its empty promises, illusions, and lies.

What about children with good spiritual backgrounds, now we have to look towards which side of the family carries a gene that may result in the same issues with their children and work from there. Parents, guardians etc., cannot close their eyes to family traits and hereditary disorders, meaning that the issues are transmitted from parents to children through the genes, just as original sin is a hereditary spiritual disorder passed along from Adam and Eve due to their choice for physicality versus remaining in a transcendental life. That is why Spirituality is seen as even more necessary today, since its uses of contemplative practices increases compassion, empathy, and attention while quieting the mind.

Today, too many people, especially young people, just don't seem to feel their life has a purpose. They no longer see a future, or, rather, they see a future where things get worse and not better. They spend the life they have been given wasting precious moments existing rather than living. Death is no longer feared, and, in fact, in many cases it is almost welcomed. Everyone needs a purpose to live, and there are so many ways to find purpose; yet few know how. That is why the secret desire of an apocalyptic disaster is played out in movies and rising UFO interest and the like. There are other life altering events, however, that create unrest within our souls.

LESSON 102

DOOR #26 DEATH

There is death by illness, accident, or old age, abuse and violence, or terrorism, which is bad enough in itself, but there is nothing worse than a pointless killing or murder especially of little ones and young people who have their whole life ahead of them; in other words: anyone. In all respects, the "thoughts and prayers" said to be offered, in many cases only agitates those who are going through the pain of loss. It is not comforting, nor is it satisfying, but rather this stirs something considered to be righteous anger and violence. Parents and teachers all want solutions. Who should these solutions come from? Many have tried to eliminate those things they feel are the problem, i.e., guns, but those who are in favor of bearing arms carry just as great a responsibility. These are the experts. These can't just defend a right by supplying other means of weaponry but THEY MUST think of solutions, which stop heinous crimes with strong preventive solutions.

Perhaps, it can start with stricter censors from manufacturers of video games, or violent movie etc. that result in making acts of killing entertainment (for all states of mind).

Where video games can assist doctors in keeping skilled and trained to the best of their ability, and the military sharp and keen minded, in the hands of children and the general public, they are too often training the mind negatively and are detrimental to procuring a peaceful and nonviolent society. Is it any wonder why the public feel they must arm themselves against criminals rather than trust those who should be protecting the public? No one can blame a person for wanting to take action on their own if those governmental agencies are dropping the ball in protecting its citizens. *Teachers, police, even parents need training on how to handle these situations.*

As with any untimely death. be it by illness, drunk driving, carelessness etc., the loss of someone you love takes a piece of your heart that can never be replaced, especially in ways, that even though it happens to others, is not the same when it happens to you. Only God knows a person's heart; people can be empathetic, but they will never know what God knows.

Next, we are faced with victims of suicide, which includes very young children. Suicidal death renders those left behind helpless and with no receptacle for the love they had for that person. Suicide is something few, if any, understand when it involves a loved one. It may appear that it is based on the choice of the individual to live miserably or end their life or an answer to what some parents feel was the end to a tormented life. A torment which they simultaneously lived with the loved one, and never knowing, while waiting for the last phone call, which they both feared and in some way prayed for. It has always been seen as murder of one's self, and, in many Christian-based religions, was viewed as a mortal sin punishable with hell. These poor souls were looked down upon by those who felt the person should be denied a funeral and gravesite within hallowed cemeteries.

Eeshans posit that though the lack of faith and spirituality are most certainly part of the cause for suicide, the mind, being so complex, it often blinds victims and distorts their thinking to the point where they feel abandoned, even by God. One cannot be held accountable for a mind which is beyond reasoning with, let alone punished after death for the act itself. Since years and years shame was what followed the family of such a victim, adding insult to injury, leaving no room for healing, or means of strengthening the human bond of love and friendship.

Suicide takes many forms. There is the end to one's own physical life. This causes confusion, resentment, hopelessness, and lifelong pain, leaving behind family and friends who can't accept the reasoning behind such a deed. Here the family and friends can't comprehend what often is deduced to be weakness, or an escape, from what could've been a promising life, to the anxiety of well-wishers who come to them with solutions to what could've been signs of a troubled mind, thus, causing the family and friends to wonder why they missed these signs, or why the person denied they had a problem or refused help.

This ultimately becomes an endless paradox, which, of course, continues throughout the survivors' lives. Finding closure often seems next to impossible.

The trauma of living with a troubled person, or a victim of suicide, may cause one to ask, "How does the individual ask for help if they haven't learned how to identify if what they are feeling is true or not?" What if the person already feels dead? What if they were slowly dying spiritually for a long time? Suppose these issues plagued the individual as well, and, thus, they learned how to ignore the problem because of the parent(s') inability to recognize or sympathize, or they themselves refused to seek help to address the same issues in themselves?

Suicide tendencies are often found where one least expects, such as a smart student, a person who always seemed so happy, a child who had a parent who excused the alcohol, or drug, abuse of the other parent, or denied they had a problem? Suppose the parents ignored the signs out of embarrassment? Or suppose the parents didn't want to look like failures themselves to other family members?

Suicides are high in places where parents were raised to see their children's issues as private, especially where other siblings and children are made to look successful or the siblings are successful.

Suicides are prominent where protests for individual freedoms usually take place. What if they are made to think that their suicide would be the one thing they could do to promote 'freedom' and finally serve as a hero for a cause? This is a very distorted version of "putting your money where your mouth is." Why would anyone consider this a valid and sane outlet for expression? What if these people felt that they would never or couldn't reach the potential they set for themselves, and never would, or reach a standard that was set for them by people they admired, or what if they simply feared the outcome of failure? What if they actually saw what other people saw about them? What if they couldn't explain, or dreaded, the possibility of hurting or disappointing someone they love, not realizing that a world without them would be worse for their loved one? This is not an alternative. The list goes on and on.

Other examples of causes for unnecessary deaths, or murders, include what has been going on in religions over the years. Over decades, mass graves of children have been uncovered, and sadly these were at the hands of clerics, priests, and nuns. Yet, no one wants to know.

Death by abortions are yet another issue. Always said to be the first shoe, we find euthanasia being the second shoe to drop, and this is now a reality. Though abortion is usually a means to handle fear, euthanasia is said to be the means to end suffering, and is also said to be the end of the economic burden on families and society. All these in their worst scenarios teach that life is expendable and deserved only by those who are healthy and can contribute to society. We are eliminating the miracle of the first inhale and the last exhale.[145] As we said, "We don't have any say in being brought into this world, it now looks as though we don't have any say in when we are going to leave either." It may very well be by the hands of our own children, if they are made to believe 'they' know best.

It doesn't matter how the terminally ill, or the deformed, or even the unwanted children, can be the balance for the healthy; this is of little significance when compared to the overall purpose of life, as defined and contrived by healthy and wealthy individuals and those in power.

Death, though inevitable, is never easy to talk about. The world is always affected, and because we are all part of the human family, we all feel the loss, even when the situation, or circumstances, seem to allude to it being the "best" thing in certain situations.

According to *Popular Science Magazine*, studies show that between ten and twenty percent of those who are resuscitated from cardiac arrest report near death experiences. The frequency of near-death experience [NDE] is 418 percent. There is a progression of stages: the person has a sense of peace, then a sense of separation from the body, where they feel that they are floating above their body, or near the ceiling in the room where the experience is taking place. The person then enters into darkness, and sees a bright light like the end of a tunnel. Then the person

---

[145] Cf. On this topic of abortion, there are two worthwhile films to consider: *You're Beautiful When You're Angry*, and *Unplanned*.

enters the light, and interacts with an entity, such as God, or a universal cosmic force.

When studied, people who 'come back' describe specific memories, and demonstrate consciousness; however, there is no measurable brain activity at that time from the medical standpoint. No one really knows if, or when, the consciousness and mind cease functioning. Is it minutes or hours later? No one knows for sure.

Eeshans believe that it is at the time when a person is pronounced clinically dead and right before the doctors quit working to revive the person, that the fontanelle opens to a small degree to prepare for the life/death decision and for access to the divine; and all means possible are called into effect in the off chance of death that will be used to release the soul at that point. Usually if the decision is to return to life, the soul, subtle body, and mind will be restored and refreshed, and the person will regain life (perhaps after fourteen paddles) to begin a conversion towards correcting those things that caused them to realize they were given another chance. If the decision is death, this will take place most likely within a few minutes afterward. If death is the decision, the soul leaves about twenty minutes after the person is truly dead, not just pronounced *clinically* dead. That is why in a near death experience it is then that God makes the decision for supramentalization, the consciousness is suspended and the body of matter dies, but the subtle body moves with the soul and consciousness. To be in the room with someone while they are dying is a privilege for it gives the person the opportunity to have someone with them to pray, and remind them, of God's unfathomable mysteries, thus, preparing them for interaction with God. Believe it or not, there were times when the soul was actually seen, and photographed as it was leaving the body. In any case, those nearby should pray for a gentle rather than stressful release of the soul. A little kiss is sometimes placed on the person's face—for love is life.

LESSON 103

DOOR #27 DEATH BY DISCRIMINATION AND PREJUDICE

There are other kinds of death. These include death by prejudice and death by discrimination, since these cut off human life in a way that mirrors what Jesus declared as wrong. These two are caused by those who kill not only the body, but they also "kill" the body and soul by depriving life to the soul of a person or people.

The Catholic church has proven itself to be guilty of many racial prejudices and discriminations since its onset, as we said.

Few know about this one that is documented in the book, *From Slave to Priest: The Inspirational Story of Father Augustine Tolton* by Caroline Hemasath and Deacon Harold Burke-Sivers, which we feel is a must read.

This is the story of a slave in the Civil War period who wanted to answer the call of becoming a Catholic priest. Augustine Tolton, a black slave, who escaped to join the Union Army and fight for black freedom, died battling for the cause. Tolton met, and found help among priests and nuns, despite the many seminaries that rejected him. According to co-author Harold Burke-Silvers, "If anyone had a reason to leave the Catholic church, it was him." Tolton recognized that Catholics who discriminated against him were violating church teaching on the dignity of all people. According to the Associated Press, however, there are only a few small signs in Chicago that say that Augustine Tolton was there. A few buildings such as a 'senior citizens' building carry his name. But, the Roman Catholic church where he preached his sermons to those who adored him on Chicago's South Side is long gone. It says few know the story of the first "acknowledged" black Catholic priest in the United Sates, and what he accomplished under severe limitations. Today, we are told that the church says that this story is a mystery, and does not have enough credible information to prove he existed.

It is not surprising that questions of gender identity were forbidden, and "fear of God" was used by the church in order to succeed in making a person, especially while young, and going through the confusion of adolescence, feel like abominations before others, and sometimes become victims of predatory religious. Rather than helping them to discover who they were created to be, some authority figures took advantage of the weaknesses of the troubled individual, giving them the alternative of having a safeguard under the 'protection of Jesus,' or a twisted version of a 'special love'? What happens if, during the psychological development happening alongside the normal physical changes within that particular child's body during adolescence, a young person feels an identification with a gender opposite their physical body's gender? What if who they felt they truly were left them vulnerable to punishment and abuse by peers and family, or religious authority, which could easily be translated in their minds as Jesus Himself, *God*, seeing them as an abomination? Do you not see that religion has caused innocents to think that they were selected by God to be *hated*? What if they felt that they had no choice than to believe that they were an offense, an embarrassment to God, and, thus, live without God's love without salvation except to live and without ever expressing their love in a relationship, and having to bear that cross alone?

Whose responsibility is it to secure a spiritually based life for everyone? Again, the desire for spirituality is within each of us, by which each to a different degree, each of us as adults, especially parents, guardian, teachers, religious leaders etc., have the responsibility to help mold a wholesome, healthy, spirituality in children, until which age they may be able to make good, balanced, and wholesome decisions on their own.

Insurance companies claim that their policy premiums are higher for teens because it was proven that the judgment part of the brain isn't fully developed until the age of twenty-one; in light of the above abuses, Eeshans wonder if some ever mature.

With regards to the dangers of not teaching children the difference between right and wrong, good and evil, and the sanctity of life, parents and guardians fail to understand that under the 'immortality of the soul,' which is destined to return to God, it is required that there be a certain degree of responsibility placed upon them to establish a solid foundation, upon which children and young people in their care learn decency, honesty, dignity, honor, kindness, and love. Because we are made in God's image, and likeness, parents and family under God are obliged to responsibly guide the children because these are the first people the child is in contact with. To not do this not only deprives their children of love of God and neighbor, but also the value of life and risking the everlasting life of the child with God.

Next, the responsibility falls on the country, state, city, etc., to protect, and uphold, the dignity of each individual, because environment affects the formation of the body, mind, and spirit, too.

For example: when a nation robs its people through overly restrictive laws and Godless secularism, or when there is no balance of spirituality with humanity, is not the 'society' guilty of not providing for its people the recognition of the true importance of life? To deprive people/souls of spirituality for what is considered secular humanism ignores the necessary component that drives the human desire for a healthy self-love and love of neighbor. The need for its people to be decent, God-wondering (fear-respect) and law-abiding citizens of country is necessary because a world united needs to recognize all human rights to protect life before it's too late. The value of life has already become diminished. We are already seeing where a deliberate intervention is undertaken with the express intention of ending a life, to relieve intractable suffering, and this is how euthanasia is defined in the commonly understood language of Wikipedia; and in most cases we are depriving the person's soul of 'assisted purgatory' here on earth and risking that person spending time *alone* in purgatory.

A person needs a reason to live and not one to die in order to put an end to their pain, especially spiritual pain. However, without the food to feed the Light Body, the Eucharist, which is necessary for everlasting life, there can be no transformation from the temporality of time.

The Eucharist is that which propels human life to everlasting life with God; thus, without it, the person cannot see beyond this life. It is never good to see another suffer, especially a loved one. It is sad, however, and one should do some soul searching for the actual reasons euthanasia, or end of life protocol is being practiced, to be sure it is not becoming the means of relieving "our" suffering because of inconvenience or financial concerns.

When the spirit of a person is broken, there is a pain that is obviously not apparent to others; but it is so deeply buried that they themselves have a very hard time knowing what it is that hurts so badly. When this happens, the pain just splinters into countless reasons too numerous for the person to explain and identify. This is often described as depression. Due to the omission of a guided path to the transcendental consciousness, these souls feel their existence will not be missed and has gone unnoticed, even by God. The mind and spirit without God cannot see anything beyond this world. Everyone, whether they admit it or not, wants to believe that God cares. The fear of being forgotten, or abandoned, renders life meaningless. Even an atheist, whether conscious of it or not, knows God exists, since the immortal soul was created by God.

Eeshans believe that the torments within a soul, and its failure to know God exists and loves the soul, is often at the basis for the murder of one's 'self,' as in suicide, or the use of drugs, due to lack of knowledge that God loves them, and death is not the end.

What has the world positively done to offer someone who needs help spiritually? The world itself has done nothing. The world is exile, and obviously holds a poor and tainted human view of it being a temporary heaven. But, it is not heaven. It is exile. Our true home is with God. Earth however, as a material world, was built to be the temporary home to physical life. It is the place where we can live to show love of God and neighbor outwardly. This world was created for Adam and Eve's descendants, due to their choice and their desire to become human. Due to this choice and obvious reasons, they, nor their descendants, could be allowed back to Paradise without God's permission and conditions met, which was, and still are, contingent on the Christs' directives.

The world is not our last stop, and though it has a tremendous pull on our choices, and false sense of entitlements we have before God, it is not loyal by any means. It places us in the position to 'demand and take' because of our ostensible definition of free will. All in all, in this world we really feel we are entitled to all we want and often can't get. It is not perfect by any means, with its ensuing trials and tribulations, but by the grace of God, and a balanced discernment, it is beautiful, and one should love life nonetheless. Just a word to the wise, do be careful who you try to rehabilitate, especially since you may very well not be rehabilitating them but rather are only enabling them.

Given the fact that the only-begotten Child of God became humans, and, as such, Jesus' life, marriage, death, and resurrection occurred here on this earth, and, as such, makes up for our imperfections, we, by our choices, can have it all ... all that is important, that is. One way, or another, our choices can give us our reward here, or when we die; or we can lose in both worlds.

LESSON 104

DOOR #28 CONSCIENCE AND MIND

Jesus gave life and merit to a desolate life,[146] as well as proof of life everlasting, "if you believe." He healed the people's minds by easing their fears, and displaying throughout his ministry the power of faith, hope, and most of all love.

That is why Eeshans teach that the loss of a rightly formed conscience, and Intuitively-balanced mind, will result in all levels of emotional imbalances. Since if a conscience is ignored, or not balanced, it will choose incorrectly, and, will, indeed affect individuals with tendencies toward mentally disturbing motives, causing the mind to act like an atypical cancer. It will cause radical changes within the mind, and, left unaided, may result in creating this mind, body, and spirit one that is terminally diseased.

We know that mental illness is very complex. It does appear in ways like a physical illness, and can often be hidden, misunderstood, and misdiagnosed. Spiritual illness is even more complicated. For example, mental illness, combined with the absence of a well-informed spiritual aspect, can be easily compared to a person with a brain tumor who may become irritable, or aggressive, uninhibited, confused, showing signs of apathy, depression, blurting/flattening of emotion, anxiety, and mood swings. A spiritually deprived person with emotional disorders, etc., can be witness to the same issues, singularly, or all.

---

[146] 'Desolate' in the sense of a person whose life was 'nothing' to them; before they felt no purpose, while after, in a relationship with Jesus, there is love, purpose, and merit that naturally arises from the relationship. – Ed.

If one does have a balanced faith, and loves God, yet, cannot reach the mind, or ease the spirit of such a sad soul, it is our responsibility to at least present this soul to God through prayer, and, absolutely, never condemn the person before God, or 'deny' them refuge in our prayers, but rather ask for their restful peace.

Finally, Eeshans feel we must at least mention yet another kind of philosophy, which is often confused as a spirituality, however, this is powered by hate.

LESSON 105

DOOR #29 THE CONSEQUENCE OF ASSUMPTION AND MISUDERSTANDING

It is said that 'assumption and misunderstanding, without a doubt, can cause not only civil wars but to also precipitate world wars,' and all because no one took the time, nor did anyone intend to honestly take the time, to seek the truth. Oftentimes, this happens because the original statement fit the mindset of a particular point of view to use, for whatever one needed, to support their agenda.

Interestingly enough, though, the above philosophy sometimes can be the origin of what seems to be Christ-centered, but can be discovered to be the case that, as Ben Franklin said, "Half the truth is often a great lie." This is reared in hate and punishment, and it is totally apart from a God of love. Crazy? To have ten percent of the truth is not truth, since we have given examples of this by pointing out the different verses of scriptures that were assembled to support the primacy of Peter's leadership; whereas, other books whose contents, which total more in number that are contrary to that deemed as Sacred Scripture, have been assumed as being the truth.

There are reasons why other religions object to Christianity. 'Misinterpretation' of Jesus' comment, "Give to Caesar what is Caesar and to God what is God's." is one of these. Where the first explanation was thought to have been the truth, further interpretation finds that it actually became an insult to other religions, since the explanation given allowed for total misunderstanding and total assumption.

Jesus always answered trick questions posed to him by the authorities in very human terms; however, his answers always reflected a higher consciousness in an effort to raise the consciousness of those who came to hear him. That was also why He often spoke in parables.

We also know that there were always people looking for fault in what He taught, or an issue they could use against Him, in an effort to stop him. The reasoning behind this was to break up the crowds, which were becoming increasingly large.

We find one such occasion in Mark 12:13-17. Jesus did not use a parable, but rather spoke directly and emphatically. As the Pharisees acknowledged Jesus' character and treatment of all people, to include the mindset of those with darkened minds, they became uncomfortable. This may have hit a nerve, since He seemed to indicate, or identify religious groups who did not know God, and used the law as if it was God's Law in order to inflict fear and secure their authority; yet, all the while they were not interested in teaching people love of God and neighbor.

> *Later the leaders sent some Pharisees and supporters of Herod to trap Jesus into saying something for which he could be arrested. "Teacher, we know that you are true and do not care about anyone's opinion. For you are not swayed by appearances, but truly teach the way of God. Is it lawful to pay taxes to Caesar, or not? Should we pay them, or should we not?" Jesus saw through their hypocrisy and said, "Why are you trying to trap me? Show me a Roman (denarius) coin, and I'll tell you." When they handed him the coin, He asked, "whose picture and title are stamped on it?" "Caesar's", they replied. Then Jesus said to them, "Give to Caesar what is Caesar's and to God what is God's". His reply completely amazed them.*

Recognizing what they were doing, Jesus was addressing not just those the leaders sent, but he was also replying to all those who were of the same mind. Contrary to how his answer was taken, Jesus was warning that when we are more focused on the body, the less the inner light of awareness shines through a human life and through the heart; thus, then, one is giving to "Caesar" truly what is desired by man; but when we govern the mind, senses, and bodily instincts properly, we give most appropriately to God what is God's.

LESSON 106

Door #30 Coercive and Persuasive Ideology

To those whose religion is their culture, this concept has often been mistaken for the separation of church and state, which to these is unacceptable since all things belong to God; therefore, any belief outside of this thought is considered to be Satanic. That is why to some, any nation based on Christ's standards is looked upon as Satanic today. Only those who had ears to hear would know what Jesus was talking about. These who were, and are, looking for fault in His words, therefore, had no clue to what he was referring.

To clarify this notion, one must remember that Jesus' teaching had nothing to do with the issue of politics, government, or religion. Essentially, what he was talking about was our purpose here on earth, aside from all these, and the need for us to reestablish the relationship between humans and God, and not becoming trapped in discussing politics; thus, avoiding confusion among his followers. Jesus, who was the Master example of 'soul governing the mind, body, and senses,' taught the dangers and consequences of the mind, body and senses 'governing the soul,' and the 'fear of not surviving' impulse, which grows until it governs not just one person, but whole groups of people, indeed, as well as nations and histories.

The fear of change causes one to fight against anyone or anything that disrupts the life they have been living. It may not be the best life, but they are accustomed to it. The ability to twist words was a weapon that was used against what Jesus said in the presence of religious authorities;

and we see it used today in political propaganda clouding truth and clarity. In religion, as well as in all walks of life, it can also be used to set the foundation for whatever agenda is trending at the moment.

Fear of commitment causes people to react because it is easier to quit if there is no commitment, and if things get too tough and they can't be blamed, since they can never be wrong. These people love to ride on the coattails of those who stand committed, and they enjoy the benefits of the success, yet can quit with no wasted effort on their part.

These are examples of terribly sad misuses of the God-given gifts of free will and conscience, but are often what makes one a target for leaders, since these weaknesses can be easily manipulated in those who are very vulnerable, meaning those who feel they have no alternative but to follow what they only know is told to them. In this instance, regardless of its flawed and godless foundation, these people believe only what they are told, and what they are told is that this particular religion is God's own.

Raised with an isolated, and, may we say coercive and persuasive ideology, this is one thing that separates a religion from the Jesus people want to love.

When it comes to this problem it's easy to point the finger at religions that do not believe in Jesus, but what if it came from within a Christ-based religion? What if this philosophy was prominent, and exposed in over eighteen orders of Catholic priests, brothers, and nuns who must admit to decades of chronic child abuse in orphanages and schools, all in Jesus' name, which was viewed with having purpose? What if, up until and including recent times, the image and person of Jesus was used to lure in innocent children only to be abused?

It's clear and easy to see how one can be ignorant of radicalized religious leaders and clergy because brainwashed members chose to ignore what transpires, and turn their heads so as not to see the obvious evil. How could no one see the difference in the above versus what and how Jesus preached?

Who is the Jesus whose name is used in the committing of these dastardly crimes? Did and does He discriminate? Is He also prejudiced? For if He is, then he cannot be God; and how much worse if Jesus would then be as evil, as defined by those leaders and teachers and civil/religious groups today, who are bad as (or worse than) those who had Him killed.

We know Jesus did not seek or teach punishment as in an 'eye for an eye,' but He taught justice, forgiveness, and love. He did not turn the 'adulteress' over to the authorities, but, instead, addressed the more important issue of clearing his wife's name and identifying himself as the eyewitness to her violators. Jesus made it known that if the issue presented to Him was the act of violation of a woman, He would not tolerate it, especially if it paralleled what happened to his wife. He also made it known that in an act of adultery, the man involved was just as guilty as the woman, if not even more guilty.

We believe that all people have the right to their beliefs, so long as their foundation poses no harm to any person, or persons or to any nation, in and of itself since we believe all life is sacred. We have witnessed how some have taken these rights and have wrongly used them to openly cause havoc in an attempt to force their belief system in several countries which are not theirs.

This type of philosophy, or similarly, this kind of religion, takes on a terrifying and radical system of beliefs contrary to all those whose faith embodies love and everything they believe about Jesus' life, and, indeed, lives it.

There are all kinds of religions and spiritualities out there. Should you encounter a religion with no understanding of human rights, remember that when it comes to a misinformed conscience, which only operates by an outside control of emotions and fear-produced loyalty, ask questions. The disposition of the soul, whose sole desire triggers it to harm, abuse, or kill others for redemption and reward for expanding said consciousness in order to correct and destroy may 'feel' right (to them), but with this kind of belief system, it is very difficult for its members to see anything but the need to take *radical* steps to please their God. Since they may also have a political ideology, or agenda, which calls for the need to 'fight for God's community,' search further. An unbalanced and spiritually deprived person can see only that God must win in the end; therefore, all must come under their control and abide by the law of God, as it has been interpreted (by them). Being unable to see, or understand, that their beliefs are not those of a loving God, shows the danger of one searching for true meaning of their life, but though they have eyes, they still cannot see.

Without having Jesus and the Spiritual Food of the Eucharist of the Marriage Feast that contains the Divine and Sacred Balance, all you are getting is a belief system connected to a very flawed human consciousness.

LESSON 107

DOOR #31 "UNLESS YOU BECOME LIKE ONE OF THESE"

"Let the Children Come to Me"

Jesus spoke these words with no hesitation. We understand that through a child's innocence, it is capable of a greater understanding of trust. A child trusts an adult who is raising him or her, a teacher whom they feel knows what is best, or any adult that seems to understand it. They have no reason to doubt. So, if this child is inclined to "trust" a human being, one can safely presume that the child would recognize God and the things of God from birth and before its soul has contact in a spiritual way with anyone other than its mother first, and then the father. Why? Simply because the mother carries the little life within her—normally for nine months before it enters the world.

When do we become aware of the supernatural? The transcendental consciousness is often seen readily in very young children, who seem to commune easily, and transcendentally, through conversation with angels, imagination focused on God, and the things of God, and various forms of creative expression. But this knowledge and a natural response relating to the transcendent is gradually covered over, when the conditioning process begins. This process has for its strength and effectiveness the age of reason, when parents or guardians feel that these experiences are purely imagination and must be curbed to strive to bring a sense of reality into the child's life. Then begins the process of curtailing imagination, awareness of the supernatural, and balance is interrupted, since adults often see imagination as an escape from reality rather than a source of creativity. There is no room for any supernatural and transcendental awareness. This brings a greater awareness of being embodied, and a feeling of more awareness, with regards to how life 'should' be. This becomes the 'acceptable' mindset, and is experienced through the mind and senses; but it is mostly felt through the process of being educated in terms of social pressures and conditioning. This conditioning includes how human beings have passed down over immeasurable periods of time, their own experience as races, cultures, and forms of materially limited and spiritually restrictive modes of thinking, feeling, perceiving, concluding, and behaving.

This is why Jesus said one must become like a little child in order to enter in upon the things of God. It requires an innocence combined with a measure of freedom from all the mental and psychological restrictions that are woven into the process of conditioning. It limits one to think inside the walls of a curtailed understanding of life, seeing life only through the lens of a particular race, creed, and culture. That lens is often carefully calibrated to deliver a form of awareness desired by the leaders of that group.

It is good to remember that teaching children about spirituality is more than giving them 'God's law,' and it is, indeed, giving them the opportunity to ask questions, or perhaps, in some ways, to even test your own beliefs as they grow to maturity. It's been said in many different ways by those from different spiritual backgrounds that in order to truly understand God and the things of God, becoming 'learned' in ways that may impress others (i.e., advanced schooling, degrees), with all the intellectual, psychological, and emotional conditioning that goes along with that, actually only serves to hamper one's true spiritual growth and awakening, as opposed to facilitating it.

Eeshans believe that when a child is very young, the consciousness easily transitions in and out of its transcendental consciousness. As the child ages, material and social conditioning takes over, and the transcendental awareness is gradually buried beneath more and more layers of material consciousness. Things become less magical as the 'reality of life and the real world' has to be embraced. THIS IS WHEN A LITTLE

CHILD IS MOST VULNERABLE TO PREDATORS, especially priests who take advantage of this time because they use the child's attachment to God as the foundation for a 'special love' as though it is what Jesus wants them to do. What Jesus wanted when he said, "Let the children come to me," was the opportunity to teach children, since at that time neither male nor female children were allowed to be taught until the male child reached the age of reason. Again, Jesus taught everyone regardless of age.

While it is still possible to open the gates to the transcendental, or throw back layers of this material and rational consciousness, the vast majority of human beings are afraid to do so, or have so little awareness with regards to how to accomplish this. This is so, because of the attachment to the physical body and mind which have been so heavily impressed upon the soul for so many years.

Too often a person comes to believe that they 'are' their body. In recent times, a person who begins to wander outside this confine of established institutionalized reasoning and thinking, and begins to question, or to think imaginatively and contextually, is often ridiculed. Physical, material existence is only one small part of a soul's experience, but it would seem from the perspective of most, that it is the "all," so much so, that many people scoff at the notion of the transcendental when it is mentioned or discussed.

Many cannot believe that it exists because of the overreliance upon the human, materially, and socially conditioned mind; awareness is for many, if not most, limited to only what the mind and senses can perceive. To perceive life even with the best intentions and good works, without God, makes one finite and incomplete; whereas, to love God makes us immortal and complete. That is why children are so precious. Through, with, and, in their innocence they believe. It is also the reason predators will experience God's wrath.

Maintaining a mind geared towards a transcendental realm, even with the pull of human nature, though it feels strongly in the physical part of the human person, the nourished soul will always lean towards God. This is what Jesus counted on when he addressed the crowds.

LESSON 108

DOOR #32 THE ETERNAL CONSCIOUSNESS

Eshans know that the consciousness of the human being is eternal, and is of the same substance as the Divine Consciousness, since it, too, was imaged, and likened, to God's. This is one of the most important truths to our faith, since it encompasses the supramentalization and divinization of our Foundress, whom we believe teaches with the eternal consciousness of the Divine Feminine, Mary Magdalen and Jesus' eternal consort.

In our mystery school, we read and researched all we could about various religions, and beliefs, and came across the best of each. Loving our neighbor obliges us to understand what they believe and why, and find most importantly their views about life, spirituality, etc ... in other words, what makes up their person and who, indeed, they are.

Why are we interested in other religions outside of ours? First and foremost, Eeshans can't imagine an omnipotent, omniscient, omnipresent, and omnificent God as not being capable of radiating truth throughout all of humanity, especially in sharing, loving, and teaching all who are loving examples of God's own love. In any event, we found this beautiful verse in a writing entitled, "An Eternal Identity," by Philamorman, who writes that the prophet Abraham recorded his vision of pre-mortality, a condition prior to creation and population of the Earth; and though Eeshans do not subscribe to most of what he writes, this passage almost confirms, and conforms, to the Eeshan version of Adam and Eve. He described the hosts of beings present in his vision as "intelligences with the capacity to weigh options, to make choices, to demonstrate faith. God intended for each intelligence to enter Earth and receive a mortal body in order to prepare for the next stage in eternity. This is who we are. In reality, we are each an eternal being made up of capacities to think, reason, believe, choose, grow, and develop. Our core identity is nothing more than this eternal reality."

"All human beings, male and female, are created in the image and likeness of God. Each is a beloved spirit, son or daughter of heavenly parents, and as such, each has a divine nature and destiny."

LESSON 109

DOOR #33 THE WHAT AND WHO HUMANS ARE

After all we have discussed so far about the transcendental, one could begin to wonder if there is anything valuable about human life?

Though it seems that God put a lot of effort into giving us a way back to the transcendental life, we don't want you to lose sight of just how special being human is.

We have the capacity to love, share love, and be loved. We can be joined together in public, officially and permanently. There are endless opportunities in which to share a life together blessed by God. Our expression of love brings not just a spiritual and transcendental union, but a beautiful physical expression which, by its joy, can be blessed to bring about the greatest fruit of love, which is children.

We can choose to share solely in a relationship with God, losing no joy and living a life mirroring one in which we shall share in oneness with God when we return to heaven. We can also choose to live a committed relationship, and/or a single life, full of adventures, meeting new people, and sharing your life with friends when you want to. You can arrange your home and life so that it becomes your escape and safe haven. You can include yourself and participate in group activities should you desire to be with others.

We are treasures in the sense that, though imperfect, we're special enough that the Only Begotten Child of God chose to become one of us.

Both the divine masculine and divine feminine of the three Persons of God became familiar with all we have to face on a daily basis that we can, thus, conversely, relate to them. The First and second Persons know first-hand birth, death, joy, sorrow, health, pain, friendship, loneliness, wealth, poverty, anxiety, and patience. They witnessed the reasons people turned away from God and also feared God. They saw corruption, breach of trust, demoralization, misrepresentation, payoff, profiteering, and unscrupulousness; but they also saw decency, honesty, honor, truthfulness, and wholesomeness.

Even in traditional scriptures, we witness the difference of fear-driven betrayal, and denial of friendship with Jesus from men, to the courage of a woman pushing passed soldiers to wipe the face of her Lord, to women who stood at the foot of the cross, willing to give up their lives if need be just to be near him. The Third Person of the Trinity has always assisted, and as God made Man, the Divine Masculine, as well as the Divine Feminine Spirit, has assisted in giving us strength to endure all that goes with trials, and shares in our joy with complete love.

Jesus experienced a human marriage, the true love of a woman, and the selfless sacrifice of marriage. They laughed together, they cried together. They ate together, they fasted together. They dreamed of a life together that would go beyond the inevitable. They experienced the agony of separation and the joy of returning to each other.

There was the adoration of followers, the willingness to give up one's life for a friend, and because of them, we know that death isn't the end, it is the beginning of yet another life, prayerfully one of even greater joy.

Human beings, despite their weaknesses and faults, were and still are worth saving.

Yeah, life is beautiful!

*May the Divine within Each of Us,
Bow to the Divine within Each of You*

THE EESHAN RELIGION AND SPIRITUALITY

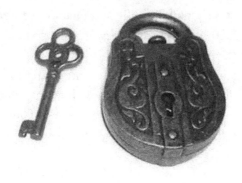

LESSON 110

WHAT IS THE EESHAN RELIGION

The Eeshan religion is founded upon what Eeshans believe is a mandate from God, by which the Divine Feminine 'returns' to the world and brings with her the Sacred Balance, as was intended by Jesus' true purpose and mission on this earth.

The Eeshan belief system accepts males and females, men and women, as equals and we believe each has an equal role in this world and in all aspects of religious and spiritual worship. Our religion is a transcendental, *ancient*, mystical, and beyond Merkabahlic and Kabbahlic[147] spirituality 'brought *back* into existence' because of the love of God, and in order to meet the spiritual needs of the people who are, whether they are directly conscious of it or not, searching for the Sacred Balance and the Sacred Food and Drink.

It is not presenting new doctrines of Jesus, but it is 're'-presenting what Jesus Christ really taught: fully and unabridged, against what may be defined as a 2000-year old ad hominem belief system.

This means that one can no longer turn a blind eye or deaf ear to the countless tireless works of those fearless and daring individuals chosen to pave the way for the Divine Feminine. Many may think that Eeshan Transcendentalism just resembles another 'variant' of humanistic religion. As it can appear that way, it does have, however, a combined theology and thealogy.[148]

---

[147] These are an integral set esoteric teachings from Judaism to its later Christian, New Age adaptations.

[148] A discourse and study and reflection of the feminine divine.

It is founded by a woman named Mary Ellen Lukas, who Eeshans believe teaches with the eternal consciousness of Christ's wife, Mary Magdalene, as self and true self by means of a process called *supramentalization*.[149] *Supramentalization* is the spanning transition between an old consciousness and true consciousness, allowing Mary Magdalen to present to the world all her husband taught, in the circumstances of today, and bringing Truth back to those seeking truth.[150]

Eeshans believe that our Foundress was given the directive, and mandate, which brought with it an understanding that Eeshans feel touches the hearts of those seeking God and a relationship with Him which was supposed to have been be carried forward from Adam and Eve.

A Brief Summary of the Controversy that Surrounded our Eesha

From the very early age of 18 months she knew this extraordinary love. For more than thirty years, she implemented and continues to teach what Jesus taught her. She worshipped within her birth religion, which was Byzantine Catholic. She lived and taught the love of God in the manner in which Jesus taught her, while yet still abiding by the restrictions of her Catholic Faith. Directed by Jesus who was, and is, the source and summit of all she believes, and taught, and along with her "yes," she began to establish the groundwork for this, His omega plan, being the completion of "Gods salvific plan."

Little did she realize that she would be the catalyst which would bring about His plan for a religion and spirituality, which commands us

---

[149] It may be important to the reader at this point to go back and review the way Supramentalization is described and discussed in the earlier parts of this book, in order to better understand the present and forthcoming contexts. – Ed.

[150] This subject might be observed from different perspectives. One such useful perspective as Sri Aurobindo might explain it, is to see that the unique identity of the Divine Feminine permeates both personalities of Mary Magdalen and Eesha, displayed at different times and in different ways, as we understand that, in a sense, the way the same actor would play different characters in different plays. – Ed.

to pass on to others integrity, character, and respect for God by teaching the whole truth and the fullness of what Jesus taught. What He had begun when He lived here on earth is what she would bring to fruition; and what is truth, and what is fallacy, would then be revealed.

Growing up, she, as did most who are part of the Eeshan Religion, was raised to believe that the Catholic faith was founded by Jesus; and that it was the "One, Holy Catholic and Apostolic Church," and that its bishops were the successors of Christ's apostles. She, as did they, believed that the Pope is the successor to Peter to whom the primacy of authority was conferred by Jesus Christ. She was taught that the Catholic church maintained the original Christian faith, and reserved infallibility, as passed down by sacred tradition. However, there were more questions than answers. There was also a signal grace placed within her, and having a body prepared by God, she received the first of many miraculous and mystical gifts. This gift, the jewels with which Jesus adorned her, were the visible Stigmata ... the manifestation of His love for her. Sharing, as one with her Beloved, caused this love she possessed within her heart to fill her resolutely and dutifully with a firm, unwavering desire for God, which was ever-present. When meeting people, this desire to tell all He was teaching her would well up within her soul, and Christ's presence would fill the room wherever she was. Oil and water were witnessed exuding from her heart.

This love rose above ordinary love and trust. In the face of controversy, and there certainly was that, Jesus nourished her privately and publicly with the Eucharist from His own hand. She witnessed His presence through her teachings, His manifestations through her healings and writings. In public forums, He gave her Communion, often, with as many as eighteen to twenty priests and twenty-one eyewitnesses looking on.

Caught in a flurry of phenomena that surrounded her, it was as though Jesus abscised her from the faith that had introduced her to Him. She was taught by, and supported, by Jesus Himself, in order to carry out his directives, even though some of these appeared to be contrary (at first) to what she was taught. She spent several years appearing before crowds, but never did interviews, and frowned at getting her picture taken. Eesha, as is her title, was subjected to ridicule and fabricated stories.

People didn't understand most of what was happening to her, to the point of saying the appearances of the stigmata were not real. One man actually accused her of being a fraud because, since the Stigmata appeared during a talk in church (it was Easter), it did not appear when she was in other places. This gift, and others, became a prison in which people's opinions were construed. Sadly, people believed that these phenomena were also meant for *them*, when in reality, she would one day find they were really only for her.

One day she was told that the Cardinal, who presided over the Archdiocese where she spoke didn't want her to talk, since the crowds were getting larger and the people wouldn't leave church. He made it a point to try and discourage all those who advocated her. Eventually more complaints were issued, mostly by priests who felt that she was embarrassing them because she received Holy Communion from Jesus, directly, and not them. Comments coming from one priest included, "What right does He (Jesus) have to interfere with the Mass?" and "What does He (Jesus) think we are doing behind the altar?" Obviously, Jesus didn't like what they were doing, nor did He like them insulting Eesha because of her reception of Holy Communion at His hands. Next, was the complaint was lodged regarding people kissing the Monstrance which housed the Blessed Sacrament, which filtered down the grapevine. After Eesha made the argument that if Communion is given in the hand without concern, how much safer is a Host safely secured in a monstrance held by a priest in a secured area more dangerous?

Then complaints about a priest, who worked with Mary Ellen, who was ordained outside the normal channels of the church, under a Sacramental seal with witnesses present, became a topic for some wealthy benefactors to the Cardinal, and, of course, that was the bone of contention that solidified Eesha being stopped, along with any other women, from speaking in a church.

After vicious attacks, where only false information and malicious gossip were presented, the priest was eventually accepted by the Cardinal, so long as he checked in with the Chancery upon arriving in town and notified them that he wished to celebrate, or concelebrate Mass, or be present for funerals or weddings.

The decision to prevent, and refrain, from receiving the Eucharist from Jesus' hands, OR so long as she also received the Eucharist at the hands of the priest at Mass, with witnesses (which would be her denial of the Eucharist by Jesus' hands) was what actually began to escalate our Foundress' problems. As complaints from the Cardinal, and the auxiliary bishop, from her own area, along with a few priests, though her own Bishop stood by her side, she actually had done nothing wrong. Needless to say, she was brought in to the Chancery, in Baltimore, Maryland, only to be interrogated inappropriately. She was then given directives to include that she could not teach that Jesus was the one true God. Not knowing that one day these directives were laying the groundwork for Jesus' plan she refused to abide by their warning. This was timely. Unbeknownst to her, that same day she was told she was in good standing, and the Cardinal widely circulated a fax containing a directive that no priest was allowed to invite her to their churches.

Were these the only reasons? Considering that the human rational consciousness governs within the church, and on a transcendental level, the answer is no. Shortly before this fax was sent, Jesus intervened, and asked the present Bishop (Eesha relayed the message) if he wanted Him (Jesus) to refrain from giving her Communion. With the Bishop's 'yes,' Jesus' response was, "Then she will not speak in 'your' churches."

Eeshans see these altercations being the means used in leading to the way to fulfill Jesus' plan. As he was accused and condemned by the chosen people who made up His birth religion, so be it, and, so, too, would be the case with His wife. The bottom line was at the interrogation where she was accused, "You are making people think." Yes, after accusation upon accusation, insult upon insult, the bottom line was that our Foundress *was* making people think for themselves.

Many priests came to her defense, as well as canon lawyers, with suggestions and advice. All the above what was documented as private investigations were made on behalf of our Foundress, and all complaints, heinous accusations, and rumors were traced back, and were found to have been initiated by a few benefactors of the Archdiocese of Baltimore. Though these events proved to be nuisances, Eesha wasn't really affected. In fact, though she was told by officials to report, and name, those in the

Baltimore Archdiocese, and those involved in this conspiracy, although she didn't do it.

Instead, Jesus continued with his directives, and she grew in love, even for those who tried to stop her putting all in God's hands. For the vengeance of God is not some irrational burst of divine anger; it is divine justice, which is perfectly timed.

All those whom God calls face, ridicule, hatred, betrayal, and rejection, but so did Jesus and Mary Magdalen.

Once she chose to stop doing public appearances, a house was purchased, which was soon called "the Place," and she founded an Order of Sisters and Brothers; in time, the Kallahs came into being. All God's plan for a change of Consciousness in an Age of Enlightenment.

Now, once again, she is called to participate in the grandest of all works, and that is to bring the truth and love of Christ's teachings back into the world. Her innate desire and love for God, without a doubt, comes naturally from who she is in relation to Jesus.

A Life Rooted in Supramentalization

Undoubtedly, what was not yet revealed to Our Eesha was that this desire came from being the vessel of the consciousness of his eternal consort. The identity of Mary Magdalen, as Jesus' wife, was not to be revealed to her until the fullness of time, when the Divine Feminine would once again return to us. That was why her whole life was about the Eucharist. When other children thought they were receiving their first Communion, Jesus was renewing his marriage vows with Eesha. With God, time does not exist; therefore, the past, present, and future are one. Now, today, she is the one who carries the eternal Consciousness of Mary Magdalen, who teaches, heals, and represents the Mysteries of God in their truest forms. Will she be rejected? She most probably will, but there will be those that will come who are called by God, and these will become the leaven to others.

That is why, and how, we can say, though Eeshan Transcendentalism is new for today, its origin is rooted in ancient times, and the *core truth* of our faith is truly, and unequivocally, based on our belief in *Jesus' marriage to Mary Magdalene at Cana*. This is the same Christ whose life, death, and resurrection story, which most everyone knows, or, has heard about, presents less than half the story and spirituality Christ intended.

In God's infinite timing, when everyone least expected it, this mandate is the one that has returned as Mary Magdalen through the Consciousness of Eesha. It is given to her, by Divine favor, bringing the wife of the Lamb back into time. Crazy? Impossible? No more crazy, or impossible, than it was for God to become human, and live among the religion and culture of his chosen people, and by their hands, to suffer and die. They are no different than those who feel that God cannot repeat that same scenario today, and this time with a *woman*.

She, by the power of the Divine Feminine, will guide God's people back in, into, and through the omega time with Christ (Revelation 22:13). You will share in the most unique mysteries intended to provide details for the culmination of the brilliant redemptive, most beautiful salvific mission of Jesus Christ.

Though many have been told that the Book of Revelation has already been fulfilled or that it is already history, Eeshans believe that though it may not be in chronological order, and though so much has been wrongly explained, there are bits and pieces that when reordered properly, and the omitted information that is put back will reveal surprising mysteries and treasures kept hidden for ages and generations.

The continuation of our journey back to the transcendental begins with the empowering love of the feminine consort of the Holy Spirit who is the Divine Feminine. She who is the counterpart to the third person of the Holy Trinity, and reveals that total equality and distinct similar character in all persons of the one true God, and by the personage of Mary Magdalen, is now guiding God's people through, with, and by discloses, as promised in the Book of Revelation, the Wife of the Lamb. She is the essential component to restoring the sacred balance between male and female in these present times.

As the divine feminine of the first Person of the holy Trinity brought us the Divine Masculine consort of the only-begotten Child, the Divine Feminine of the third person of the Holy Trinity, as did her Divine

Masculine consort, the Holy Spirit, brings the strength and wisdom necessary for God's people who seek to understand and follow the Wife of the Lamb. Having given us the means of salvation from which we were turned away, Jesus now presents Mary as the active consort to bring to fruition the promise given to our first parents, which are hope, love, and salvation.

This wholeheartedly differs from the traditional version, and teachings which Eeshans believe have been unquestionably altered, destroyed, or lost since the 'beginning of the creation story' has been handed down, through human history. Whereas, this plan connotes a doomsday consequence for a people who turned away from God, we see the co-Savior here to ease our pain and bring joy in establishing order and faith once again.

Eeshans' foundational beliefs will be found to emphasize that Jesus manifested Himself as true God and true Man, and that God never fails, as deemed by a human consciousness; thus we are not left with an option, which allows for a turning away from a God who is Truth and Love, especially in light of God's love and promise. Because of Jesus, and his divine consort, we are given another opportunity to return to God, as originally intended. Those who want to follow Jesus, but don't agree with the church, and its corrupt history and teachings, are no longer in a weakened position and disadvantage to counter these people who consider themselves the 'true believers' of Catholicism; previously those who wanted to know Jesus and to follow Him didn't have anything else before; thus this book helps us all.

LESSON 111

QUELLING THE TERROR

It is obvious that the world around us, in too many places, is spinning out of control. We say we are fighting discrimination that exists today, yet all that we witness in these times is the fight and the hatred that exists for anyone who goes against the status quo for the sake of what is good and right and true, and, thus, they are stifled in their tracks. Are we really fighting for equality, or are we confusing discrimination, as a means to maintain the status quo and allowing political parties the opportunities to not right the wrongs, but to use discrimination and prejudice, as platforms for "gaining and empowering themselves" among the masses, with little to no change in the lives of their constituents? For example, are we really being represented towards good change, even if it involves accepting good advice from another party? Or are we just being led around like sheep?

For many politicians who feel apathetic towards the great degree of injustice and suffering in the world today seem to exhibit no God at all in their life. God has been truly misconceived and dealt a "bad hand" each time their only conclusion is that if there is a God then 'He' is responsible for this outrage, i.e., "If God is all good, why is there such evil in the world?" We forget, however, that what 'they' are seeing *are the results of the choices human beings have made.* What 'they' are saying is the result of the people seeing only issues and no solutions. It's like taking something good that was created and finding a bad use for it, and then blaming God for the harm that resulted.

From the Eeshan point of view, God gave the answer to this ancient problem. We received the template from which we might learn how to build a peaceful world, starting with one's own self, by simplifying how we are to live when Jesus took the Ten Commandments and narrowed them down to his Two Great Commandments. It is time to witness to the truth, and bring love, hope, and trust back, again, first in God, and then filtering down to our neighbor, whom He taught are His children, and as Jesus welcomed everyone, no matter what religion, race, color, or creed into His presence.

Jesus said, "Blessed are the meek, for they will inherit the earth." (Matthew 5:5).

This is foundational to what Eeshans teach. As Jesus is meek, we too must present ourselves as meek. This does not mean that he wants us to be *weak, tame, or deficient in courage*. What Jesus meant, was that *we must exercise power under God*, and not based solely on our own human standards. Jesus portrayed this in the cleansing of the Temple where he actively and publicly exhibited his strengths and abilities exercising his power for God's benefit. As God's people, we have an obligation to respect, and revere, the things and places of God along with the directives given to us in order to see results.

The core of our beliefs, which are the foundation of our Spirituality, are built upon the Marriage of Jesus and Mary Magdalen. We believe the hidden truth about the relationship between Adam and Eve, and, then, subsequently, the love between Jesus and Mary Magdalen, is key to why there is such misunderstanding and disconnect in the minds of people towards how God sees, hears, and answers prayers. To this day, no one has linked the mystery of marriage with the reason Jesus came to earth, let alone the power behind this mystery in dealing with all the issues we are faced with today. Everything comes back to 'love,' and how to solve the plights we face today: divorce, gender discrimination, drugs, and a world in turmoil. The impetus in the preceding is not knowing the why, the who, what, where, and how of all things spiritual, and how they relate to daily life.

By the elimination and omission of Jesus' marriage, and the furthering of the one-sided, goal-oriented misinterpretation of his mission and teachings, and presenting the familiar traditional scriptures, which were tainted, it is easy to blame God for all the pain, suffering, and wrongs in the world. Eeshans believe that these, most assuredly, are what has given place to fear, and rejection, of God rather than respect and love.

What about the Bible? Backed by many, scholars claim that the stories in the bible should not be taken literally *because they have only the smallest possible quantity of adequate and reliable information.* Aside from the wisdom writings and prophets, there are many questionable accounts in the Bible that don't seem remotely compatible with Jesus' teaching, or seem as though passages were altered to suit a political objective. Instead, scholars are able to point out many different writing influences and signs of editing, and Eeshans believe this about the Bible, and how it was written, and how it was put together to appear in its present form, and in light of how Eeshans believe that the New Testament writings were 'remembered' and edited/revised, or omitted etc., there is agreement with much of what scholars recognize about the Bible, and how it was written and composed. What Eeshans know through their studies in Mystery School with Eesha only affirms this.

Throughout recent decades, many experts studying scriptures found stories that have been altered, or endings that have been added, as there are too many inconsistencies and proof that many parts of stories, as well as endings, were missing, or inconclusive and one-sided.

Eeshans feel that a lot of these inconsistencies had to do with the elimination, omission, and denial of Jesus being married. Eeshans hold that anything written about Jesus without mentioning Mary, especially as His wife, is likened to a story about Adam, without Eve being mentioned, or better, putting the brunt of the blame for our suffering on Eve.

In an effort to cover up the truth are the poor attempts of religious leaders to replace, or disguise, the place of Mary Magdalen with events that warrant a wife's place, not Jesus' mother Mary, who Eeshans yet hold in highest honor among women. With God, the Almighty King and Father and his wife the Virgin Mary Queen and Mother, once Jesus took his place as King, so His wife would become Queen. Presenting the Virgin Mary as Queen of Heaven and Earth is true if her true Husband was revealed as God the Father Almighty. This is another excellent example of a half-truth being used for centuries. How can Jesus replace his living Father as King, and rule with his Mother as Queen? How did this "arrangement" come about? It happened by means of a kind of expungement, which we have discovered by the urgings of persistent memory, what we believed was revealed. There *was* indeed a hidden queen, and it is Mary Magdalen.

The bible and traditional scriptures were, and did, serve to produce a cathex is result, meaning that Christ's followers entered into a tremendously significant emotional investment. Why and how? First and foremost, because they were told they had to conform or be condemned to Hell; and, secondly, they had no reason to doubt. nor could they, for reasons found in number one.

There was also a period of time in which God's people were told not to read the Bible for they would not understand it. because most people at the time were only functionally literate, if they could read at all. Later on, as bibles were being printed, there was a fear that the vernacular bibles carried anti-Catholic notes. The Latin version was available with no restrictions, however, you needed to be able to read Latin and accept what was written without question.

In more recent times, and as people became more educated, and as fear could no longer be used as a tool to control people, and deflect questioning, another method was instituted and called "the deposit of faith." This means that the church claims all faith necessary for all men at all times (*pretty sure this is supposed to be inclusive however it is not, i.e., the case of ordination of women*), and all places, and if a true saving faith demands a clear knowledge of what we have to believe, it is clear that an infallible teaching church is an absolute necessity. By establishing itself with this unquestionable authority, the ability to control *could well seem assured.*

The church has over so much time gathered the momentum of authority over the masses that it seems to be able to say that it alone can speak to "men" of all classes and at all times. It alone can, by reason of its perpetuity, and ageless character, meet every new difficulty by a declaration of their soundest form of doctrine (they have to own it), which is to be held. If the teaching is distorted, none but the church can say, "*This* is its true meaning, and not *that*, I know that it is as I say the Spirit which assists me and is One with the Spirit which rested on Him and them."[151]

This statement ends all discussions on topics presented to them that they do not wish to entertain issues such as women's ordination and the true account and meaning of the Marriage Feast at Cana, about which the church has no answers.

In the following sections, we present earnestly *our* fundamental beliefs in such a way as to cover all those areas in which to show what we as Eeshans believe, agree with, and don't believe, as well as plausible reasons to support each, as best we can in this book. What was presented to you up until now, should help support what we will present to you from here on.

Again, you are under no obligation to accept our beliefs. We ask only that you respect ours. Remember, this book provides the opportunity for you to see some of our views of what we feel Jesus intended for all of us, and to reintroduce the Divine Feminine in a way which has always been previously skewed through the eyes of humans under the guise of a directive from Jesus with a purpose to maintain a patriarchal world.

Eeshans believe this world we are living in has been thrust into chaos because it has been devoid of knowledge regarding the female consorts of the Triune God, who makes up the Sacred Balance of all things God. Without balance, facts, ideas, and teachings about God can be exaggerated, or distorted, and human power and authority could and would use its influence and leverage over interpretation, and speak for God to suit its own agenda. For example, as we noted earlier, being meek does not mean being cowering or weak, but being strong in doing what God asks, and this not in a radical sense, but by being strong under God's control. This does not mean taking matters into one's own hands in order to hurt another. It simply means aligning one's life with Jesus' teachings of kindness and love, yet, still being firm against any wrong doing.

---

[151] Pope, Hugh. "Catholic Encyclopedia (1913)/Rule of Faith." Catholic Encyclopedia (1913)/Rule of Faith—Wikisource, the Free Online Library, 1913, en.wikisource.org/wiki?curid=99061.

LESSON 112

'REPETITIO' OF THOUGHTS: A 'KIND' DISCLAIMER

You may have noticed, thus far, that we have repeated some teaching points several times. In doing so we feel we are providing some additional thoughts sometimes, coming with different perspectives, such as found under the Eeshan Salvific plan section. Other topics may be broken down into sections to further explain a specific point or belief.

The words **REPITITION–REPITITION–REPITITION** herald the title of this section.

You've probably already noticed that we make use of other writings, books, media (social or otherwise), to accentuate our point of view, drawing on claims pursuant to information deemed accurate, etc., or, which are used to get people thinking again. By providing other people's thoughts, various translations, findings, arguments, perceptions, understanding and opinions. These are used as references in an effort to show a God who is not limited to one particular religion and culture, but is rather part of all of us. Also, you will find references and points of view that to some are not 'credible' enough to hang one's hat on (such as Wikipedia, for example). Our reason for doing this is to encourage the reader to go to these sites, and think for themselves, and 'do their own homework.' Sometimes it happens that expressions, or quotes, and other forms of useful information comes our way without an author's name attached to it. We have and will always encourage our readers to seek more information for themselves. Because people identify with different points of view for very different reasons, we purposely try to include those varied points of view, all the while trying to retain and underscore those that most closely align with what we believe as Eeshans.

We stand by this approach, even while some may dispute it with purported facts or references that may contradict our view points. That's alright. It's alright to refute our findings, beliefs, and information, etc., and reject it. We are simply laying it out here as to why WE believe what *we* believe. Try not to take offense to our 'fault finding' opinions of the church, at large, since, again, we are simply trying to present our reasons for the bringing back into existence the viewpoint of Eeshan Transcendentalism.

The God from whom Jesus was begotten is truly, and always will be, identified with extreme love and devotion. We hope we provide enough external material, which you too may find helpful in securing and developing further your love for God, since it, and more, has played a tremendous role in influencing God's people wherever they may be, whatever culture they are, and no matter their views, or beliefs, on religion or spirituality.

We feel these references are not only necessary in order to being forth the most fruitful and richest, most sacred, ways of God, but they tie in so perfectly as to how God is *not a religion*, but, in omnipotence, shares love with every human being in the world in one way or another, allowing for culture, individuality, and expression to grow.

That is why we try and emphasize our use of the term "religion," as not being in the context of what people think, but rather in light of the definition as we had in the beginning of this book.

We don't want Eeshan Transcendentalism to be confused with how others have defined, and commonly think of, religion. We feel it is better defined as our attempt to represent the true teachings of Christ and the real reason for the Messiah(s); we want to reorder feelings, imaginings, actions, and beliefs that have arisen in response to the direct and mandatory directive of the sacred and spiritual. As this attempt expands in its formulation and elaboration, it became a process, which created meaning for itself in an effort to deflect what we as God's people have become accustomed to when thinking about religion. We want Eeshan spirituality to become a sustaining basis for understanding wisdom and truth by its originating and representing the transcendental experiences, and, thus, continue to sustain a faith that will continue to grow, so that when Jesus returns with His Gift, He will find FAITH. We want to raise the bar for our humanity, and help all who desire to find completeness in the intended transcendental meanings we provide.

Still, no one is pressured to agree with us. If you are happy with your faith, be happy. Not everyone agrees with everything regarding religion, faith, or spirituality, fact, theory, or otherwise. We believe that whatever path one takes to find, renew, or grow toward one's relationship to God is profoundly personal. Eeshans profess that whatever Absolute or Higher Being that you are searching for, or need, to become a better person, or become the "you" you are searching for, Eeshan spirituality could compliment and aid your search.

We are always open to sharing our timeless spirituality to serve the need of all those souls who seek and ask questions for their own spiritual betterment. We want to make the world we live in a better place. We want to spread the true teachings of Jesus and His wife so that something can be done about the problems we all face as a people created by a loving God. Our faith, trust, and love of God strengthens us, allowing us to never be discouraged but to see beyond whatever apathy and cynicism people send our way.

Though we have taken the time to present our views and conclusions, and substantiate them with our understanding, or, perhaps, even by asking rhetorical questions, it is not to be misconstrued in feeling that the burden of proof is essential to our existence. It is not our intention to have to explain to everyone's satisfaction why we hold this belief or point of view, nor do we feel the need to have to try to prove what we believe.[152]

We will not enter into useless arguments with others who have no intention to seek enlightenment our way, and we offer no argument just for the sake of arguing; but we do desire that you continue reading with an open mind and heart, since it is better to build up the love of God, instead of breaking that love down by engaging in pointless debates.

---

[152] When someone doesn't 'want' to believe, there is never going to be enough evidence to satisfy them; again, the person doesn't 'want' to accept something, and so they won't – not truly. Thus, the issue comes down to faith. What do *you* believe? – Ed.

What you have, and will, continue to read, is solely for the purpose of explaining our reasons for introducing the results of our responding to God's mandate, especially since it may not be easy for members of Catholic and Christian denominations, as well as other faiths, to understand.

Being in the fullness of time, we believe that the revelation of God's full intention brings to light the return of the Divine Feminine, to complete Christ's mission as intended, originally thus, calling out that catalyst that reared its ugly head as the source of hatred, unrest, and failure in order to move humankind in a positive direction.[153] This catalyst causes discrimination; and discrimination is the cancer which grows at a rapid speed, and is aggressive and metastasizes regardless of color, creed, gender, age, etc., each time people judge other people by personal, or human, standards and not by God's standards.

We believe that Jesus revealed, by his single and married life, his teachings, and his death on the cross, that we are to love God first. He showed how God is our Father, and how the love of Mary, his Mother, for the Father was expressed in her 'Yes,' to do as God, her husband, desired, as it is written in Luke 11:28, "Blessed rather are those who hear the word of God and put it into practice." Furthermore, we see how this love was, and still is, found in the love of his own wife who stood by His side, fearless and strong. In these present times, we are given another chance where we are all united once again when we hear the will of God and do it.

We, as Eeshans, believe that the Eeshan religion, and spirituality, is an integral truth and that the Sophia Perennis is guiding us. We believe that it is God's will to introduce our religion to the world; though we may be going against the grain, we, like the 'Marys' (Mary Magdalen and Blessed Mother Mary), wholeheartedly give God our 'Yes,' and will stand strong and fearless before Jesus, who is our everything.

---

[153] *Duhkha* is the Sanskrit term for 'suffering'; perhaps the best way to understand the term, especially in the present context, is "suffering as opportunity." All difficulties can be turned around and used for a positive spiritual end. – Ed.

A SUMMARY OF EESHAN BELIEFS BASIC TEACHINGS

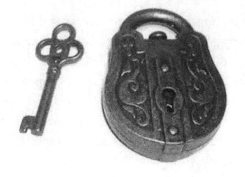

LESSON 113

SPIRITUAL TEACHING ONE: AND GOD SO LOVED US…

It is said that God so loved us that He sent his only begotten Son. Honestly, 'God' so loved 'us' that the Divine sent the only-begotten Child. When God corrects, or chastises, it is always out of love and not out of rejection; and Jesus gave many examples of this.

Though we all were taught this, this opinion changes, however, when one is not willing to accept discipline. In this case, the individual will not see love, but judgment. Today, more than ever, correcting one who does not desire to be enlightened, only causes them to grow darker. Why? Because, today, to seek to become enlightened, or spiritual, is frowned upon, and seems to equate with being judgmental. Thus, the kneejerk reaction to the truth, for many, is to turn the table and seek defense behind the response, "Don't judge me!" Many of these types of people also resort to criticisms of spirituality, such as "I think for myself, and I am not swayed by group think," especially when the truth is they don't realize how their own mentality is very much tied to the groupthink of the World in the very manner they superimpose upon a person sincerely seeking God, who is trying to align their life with the things of God. This sort of dynamic is especially prevalent in politics, where you find such degrees of criticism from one party against the other, when in plain sight you see that the accuser is most guilty of the precise thing in which they themselves sit in judgment.

To attack, even those who are against our beliefs, does not allow us to correct, or bring truth to, often erroneous and disconcerting remarks, and presents no opportunity to bring God's better judgment into play.

However, to be meek as Jesus is meek, allows us to stand firm on what we believe, and to not be a doormat.

It was because Jesus loved us that he taught by his word, life, death, and resurrection. It was for this reason that he identified himself as God "before Abraham, I Am" that we, as humans, would recognize that he wasn't just teaching from a human perspective, but as, indeed, God. Yet, he was certainly concerned Himself in addressing hypocrites and liars when necessary, even in public. He did this because He was God; and He demonstrated what was right by having His wife accompany Him, as well as other women, and, sometimes, children.

LESSON 114

SPIRITUAL TEACHING TWO: BATTLING HYPOCRISY

Jesus was leading people away from a fear-induced religion to love of God—and making them think.

We made the point that we feel the teachings of those authorities, who knew, taught, and continued to teach in Jesus' name only, were guilty of presenting only half of His story. In doing so, they not only failed to see the consequences, but rather than provide spiritual growth, they instead contributed to the collapse of the human heart's belief that God exists.

Jesus was the end of the old covenant and the beginning of a new covenant; and *our faith* is based on the new covenant. Eeshans feel that no old testament book, such as Leviticus, should ever replace Jesus' teachings. It has continued to be used for purposes and points made on issues that do not reflect Jesus. To constantly use Leviticus' reference only shows that there is not enough understanding of Jesus' poignant views, as if He never addressed issues relative to recent times. It is said that Leviticus' obsessive detailed account of sins, especially after having been given the Ten Commandments. points to man being the author of these laws of such earthy and often hair-splitting tones. Moreover, there is much in the Old Testament regarding God, and God's directives, that deeply conflicts with what was taught by Jesus.[154]

---

[154] Again, it becomes an intriguing question as to how much of the Old Testament writings, aside from the Wisdom writings, were the unvarnished Word of God and

This is what Jesus meant when He said to the crowds, "The teachers of the Law and the Pharisees sit in Moses' seat. So, you must be careful to do everything they tell you; but do not do what they do, for they do not do what they preach. They tie up heavy, cumbersome loads and put them on other people's shoulders, but they are not willing to lift a finger to move them." Remember they may have interpreted the law to the letter but *not to the spirit*, and this *led to a whole lot of perversions and distortions* of what the Law actually said and meant. A perfect example was the Pharisees telling Jesus that it was unlawful for him to heal a person on the Sabbath (Matt. 12:1-4). They quoted a very long and complicated oral law, which was to them an authoritative tradition, to what is known as a block, or fence, around the written law. Though if they were addressing anyone other than Jesus, one would say that they didn't really do anything wrong, *but it was Jesus*. Hence, because Moses' presence was representing the Mosaic Law, and was being fulfilled by Jesus in the Transfiguration on Mount Tabor, and *as Messiah*, in the presence of Elijah, as the prophet in the fulfillment of Prophecy (Luke 24:44, John 5:46; Matt. 5:17), then Jesus had the right to call them 'hypocrites' because they were denying him and undermining him on purpose and with full knowledge of who he was. 'This' also meant that any objection to Jesus indicated they did not know the spirit, or the heart, of the Law. This simply means that to 'hatefully' reject Jesus is clear proof that they could not be trusted, and, thus, it is much the same which applies today.

To not accept, or deliberately, refuse to teach, or to acknowledge any teaching, especially with regards to his wife, Mary Magdalen, is ultimately wrong and dangerous. We feel that these reasons, in particular, point to those in authority today who are guilty of the same hypocrisy, since they have taken God's law and made it their own; *and they know who they are.*

---

how much were the product of men overlaying a revision on that Word of God in light of a fear-driven or greed-based driven political agenda. If it was that way with Jesus' teachings at the hands of Peter and the human consciousness ... is there any possibility it was this way after Moses, through the times when the Old Testament writings were composed? – Ed.

Jesus taught love of God and neighbor. He vindicated sinners and never spiritually imprisoned them. He opened the heart and released souls from the darkness of hatred and fear, and led them to love and life.

The success of the goals of those in false authority (who came later on) was guaranteed when followers of Christ were made to feel that to question this authority was to question Jesus himself, as in "To question my authority is to question God's authority and law."Therefore, what was taught by the Jewish authorities, at that time, was easily accepted, yet it was devoid of the actual *complete* teachings that Jesus taught (i.e., when Jesus taught a balanced, common sense, and complete understanding of the law, as when one's ox, or child, falls into the ditch on the Sabbath, or how to live the balance between the sacred and the secular, as with his example using the coin with Caesar's face on it).

We present that. in a way, it is easy to make a Gnostic writing look heretical if you wanted to, perhaps, much in the same way that an Orthodox Jew could point out the Gospels are utterly heretical on any number of points. The key is that it would be so only *'from their perspective.'* So, if and when, people argue 'from scripture' that a Gnostic text, or even the Eeshan writings in this book are 'heretical.' it is only in relation to the point of view they have been conditioned to have in place, a set of lenses they view and evaluate by. What they don't realize is that their conclusions are just something they have chosen to agree with in a group context, and these perceptions, and conclusions, change from group to group, and time to time, depending on what the commonly agreed upon priorities are. What should also be considered is that when speaking of the mainstream accepted Gospels, and other New Testament writings, most people actually don't even know what the scripture passage really said in its original language, let alone understanding anything about all the stages it may have gone through just to bring it even to a primitive form in an ancient language that had to be copied multiple times and translated into other languages.

So how can Eeshans say that what *they* have is the truth, when the church teaches that the gospels written were conceived from 'divine inspiration' in lieu of the above? Well one should remember that in the beginning, only a few Jews who were 'inspired' by the Divine wrote down what they *experienced*, and only a few early followers of Jesus who were 'inspired' by the Divine wrote down what *they* experienced. It wasn't a common thing to write journals and 'complex treatises' and explain all about what went into the writing of these documents. Similarly, what is in this text you are reading is certainly no different.

Eeshans explain that if one views religions as beginning with Light, that due to human corruption over long periods of time, these religions become increasingly darkened. This Light is the Primordial Wisdom, or the Perennial Wisdom, or Sophia Perrenis; it is all knowledge and all wisdom (feminine), and when spoken, is the "Word," or Logos (masculine). The female encompasses the male.

The Eeshan path is not new. Being as that it incorporates Merkabolic and Kabbalic energies, it has throughout humankind, returned to restore the Light when it is required, and that is what you have here in these times. Because it is a living Light that connects to the Light Body found within each person, the 're-opening' of the Eeshan path is, thereby, identified when Jesus, who is the "Light of the World" said, "My sheep will hear my voice." It is this "Light" that was there when the Mosaic religion began, as well as when the early Christian sects began, or with any other faith that began inspired by this Light. In the same way, this "Light" is what animates the Eeshan perspective and religion, but it should be underscored that this Light currently in question is also that very same Light at the beginning of time. What human beings inevitably build around that Light that originally spoke, and inspired, and gave life, may well often turn towards corruption due to the human tendency towards choices leaning in the direction of, or under, the influence of illusion.

For one to base what a tradition hinges on, and its power, and the truth found in it, purely on how long it has been in existence, is a mistake. The power that results from the snowballing effect that institutions tend to create around themselves is not necessarily an indication of divine appointment ... or that the stamp of God's approval is upon them; it is just the illusion of power, this mystique, that powerful institutions inevitably create in the minds of their subjects, and it is this powerful effect that can be used to maintain power and control over minds. When this problem reaches its fullest measure of epidemic proportions it is then that nothing can be seen any longer, God intervenes by way of this Light. This Light penetrates everything and illuminates the darkest areas (cf. Ephesians 5:13, "But everything exposed by the light becomes visible—and everything that is illuminated becomes light.") and 'sunlights' those agencies that continue to exist and spread under the cloak of darkness to include all that is necessary in order to bring about the true teachings of Jesus, and to correct the errors in interpretation and by omissions, etc.

The above all leads back into a basic premise of this book, which is that Eeshans present their religion as being specifically that Light that Jesus spoke of that 'cannot be hidden under a bushel basket;' and God will bring about its resurgence in order to return faith and spirituality back to the Consciousness of God.

Thus, it only makes sense that the church chose certain gospels and not others, and included certain writings while rejecting others, while branding yet others 'heretical' if they were known about, in order to give the people only what the church wanted them to have. The problem has only been perpetuated, serving to further embed the cancerous growths of discrimination and oppression in the official teachings of institutions that supposedly are founded on divine authority as so much of the Christian world reimaged Jesus to supposedly give them exclusively.

Back then, even though given what Jesus taught encompassed was truth and love, it was still deemed as having a *"radical component"* because it went against the establishment of his time. All the people knew was what they were raised to believe. and that all that was from God was under Mosaic law, and their culture and religion were one.

One must remember that's how Jesus was *living* and what He was *teaching* was, in fact, making too much sense. He also spoke publicly what *the people were thinking interiorly*. It evoked the respect of most all of the people outside the religion and culture of the time, for it revealed a balanced ego, and the disparity between man's interpretation of God's law and the spirit of God's law showing a loving forgiving God. In other words, *he was making people think and rethink what they had been told.*

Couple the above with His being married to Mary Magdalen, sitting, talking, and teaching women; and now we have a serious competition rising against the established religion and culture of the time.

Yes, Jesus was successful because what he was doing was leading people away from fear-induced religion to love of God and "making them think."

Hmm ... who in these days was accused of exactly that? Oh wait, our Foundress was. This is what would eventually make Him appear to be dangerous to the established religion and culture of the time and an enemy and threat to all the authorities and laws of that time and perhaps over 2000-plus years. That is why we believe that at the onset of Peter's self-appointed leadership, via the human consciousness, this is what continues up until today.

The same issues addressed by Jesus as wrong at that time are the same issues we find wrong today within mainstream cultural and traditional church teachings. This includes the refusal of spiritual authorities of today, to see and accept *his mastery* of spirituality. One such issue that immediately comes to mind is the refusal to accept women's involvement in church leadership and officiating in worship services.

As we said Jesus kept His wife close, and treated women as equals. Not only had He talked to the women who surrounded him, but He spoke to and taught those women whose cultures were shunned by the religion of the time, as was the case (John 4:4-26) of the Samaritan woman. He did the same regarding the acceptance of all genders, colors, races, and creeds.

Yes, Jesus taught everyone, sat with everyone, ate with everyone, especially sinners, you know, people like us ... and discriminated against no one, despite their person, cultural, or religious background.

He was guilty of making people think because of a 'certainty' found within them, a kind of infused knowledge, already ingrained, just deeply buried, but which was now being brought to the surface. What He told them just made sense.

Fearful were the minds of the authorities, as the people were on the verge of *waking up and beginning to think*. The religious teachers, the Pharisees, and Sadducees, realized that these kinds of teachings could bring about the demise of a culture they had cultivated and enjoyed by centuries' worth of religious 'experienced' authorities. They, alone, were the spokespersons for God. They believed they were chosen to make and enforce the laws, both in their immediate lives, and in the history of their traditions going all the way back to the beginning of creation.

Who was this man to question the law? How could He say, "Before Abraham, I am?" In other words, as Abraham lived some four hundred years before Moses, he (Abraham) was progenitor of the Hebrews and founder of Judaism. Jesus used this comparison for that reason. That He existed, as God, before the Judaic religion. If Jesus said these words today it would be for people to realize that the world's three largest monotheistic religions may have been founded by Abraham, but the Son of God (now in the human/divine form of Jesus Christ) not only existed but *was God* before all of them.

As important as it was for Jesus to identify himself back then, it is equally important for Eesha to be identified today as the one carrying the consciousness of Mary Magdalen. In other words, to mark the continued mission of her Husband, Eesha not only says, "Before the Catholic church, I AM," but also that Mary Magdalen was eternally married to Jesus Christ and, thus, has the authority to identify herself as His eternal consort.

LESSON 115

SPIRITUAL TEACHING THREE: JESUS WAS NOT GENDER CONSCIOUS/EXCLUSIVE

Actually, He was not prejudiced culturally, racially, with regards to creed, or age, nor was he against any people.

The Pharisees said in Luke 20:21, "Teacher, we know that you speak and teach what is right, and that you do not show partiality." Everywhere the translations indicate Jesus wasn't swayed by others, He paid no attention to the social status of the person, and thus He was impartial and didn't play favorites, and didn't care about anyone's opinions, since He was not swayed by appearances. In other words, Jesus was an honest man, and taught with the truth.

Can you imagine, then, God created "you" to be a 'certain way,' i.e., female, a different color, or different in your sexual orientation, so that He may have others not accept you? Can you see yourself perhaps a white Christian, Irish Catholic, a Jew, Muslim, black slave, or a deformed, poor, too old, or a terminally sick person? Or, perhaps, you were made to feel worthless, and expendable, because you can no longer contribute to society, and further, that you are a drain on the economy? What if you were told by a particular person, or group, that because you are one of these you were an abomination to the God that created you? Because that is what discrimination is, the finding of 'any' reason to hate and reject a person created by God, loved by God, because 'someone,' or 'some group,' doesn't like them. How would you feel if people treated you badly, and unjustly, because *they decided* God hated you? Sadly, this is a flawed human mind that could change on a dime. and one day they don't like Catholics, then the next day they hate anyone who lives in a brick house. What it boils down to is discrimination is the result of anyone, or any group, that has no inner sense of what is right or wrong is motivated by fear, and who uses a dominant personality (political, religious) as an authority and an example for wrongful conduct, or presents motives to satisfy their own insecurities. It impels one towards wrong actions, in that hate has no moral principles, and goes against all that is in harmony in the universe. It is when one has not figured out that it is yet through another way that the divine works, and that the human conscious is even with those who do not believe in a God, or have a religion or spirituality.

Jesus so clarified the 'true' Law, and in doing so, automatically abolished those historical, and cultural, accretions arising out of irrational fears, fears that were created by men, and over time gathered momentum, which now even today serve as the basis for all kinds of discrimination and violence, and was sometimes even codified as officially 'coming from God' i.e., IN THE OLD TESTAMENT, and, so, therefore, it can reach a point where what is so very wrong cannot be amended or even questioned.

Jesus revealed the truth about the Old Testament Law, and revealed the kind of Law that God *actually* taught from the beginning, and not what men interpreted it to be; He was able and authorized to do this because he was God. On the other hand, man, after he took over when Jesus was gone, recast what Jesus taught. and meant. and changed it back to the *OLD LAW*. To keep going back to the interpretation of the Levitical Law, and make Jesus' teachings conform to it, a law that was written and interpreted by men that Jesus (as God) rebuked, and that goes against Jesus' commandment to love, basically is to put God (Old Testament) against God (New Testament).

Eeshans believe that physical body gender is a covering for the purpose of distinguishing the physiology of a person, but is not always the same as one's gender *identity*. In some cases, the gender identity is in consistent with a person's biological sex characteristics. Gender dysphoria is when the biological gender of the person does not match up with gender identity. This is not the person's fault, or choice; and it is not who, or what, makes up the person. We are not responsible for being born, or how we are born, or we look, or to whom we are born, as a human family we should be there to help those who need help and welcome each as family.

Who and what the person is, is much deeper than the body's covering. Just like you can't judge a book by its cover, you cannot expect people to fit a particular template, and so on.

God designed us to love each other and not oppress one or another; but to unite with talents and skill, not for just within one owns culture, race, color, religion etc., but for a better life in this world and a better tomorrow. Because we look, or are made differently, or because we are male, female, or prone to feel male, while in a female body, or female in a male body, or androgynous, gay, lesbian, or intersexed, these things should not ever be a cause to hate, harm, or reject someone; and most definitely *no one has a right to keep anyone from Jesus and his Mysteries.* Though we may not understand the why for those things we feel are punishable, we must understand that these are human beings and judgment should be left to God. To be clear, discrimination, and prejudice arises out of fear, and this is the seed of all oppression and suffering.

We were always taught that it's what is inside that counts, and not to judge a book by its cover, and that beauty is only skin deep; so, why can't we remember that this is a reference to all things under God? We are obligated under God's law to find what is beneath skin color, gender physiology, and gender identity, and love the *person*. As beauty is only skin deep, so the person is just beneath the covering. Accidents deform people, so if a fire disfigures a loved one, do you not love them anymore?

Wouldn't the greater test of revealing discrimination be found in this little allegory. God gives some angels a new job to learn a different skill. The newbies were trying to meet the quota and looking to God to be surceased, and so began to get careless. They started to put a male in a woman's body and a female in a man's body. Once they realized the error, they went with bowed heads to God and explained. God being all loving, smiled, and said, "I have all kinds of angels. I have two-winged, six-winged, many wings, those with faces of animals, those of all colors, etc., and I love them all. The same should be with all my children. To love me above all things with one's whole being, and to love their neighbor as one's self, this should not be an issue. Let see how my children respond and treat these whom I love as I love them?"

How should one judge these? One must be careful not to judge by man's standard, as if speaking for God; God may then judge us by our own standard. To God, we are all made in goodness and love, and our outward appearances and personalities are as special, just as all little children are, indeed, good.

Another striking lesson we feel is important, is with regards to two of the most impressive examples of the person of Jesus, and how He lived, what He taught, was how He spoke and shared the 'most unfathomable truths.'

We all know about the account of the woman in Sychar, Samaria, at Jacob's well. This is unique because not only did He talk with a woman, but she also originated from a culture that was shunned by the Jews. She knew this, and said, "You are a Jew and I am a Samaritan woman—how can you ask me for water?" Jesus answered, "If you knew 'the gift of God' and who was asking you for a drink, you would have asked Him, and He would have given you living water." He also told her, "A time will come when the true worshippers will worship the Father … in Spirit and in truth for they are the kind of worshippers the Father seeks. God is spirit and the worshippers must worship in spirit and truth." The woman proclaimed, "I know that the Messiah (called Christ) is coming. When He comes He will explain everything to us?" Jesus answered, "I, the one speaking to you, I am He."

The second most beautiful verse is found in one of Jesus' parables. This time it was about a Samaritan man [Luke 10:25-37]. This parable is about a traveler who is stripped of his clothing, beaten, and left half dead alongside the road. First a priest, and then a Levite, came by but both avoided the man. Finally, a Samaritan (who was from a culture prejudiced by the Jews) happens to come by. The Samaritan, despite the fact that they did not get along with Jews, and vice versa, helps the traveler, and pays an inn keeper to watch over the injured man until he is well. He promises to come by later to see if more money is needed for the man's expenses. Jesus was showing here that we are all children of God, and we should rise above our differences, since we are all neighbors and human beings. Therefore, we should have a sense of responsibility, commitment, concern, and, most of all, love for each other.

If Jesus was not prejudiced and did not discriminate, how dare we? Are we above God? By discrimination are we not presenting our rules as God's, when in fact they are human's? When did discrimination first show its ugly face? Before we Eeshans talk about how we believe it originated, let's examine the following. God's plan for the entire universe is imaged in duality, so that each part is balanced by a counterpart, and where the inner Light within the body radiates, and connects us all as one with God, and who and what we are before God is not exclusively defined by the outward shell of the physical, material body.

LESSON 116

SPIRITUAL TEACHING FOUR: LOVE THY NEIGHBOR CONTINUED

Have you ever believed a person to be one way, then you met the person, and found they were nothing like you were told, or thought? They were actually wonderful and kind etc.? Being human, we are always prone to error, especially in instances like this. Yet rather than learn from our mistakes, we continue to make the same ones. We judge by other's opinions, we judge a book by its color, and, for the most part, we are always proven wrong. Why is that? Recently on the news, a panel of commentators were talking about this very thing. Though they were rivals in politics and argued, and debated on radio and television, outside of work, they have dinner together, travel, and go to games and parties together.

We often find ourselves in positions where 'loving one's neighbor' doesn't seem to matter. This happens on a daily basis when we begin judging those whom 'we never met,' whether it is politicians, celebrities, or people at work. We don't know these people. We forget that in politics and television, it is their job, or career, that requires them to keep ratings up. These have reporters, speech writers, public relation people, all who for the sake of keeping their names alive use any tactic necessary, i.e., tabloid material and gossip, to accomplish this. We don't have to like their methods, policies, or antics; and of course, we can discuss, and give our opinions, too; and, as we should never wish ill upon them, we often find ourselves doing just this.

How often have you found yourself taking the word of a person, or persons, who are not credible sources but rather 'have a history of lying,' or making more of a situation than there really is? Or how often have you had the experience of knowing, and finding, they only prove that they lie, fabricate stories, gossip out of jealousy, or just to hurt the good image you may (or may not want to) have of another person? Perhaps, you want to believe what you are being told, and, therefore, keep going back to hear what this unreliable source is saying as though they are a credible source. There are also those people who preface what they want to tell you by saying, "I can't lie," since they really enjoy spreading gossip and causing dissention. They obtain enjoyment at telling you all those hurtful things someone said about you, for no good reason.

Our fallen nature enjoys hearing bad things about people we don't like; and will believe anything regardless of how far from the truth the facts are regarding them. Then there is the plight of embellishing additional details to make the story much more interesting, hurtful, or to gain some kind of credibility.

Where there is fallacy there is also an opportunity for truth. When you go wrong, you can correct yourself, and get back on the right track. You can correct the gossip about someone, or, in many cases, end it by telling the 'gossiper' they shouldn't be spreading information like that.

All of us truly make up a rainbow of race, color, ethnic/cultures, beliefs with an array of beauty, if we could only take off the blinders of discrimination and prejudice. We should, for humanity's sake, see each gender, age, race, and culture contributing to a vast bounty of all kinds of things that opens up the world to us. These are the endless possibilities of experiencing what God gifted us out of love. The enjoyment and pleasure of eating and experiencing food, talent, skills, thoughts and science ... the uniqueness of tradition and folklore, which we should thrive to enjoy. The beauty of other cultures and countries and customs that we can delight in and by which we can be enriched.

This is what Jesus taught, and that is in those things we allow others to use as tools of discrimination should be turned into tools to teach and bring joy and longevity. No person is an island. No individual group holds all the keys. The United States is powerful in its multicultural strength and acceptability and under God has been blessed. It is only when politics and the powerful enter the picture that a people learns imbalance and ignorance. Everyday people understand culture and customs, and see no difference in their fellow human beings until they are told to.

Still, we are against blind acceptance, but are praying for this world to find the ability to build a culture built on a foundation towards a goal to become the example of a culture that enables everyone to contribute all they have that is good. In this way, we become one body, one spirit, one mind. It is not in conquering, or isolating, the people of any nation from other nations, or in forcing one's own belief on others, that represents Jesus, for that is contrary to everything he taught, was, and is.

He would not be in favor of, nor would it be acceptable to him, to allow those policies to take effect that drain the economy, or seek entitlements. or restrictions, and regulations that break down a country's backbone, such as with the natural resources, agriculture, or industry, in attacking the very fiber and integrity of the country.

Consider the following scriptural passages:

James 4:1-12

> What causes quarrel and what causes fights among you? Is it not this, that your passions are at war within you? You desire and do not have, so you murder. You covet and cannot obtain, so you fight and quarrel. You do not have because you do not ask. You ask and do not receive, because you ask wrongly, to spend it on your passions.

2 Thessalonians 3:10

> For even when we were with you, we would give you this command: If anyone is not willing to work, let him not eat.

1 Timothy 5:8 (Especially for husbands)

> But if anyone does not provide for his family, and especially for members of his household, he has denied the faith and is worse than an unbeliever.

Galatians 5:19-21

For each will have to bear their own load.

Politicians who are supposed to work for the people but often begin to use the people to attain their own 'objectives and goals.' They seem to lose track of why they were elected and why they are in office. They are there to find solutions and the means to make things better, and should be held accountable for their promises. The overemphasis on who's right and who's wrong, while exploiting the weaknesses and faults of each other, coupled with the constant attacks and debates, which paralyze any effort for compromise because of political party issues, proves only that they are not interested in bettering humankind. and are weak in their childishness. Jesus' way does not stifle reaching common ground as a foundation to a greater humanitarian goal.

It's sad that the only common cause to bringing people together, regardless of any prior prejudice, is catastrophe.

When Jesus spoke of building a house on a poor foundation, it is as though people lost the ability to see we all need each other. If all kept their talents and expertise to themselves we would cease to exist; yet, this is what is happening as there is always someone pointing out who should be getting more, who not to deal with, since too many times it involves the loss of power, or money, due to padded pockets, etc.

Not everyone is going to like everyone; but everyone should be trying to find help in efforts to balance the needs, desires, and goals of the children created by a loving God who loves all the children equally.

There is a picture painted where many people were seated at a banquet table. Everyone there had very long arms, and too long for the fork they were given to obtain food in their mouths. It was called "HELL," because though there was bountiful food of all kinds, no one could eat. Next to it there was an almost identical picture, except in this picture, the people were shown using their long arms to feed a person further away. This picture was titled, "HEAVEN."

Eeshans teach that one, or, another, often forgets that there is a common component binding that exists in real time. This component is that we are all human, and are all God's children, and we are all responsible to do what's best for all of humanity, and not just for ourselves. Unless we use a knockout component, which is "Metta or love," we will continue to reside in the picture labeled "HELL." To find the best means to help others, and, in turn, each other, we MUST begin by breaking the bonds of hate, dissention, and radicalism. We must learn we have to stop taking, and start giving back, too. Everyone is obliged, and should be inclined to do their fair share.

Entitlement should only refer to freedom of human rights. and not to money for doing nothing. It should not be used for illicit and recreational drugs, or anything that weakens the source of the funding, which can be put to better use, such as for prescriptions and for medications to treat illnesses, and towards the lowering of pharmaceutical prices for those who cannot afford them. as we; as towards the continuing research for heart disease, lung, and pancreatic cancers, and diabetes, to name just a few. The first picture titled "HELL" is the refusal to help individuals who could become helpers and contributors to a society, which, in turn, may help those who "actually need care and guidance." If we accomplish random acts of kindness and move forward towards loving all people, as God loves, we will virtually become the human picture of "HEAVEN." Any country that works towards this goal will be blessed and will flourish, and peace will reign.

One the other hand, for anyone to take financial assistance when one is capable of work, or bettering themselves, is to steal from God. To use what could've been given to one who really needs the help is a grievous sin. To feel that you are 'due this' does not bring us together as a family, but, instead, divides us as we are making it more difficult for those who have little and must share what *they* have to support you. It is a known fact, that one who will witness this are those who have little that and who are the first to run to your assistance. These give out of their need not out of their excess. These are teachings of Christ. These are the building blocks to our salvation, along with the Sacred Eucharist, which is the leaven from which we love and what unites us as a family before God.

Young able-bodied people should desire to work to their fullest potential. They should be drawn to help the needy and elderly by doing things for them, not taking advantage of them, especially in family situations; and doing so without being asked to help, since we know when they can no longer do for themselves.

Profit is good. God does not frown on the rich; God blesses them with riches that they may help others by contributions, donation, providing affordable housing, better water, food, protection, and friendship. God did not intend for the rich to replace employment for those who they have continuously helped and see no improvement. For those to rely on any individual for money just because said person has money is wrong. God warns those who take advantage of other's kindness and generosity for these who were helped, and don't see the generosity given, but see only what they weren't given deny God's generosity. These people expect more for doing less to nothing; and are usually envious of the giver and are never appreciative or satisfied. Rather than thanking God, and the person for their help, they turn on one who stops giving. People of this sort will never be grateful for the help that they received, but, rather, feel they are actually entitled to more, because God didn't give it to them first, and rightfully should have. People like this may not at all deserve what they crave, yet they will find a way to get it anyway, and justify whatever means will secure the ends ... whether illegally or legally, morally or immorally. They will stop at nothing to destroy the person who stops giving, once they are sure they have no further recourse to them. A truly bad and calculating person wants what they want, as opposed to an "ignorant" person who behaves obnoxiously, and causes damage without being aware that their actions are harmful. If they don't get what they want, they will strike the heart chords of whoever is their target, threatening suicide, if necessary, to ensure a reaction. When their threats don't work, they resort to anger and character assassination of the one who previously may have helped them, by using lies and threats, and turning the tables to make that person look like a monster ..., i.e., that the person being attacked has the financial means to support and cover all the debts but won't. Bad people are in the situations they find themselves in not because of 'anyone else's' fault, or because of their 'bad luck.' They are there because of the succession of their own choices. They refuse to see that it's no one else's fault but their own.

God did not give us all the same gifts. If we were all rich there would be no need to help others, and, therefore we would not possibly know love. If we were all poor there would be no means to better ourselves and our neighbors, as well as all of mankind. If we all were ill, we would not appreciate health, etc. However, to allow anyone to take advantage of, and to use people in any of these situations, breeds the worst actions in humans, to include drug and child trafficking, and this enables any other number of illegal activities to continue to flourish. By allowing, or not stopping crime, domestic violence, or any horrible action for personal gain is a grievous sin. To protest or ignore immigration laws set up to protect the security of citizens, and to protect their health by preventing the onset of disease, in the name of 'freedom' or 'compassion,' without any regard to the populace of one's own country, is wrong. Today, especially with child trafficking, to enter any country illegally allows for no possible way for one to find their child, or even an adult for that matter, as there is no record of them entering the country.

To feel that you are not directly hurting anyone with wrongful, uninformed decisions, or opinions that generate hate, or violence, or by just burying your head in the sand regarding the human family and the environment, thinking that it's not your problem, is inhumane, and, certainly, not of God.

Misuse of something as simple as food stamps, or any other government assistance, and/or not preventing others from using them for alcohol, cigarettes, beer, drugs, etc., is taking food away from an elderly person, or begrudging someone who actually needs help. This is looked upon by God as starving the hungry. Letting someone "you know" walk with difficulties, while riding in a warm car, or not walking an elderly person to safety, well, you get the point. These were the very things Jesus was talking about when he taught the corporal works of mercy, which simply were:

1. feed the hungry (not supply food stamps or government programs allowing assistance for alcohol, cigarettes, and recreational drugs),
2. give water to the thirsty (enforce laws supporting better drinking water),
3. clothe the naked (not with designer clothing),

4. shelter the homeless (not without providing them with a means to work and help contribute to society by getting training for jobs),
5. visit the sick,
6. visit the imprisoned,
7. bury the dead.

We are obliged as human beings to:

1. share knowledge,
2. give advice to and challenge those who need it,
3. comfort the suffering,
4. be patient with others (not to be confused with *enabling*),
5. forgive those who hurt you (you don't have to like them, but you shouldn't wish harm on anyone),
6. give correction to those who need it (even if not solicited or appreciated) for their own good,
7. pray for the living and the dead (and for oneself).

To end corruption, discrimination, and prejudice we must unlearn past mistakes, and relearn what family is, and not how it is defined by family members. Under God, we are the children of one family. We must learn to think of all people as our family. and not as a race or creed, religion, or political party, but a FAMILY, under God, a God who is Truth, and not a fool.

If we don't have people representing all of us in government, we must do our best to get representation, or at least back up our leaders by applauding their good work, and helping resolve impending issues, and to move forward without pointing fingers and remaining stagnant. We, the people, know the issues, now it's time to fix them, and not fixate on them. When one is cheated, we are all cheated. When one is healed, we are all healed.

We must be the eyes for those who are blind, the ears for the deaf, the hands and feet for those who need these, and the heart of the world, but not the enablers of false entitlements, being tolerant of wrongdoers, or the receivers of kickbacks, whether it be related to subcontracting, government agencies, or numerous other sectors, with the intent to influence or gain.

When one hurts, we all hurt. We need decency restored. We need to understand that all the Millennials have to work with, is a bill of goods, which becomes the basis for their emotions. This is what confuses them in their attempts to move forward. As they want to correct injustices, and live without fear, and with support for bringing decency, kindness, and love of neighbor, baby boomers often fight those things, ideals, and efforts to rid our world of stagnant opinions and fear.

That is why young people are so easily led astray. Those who have experienced violence feel that violence is the answer, and that makes those who are deemed vulnerable, strong and respected. The mindset which says, "If its violence you want, it's violence you'll get" solves nothing (what Jesus meant when He said, "To live by the sword is to die by the sword.") This is why thinking that an 'eye for an eye,' is the only method one has to get others to listen to them has become a tool used not just by those who want revenge, but by those who have no one to represent, or worse, no one to guide them. Getting laws through Congress, for example, seems to take forever. A person's life is short. When crimes arise, people no longer believe in the 'system,' since by the time the 'system' gets anything done, someone else dies. For those who have lost loved ones, the only thing that eases the pain is to find and punish the guilty person. To them, time is of the essence, since their pain is too great.

Though this seems to make no sense there is definitely a prejudice toward age. Waiting for some good to happen after a catastrophic event, with the way laws are brought into effect, leaves little hope that grandparents, or elderly relatives, will ever see justice. So, when there is someone who listens, that person becomes their hero. Sadly, all age groups are vital to the existence and continuation of all our human rights. The experience and life of an elderly veteran, doctor, fire fighter, mechanic etc., measure the technological advancements but the pride and experience of life they offer surpasses those advancements. From them we learn the mistakes, and consequences, that help us to do better. We learn the whys of their methods based on the circumstances that surrounded them at the time.

Yes, everyone can, and should, be heard in an effort to make this a better world; but no one group has the right to force their own agenda on another.

Eeshans believe that the Divine Feminine is behind evoking change and a return to balance.

> When Jesus spoke, He said he did not come to bring peace, (Matthew 10:34) but as word! (but before you confuse this statement read on.) "Then he called his apostles—male and female—and said He gave these the power against unclean spirits—to cast them out, and to heal all manner of sickness and disease. He bid them to go to the lost sheep. To go teach those who would listen. To go and heal the sick, cast out devils, and freely give what He gave to them. He told them to be wise as serpents and harmless as doves. He instructed them to beware of the councils, for they will scourge them in their synagogues (and today in their churches and places of power). For if they criticized and accused Jesus the same will be done to those who try to do as Jesus did."

LESSON 117

SPIRITUAL TEACHING FIVE: GOD

How many times have you heard, or may even have asked yourself, "Who is this God"? Standard answer is, "God made us." 'He' made us to know, love, and serve 'Him'. As we already covered, the who, and the what, we know God to be, it is important to know that it is in the unpacking of our beliefs that one discovers *more than what most were told to believe*. Since it is in what we are told that we should find contentment and peace, and most assuredly satisfaction, deep within our soul.

Yes, God is the Creator, an infinite, all-knowing, all-present, Sacredly Balanced Deity. Eeshans believe that without a doubt, without an infinite Creator, there would be no laws of physics, and in fact, without a Supreme Being, life as we know it would not exist. With that said, Eeshans also believe that as there is no suitable scientific explanation to the origin of all things. this is proof enough of as to a 'who' and a 'what' to God; since there is no way that anything can come into being without a source, origin, or cause of each, or for any of these coming into being by itself. There are three topics we would like to bring into your Consciousness.

If one accepts, for whatever the reason, that there is a God, it is usually followed by a slew of objections, as faith is not a 'fact' that is acceptable to everyone, nor can it be explained. That is why, in a transcendental writing, you find boundless ways to talk about God, for you are not limited to logic and fact, and, in addition, you are guided by love.

Since as long as there have been discussions on God, there have always been those who feel that God's existence will be proven through, and by, mathematical arguments and equations because for them everything revolves around math, and math is 'provable.' To prove there is a

God, is by far, a task, which most intellectuals feel will define the origin of the human race and natural laws. If there is a God, it would mean that the human race is not superior in itself, and that we are actually accountable for all actions and decisions in this material world, and that death is not the way out of the question. Yet, something like love does not reduce to mathematics, since love is not logical, and therefore, cannot be explained using logic. So, Eeshans, holding that God is love, show, plainly, that God, who is the author of love, also cannot be explained, proven, or disproven, using the human science of mathematics and logic.

We are trained and groomed to be what we are told we can be, so long as we do so by human governing laws and philosophies, but the moment we include a divine factor, or right, our thinking becomes 'irrational' to those who would rather not feel accountable or judged.

We believe that all we witness must be balanced to work. If humans are the superior beings, then there must be a lesser balanced nature that is created by humans that is its counterpart. If humans are the creation, then there must be a nature that is superior to humans, making that nature divine, and, thus, the creator of humans. Since there are two genders then the Superior Being must be perfectly balanced, and, thereby, must be wholly masculine and feminine, not masculine with feminine attributes. Then what are they saying? If this Superior Being is just masculine, without an equal counterpart with just feminine attributes, then all else in nature is imbalanced from its origin, and source, since everything in creation is wholly balanced, such as masculine/feminine, positive/negative, etc.

If we claim God is genderless, this would definitely negate balance, and the laws of the universe. That is why factoring Jesus and His wife into this equation is important. Since Adam and Eve, the human and Divine Masculine and Feminine, after the fall, must quantify a reverse image, just as before the fall. Therefore, God is Redeemer/Savior, too.

According to the Old Testament, God was not supposed to have a human gender, but the personal pronouns used are always in the male gender; however, even here one can find rare occurrences of female imagery with regards to God, which exhibits there was more than just a masculine attribute to God. Primarily, though, the scriptures as we have read countless times cannot help but convey a clearly reimaged masculine God.

Thirdly, in the Psalms, and other Old Testament books and writings, one finds such nomenclature as "husband" and "wife." We are told, however, that the reason for the more prominent masculine pronouns stems from the all-inclusive etymological noun, "man," meaning human being, which encompasses both genders. Surprisingly, the Third Person of God is called Emmanuel, as the Divine Masculine of the Spirit of God became Man. The Divine Feminine takes on her form in many ways.

It seems however, that the above text, which at its onset may look like a well thought out plan bordering on sexism, is that which can be loosely used for whatever a future need may be with regards to women's rights. Articulation of the term 'mankind,' which was supposed to represent 'all humans,' has become a bone of contention with women over the years, for obvious reasons, one being that it has not been played out with regards to equality of sexes, or genders, in any capacity. More acceptable nouns, such as human, human being, humankind etc., are now being used to replace what was supposed to be representing inclusivity in the past; and now these words are considered necessary to reflect that inclusivity these days. Petty? Well, not really, but it is just more equal.

We believe that this pervasive use of the masculine noun, or masculine pronouns, with regard to God's gender quality found its beginnings, and, was ultimately linked to the traditional story of Adam and Eve. Words are often be manipulated, by using whatever definition suits the intention; but when the definition fails to accomplish a positive end to a God given right, it is most likely that there's human error involved.

Beginning with this thought, we find in one particular version of the story in the bible (called traditional) that God created man first, and female second. Woman would then be the afterthought. To further this assumption, we read that she was created, or formed, from the rib of Adam, and, more or less, owed her existence to the male/man in a very submissive way, attesting that man was the first dominant gender made in God's image and likeness.

We have been taught that Eve was put here to delight, accompany, and serve as a helper to Adam. It would appear then that God, being the perfect androgynous being, is not only imbalanced and imperfect himself, but the cause who secured discrimination and not gender equality.

Eeshans see God as a perfectly bigender being: holy, almighty, immortal, transcendental, and totally and Sacredly Balanced.

God is a Oneness, merging of selves: male and female, triumphing over deceptive duality, eternal and infinite. God comprises three complete and Sacredly Balanced Persons all equal to, and as, One Being. God's perfection triumphs over mind and ego, and the accord between sameness and diversity, particularly duality. God needs nothing else but itself to produce a royal Child. God possesses two gender identities, either simultaneously, or varying between the two. God has the ability to present dysphoria, where each gender may reflect traits from two distinct sexes: female grace, male force, and the two sexes' other distinct qualities.[155] This would be explained since the male traits of God would become apparent in the body of Christ's wife in these present times, further accenting the meaning of the 'woman encompassing the man.'

Eeshans feel that this prophecy was obviously kept from humankind as far back and further in history than the uses for the word 'mankind. 'How far back? For reasons upon which the Eeshan religion came back into our awareness, we reach back to a very familiar story to search for answers, and ask, "Could 'man' have altered the original story of Adam and Eve to suit his own designs, standards and goals, not God's?"

---

[155] Some expression adapted from symbolisms.net

LESSON 118

SPIRITUAL TEACHING SIX: ETERNAL CONSORTS AND THEIR LOVE FOR EACH OTHER; CREATION OF PARADISE AND THE FIRST HUMAN

As God is three Persons, undivided unity, each person is also two in one, begetting the Fruit of their love, which is, ultimately, the achievement of the Philosopher's Stone.

Being all-loving, and desiring to have a witness to perfect love, God the first person of the holy trinity, with his eternal female consort, both being formless, and through a transcendental process, begets the extension of their love unlimited. Next, we have the second person of the holy trinity, the philosopher's stone, mirroring the first person and equal in every way, who is transcendental, and, by will becomes the transubstantiated gender, also. The identification of this being, who is the Only Begotten Child of God, is also, perfectly, and Sacredly Balanced. This beautiful infinite being was truly the desired fruit of God the First Person's oneness, who being God, by prophecy. in end times, shared in the fatherhood and motherhood of God (the first Persons also).

Being captivated by such joy, and the love they shared through their oneness, the Second Person as Divine/Human Father and Divine/Human Mother's love and desire brings about the Fruit of their love, another being, a divine/human being. This being would share in the oneness of the love of the Soulmates/Twin Flames, since they, too, would experience this same joy and love of the fruit of their love, just as God, the first person, experienced their oneness and love by their begotten Child.

God's desire would bring about the manifestation of the first Divine Family in the 'creation' of the first human being.

First, however, with the creation of the beautiful beings who would become Adam and Eve, God had created a heaven, one in which such a divinity, as God lived in, but this place would be called 'Paradise,' since it could not be heaven, but a mirror image of heaven, since unlike heaven, it did not already exist, it would have to be, indeed, created. This Paradise would, however, be connected by a kind of bridge to Heaven.

The infinite Creator took from nothingness,[156] and began creating the laws of physics. In the big bang theory, we find a definitive truth, and strong indication of the existence of a Supreme Being. One extraordinary fact is that with the creation of this Paradise, there is what is called "the virtual particle," which is both creation and annihilation, for God, as omnipotent, can, indeed, do all things.

Paradise can be described as a cosmological place,[157] meaning a place within the cosmos or universes of timeless harmony, which and was perfectly designed to reflect all the beauty and love God has to offer. Though there are still some who believe it was simply a story designed to show the progress from innocence to the now present time of knowledge, which was responsible for the learning of sin, and the cause of suffering and misery today, Eeshans don't agree with this notion. Because humans draw from a material world, with no real sense of the transcendental, they often believe in their limited capacity that because they can't prove something with their senses, it doesn't exist.

Eeshans can, and do, understand those who present, with a mythological mindset, the case for whether or not there is or was a place called paradise, where the events that took place warranted the acceptance of the consequences of sin[158] by the choice that was made by Adam and Eve.

---

[156] Term chosen from a western scientific basis, but which is not intended to exclude other cosmologies. – Ed.

[157] A place that came into existence by God's design found within the studies of the origin, structure, or dynamics of the Universe. – Ed.

[158] As in the sense of entering into compounding illusion, leading to grave consequences. – Ed.

Much of what was known about this Paradise came from Sumerian texts, or the mythology of the ancient Middle Eastern and Far Eastern writings. In some descriptions, it is said to have every tree rich with fruit, all kinds of animals, five beautiful rivers, and flowing streams. This mystical place, as you will find in our writings, is where God and the first human(s) lived in harmony.

Paradise was a sum of all mysticism. Its four rivers, often whose names vary, watered the Garden and seems to have the curiosity of all humans today. Just as Paradise reflects a possibility of a greater place than earth itself, explorers have gone in search of it, using the existing rivers today to identify, in this world, where Eden is purported to have been. The Pishon river circled Havilah; the Gihown, the Hidiqel and the Prat.

Eeshans feel that more important than 'where' this Paradise was said to have been located, is the *meaning* of what happened there.

LESSON 119

SPIRITUAL TEACHING SEVEN: THE FIRST TRANSCENDENTAL HUMAN

Within paradise, there was an extended garden on a level higher than where the first human would commune personally with God, and spiritually break bread with God. To eat of the "manna" provided by God filled the being with the light necessary for eternal life.

This being, who would be the extension of God's love and life through, with, and in a transcendental state, would exercise dominion over all that God created. It was a beautiful being, and as it was formed in God's image and likeness by God's own hands, it reflected all the beauty of God, and all the love and oneness shared between the male and female. It would enjoy all the goodness from God's imagination.

The first bigender/androgynous being, with male and female gender traits, that reflects of all qualities/natures of God, was created. As God's nature is ever-creating and expanding, God desired that the being would uniquely embody the same traits which would also be capable of receiving what God wanted to share, such as a vessel which wanted to receive all that it was offered.

Eeshans believe that the Creator decided that this being would be a spirit of a cosmic, vibratory nature, who cloaks with a portion its own unmanifested consciousness, and with the illusion of differences or particulars.[159]

The Spirit began with the empathic forms, first with positive and negative elements, meaning male and female, and, thus, mirrored God's self.

---

[159] Adapted from The Second Coming of Christ by Paramahamasa Yogananda, Discourse 62.

Next, God used the law of duality and relativity to differentiate the one consciousness and cosmic energy, which embodies the law of Divine Oneness, the law of vibration, the law of action, and the law of correspondence, as applied to blessing and abundances, the law of cause and effect, the law of attraction, the law of perpetual transmutation of energy, relativity, polarity, and rhythm, thus, giving this being everything to make it perfect in every way, so that it may glorify God. This made it necessary for the being to be embodied with the universal laws only on a cosmic level.

God then covered the soul and light body with a Subtle Body, and next with a kind of vegetative skin, which stayed harmoniously intact with those foods that broke down into light. This enabled the being to have form, but not be limited, or bound like the laws of a physical universe, *for theirs was not a physical universe.* This body contained within itself three divine potentials: reason, or discriminative will, the feeling that which one is conscious of and able to delight in enjoyment, and, lastly, as Paramahamsa Yogananda describes, (the) energy, the substance that creates and activates the body.

We understand a soul to be the spark of the consciousness of God, and it is at the foundation of our conscience since the 'fall' of Adam and Eve. It is individualized and capable of expressing God's image. It is also immortal, meaning it will never die, unless it *'chooses' mortality*. To choose mortality would be to enter into a mortal *sin* state where one is totally separated from God, and chooses to ignore God's directives for everlasting life, and thus finding itself in 'eternal death.'

Despite the fact that this being possessed everything, *it was still imperfect, since it was created and had a beginning, so it was not infinitely in existence.* God decided to separate the 'imperfect' being, since this would further show the unique ability for the one to become two to reflect the male and female genders of God, and, thus, relate each to that gender relative to itself, thus magnifying even more God's duality, as soulmates in itself. It would also prefigure the future of the creature in times to come; however, the two would experience the companionship *the infinite* enjoyed.

One must remember that another reason the perfected being could appear 'imperfect' was that it did not exist of its own, but rather *'resembled' and 'reflected'* God in all things to include a perfect life, even so far as begetting children as extensions of its life.

Now we are getting into beliefs that are most sacred to Eeshans.

LESSON 120

SACRED WRITINGS OF EESHAN TRANSCENDENTALISM: WHAT ARE THE SACRED WRITINGS

The term 'Sacred Writings' are those most sacred scriptures, hymns, and any collection of texts written, and regarded, as the absolute authority for Eeshan religious knowledge. It is upon these stories and writings that the Eeshan path is founded and based upon.

PART I

MANIFESTING GOD'S DUALITY

LESSON 121

Section I: A Summary of the Creation of Adam and Eve the First Human Marriage True Love

To better manifest God's duality and love between the Divine Masculine and Divine Feminine, God decided to it was time for the most perfect creation ever. It was time to separate this beautiful being into two in order to love, honor, and cherish one another.

Using vibration (that's what the word 'rib' means) the being was then separated, just as it was formed, in order to create a relational complementarity, and reciprocation, as with all things in the physical universe that surrounded it. Replacing the altered text with true text we present the combined scriptural verse with added Eeshan texts.

> "God created mankind [humankind] in his [their] own image, in the image of God He [they] created "them;" male and female He [God] created them."
> —Genesis 1:27

Eeshans believe that Paramahamsa Yogananda was almost correct in saying (paraphrasing) that due to the attraction of the divine soul within, when separated they became husband and wife, and even though they were transcendental they were in an extraordinary way, as one, in 'one flesh.' They acted in harmony, and in unison, in body, mind, and soul; even though they each had a body (as we described in the section above, not to be confused with a gross physical body), a mind, and a soul; they lived as with one ideal. What he didn't say was that this was perfection in the sense that they reflected God as perfectly as transcendental beings may, despite the fact they were created beings, with a beginning but subject to a spiritual nourishment necessary for eternal life, without which they would die.

God smiled, and blessed the two as one, and told them to go forth and love each other as one never separated, since one who depends upon the other for strength, especially for balance, as each is sacred and balanced in the other. God told them to bring "the fruits of their love as extensions of themselves," as they were extensions of their Creator. This was to evince thanksgiving, and that they would all be blessed by the one who gave them life. God provided them with the food for immortality: so that they would be nourished and remain in the light. This was the first 'marriage' called into being, and mirrored God's perfect and sacred image and likeness, while sharing by being, with and in God.

These beautiful transcendental humans now had the capacity to use reason and free will independently and together as one being. Most importantly, they could "love." Love was the greatest treasure and power of all they possessed. Since it is love which bound their hearts together in perfect harmony. Love is patient; love is kind. It does not envy, it does not boast in the sense of hurting another. Love is not hurtful, but is empathic. Love protects life and innocence. Love is the most powerful weapon against evil and evil doers. Love is sympathetic, but not naive. Love shows balanced judgment. Love is guileless, candid, and honest. What is the point? The point is that as transcendental beings, or human beings, we are created by God; and God is love. This is key to understanding the misleading and deceptive stories of a punishing God we came to fear according to Christian denominations, the very God Jesus told us to call Father. (Eeshans believe He taught us God is our Father and Mother, as he introduced the Virgin Mary as his Mother, connoting a marriage between his father and Mother.)

Perfect unconditional sharing of love, which comes from the heart consciousness shared between transcendental human beings, would bring to the heart an overwhelming, irresistible and feeling of gladness, witnessing to the same perfect exchange of love that God enjoyed with their eternal oneness and love of their consorts.

The separation of the genders called for a safeguard, or directive, which would result in initiating an immortal love between the two, which was not necessary with the singular being. As two, they reflected the wholly sacred balance and love of God, the Divine Being, but because they were 'created' they could only 'mirror' the divine completeness of God in their shared oneness; whereas, the divine consorts were 'eternally united,' without beginning or end. This means that as long as they did as God directed they would enjoy what the divine consorts enjoyed. God planned that the oneness of this being when it was separated into two transcendental beings would come about only through the sharing and experiencing of giving and receiving the love from each other through, with, and in God. Being they were the extensions of God's love they couldn't find total oneness as God intended without involving *the God particle as the catalyst.*

LESSON 122

SECTION II: THE KEY TO ETERNAL LIFE AND ETERNAL LOVE

This catalyst came in the form of a Sacred Bread and Drink, which provided nourishment for their immortality and God's presence for their perseverance and love. God imparts everything to the human heart. It is in the heart that God is said to reside and anyone desiring love needs only to go there.

Especially after the fall from grace, this Sacred Food and Drink would become what was/is necessary for salvation. Since this is the part of God, when consumed by a human being in union with the soul, and when that human being in union with the soul nourishes it with light so that it does not darken. This nourishment can only be God and come from God.

That nourishment necessary for eternal life came in the form of a Sacred Bread, which was 'light' as air and a Drink made from the pure "blood" of the grape. Why wine?

> How God has blessed us! He will tether His donkey to a vine, His colt to the choicest branch; He will wash his garments in wine, and His robes in the blood of grapes. (Genesis 49:11) The greatest blessing is to drink the pure blood of the grape, which will become a symbol of the perfect shed blood of Jesus Christ, Messiah. (Deuteronomy 32:9-10)

It was most important that our First Parents would always partake of it.

Each day they would share this "Light," or transcendental Sacred Bread and Blood Drink, and their hearts would be steadfast in their love of God and each other. It is this Bread and Drink that is of the upmost importance. Let us pause here, that we may explain, outside of time, the reasons we claim this. Jumping ahead:

The whole purpose of Jesus and his wife's coming was to restore what was lost by our first parent's choice AND yet raise their human physical life to the highest level of life imaginable by an unconditional, sacrificial love, bringing the Divine to Humans and Humans to the Divine, as it was in the beginning, is now and ever will be. Since this to take place it was necessary to reverse the adverse effects of original sin; yet, we were given a conjecture based on only part of Christ's mission. Eeshans hold that the consequences of the ingested forbidden fruit (the apple), would be obliterated with the consumption of the Fruit of the Marriage Feast of Jesus and Mary's love and sacrifice. Why not an apple for an apple? Jesus Christ is the Apple tree.

For over 2000 years we were taught that the Holy Eucharist is Jesus Christ body, blood, soul, and divinity, and the Fruit of his passion, death, and resurrection was what was necessary for salvation. Though this is true, from the Eeshan perspective it is not complete because it doesn't have all the necessary components making up the total Eucharist as God intended it to be. This in itself makes it incomplete and insufficient for what is necessary for salvation according to all of Jesus' teachings and directives. Regarding these, one must understand the connection between Adam and Eve, and the sacred light Food and Drink which they consumed before their fall to physicality, and how it differed from the sacredness of Christ's marriage and the bread and wine they consumed once they became totally human. Afterwards, you see, it was nourishment only for the body.

That is why the Wedding Feast of Cana was so important. It was the true initiating of the Eucharist, which had been wrongly attributed to the Last Supper (continuing up to and including the Crucifixion).

This mystery of the Holy Eucharist would begin with the basic alchemy of Jesus turning the water into wine during their Marriage Feast, which would effectuate the ultimate transubstantiation of the human Jesus and Mary Magdalen, which would then fully embrace their Divinity once again on their wedding night, whereas, upon through their non-bloody union, they will transubstantiate from their human forms back to the Divine, in order to consummate their marriage. Though they would show no apparent change in their beings, this oneness was the key component for introducing the 'Way' back to God, which would come later when both endured the most horrible sacrifice for humanity.

For even though they both were fully Divine at this point, it was their fully human sacrifice that they shared that was necessary to bring back into existence the Sacred Bread and Drink necessary for life everlasting, which was lost. These Sacred vows exchanged on their Wedding night became the timeless alchemy, which provided the salvific sustenance to regular bread and wine at the Supper, as received by our first parents before their choice for physical love over a transcendental love, through, with, and in God; whereas, the food for the body, transubstantiated into food for the light body. Before this could happen, however, the purely human sacrificial act was necessary to satisfy that consequence which caused mortality.

It was here after the Supper that, knowing the hearts of men, the Kallahs were given a directive by Jesus along with Mary, to hide these sanctified gifts, foreshadowing the rejection of the divine feminine, which was, sadly, at hand.

To *intimately and thoroughly* understand the Eucharist is complicated, but in a few words, it is God, Divine Masculine, and Divine Feminine., who nourishes our souls and gives us life everlasting. We know that the Eucharist was intended for us to consume and it causes us to be ushered immediately into God, and, God into us, simultaneously. When we consume this precious Spiritual Food, as intended for us by God, it contains within it all the 'Mysteries of the Marriage Feast of Cana,' to include the wholly mystical duality and love of God as soulmates, all intended for our salvation. That is why the emphasis on the foreshadowing of the rejection of Divine Feminine *is critical to mention here*.

The Eucharist, therefore, affects the energies of mind and emotion that we call thought and feeling ... Through this introduction of spiritual [Divine] Light, these energies not only become one, but also bring about a new energy pattern. This energy pattern resonates with, and increasingly conforms to, the Divine inner nature of each human being.[160] That is why today, though one is vouchsafed with the Divine Masculine in what the church calls the Eucharist, without the Divine Feminine, their Eucharist, as we have come to know it, is not in its complete form, and, thus, the new energy pattern that resonates lacks the conformity and balance that God intended.

In order to restore the Spiritual Food that was lost due to Adam and Eve's choice for physicality, it would take the Marriage of Co-Redeemers for the choice was made within their marriage and with mutual decision. That is why, **even with the Real Presence of the Divine Masculine of God in the world, and the reception by the faithful, the world has not been affected in the ways it should have been.**

Secondly, to teach about the Eucharist being instituted at the Last Supper by Christ, *as though it was the event which brought it into existence*, was detrimental to salvation as it presents no origin, or link, to the duality of God and the Sacred Balance, which would have had the greatest impact upon all of humanity, and its belief in God. God's love for us, true love/marriage, and the value of life as the fruit of the love between human beings, depend on this.

The teaching should have been that the Eucharist was once again 'returned,' and once again 'restored perfectly,' as it was complete, in that it included our humanity this time, thanks to the *Christs' plethora of love*, perfectly demonstrated in their timeless sacrificial marriage, passion, and death. This Eucharist, of course, required the perfect Sacrifice, the perfect Altar, and the perfect Victim, because it is Christ and His wife who are the Eternal consorts.

The second reason why Eeshans disagree with what is taught by the established church is that the church indicating that Adam was the first high priest. We disagree because before Adam and Eve chose the

---

[160] This insightful highlight is drawn from newlightbody.org.

physical, they were in union with God, therefore, they did not need a 'sacrificial' Bread and Drink in their transcendental life together. It was after their choice that the Salvific Eucharist that came from Jesus and Mary's Sacrifice would be necessary. Adam's toiling was not for a sacrificial bread or drink, nor was Eve's new reproductive system a curse. The bread and wine were merely the consequences of their decision, which was sustenance for their *bodies*. Remember, the sacrificial bread and wine was promised.

The first Divine/Human priest was, for all salvific purposes, Melchizedek, who was God the Eternal Divine Masculine and Father, King of righteousness and true High Priest. He had a tent open to travelers where he taught about God and then distributed water, bread and wine and carried the blessing which he gave to Abram. The Eternal priesthood began with him and would be that order from which Jesus' Priesthood would continue, and who would be his sacrifice of love. The First Divine Priesthood had fallen under Lucifer.

It would be he as the 'Divine Masculine' of God, the first Person of the Holy Trinity, who would prepare the way for his son Jesus' mission for all of humanity's salvation. Together with his wife, who is His Divine Feminine and eternal consort, He shares as the first Divine/Human Feminine Priestess, Mary the Virgin Mother of God, who brought the Divine Masculine male of the only begotten Child called Jesus, into the world, as her sacrifice of love. This would be the beginning of the plan of salvation for all created children of God.

Jesus would be the perfect Divine Masculine, being the second Person of the Holy Trinity Divine Masculine, perfectly human, who would, along with his eternal consort and Divine Feminine, replace the first created children known as Adam and Eve. 'After the fall,' being perfect male/female Divine and Human, Jesus and His wife were the perfect priests, since they represented, by their Divinity, the first Person (the Father/Mother) of the Blessed Trinity. As Divine/Humans, they represented Adam and Eve before the fall; and by their humanity, they alone could be the perfect human representation to offset the fall of Adam and Eve to the physical realm. They became the perfect victims, and by love gave the perfect sacrifice. The perfect altar of the Co-Redeemers was, indeed, their bodies, which suffered horrendous pain, and death, at the final moment of Christ's capitulation on the cross. All this to 'reverse and align our lives' with God once again.

In conjunction with this teaching, one would still have the choice to grasp the need and have the desire to be saved. Yes, it is indeed a choice of free will, but it's also a directive by Jesus in order for the salvation of one's soul to take place.

In hindsight, that is what Jesus knew by His command to all those who heard His Bread of Life discourse. There is no other way than this Sacred Bread and Drink if you believe in Jesus Christ. Because this Sacred Bread and Drink are truly the bodies of Jesus and His Wife, keeping the Blessed Sacrament on reserve reconnects Adam and Eve's daily encounter with God in the Garden. Being in God's Presence gives one a way to identify with the Christs as having a personal relationship. The importance of and the need to spend time with the Real Presence is to receive strength in confusing times, or when under tremendous temptation, or when one wants God's guidance in making a choice, or to just offer thanksgiving, since it was for all those who desired to be with him.

If gone according to plan, it would be deemed a necessary joy to not only spend time with God as it was for Adam and Eve, but to be in the Presence of God meant sharing and enjoying reciprocal love of each other through, with and in and for God, while knowing the ultimate union of their whole being with the whole being of God.

Remember, Adam and Eve were the created extensions of God's love in God's intimate consort marriage and as soulmates, so they could never find total oneness as God intended *without involving God as the catalyst for love.*

Spending less and less time in the Presence of God, and lacking the Sacred Food and Drink necessary for the nourishment of their souls and light bodies, began the weakening of their spirit, subsequently, leading to a choice apart for God. This is why as humans, God deemed it a 'directive' to eat and drink his Body and Blood, and spend time in the Real Presence, since the goal and consequences would be the same in our life here on earth.

This Sacred Bread, which provided nourishment for their immortality, of course was God in a transcendental light food (that is where

Jesus' words, "Give us this day our daily bread" came from), and, by faith in his words, being a consistent reminder and connection to his bread of life discourse and identifying one's acceptance of Christ's directives. Everything Jesus taught, and lived, had to link and conform to the plan of salvation.

God's daily presence moving about with them provided them with wisdom, understanding, counsel, knowledge, piety and the wonder (the true meaning of holy "fear") of God. It is through love, after the fall from grace, that God imparted everything to the human heart. It would be *upon its awakening that enlightenment would blossom.* That is why we say, "it is in the heart that God resides and anyone desiring love needs only to go there."

That is why, too, that after the fall from grace, by 'God's promise,' these truths, 'by Christ's directive,' were sure to occur, especially as His wife attempted to continue His work, after his ascension. If these truths were taught, all who believed in Jesus, be it Catholic, Christian, or any other, when upon hearing this command, would absolutely deem them automatically essential and unavoidable for salvation. One would have known from the moment they learned of this directive, that without a doubt to not "eat, or drink, of the 'Christs' body, blood, soul and divinity," everlasting death would be inevitable.

This is why Jesus' Bread of Life discourse was not an option but a commandment, since soon the sacrifice necessary for 'everlasting life' AND the means by which one would partake of this Sacred Bread and Drink would come to pass. That is why he would not/could not compromise with those who walked away from Him. Jesus taught this unfathomable mystery as the God/Man, or the liaison, the link between God and humanity as the Divine Masculine Savior/Redeemer. That, too, is how Jesus could teach and love, and never discriminate, or be prejudiced, as the Plan of Salvation does not discriminate, since all are God's children. Salvation is, indeed, meant for all, but free will is the deciding factor in whether one believes, and accepts, or denies, and walks away.

You must understand that the Holy Eucharist, being God, when consumed by a human being in union with the soul, is nourished with light, so that it does not darken; however, if the Eucharist is deliberately changed in any way the result is devastating. By change we mean if *all* the components of the Marriage Feast are not present, or if any of the following conditions are found to apply:

- Presenting Jesus as being alone in the Eucharist in a dimidiated way, so that only half is visible, meaning that one of the Redeemers is not included,
- Jesus' wife is not believed to be subsumed, as in supramentalization, and Ishvara, or water into wine,
- Saying the Sacred words without Ordination by, in, and through those who alone are the rightful, legitimate, and sole authorities.

Thus, once the truth is revealed and the means to correct the error is presented, and yet rejected, those in darkness and the sins against God and humanity would prevail.

The Eucharist provided by the Co-Redeemers would take the darkness out and put light into one's soul, mind and body, so long as sins and/or offenses against God and neighbor were not mortal, meaning that they did not cause death, or rob the soul of everlasting life.

What we know to be true is that the 'Eucharist' that Adam and Eve consumed before the fall was in its purest state; it was complete since it contained the duality of God, which reflected the love and Sacred Balance of the Divine Masculine and Divine Feminine. Eeshans believe that what has been called the Eucharist, since Peter, and by the church, at large *is not complete and carries with it a moral taint*. In addition, because of those who were responsible for continuing Peter's failure to follow Jesus' specific directives regarding the Bread of Life, all subsequent followers of Jesus were robbed of the fullness of what He (Jesus) commanded was essential for salvation. Thus, the whole ritual of the Mass became JUST a memorial, and not a ritual that connected a participant to the fullness of Jesus' sacrifice in that "time immemorial." And Eeshans believe that by not reflecting the duality of God, but, instead, filling the vacuum with truncated religious doctrines and beliefs, it thus appears that they defile Christ's intended plan with a minimalized 'replacement' doctrine that only partially nourishes the soul, instead of satisfying it. Because of the dimidiated Eucharist,[161] consequences are manifested everywhere in human life, but more specifically we see the evils of this deliberate, devolving spirit made known:

1. By priests living in mortal sin based on their negligence of duties,
2. In the many sex abuse and pedophilia scandals ignored, and allowed to permeate and pervade the priesthood and religious communities, and other ministers, etc., who claim to be of Christ and His work, as well as other religions who teach and feel that this outrageous act/belief is 'a special love' or is of God,
3. In the sinful, unconscionable abuse of women at home, in the church, workplace and in every profession,
4. In the many who Christ would consider neither hot nor cold, who do nothing by sitting back, and ignoring, or not reporting, and stopping such acts within the churches of God, the priesthood, politics, professions, workplace, and relationships, by not bringing the perpetrators to justice going to be as God says, "because you are lukewarm—neither hot nor cold—I will spit you out of my mouth" (Revelation 3:17),
5. When sitting back, saying, "I have everything I want, I don't need a thing!," but you don't realize you are wretched, pitiful, blind, miserable, and naked." (Revelation 3:17)

Without a doubt, these, and all those who played a part in not protecting the innocent, points to what just may have been found to be coercion at the highest level, in order to keep alive patriarchal leadership.

---

[161] When those under the spirit of the human consciousness devolved the fullness of the truth to a 'half-truth,' and then canvassed that half-truth as the whole truth, Christ's true mission regarding human salvation was neutralized (temporarily); but even when a dam is put across a powerfully flowing river, the waters will find a way around. – Ed.

By today's standards these could, and should be, defined on the order of infidels against Jesus' true teachings and directives. They are also guilty of:

1. Reimaging not only the three Persons of God, but
2. reimaging and betraying Jesus Christ who they declare the founder and head of their religion and
3. substituting and teaching man's law as though it was God's by declaring their religion and only their religion as having the 'truth,'
4. and covering up such, then using the people's money to pay for legal fees
5. and reacting with distain to women's place in any official status and worship.

LESSON 123

SECTION III: EUCHARISTIC BELIEFS

The church overtly teaches that at the last supper, Jesus took bread and wine and offered it to God saying the words of consecration, whereby "the signs of bread and wine become in a way, *surpassing all understanding*, the body and blood of Christ," with the appearances of bread and wine still remaining. They teach that afterwards He gave the directive for his apostles to do as he did.

Later on, through the years, based on the above beliefs, debates arose, and some did not believe in what was declared as transubstantiation but rather it was 'consubstantiation.' Transubstantiation, unlike consubstantiation, is where the Real Presence remains, and can be put on reserve. Consubstantiation means that the Real Presence of Christ is present *along with* the bread and wine, but Christ's presence does not remain after all have received. In Consubstantiation, there is no Blessed Sacrament on reserve.

In Eeshan Transcendentalism, we say that neither reflect the truth, in these ways:

First, neither reflects the duality of the Eucharist. Even as Jesus was the active Consort at the time and His wife was the passive consort, together they gave the words at the supper, and these words were vital, since they were part of their Marriage vows to each other, and necessary to offset and restore humanity's salvation. Both had to speak them in order, and this was the directive of Jesus.

These words were, and are so sacred and powerful, that they can only be spoken by the Co-Redeemers through those priestesses and priests who are in succession of the apostles present at the time. For only by their own organic voice can these words turn the gifts of human hands into the body, blood, soul, and divinity of Christ and His wife. These words of consecration are capable of transforming whoever held possession of them. (This is why Lucifer wanted them so badly, because of the power within them. They would give back whatever was lost and more; these words were hidden away so as not to get into the wrong hands because they are dangerous if used the wrong way, and, were, thus, forbidden to be spoken if found).

Long before Adam and Eve, these words were inscribed in an emerald, and secured and guarded, as they were destined to only be spoken by the Chosen One. Once Lucifer fell under the influence of corrupt power, he stole them. When exiled from heaven, as Lucifer fell the emerald was shaken loose and plummeted to earth. When the emerald hit upon the earth, it broke into two, and the one half revealed the Chosen One and the other the Words that would restore to humanity those things lost due to Adam and Eve's choice for a physical life. These two halves were hidden away until the ancient prophecy of the Chosen One was fulfilled. In turn, the timeless words would then be spoken to restore all that was lost and to light the 'way' back to God. This prophecy was fulfilled when the Co-redeemers left heaven and were married on this earth—becoming One.

After Jesus ascended, Mary Magdalen, and the other women continued teaching and healing those who followed, or came to them. Eeshans contend *Ishvara* (the presence of God) left immediately after the men under Peter tried to force God's children back to the way things were before Jesus, not allowing women to continue as equals and taking away their rights to officiate at worship services. As a consequence, to the men's blatant rejection of the Christs' new way and women's rights as ensconced by Jesus, the words of *transubstantiation were altered to reflect only a half truth about the Divine Masculine.*

The established church never had the actual alchemical words of transubstantiation, but rather continued to use those which in no way would acknowledge Christ's Wife. So important is her role that by Divine word, the identity of the Lamb's Wife in end times was given and witnessed by John in the Book of Revelation.

This is testimony as to why our foundress had been given the Eucharist publicly, and witnessed by countless people at Mass and at the Consecration.

The better part of all of this is that those men AND women who loved/love Jesus, and believe what they were told, received 'all' the benefits, though not the '*fullness*,' of what God wanted for them. In other words, they received the fullness of the Divine Masculine, and that is what we give thanks for to God.

The actual words of transubstantiation were hidden away by God; and would remain hidden until which time only the Chosen One who is 'One' and 'equal' to the Divine Masculine would, rightfully, possess the seared and alchemical words of transubstantiation in their entirety once again. That person would be the Wife of the Lamb, since there is no one who compares.

Now, with the return of the Divine Feminine, and through the (unrequited)[162] vows of the Eeshan Mystery of Ordination, which Jesus and Mary Magdalen speak through the Kallahs, can transpire, only through those priests who have undergone 'a Subsumation Ceremony' in which the priest is subsumed into the Sacred and Divine Consciousness of the Eeshan Priesthood, who is then identified as an Eeshan *Chatan* (Bridegroom) ordained, can they be allowed to carry within his person the bodies of Christ and Mary Magdalen. At consecration, the Kallah (or Chatan) gives way to Christ and His wife to speak the precious, sacred and mystical words through her/him, so the Co-Redeemers become once again the 'Bread and Drink come down from Heaven.'

Those 'invited' to the Marriage Feast of the Lamb and His Wife, by consumption, will receive back from God everything that was lost, and will gain access, once again, to their lost inheritance.

Eeshans believe that God allowed for the denial of the Marriage of Jesus and Mary Magdalen by man's choice because of human free will.

---

[162] The word 'unrequited' refers to all the vows in the hearts of women through the ages who were drawn to the voice of God in their hearts, to take their place at Jesus and Mary's side as the Kallahs did but were prevented from doing so because of the leadership structures the men had put in place to secure a point of view rooted in the human consciousness. – Ed.

Further, it would not be made known until all efforts to deny this truth were exhausted, the concept of the only begotten Child versus the identity of the only-begotten Son, would also not be rectified until these eschatological times, where it would be witnessed in the 'fullness of time.' That is when Jesus, together with His wife, will re-introduce to the world the true alchemical process which will ensure salvation for all who believe. The time for this is now.

PART II

TIMELESS LOVE

LESSON 124

SECTION I: LOVE: ORIGINATING FROM A TIMELESS GOD

God blessed the transcendental Adam and Eve to enjoy the love from their oneness. The two shared a perfect love that mirrored God's love, and they begot many children. This pleased God, since, it showed how by separating the being into male and female, this would become the outward sign of their own interpretation of divine love. It not only mirrored, but witnessed the desire for love, and lovemaking, of the male and female and God initiated this by placing a part of each gender in the other, initiating a flawless attraction for each other. Thus, the female had a male component and the male had a female component; and, thus, 'found themselves in each other.' Recognizing they were one that became two, and, then, one again, through, with, and in God's love, only solidified their being soulmates.

Looking ahead, God saw that as a result soulmates will always find each other, since this provides for the underpinnings of true love, since the true male soulmate will be united to his true feminine soul companion by virtue of this 'spiritual' union that perfects the expression of the complete spirit nature of each soul according to divine decree; and since they shall have the purest love that God placed within their hearts and souls.[163]

---

[163] Cf. Paramahamsa Yogananda, *The Second Coming of Christ*.

LESSON 125

SECTION II: BECOMING MAN AND WOMAN

As it happened, once the being was separated into two, they were filled with divine magnetism to reflect God's own wish, which was the supernatural demand to know reciprocal love according to God's specifically ordered divine plan so that they draw each other unto themselves. According to Eastern teachings,[164] 'They were to lead natural lives with uplifted spiritual consciousness free from the dangers of sex-motivated mis-mating, as necessity of separation for sex-motivated love is a physical act which may, or may not, involve love.' This point is of the utmost importance to remember.

So before as well as after the fall, be it transcendental or human, by God's design, when the one becomes two, and the separated beings who are equal to each other manifest as one, this witnesses is to the 'power' of love, within the mystery of marriage and the Sacrament thereof.

Once separated, yet still maintaining the transcendental state of life, the one with dominant male attributes was named Adam, meaning 'of the earth.' This means he was the masculine part of the first being 'created on earth,' in the Garden of Eden, and did not infinitely exist in heaven. He would be one of the two progenitors, which would beget children. He witnessed to the masculine attributes of the Divine Masculine of God. Now, we have a male gender, which would come to be called 'man.'

Once separated, his male attributes became more and more pronounced, but as we said, he actually carried a part of the female gender

---

[164] The following is drawn from Paramahamsa Yogananda's *Second Coming of Christ*. It is the closest to the beliefs of, and frequently parallels, the Eeshan perspective. Sections and phrases were borrowed by the author for this reason. – Ed.

within him. He used reason and cosmic energy. He had feeling, but God kept it uppermost and hidden, and, thus, we have the familiar version of man, but as an enlightened being who is not limited to a gross 'physical' body. He now demonstrates all the masculine attributes complete, with a total innocence with regards to good and evil. And why not? There was no desire to go against God, especially since he had all he needed and enjoyed it all, thoroughly.

Adam continued to become more identifiable with respect to gender identity, and gender expression, to include linear thinking, that is logic and reason. He was more inclined to demonstrate unflawed strength, rationality, loyalty, and healthy competitiveness, to name a few characteristics important to his gender identity.

That the separation of the original, being by vibration, which was, and is efficaciously duly noted, was the means by which the one, uniquely beautiful, androgynous being became 'two,' and the female would have to be the male's equal in every way, as his counterpart. It was not possible for her to be lesser or subservient; rather she was uniquely patterned for being Adam's counterpart and opposite. God so cleverly brought about the means for both genders to remain balanced, so that one would not become predominant, but that they would be complementary, by having both the male and female demonstrate, and use, the strengths of one another to offset, or supply, what the other needed.

The process used to separate the original being was called "rib," meaning 'vibration.'

That is why you will find that the use of tones and vibrations can have a positive or negative effect on us. You will find later on how scientists, and those in the medical fields, are finding that using tones and vibrations have been beneficial in working with the deaf, and with autistic children. Vibroacoustic therapy is a field exploring the use of tones and vibrations in both alternative and conventional medicine.

Scriptures do not mention the 'rib' as a process for separating the androgynous being, since they won't even acknowledge said 'being,' at all, for obvious reasons. The confusion to many was that (according to the original Adam and Eve Story), the only 'rib' they were told about was the one made of a kind of cartilage which gave form to the man, and it was written that it was removed from the man called Adam during the creation of woman, which was then permanently affixed to the female.

From a scientific point of view, the number of cartilage 'ribs,' all of which formed at the beginning of entropy, were equal in number when the physical bodies were being formed. If indeed, there was the so-called "rib from Adam" in the woman, which there was not, since it certainly did not indicate superiority on the part of the man, so then why would God choose this, if God did, to show superiority? Rather, we would have to say that God planned in the evolutionary process of 'human' beings that this particular 'bone' be used to establish, or witness, to an original connection of some kind; and, that since the couple no longer had a transcendental body, it would make more sense as to what would the purpose would be in a rib being drawn from the male side, like a puzzle piece that connected to another piece of the puzzle. Well, it would seem this is not a good foundation for us all being equal in the eyes God. This 'rib,' and the written text accompanying it, would be by today's standards, translated into "woman came from man," which would be a throwback to the mindset at the time of Jesus where women were not equal to men or even "worthy of life."

Today, the Eeshan religion would declare that one may interpret the above story and text in this way: Man, being linear-minded, would denote that if the 'rib' story was true, it would appear that men would indeed feel themselves superior, and made in God's image and likeness, and have the right to demonstrate all misconduct privately and publicly towards woman and children, especially female children. It would put credence behind those familiar words, "if it wasn't for me ... !"

Truth is, when the consequences of this 'foundational text' of the 'rib' via the Divine Feminine is fully realized, *those males* who consciously, and without remorse, lived and acted out of this superior god-complex in any way for any reason, will now stand out and be seen apart from decent men, as examples of a failing model of oppressive chauvinism, comprised of perfect and complete godlessness; they are outward examples of the unconscionable, lowly traits witnessed in themselves, and shared among those of the same mind.

We are often judged by those we associate with, whether close up, or far away, when we subscribe to any group, or when we sit back and watch with comfort, or in harmony with any individual or group displaying irrational, dysfunctional decision making, or actions toward a particular outcome, usually sexual favors, and minimizing the accountability of those individuals involved in such behaviors, and in some untoward way justifying these things without critical evaluation, and allowing it to continue, if we condone such practices, since we are equal to, if not worse than, they are.

Eeshans regard healthy relationships in the highest regard, with Marriage being the most sacred of all of God's mysteries. 'If' the androgynous being didn't exist, and there was a 'true rib' involved, it would have to prove that with the extra rib, a husband was only 'perfect and complete' in his wife, like a piece to a puzzle. Sacred Balance of God makes it necessary, and desires that this perfect and complete balance can only be attained when both male and female shared this mystical and mysterious connection via the 'extra' rib being a symbolic connection to when they fall in love.

Sadly, this rib- has been a 'bone of contention' from the start. Eve being tied to Adam this way safe-secures and safe-guards viewpoints that are not wholesome. It does not allow for the transcendental life that this beautiful separated androgynous being, who became Adam and Eve, enjoyed. It affirms that the male was first, and the woman's body was, in effect, his rightful possession, and, thus, depended on him.

We wholeheartedly stress the separation of the beautifully androgynous being blessed by God to become two individuals equal in every way, to counter what is written in the Bible regarding Adam, saying, "She is bone of my bones and flesh of my flesh and she will be called woman." Realistically and truthfully speaking, 'both' were of the same bones and flesh as in the original being, so why is an extra bone added? Hardly. Perhaps, the word woman in and of itself carries the answer to this mystery: <u>W</u>ithout <u>MAN</u>. She was formed just like Adam was, as one part of the division from the one being; she was not 'from' man, only as an afterthought. Perhaps, this is how God encrypted the truth, beneath this wording and in these times.

LESSON 126

SECTION III: LAW OF ATTRACTION, LAW OF OPPOSITES

The female was given the name "Eve" by God, meaning 'life,' or 'enlivening,' since she was the representation of the Female part of God and Mother of souls (her begotten children) and stewardess of the created order. Being totally enlightened, she demonstrated the feminine consort attributes of the Divine Feminine of God, becoming a complete version of woman with a more cyclical way of thinking, having an intuitive nature, and an attraction to nurturing. Eve shared the same feeling, reason, and cosmic energy as Adam, but reason would 'APPEAR' to be the uppermost and hidden within her nature. She was softer and expressed more feeling.

As the man was drawn to reason, and being aggressive, he possessed a positive transcendental processes, meaning he would desire the woman/female, who had deep feeling and *negative* transcendental processes. This explains the Law of Attraction in the Law of Opposites. One must remember that the laws of physics had already been set into motion. So, the positive and negative processes we are talking about refers to this Law within the Law. This means that the original being was perfectly divided, and positive and negative processes were placed within each of the two, respectively, causing this powerful euphoric magnetism. Having negative processes caused the female/Eve to have deeper feelings and recesses, which enhanced her desire for the man/male. Having the negative processes does not mean that she was 'negative' in her beliefs or emotions, but, rather, it made her more cyclical in her thinking. A perfect example of the two ways of thinking is in cyclical thinking we are thankful for the 'opportunity to experience winter.' It would be different than what was experienced before, and one would feel the falling temperature as it turned cold, and that as the temperature rises it will get warm once again. Going within that feeling and thinking provides opportunities to experience something new. In linear thinking, one would fear that the 'summer will never return,' and be 'positive' that one was right. Together, however, we find that they must seek the other to be balanced.

> *The ideal spiritual union between man and woman (male and female), was ordained that man/male might bring out the hidden reason in woman, and that woman/female may uncover the hidden feelings of man. Together they had the perfect sacred balance.*
>
> —Yogananda

By aiding each other to develop perfect balance of these pure divine soul qualities, they realize their true nature as inviolate souls. Eeshans agree that liberation was to be accomplished by their becoming united, first to each other in divine friendship, the purest expression of God's love between two individuals, and, then, when perfected, ever ready for the ultimate union with God. That is why what Jesus taught, in John 15:1, is so noteworthy, *'There is no greater love than to lay down one's life for a friend.'* The reason being that their love was not sex/lust-driven but was a mutual love for each other with a desire to share that love, which was above just the physical act we call sex today.

LESSON 127

SECTION IV: TRUE LOVE THROUGH, WITH, AND IN GOD; AND IT ALL BEGAN WITH A KISS

The love that Adam and Eve shared did not lack emotion or gratification. In fact, it was a far greater experience than the physical love humans enter into today, solely because they entered into their lovemaking with a pure transcendental love, which was totally focused, innocent and pure. This was true love, for it was through God, grounded in God, nourished by God, and originated in God, with a selfless, genuine, desirous love totally connected to God. It was so powerful a love yet with all its intensely mystical, self-transcendent experience, each time it began with:

a "kiss," a pure and sacred "kiss."
Yes, we are all familiar with the kiss.

We can all agree that a single kiss can express sentiments of love, passions, romance, sexual attraction, or arousal, affection, respect, greeting, friendship, peace good luck,[165] and more; but, the Sacred Kiss *is so much more*.

---

[165] "Kiss." Wikipedia, Wikimedia Foundation, 9 Dec. 2019, en.wikipedia.org/wiki/Kiss.

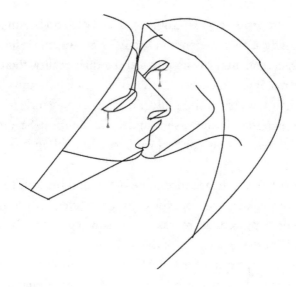

SECTION IVA: THE SACRED KISS

Oh the "Sacred Kiss!" Did you know, that the fingertips and lips transmit more 'light' from our bodies than any other place? So, to kiss one on the lips is to transmit, exchange and share light. As you become enlightened, and move from the human to the transcendental consciousness, you will better understand how powerful these two images are separately, but how much greater the power when the two become one.

Eeshans present the 'Kiss' as God's first expression of the purest, holiest, most sacred of all acts between two beings.

To Adam and Eve, the kiss was a ritual. It was designed by God, and was an outward sign of grace, upon which flows true love and devotion. It was their Sacrament.

This sacred kiss they shared would cause them to go into a state of rapture, or ecstasy, and they would be drawn out of themselves and into a transcendental feeling, or an increased awareness of *each other's* energy. They would then share this energy of the two combined with what is called an esoteric energy, which was the energy that surrounded them.

They entered into what resembled a dance with no beginning and no end, particularly as they were not in "time." Time was the result of the fall from the transcendental to the physical. In their reality, there was only eternal lovemaking, which was meditative, expressive, and intimate. It enhanced their love, trust, and mutual respect, using gentle touch, loving words, and extreme kindness, surrounded by the most beautiful music. It was the fullness of how you feel when you first fall in love, only more perfect and forever.

It caused them to experience more depth and breadth to their love, since their lovemaking was not subject to age, gender, body looks, control, or how the body moved. There was no focus on a goal to achieve, or anything outside of the experience of the moment.

There was no pressure for satisfaction for both lived for each other. What they experienced was exhilaration, and it was luminous, since they were suffused with, and shed, a bright interior light. It expanded their consciousness and weaved together the polarities of male and female into a harmonious wholeness, thus, their hearts were as one. Most importantly, it opened the doorway to the Divine, who blessed this union, unconditionally.

LESSON 128

SECTION V: SACRED BREATH

Without a doubt, breath is sacred. As an example, Wildspeak.com had this to say about Sacred Breath:

> Breath animates our body, gives force and power to our words, chants, and songs, and it enables us to purify ourselves and cells. It is powerful. It gives meaning and language. It can carry wisdom or foolishness, and it can store power or send it outwards.
>
> Breath in some cultures is crucial in soul retrieval. It is how we draw in a missing soul fragment, and how we give it to the person in need of healing. It becomes a powerful healing tool. In some Siberian cultures, it was the only way the soul could be placed back into the body.
>
> It says, in the author's practice, 'a missing soul piece is cradled in the hands of the Oraite (shaman) and placed into the region of the heart for safe-keeping.' There it knows that it is safe and protected, while we negotiate our way back to the person in need of healing. Once there, the soul piece is concentrated into the breath, and then 'blown' into certain places on the body, including the forehead (or crown of the head), and the heart. It is a special breath that carries the soul, it can be taught, or it can be innate and learned through instinct. Only one of these breaths is needed, and then one more to seal it in.

In some cases, we are able to bring back our own spirit while meditating, or simply by going on a spiritual journey. We might notice that we breathe easier, or that suddenly we take a deep breath or a long exhale. It is our own soul recognizing how to integrate what was missing that becomes found. We breathe it in, and so circulate our spirit back through our body again, and likewise we can breathe out negativity.

It is common in many visualizations to imagine all the negativity of the day, including bodily tension, or mental anxiety, to leave the body on each exhale. This acknowledges the innate power of our breath to heal ourselves. Whether you are a spiritual animist who believes in soul retrieval or not, our own breathing is a sacred and healing act.

Eeshans believe that the breath is the exchange of light which similarly occurs through the lips and fingertips. Along with the Sacred Kiss is the purifying breath that dispels negativity that was one of those effects of entropy.

Can you imagine the power of the breath, which was exchanged between Adam and Eve, who, though transcendental, were still *created*? And now compare theirs to the intensity of the breath exchanged during the *Sacred Kiss* between Jesus and His Wife for the first time?

LESSON 129

SECTION VI: SPIRITUAL FOOD FOR ETERNAL LIFE: LOVE VERSUS SEX

As their love was truly a gift from God, Adam and Eve entered into this mystical euphoria that sealed their bond of love and continued to influence them until the next kiss, whereupon they would once again enter into a very sensual, tantric lovemaking filled with light energy and vibrations of the purest and most perfect expression of Kundalini.[166] In fact, it is believed to have been imprinted in each of us; however, in most it is rarely, if ever, attained, and thus remains dormant throughout life.

This love, along with the Spiritual Food and Drink God made available to them, literally gave them the means to live forever. That is why Jesus taught about love for what they had, and linked their love to God's. Just as Jesus' Bread of Life discourse was such a profound teaching, we see why his identifying Himself as the "Light of the world" was so imperative: since it showed how a marriage of true love seeks to unite this love through, with, and in God by means of the sacred food of Holy Eucharist, which shares God's love for us through the spiritual, and sacramental, intercourse with the body, blood, soul, and divinity of the Divine Masculine and Divine Feminine of Jesus and Mary; thus, awakening and uniting our light bodies with theirs once again, for life everlasting.

This mystical union of Adam and Eve's love, via the sacred kiss, in conjunction with God's nourishment, is what literally gave them the means to live forever as 'pure organisms,' and kept their genetics pure

---

[166] In an Eeshan context, the energy of life that rises in the soul to the point where it can result in spiritual enlightenment and/or supernormal abilities. – Ed.

and alive; but both were necessary, since without nourishment from God, or without a true relationship with God, who is without beginning or end, there would be no eternal component through which life could be extended.

The immortal and the transcendental life then gave way to the begetting process, which is how, as pure beings, they reproduced through desire. Through this transcendental union, they fulfilled God's command "to go forth and be fruitful and multiply," according to their transcendental natures bearing 'God's' imprint.

Remember how we discussed about how within the Garden of Eden there was a bridge which had a gateway that opened to a path, which led to another garden filled with beautiful flowers, herbs, and countless kinds of trees, especially flowering and laden with fruit. There were alluvial fans, which resemble giant sea shells, and are formed by sediment that forms a cone shape, which transports a rush of water, which then flows into small streams of water, like tributaries, that all come from the flowing of waterfalls and yet even more beautiful streams. These were separated at the time of creation when God made a space to separate the waters of the earth from the waters of the heavens. It is within this Garden where God would walk and talk with them, and share with Adam and Eve, a very unique food and drink. The food was very similar looking to a manna, but filled with delightful taste, a blessed heavenly oil, as sweet as honey, with a dash of salt; and on an altar, sat a cup of wine 'in a glass made of water.' It was very light and very delightful, providing the light, which kept their souls nourished, their bodies transcendent; and with love they received these victuals, since they were from God for eternal life. This food was given to them by God with joy. Though the Origin of this 'spiritual food' is how they shared their love through, with, and in God, it would also strengthen their desire for God, as well as the love and the desire for each other.

There is nothing more powerful than love. Love fills the heart and soul beyond human comprehension, and is not logical. It is the most powerful of all human experiences, and contains within it the propensity for living for another rather than for oneself, encompassing the desire to take care of or protect. That is why they were filled with pure love, and not a sensual desire, since sex is purely physical and temporary. Love is shared, while sex, by itself, is a selfish act, solely for the individual's pleasure. Love may involve sex, but sex alone never involves love. The transcendental love as Adam and Eve shared caused them to grow even more in love, along with the desire increasing to share love as God shared love.

LESSON 130

SECTION VII: THE LIFE WITH GOD IN THE GARDEN

God spoke to both Adam and Eve in a language tailored to each nature, with the attributes of the male relating to the attributes of the divine masculine of God (though very comfortable with the Divine Feminine) and Eve to the divine feminine of God; yet, God was most gifted in speaking to the Divine Masculine, since both, however, still contained the attributes of the other, even though each was 'separated.'

Adam and Eve were both inclined to speak to God in a language of love also unique to their gender, but not necessarily in mutually exclusive ways. In other words, Adam would speak in a more masculine, linear sense, being male dominant, coming from a man's perspective, and Eve would speak, likewise, from a woman's perspective. Thus, both could speak to God differently, as well as independently, while at the same time with equal dignity, mirroring God's own dignity, as divine male and divine female, reflecting the same 'as it was in the beginning, is now, and ever shall be.'

It is important to repeat that they possessed, and exercised, *free will*. For example, even though we are obliged to know, love, and serve God, we do have a choice. Our obligation to know, love, and serve God stems from the fact that we are the creatures created by a Creator, a higher being, God.

They were also not alone, as the children they had begotten lived in the Garden, and angels, and other beings, lived, or visited there, too. It would be foolish to believe that Adam and Eve only had each other to talk with.

Adam and Eve were, however, the only beings designed, and created, to manifest God in image and likeness from the "one" separated into "two," and, one again, in their marriage to each to each other, making them the first of their kind, as well as being the extensions of God's love for the eternal and life creating Consorts.

It's hard for us to imagine what life was like in this astonishing Place Adam and Eve called home; but they did have their responsibilities. Adam had dominion over all that God created, and Eve cared for the new growth and birthing of the animals. Adam was indeed the first man ("Ish"), and Eve, was, thus, was the first woman ("Isha"), and the two enjoyed their home and the beauty within. They shared their time together walking and talking to their children and their children's children. They talked about God's glorious creative powers which they both possessed to some degree. Fascinated with the children, they would watch, as they interacted with the angels.

It was Adam and Eve who alone had admittance into the Garden of God, or Heaven, as it can be called. It was also Adam and Eve who would bring the Sacred Food to their offspring, and would share stories of their time with God, though God would come and visit with the begotten children and bless them with sharing fruits and vegetables, and water and wine, which gladdened and enlivened their hearts.

The begotten children were also not without talents, and would present God with gifts they had made and bouquets of newly created flowers, with fragrances that filled the air. Jugs of crystal-like water from the streams that fed all vegetative life within the garden quenched the thirst, as light quenched their bodies.

LESSON 131

SECTION VIII: THE BLESSING, THE PRIZE

This unique relationship that the couple had with God was made possible by the 'God Particle.' That is what caused them to experience a true joy found only through, with, and in God, unlike any other being. This 'God particle,' or inner Light, was sanctioned, and contained and shared, only within the bodies of Adam and Eve. So sacred was this "God Particle" that, after them, it would later become known as 'the Blessing,' and would be passed along through human history, beginning with Melchizedek, then to Abraham, whose meaning, until this day, has not been revealed, except for the necessity of it for formation of countries, and how they would be populated. In terms of descendants, and division of lands and wealth, the 'blessing' was most desired. In other words, whoever carried the blessing was like a 'king,' but its actual value and meaning would remain hidden until the Chosen one returned. That time would be linked to the time of the Messiahs, upon which it would be shared between the eternal consorts once again by their divinity. This blessing was, and is, in every respect, a 'tangible' covenant between God and humanity. It carries with it the power to give everlasting life as it was shared by God, who is infinitely eternal, meaning without beginning, without end, and who cannot be destroyed.

It could also be *a source of contention* to one who covets God. This blessing brings with it endless unimaginable gifts, and, especially, for one who is not complete in oneself, it pushes them beyond their wildest dreams as humans, especially humans who never knew truth, or never believed that such a thing could exist. To humans such as these, one just 'exists,' and, in all that, one that goes along with the blessing is outside their awareness and concern.

That is why, without belief in God, we actually disbelieve even in our own existence, for nothing outside of God really lives, because, as we said, God is life. Life entered into this world in the most unique way.

This blessing bequeathed with it the divine component and the blessing of God's marriage in its fullness, upon human marriage and human love.

PART III

LESSON 132

SECTION I: HUMAN LOVE BLESSED BY GOD

We have been focused on, and speaking about, transcendental love; but at this time, we want to bring to light that because of God's love between the divine/human consorts between the marriage of Jesus and Mary Magdalen, human love is that which even the angels are in awe. Since the human expression of love, 'grounded in God,' transforms the human heart, with such joy and gladness, that a person actually comes out of themselves, which almost sounds counterintuitive, but it's true.

Human love in a committed relationship and marriage is blessed by God. Since we have been focused on transcendental love, we want to bring that to light, that because of God's divine love, and the love between the divine/human consorts between the marriage of Jesus and Mary Magdalen, *human love is that which even the angels are in awe*. Since the human expression of love, that is 'grounded in God', transforms the human heart, with such joy and gladness, that this is actually a perfect example of what Eeshans mean by the expression, a person actually "comes out of themselves." No, we are not talking about the physical component, though it is encompassed within human love, as it was in the marriage of Jesus and Mary Magdalen.

It's when two humans live for each other and would die for each other. This human love transcends logic since it is illogical in every respect. This love is not abusive or jealous. It is not hurtful or subservient. It is not taken for granted or betrayed. It does not have to seek self-gratification because it is already acknowledged and shared in the other.

In a God-filled marriage, each lives for the other and derives strength from the Spouse. There is a deep emptiness, and void, when separated.

There is no longing like the longings and caring for each other. All of life's beauty is seen, and shared, in ways that confound the mind. It's abiding and makes the best in life better and the difficult easier to bear. Each spouse finds purpose living for the other. It's a sacrificial love, and each person would rather have the other happy, rather than one's self.

> "So this is love. This is what make life-divine! The key to all heaven is mine."
>
> —Disney's Cinderella

PART IV

LUCIFER

Tracing Religious Corruption Back to Lucifer

LESSON 133

Section I: An Introduction to the Religious Corruption

Religious corruption has been exhibited in recent times in very open and shameless ways. It became obvious that corruption was/is responsible for doubting the sacred, or holy, as is prevalent in a lot of humans today. Since what is sacred and holy? How did this happen?

First, we have heard of the destruction by evil, or, what some would rather call, the 'brainwashing' brought about by religious doctrine, which was a guise used for the retention of God's, or Jesus', followers. Through the years, it became common to disregard everything once held sacred because one would look fanatical, i.e., such as genuflecting too many times. In recent years, it was witnessed by the lack of reverence in handling the sacred, followed by the disregard of casual behavior before the Blessed Sacrament. Also, there was the insolent behavior of the clergy towards the Sacraments and towards those who wished to go to confession, or refused to hold the Sacred Eucharist in their hands.

How could this happen? It was always understood that when those in religious authority claimed, that they spoke on behalf of God, one believed. Banking on God's people of this same mindset even today, authority(ies) treated the congregation as though they were all uneducated, unsophisticated, poor, or socially unaccepted, and labeled them "pockets of the traditionally minded faithful that had to be broken up." These became targets for attacks by religious liberals, and, yet, still they needed to use whatever means they had for the retention of followers. With the onset of Medjugorje these 'outcasts,' unknowingly, became victims of religious abuse and slavery.

Jesus used the terms 'stumbling block' and 'whitewashed tombs' to describe Peter and the religious leaders/teachers, respectively, back then, for denying God's people the truth. He made it a point to throw out venders, and those who were taking part in insulting God, by making the Temple a place of thieves. Today, we can see, once again, that He was also looking forward to those institutions, which would be responsible for the blatant abuse of power in His name, and the lessening of the reverence, within the churches.

Regardless of what they claimed or claim, again, respectively, God continued to protect the innocent, as none of those mentioned above ever held the hidden 'unfathomable secrets and mysteries.' Seeing that even the Presence of God, in what was considered the Blessed Sacrament, was being removed from the high altars, God decided to send One who would teach right and wrong to those who were still believers. The Stigmata and fragrance of roses she possessed brought an awareness of the sacred and transcendent back to the people who had been deprived of these things, which brought them back to God. This, however, was not what the church wanted, nor those who sought recognition for themselves, but, rather, received none, after their support from cardinals and bishops.

Just as Jesus knew Peter's intentions, and called him a 'stumbling block' (because he lived and taught by the human consciousness), He proved time and again that He was correct, since Peter displayed his inability to transcend through his behavior, as well as in his letters (said to be authentic). What was written by him, shows no record of Peter ever having an understanding of the Bread of Life discourse, even after Jesus explained it. Obviously, he had no understanding of what was meant by Jesus 'teaching about this "Bread of Life," as being himself, let alone Jesus and His wife. Truly rigid attachment to his birth religion would not allow for Peter to enter into this mystery, or the importance of Jesus' directive that *we must have* the Eucharist for Salvation. Peter didn't understand Jesus at all, and didn't understand the mystery of salvation. He just saw it as a set of new rules for a new law. And, thus, truly all Peter got from Jesus' teachings was for one to do good works. Without a doubt, he could not see beyond what his human rational, logical mind would allow him to see.

LESSON 134

Section II: The Need to Destroy the Sacred Food and Drink

Now let's take a look at another 'being' who possessed the knowledge and understanding of the great power of the Sacred food and Drink, but because of corrupted reasoning desired to destroy it. The inability for Adam and Eve to never have access to it again is not only incomprehensible, but did not even seem a possibility to our first parents. They couldn't see this as a consequence for listening to this being.

In this instance, one can predict the extent of means Satan would have to exercise to destroy this nourishment for immortality and cause separation of the humans from God.

Despite the insurmountable punishment he would suffer in attempting to enter into such a deed, one such as this, one so filled with darkness, will not stop until he brings his plan to fruition.

One cannot fully realize Satan's goal, let alone his strategy, in accomplishing this plan. Adam and Eve had no reason to question a newly formed relationship with yet another god-like being, but they would find that their relationship with this one would be their downfall.

Here we want to present some background information we feel is necessary for you to have a better picture of Lucifer, who became Satan, and the events that took place at his hand.

One should bear in mind also, that Lucifer's corruption began before Adam and Eve and continued during Jesus' time, up to and including today and will continue until the end of time. His plan to destroy Adam and Eve's relationship with God on a spiritual level marked a series of future events that unfortunately will lead us up to the third and then final phase of God's plan for our salvation.

LESSON 135

SECTION III: THE LEGENDS AND FACTS REGARDING THIS BEING

Though there is limited information about this being we know as Satan, there are many opinions about the sentence God passed on him. Over the years some cults were formed solely based on pitying Satan as though he was judged unfairly. There are people who even pray for his conversion or for God to forgive him. Some have gone so far as to say he is Jesus' brother, a relative to 'as above so below' or 'where's there's a positive, there's a negative.' Others claim he is the prodigal son Jesus talked about, believing that Satan's choice to go out on his own [to go against God] can be seen as his being punished for exercising his choice of free will. There are even those who believe that because he was so powerful a rebel that God gave him the earth as his kingdom to prove himself, and in the end, will welcome him back (again, as in the prodigal son parable). The reasoning behind this thinking is because too many it doesn't make sense that God would punish Lucifer with a kingdom to rule then why not subject him to imprisonment for eternity in hell? Or wait, maybe *this* is hell? And, maybe, this is why Satan has such great influence and why so many of us have become so delusional?

This is what we know. He was 'created' Lucifer, the most beautiful of all angels. The Son of God was not 'created,' so the legends about the two being brothers is preposterous.

Before Lucifer made a choice to rise up against God, he was the model of perfection, the sum of all things good, full of wisdom, perfect in beauty, and was very intelligent. He had to be in order to be persuasive enough to convince one third of the angels to follow him and to join in the rebellion against God.

He filled heaven with his music like no other. This is why music has such tremendous effect on us. The rhythm of music actually affects our blood. Music also heavily influences our spirit either towards the good or towards the bad. That is why we warn that it's the beat and rhythm that causes one to react, and when our subconscious engages that's when we begin to remember the lyrics. Did you ever wonder why you knew the words to those songs you don't even like? We know that music is so powerful that it is very effective in raising or lowering blood pressure, lowering heart rate, and that music aids in sleep.

According to one legend, there was a light that shone so brightly on Lucifer, and three others, that had this place before God's throne because of their love and zeal for God. It shone so bright that even other divine forms, meaning those who were of and from God, could not look upon these four but that Lucifer's was the brightest of the four. Some who are aware of this legend, and know that Jesus is the 'Light of the World,' might mistakenly think that Christ was one among these four beings, and, thus, might infer from this that Jesus had "brothers."

We know Jesus, of course, was not one of these, but was and is of Himself. The Son of God was begotten of God, and so was not created; thus He would therefore not be among these three beings with Lucifer mentioned here.

It's also been thought by some that Jesus and Lucifer were somehow 'brothers' because of the association of "Light," as in Jesus Christ is the "Light of the world," where Lucifer was known as the 'bearer of Light' ... but were, indeed, opposites, as in one is good and the other is bad. Also, there could be the parallel in some people's minds with the story of Cain and Abel, one being good and pure before God, and thus favored, while the other is rejected because of his jealously, envy, and hatred. Still, Christ and Lucifer are not brothers, and never were. Again, Christ is begotten, while Lucifer, even though an angel occupying the highest place in heaven, was still *created*.

We are told that Lucifer always had access to Eden, the Garden of God, for he had the power to come and go anywhere he chose—up and down the mountain of God, amidst the stone of fire. He wore the breastplate of every precious stone and had a voice which filled heaven with music unique to any other divine being. He was anointed and placed on the holy mount of God. He was blameless, and was the highest guarding Seraph around the Throne of God.

He had twelve wings compared to the others with six. It is said that he wore the first breastplate until unrighteousness filled him with violence and he sinned. From the stones of fire, his heart was lifted, and because of his beauty he corrupted his wisdom by reason of his splendor.

"How you have fallen from heaven, O star of the morning, son of the dawn! You have been cut down to the earth, you who have weakened the nations."

"But you said in your heart, 'I will ascend to heaven; I will raise my throne above the stars of God, and I will sit on the mount of the assembly in the recesses of the north."

"I will ascend above the heights of the clouds; I will make myself like the Most High.' Nevertheless, you will be thrust down to Sheol, to the recesses of the pit."

(adapted from Isaiah 14:12-15, Ezekiel 28:12-17)

God therefore cast him out as though he was a curse from the mountain, and by His 'Word' would destroy him. Lucifer had defiled the sanctuaries, and because he will continue to defile sanctuaries God promised to bring him to ashes upon the earth in the sight of all them that give him honor.

Most of these topics are found encompassed in the bible, some in legends, and others in books.

You will find that in order to give a clearer picture of the origin of God's salvific plan for us, we felt we should present our sacred story with a 'simplified' version of what happened in the very beginning with Lucifer.

LESSON 136

JUST A REMINDER

Since this is a transcendental document, we feel it is important that we weave pertinent information and facts, back and forth, aligning the past, present, and future, since all that is spiritual is outside of time in a kind of subjective time orientation. In other words, being time-oriented creatures we look to the past to determine what we need to do, and then we look to the future to see how our decisions will play out. Without time, past, present, and future events have no boundaries, but are happening simultaneously. How does one understand something spiritual and timeless playing out today? First, try and rid your mind of any preordained impressions and facts you have been entertaining up until now, and allow your mind to rest; your transcendental consciousness will eventually take over and your heart will succumb to becoming enlightened.

It is also important not to try to absorb too many topics at a time. This will cause fatigue and confusion for these are inherent of the human consciousness' need for information and does not facilitate transcendental enlightenment. These next few sections contain a lot of knowledge important for unlocking the mysteries of God and the entering into the compelling saga of epic proportion of life beyond human understanding.

PART V

THE CHURCH HYPOCRISY SATAN'S INFLUENCE

LESSON 137

SECTION I: MAGIC/WITCHCRAFT VERSUS MYSTICISM

In the wake of fading Christian civilization, some see that Islam is the fastest growing major religion in the USA. Though this may be shocking, you may be surprised to find that magic and witchcraft (i.e., Wicca), are religious practices that are growing even faster. However, though it has its roots back to ancient Babylon, and is just one form of ceremonial magic, it does not follow that all those who practice Wicca, and the like, are 'evil' or bad. It is predicted that such practices will become the third largest religion in the USA after Christianity and Islam. According to *The Guardian*, there is an explosion of interest in witchcraft occurring now in the UK.

One has to have noticed the extreme emphasis on Halloween, and how it is actually becoming more of a celebration than Christmas.

Why is this happening? Because faith is diminishing. Without faith humans become the judges of their own actions. The soul naturally seeks spirituality. A significant focus, as an alternative to Christian religions, also occurs relationships with angels. Angels are powerful, and people feel they can have and share much spirituality with angels as they might have with God, or perhaps even more. Angel sightings and teachings are poised perfectly in the bible; there are books galore out there about angels. Tarot cards, psychics, mediums, and others have eased pain and have lifted burdens from those who went to seek them. People no longer see evil, or feel suspicion, but do look for comfort.

Since God, who is seen in established religions as not giving them "this happiness," people turn away. Apparently, in this way, God, as defined in Christian religions, is no longer the center of people's lives; thus, people become vulnerable to the influences of the world, or spiritualisms that reimage a God, or a deity, people can relate to. The more desperate we become for this happiness nothing else matters when we then seek peace; nor will we let 'anyone or anything' get in our way.

But, as we stated before, the soul needs spirituality to nurture itself. The soul will use whatever logic, or rational reason, to indicate it doesn't, but because it has that spark of God within it that makes it immortal, it will 'seek solace' wherever it can. Witchcraft and magic might seem to provide that satisfaction without the guilt imposed by a 'judging' God.

As we mentioned before, and probably will 'repeat' again, horoscopes, astrology and sciences do have a connection to our interior and exterior dimensions as human beings, and may be very helpful to our evolving understanding in discovering ourselves and our place in a universal realm. In many ways these are helpful in discovering the different pieces of the puzzle of our physical, as well as emotional and psychological wellbeing, whereas before these were considered taboo. We believe this is because we, as humans, are made up of energy that affects our blood, and water and light, which are carried throughout the mind and body, which ultimately affects our spirit. It is important, however, to understand that God must still be the center core of our lives. These are all important and helpful, but they cannot replace our relationship with God.

For example, though some say neo-Paganism is safe since it worships nature and the 'gods' of nature, one still must be guided to stay balanced and must still enjoy God with a healthy acceptance of Jesus. Does this sound like a contradiction? Given the fact that so many teenage girls are attracted to New Age teachings, and lining up to join in Wicca practices, it isn't.

We want to establish that teenagers are very attracted to the Divine, just by their own definition of it, through an innate cosmic and universal sense. If there is no way they feel they can relate to God at this time WE MUST TRY AND GIVE THEM A LIFELINE BACK to Christ. However, on a salvific level, it is important that they love Jesus and hopefully regard His and Mary's directive for the Sacred Bread and

Drink under 'their guidance,' meaning what is provided by the Marriage Feast celebrated by a Kallah, Chatan, or Eesha, under specific conditions and requirements. They must understand that only the preceding could transubstantiate and no other. This is because 'no other' has the unspoken words, and these are highly secured.

Wicca may also be confused in celebrating the Divine Feminine and female goddesses, but remember usually there is a form of lust attached to some of these ancient deities.

Without a doubt people need 'something' spiritual to nurture them. Faith no longer suffices since they have been let down too many times. As a result, many non-religious people want instant gratification, since they live in such a volatile world such as this one, the pursuit for happiness and enjoyment of life is critical. In fact, it's absolutely *vital*.

Turning to 'alternative religions' is tempting. Although we mentioned those Wicca variations above, there are many others. One must be aware that there are others which are 'dark' religions which people confuse as Wicca. For example: Occultism, Satanism, Luciferianism, etc.

This mindset leads to actions which provide pleasure. When asked how one makes life altering decisions, the comment is: "God *wants* me to be happy." The truth is, God *does want* us to be happy; however, people define happiness themselves, but not necessarily with that happiness that is derived from God.

The greatest of these misconceptions are those that involves lust. God, indeed, wants us to be happy, but does not approve of seeking happiness outside God's Law. One can be assured that if what one is desiring is outside of God, it is definitely leaning towards "Satan's argument about everyone else being happy then why shouldn't you be?" Or, "You never stood in his/her way of happiness, why should he/she?" Lust, or the desire to seek pleasure outside of a committed relationship, or outside of marriage, is pleasure without responsibility. These kinds of actions within any religion outside of God and the Mysteries/Sacraments, which people claim as 'reasonable choices for happiness,' are delusional; and in turn makes us all susceptible to the delusions of 'Satan.'

Over the centuries, humans have felt they were so duped and continuously deceived by established religion that there is an air of a newfound freedom. This freedom is defined as 'being happy.' It is also using free will in making a choice between being happy or holy. Those who want to be holy should be; and those who are not religious, and just want to be happy, should be also. It's like a man who loves God finds a woman in church, and though married, he believes God put her there to make him happy. He divorces his wife and begins his newfound freedom to love the woman who 'completes' him.

Where fear was once the tool used for the retention of Christ's followers, we see now that it has led to a generation *who doesn't believe, or can't believe in the kind of God that not only appears conflicted but that 'He' is a self-centered, discriminating, and a punishing God.*

In taking Jesus as a shield, many people have begun to take 'Christ's' teachings of love in a whole new direction. There seems however to be conflicting stories, and with Catholic schools and Sunday schools teaching from some pulpits how Jesus loves us, and with the Pope saying there is no purgatory or hell, and that they are just a state of mind, morality and decency go out the window. Sin abounds, as does also discrimination.

On the other hand, some teach that if you aren't on board with the 'standard' from Leviticus of the Old Testament, you are an abomination to Him; yet within so many Catholic seminaries, parishes, and among the hierarchy, we find something quite different. Could this be another example of laws that benefit those in authority, but the people are supposed to live by only what they are told to do?

As a result, many people no longer feel that a Jesus-based religion, or spirituality, is necessary, for they have been made to see religion and spirituality as one and the same.

That is why spirituality has been replaced with Wicca, the Occult, and other beliefs that use pagan rituals. There are groups actively leading people into the occult by using feelings and emotions based on the tools of complacency and doubt. There are those who feel they can only believe in themselves. There are some who want only to believe in a punishing God, and frown on any kind of happiness as a means of satisfying a very deep 'seeded' pain, and they take this pain and their judgmental hearts, and, in Jesus name, disgrace and use inflammatory hate speech against other people in another way to subjugate them. These people actually can be brought to hate anything good or kind, and anything having merit, which is aligned with Jesus and his teachings, even though they call themselves Christians and believe they are doing Jesus' will. That is how Satan can get into one's head.

To be clear, **it was and continues to be the wrongs of the authorities and religious leaders and teachers** that are responsible for blurring the lines of faith and spirituality with the ongoing imbalance, sin, dysfunction—**not the members**. The members usually find solace in going to their churches and believing that they are there only to worship and love Jesus. These people lay claim that they don't pay attention, or get involved with political antics or religious scandal, they just want to pray and spend time with God.

How sad that they have been deprived of the true faith. God bless those who ever fell for the lies, and because of an innate love of God, know and love Jesus in their own way; and are trying to live out their lives as they believe Jesus intended, even if their faith has been based upon those erred doctrines.

As we delve deeper into the cause of why humans fell from grace, it is a good time to point out that though no one wants to believe it, Satan, undoubtedly, is at the root of the problems we are facing; and he is not going away. Even though Wicca, and other practices, claim to not believe in Satan, not having God included in any aspect of a religion initiates a slippery slope to those who want to fill the void deep within their heart.

If anything, one should be aware that Satan is the supreme narcissist,[167] and what a delusional being he is. He was, and always will be, in pursuit of self-gratification. This stems from vanity and egotistical admiration of his own attributes. There is a short list below to describe this being, who is as real 'today' as he was then, since Satan can't die. The danger with not believing in God is the off chance that you do not believe Satan exists either.

---

[167] It may prove useful and insightful to the reader to research this term and keep the results in the back of one's mind while reading on. – Ed.

The power behind the evil is demonstrated through these various degrees of personality traits which taken together are the foundational basis for the tactics used by him today:

1) sin or disbelief in sin against God
2) thinking that sin is merely exercising your free will
3) a growing hatred towards anyone who loves God
4) rejoicing at the success of causing anyone to fall from grace

These pitfalls that were evidenced then are just as real today, with one exception.

As we stated, in the aforementioned, fewer and fewer people believe that Satan exists, and those who mistakenly see him as powerful, or with horns and a pitchfork, or view the image which most people are familiar with in movies, such as *The Exorcist*, where Satan, or a demon, possesses people by wreaking havoc within them. Though these things can happen, as there have been documented cases, wherein these instances, Satan, or demons, and there is a difference between the two, attack viciously not just the victim, but also those around the victims themselves. Possessions are rare, and, subsequently, are usually surrounded by highly unusual phenomena. Though these attacks are rare, they do happen. There are attacks on people today which are of a subtler approach, and though there are signs of mental and psychological trauma, when it involves a subtle, weak-willed, or spiritually-starved individual, one must be wary. By this we mean that these poor individuals, if left unhelped, can become, or be used, as an instrument of harm. The truth is the greatest tool of Satan is for people to deny his existence. Yet, if you believe that God, or a Supreme Being(s), or that angels etc., exist(s) then by universal law, there has to be a Satan and/or demons, too.

Without spirituality, and faith in God, we as humans are very susceptible to Satan's traps, such as delusion. Remember, taking over souls is his goal. With each soul, he becomes more powerful.

Here are some of the ways Satan can manipulate humans. He can attack the soul privately through thought, and, even publicly, through social media and many other means. For certain:

- He has the inability to process shame.
- He sees himself as perfect, using distortion and illusion to 'prove this.'
- He uses projection to inundate shame on anyone, including God
- He cannot feel deflated, and so becomes arrogant; he reinflates his sense of self-importance by diminishing, debasing, or degrading others before God.
- He secures a sense of superiority by saying he is in his own way a son of God.
- He is filled with contempt towards God, and holds unreasonable expectations of particularly favorable treatment and automatic compliance because he considers himself special,[168] and believes God thwarted his Plan; and he considers this an attack on his superiority.
- He exhibits rage if questioned about sex as being selfish.
- He causes one to feel subservient.

With God in one's heart, these issues wouldn't exist in a person, but, without God, these actually become personality traits that lead to anger, abuse, prejudice and discrimination. To further elaborate on this teaching, Satan was never more dangerous than when people don't believe he exists, because they then subject themselves to his attacks on their mind, spirit, and conscience, as well as their body, while they think, "This is just who I am."

Satan, and his wicked deeds, are found where love is not. He is found wherever there is a void in human life where love should be. When this love is absent one's mind and senses are inevitably focused on what apparent pleasures the world of nature (prakriti) might thus provide, and the experiencing of these pleasures, apart from God, is recreated in the mind to mean 'love' along with the sensation of apparent 'peace.' From here, life easily becomes a pursuing of pleasure and the avoidance of anything unpleasant or painful, and so the world of "prakriti" becomes to such a person synonymous with "*purusa*" (the inner light of awareness) just as a

---

[168] "Narcissism." Wikipedia, Wikimedia Foundation, 9 Dec. 2019, en.wikipedia.org/wiki/Narcissism.

person begins to see the body as the same as the "I." "I am my body," or "I am my mind," when in truth, the integral person is neither, since the mind and body are the vehicles and devices of perception and experience in the material world for a soul and is the natural result of the 'choice' in the Garden by Adam and Eve.

Yet while it would seem at first that living merely in order to experience only the pleasures of material existence is fulfilling, such as a focus on living as 'one' with *prakriti* under a false guise of 'love' is actually suffocating and affects the subtle body, which is not outwardly felt, but interiorly felt as a false peace and a false happiness. The subtle body, not actually being 'satisfied' spiritually, demands more and more. However, the mind and senses are lost in the external environment of people, situations, and material possessions. This is especially problematic when a person is narcissistically inclined. The more one is 'suffocated' under this counterfeit 'spirituality' of the world, the more one is capable of falling victim to Satan's traps, and thus we see why today more than ever God is needed in day to day life.

This thinking is precisely the 'evidence of control' the *other one* has over people. What happens is that his spirit totally convinces a person that their mind, which is consumed with harmful thoughts, is justified, and then the person rationalizes their feelings accordingly, defying any healthy intervention whatsoever. But all is not lost. God offers many opportunities to come back. One needs only to remember: **LOVE CONQUERS ALL. God, being love, never walks away on us, it is we who walk away from God.**

Love being 'the most powerful virtue' one can experience, it is without a doubt that *you can have everything* else, but without love, *you have nothing*. That is why to love is the weapon of weapons in defeating bad, evil, and destructive powers. Remember though, love is a double-edged sword and a two-way street, since it can be used to create; although, in human hands it can also destroy. Only by being God-centered, can we know which is the right choice.

Satan and demons cannot experience love, nor can they conquer it. It is the most powerful weapon one can use against them. That is why the transcendental union so closely mirrors God, and 'any human union without, or outside of God,' does not.

MYSTICISM

Many people confuse Mysticism with Magic or Witchcraft. Mysticism is defined as the belief that union with, or absorption into, the Deity, or the absolute, or the spiritual apprehension of knowledge inaccessible to the intellect, may be attained through contemplation and self-surrender.[169] Religious ecstasies (religious experiences during alternate states of consciousness), that are practiced together with whatever ideologies, ethics, rites, myths, legends, etc. are what are indicative of mysticism.

Mysticism has ancient Greek origins, along with various historical meanings. In this text, however, it is the biblical, liturgical, spiritual, and contemplative dimensions of early and contemplative Christianity, as well as the early modern period, which included a broad range of beliefs and ideologies that are related to 'extraordinary experience' and states of mind.[170]

Saints such as St Theresa of Avila, St. Theresa Little Flower, etc., and also stigmatisms such as St, Francis Assisi, Theresa Neumann, and Padre Pio are among the most noted. Mysticism was very popular again in the 1980s and the 1990s, where many so-called mystics and visionaries abounded.

All religions include mystics and saints with mystical powers, and were always well known within the Catholic faith. Public apparitions permeated our faith and most popular among them was the Virgin Mary's apparition at Lourdes in 1858, which declared that she was the Immaculate Conception; and we also have the apparitions at Fatima where she warned of significant danger from enemies, which some say were Islamic forces. Next, we had Medjugorje, and the Virgin appearing again with messages for people to turn back to God. During the onset of our Foundress' speaking engagements, tremendous phenomena surrounded her, to include levitation, Stigmata, and a miraculous Host in an effort to draw attention back to the Eucharist.

---

[169] "Mysticism: Definition of Mysticism by Lexico." Lexico Dictionaries | English, Lexico Dictionaries, www.lexico.com/en/definition/mysticism.

[170] Wikipedia.com on mysticism.

In other words, mysticism includes all you ever read about the saints and private and public apparitions, including claimed locutions and mystical unions with God, Jesus, the infinite, and the Most High God.

The difference then with Mysticism and Magic (i.e., Wicca) is that Mysticism deals with transcendental energies that seeks theosis, or unity, and conformity with God. Theosis is found in ancient times as well into biblical times and on through to present times, and is a form of 'deification' which keeps the lines of communication open between humans and God. It is all about one's sense of being that draws its life and meaning from a relationship with God. Magic, witchcraft, and sorcery, on the other hand, are distinct from this understanding in that it is one's 'self' that is the center and beneficiary of all practices with the result that one becomes more 'powerful' in and of oneself, *but apart from one's personal relationship with God*, regardless of the means chosen to acquire powers such as this. This is where the reality of Alchemy is split, since it can be utilized by both mystic and magician, or sorcerer; however, what is in question is the end for which it is used. Transformation is sought in both instances, but it is in the substance of the motives and goals that they differ.

Though the church has a history of mystics, during the time our Foundress was made public, there was an immediate attention drawn to her, and the church seemed to be concerned with proof that she was fulfilling prophecies that were once considered hidden away. This time the mysticism involved not just a threat of war, or of an enemy, but the fulfillment of a prophecy that would change the course of religion and spirituality familiar as never before with the reintroduction of the Sacred and Divine Priesthood, which would rise from the ashes of hopelessness and bring with it the promise of Salvation.

LESSON 138

Section II: Satan's Hatred of Love

Satan and his demons do not love. Even though they are beings like angels with intellects and reason, they have FORFEITED their free will. They cannot reproduce either by begetting or through sexuality. Their will works through hate and their choices are against God; and they have chosen to hate God, eternally. That is why their punishment will never end.

Angels love. They have reason and free will, which is exercised in their desire to know, love, and serve God and humanity. God has a set number of angels desired, and even though these other angels rebelled against God, all these beings, good or bad, are immortal. That is why there is no reason for them to beget others like themselves. They can only take on physical forms by embodying other humans who 'willingly' give themselves to them. Angels have done this, and that is how Satan, and those who follow him, had and have the ability to take advantage of other forms from those who are willing.

After his rebellion, Satan's envy of what God had increased, as did his hatred for the transcendental beings God created, as well as their transcendental offspring, and he desired the power to beget just as these 'lower beings' had. As a spirit, he also didn't possess duality as God created only a certain number of each male and female; and because angels and demons are immortal, there is no reason that they need to beget a child. He could not see that children were the fruit of love but only as worshippers and adorers.

LESSON 139

SECTION III: THE FALL OF THE HEAVENLY PRIESTHOOD: LEGEND OR ENDTIME PROPHECY?

Power is addictive. It is having great ability to do and act greater than anyone else. When put into the hands of a 'perfect' narcissist it becomes a tool of strength, might, force, and control. The narcissist believes that all those under him must serve him. That is what happened to Lucifer. One day, Lucifer decided he was not going to be a servant any more. He waged war on God as we said earlier, with his refusal to worship God. Why did he refuse? Because he wanted to be worshiped himself. He confronted God saying, I will ascend to heaven and place my Throne above the stars of God, meaning above all who were in heaven. He said that he would sit on the mount of the assembly on the heights of Zephon; he said he would ascend to the tops of the clouds and make himself 'like the Most High.' He continued, "I will take over heaven, I will be God." He refused to do what he was 'created' to do. It should be remembered that Lucifer, regardless of his talents and abilities, was still a *created* being.

Studies of Lucifer show that it was apparent that he was initially garbed as a high priest similarly to the Jewish high priest, complete with a breastplate and knowing that he was in charge of the worship services, which included protecting the holiness of God. Lucifer held the highest and most exalted position of a created being in Heaven, but it was not enough; so he decided to follow through with his rebellion. We now have the beginnings of the fallen priesthood.

At this time, it is necessary that we mention that before Jesus what existed was the Order of Levi and Order of Aaron priesthoods. These lines of the priesthood became corrupted after which God made it necessary that God the Divine Masculine of the First Person came to earth and establish a new priesthood to which even Abraham paid tithes. That is why Jesus said to the Pharisees, "Before Abraham I Am," because being the Divine Masculine of the second Person of the Holy Trinity, He is identifying Himself first as the son of Melchizedek but most importantly as the Son of God. This is most important to the Eeshan Religion as you will come to see that only by establishing a new Priesthood not under the Law of man, but According to God, so to identify the Lamb's wife. **"For the priesthood being changed of necessity there is also a change of the law. For He of whom these things are spoken belongs to another tribe from which no man has officiated at the altar. For it is evident that our Lord arose from Judah, of which tribe Moses spoke nothing concerning priesthood. And it is yet far more evident if, in the likeness of Melchizedek, there arises another priest who has come, not according to the law of a fleshy commandment, but according to the power of an endless life. For He testifies: 'You are a priest forever 'According' to the order of Melchizedek.'" [Heb.7:1-17]**

As no Man had officiated at the altar, Jesus and his Wife would be recognized as co-Saviors and Redeemers and the Kallahs and other women could officiate the worship services and not be "breaking the law of man."

LESSON 140

JESUS' PRIESTHOOD

Another reason why Jesus had primary control over his Priesthood was because he was not of the bloodline of the established priesthood. His was from the Order of Melchizedek, King of Salem, priest of the Most High God, or simply saying Melchizedek *was* the Most High God. By the mere fact that Jesus was God and man, a definite downward spiral was initiated, and men began turning away from God from early on; therefore, God the Father (Divine Masculine of the First Person of the Holy Trinity) deemed it necessary to establish the Order of Melchizedek prefiguring the unbloody sacrifice which would follow the bloody sacrifice of the Son of God, from which Jesus' Priesthood would be destined to continue (and which disconnected Him from the established priesthood of the time). It is important to note, however, that to claim that as he was God the First Person Divine Masculine and instituted this Eternal Order of Priesthood, Melchizedek, "king of peace," would have to be without genealogy, nor Mother or Father, or beginning or end of days. In other words, all that was written about Melchizedek provided enough proof to show that he was in fact God. As God, He would never allow His Son to enter into a corrupted priesthood (corrupted because women were not viewed or treated as equals; thereby denying the duality and sacred balance of God). God cannot tolerate corruption.

His reputation was said to be so great that he was feared among men and that the Patriarch Abraham himself gave a tenth of the spoils to Melchizedek. Those who were the sons of Levi who received their priesthood under Abraham, had a commandment to receive tithes from the 'people' according to the law, that is, from their brethren, even though they had come from the loins of Abraham. But Abraham, whose genealogy blessed them (his priests, and through them, the people) and who had the promises (the blessing of his seed by God) paid homage to Melchizedek. In other words, Eeshans believe, that beyond all contradiction the one who one would think is the lesser (Melchizedek) is blessed by the one who is believed to be the greater. Why? Eeshans believe that Abraham was drawn to meet with Melchizedek in the desert. Upon his arrival he recognized Melchizedek as the God who gave him the blessing. Abraham therefore was awakened to the unfathomable Paschal Mystery of God's love and his role towards the coming of the co-Redeemers. One must understand the importance of this revelation since the Law in place would cause mortal men to receive tithes, but here, *Melchizedek* receives them, by Abraham, who by giving of his tithe to Melchizedek, witnessed that God lives. Even Levi, who receives tithes, paid tithes through Abraham, showed that before Abraham was the 'I AM' Melchizedek. So Eeshans believe that before God, so to speak, even Levi was destined to understand this Mystery even though he was still in the loins of his father when Melchizedek met him.

In summary to this point, we want to remember that Abraham was blessed by God so that his seed would continue a line specifically ordered for the purposes of God; Melchizedek, being the Masculine counterpart of the Divine First Person, came into the picture, to deliver to Abraham the "Blessing," which in effect couples the masculine blessing of Abraham's seed with the feminine blessing of the Divine Presence. This balance would then be gradually strengthened even up through and beyond the Exodus event, when the tribe of Levi (set apart by God to serve as priests) would serve before God on the part of the Israelites; however, as one will see in Israel's history, due to corruption, the angels came down and removed the "Presence" (Divine Feminine of God) from the Holy of Holies in the Temple. Without this Sacred Balance, it was certain that Israel would go astray so that by the time Jesus came into the picture, the entire nation of Israel, as intended by God, resembled nothing of that original Divine Plan.[171]

It was thus God's plan by the coupling of Abraham's seed with Melchizedek's bestowing of the Divine Feminine that the Sacred Balance would begin to take root and build, through time, a new and enlightened humanity that would have served as the Light for the world placed on the stand; however, due to willful corruption and stubbornness, the Divine Feminine Wisdom, was taken from Israel as a divine punishment, which in turn led to the patriarchy taking deeper root and affecting all generations to come, throughout the world.

Eeshans then present the following question: if perfection was through the Levitical priesthood (for under it the people received the Law), what further need was there that another priesthood would rise "according to the Order of Melchizedek,"[172] ignoring the order of Aaron?

The answer, according to Eeshans, is that it would be the basis for the future acceptance of Gentiles, men and women. Eeshans clarify that, at that time, though it was said that Gentiles were included, it was only under the Noahide Laws, which were not equalizing, but gave of an honorary but subservient role. Women didn't have the place to be recognized, in any case, except by way of the judgment of the husband with regards to politics, religious organizations, and laws. That is why for the priesthood to be designated by God it had to be originally

---

[171] We find here that Eeshans conclude the following: That the "Divine Presence" is the Divine Feminine of the equation, which is the Eternal Wisdom, the Sophia Perrennis; this element is essential to live by and without it, only the male human consciousness will lead and create inevitably an unbalanced patriarchy. Without Wisdom to balance and provide light to guide the way, Israel founders on its own and falls into further corruption. The Urim and Thummim cannot be any longer understood, the prophets are not heeded, and this is how Jesus came and found an Israel hopelessly misguided. This needs to be kept in mind when we see how Peter, who rejected and sought every opportunity to deride Mary Magdalen—Wisdom/Sophia Perrennis/Divine Feminine—he would thus be confined to his own rational human consciousness and be subject to all the errors of mind he was capable of, including being at the mercy of his fallen nature. – Ed.

[172] Hebrews 7:11.

changed, since it had to come out of a necessity, and this would also denote a change of the law. Thus, we have the new law under Jesus, which serves as a liberating dispensation from what had become of the Old Law; this is where and why Peter was hesitant to follow Jesus' specific instructions and teachings regarding the Old Law.

Coming full circle, He of whom these things were predicted (Jesus) would have to fulfill scriptures, and likewise He would, in fact, identify himself with the words, "Before Abraham I AM." Whereas, the correction and Sacred Balance would have to begin with the return of the Divine Feminine. She would, therefore, come as the one who would be the perfect Altar, and an Altar at which *no man has officiated*.

It is evident that our Lord arose from Judah, of which tribe Moses spoke nothing concerning priesthood. This is because, Eeshans believe, Jesus came from the Order which is transcendental to the twelve tribes of Israel, which would be more than fitting for one who was the author and creator of the tribes in the first place (God). And it is yet far more evident if, in the likeness of Melchizedek, there arises another priest who has come, not according to the law of a fleshy commandment, but according to the power of an endless life. For He testifies, "You are a priest forever 'According' to the order of Melchizedek." [Heb.7:1-17].

This is all very important to remember as even though Jesus' Priesthood originated in the pure eternal Priesthood of Melchizedek, and once corruption appeared on the horizon of his own Priesthood, via 'Peter and his succession of apostles,' *the Order of Melchizedek was withdrawn from the world as was Ishvara.*[173] Only upon the fullness of time, when (also, in End Times) the Divine Feminine returns, will she re-establish the

---

[173] Eeshans maintain that history repeats itself, for as we see, as mentioned, that the "Shekinah" or "Wisdom" was removed from the midst of God's people in the Old Testament—and mirroring, or rather, *'foreshadowing,'* the crisis to come in the wake of Jesus Christ. Once the decision is made to 'put the hands to the plow' living in full responsibility 'for' the life given one by God, it should never (indeed 'must' never) be withdrawn. Just as the corrupt Old Testament authorities and teachers withdrew unto themselves over time, Peter followed suit and with disastrous results, despite Jesus' attempt to change his focus. – Ed.

Timeless, Divine and Sacred Order of Melchizedek, and this will continue with a priest who was chosen to carry on the Priesthood alongside the Kallahs, since it was intended to be 'According' to Melchizedek; and bring back the Sacred Balance to God's people. This Priest will "not" be of the blood of Peter (which was poisoned), but from the bloodline of Melchizedek and under the auspices of the Divine Feminine, who encompasses the Divine Masculine.

Though Lucifer's breastplate was the first, it was designed to protect God's plan for humanity, proving God's omnipotence. Interesting to note as proof of God's[174] love was that Lucifer's breastplate had only nine stones, whereas the High Priest had twelve gems. Lucifer was, indeed, missing the fourth row.

Since each gem was for a specific purpose, but unknown to him, there was a fourth row, which would never be put on the breastplate. The stones from the fourth row of the breastplate held specific powers. God, all-knowing, saw it fit that this row would not appear on the breastplate. This row had jewels that by God's omnipotence were safely secured and for good reason. The jewel for Issachar was deliberately taken away since this was the jewel of burden bearer, and this was already earmarked for Jesus. The jewel of Gad was missing and thus Satan's future punishment was secured. The jewel for Asher was also missing, which meant Satan will never produce royal seed. So, you see, God, being all-knowing, allowed Lucifer to exercise free will, but being omniscient, as well as omnipotent,[175] was already steps ahead of him.

---

[174] Because God never placed it in the breastplate, knowing what Lucifer was going to do.

[175] All powerful, because this subject matter became the substance of a power play between God and his former highest-ranking angel.

LESSON 141

Section IV: The Emerald

The story of the emerald is almost as fascinating as the previous chapter because it mystically connects to the rising again to life and the resurgence of the Eeshan Religion. *The emerald gem is the most interesting of all the precious stones.* Originally, this gem was placed in the furthest place in heaven, encased and guarded, since written upon it were the words capable of transforming[176] whoever held possession of it. It is said that if given to one who lost everything given to them by God, they would gain access once again, to their lost inheritance.

It is said that when Satan found out about this gem, and about its value, he immediately believed it should be his. He believed that if he succeeded in replacing God, he could use this to gain access to God's inheritance, which he believed was due him. The emerald, however, held unfathomable secrets unbeknownst to him. Aside from it being the source of extreme power, it had ancient alchemical words inscribed on it, and when those words were spoken, they gave the power to change a substance into a living thing, even a physical being without change in appearance to the original substance. This would later become known as Transubstantiation, but not as the church teaches; it was rather, by a similar process, how Jesus turned water into wine in Cana that brought with it a quickening of chemical, distillation, and fermentation contained in His breath. This process, and the most sacred alchemical words, when completed, touches on the operations of God. These words, if placed in

---

[176] One might add 'transmuting,' 'transcending,' 'transubstantiating,' since it includes all of these. – Ed.

the wrong hands, are so dangerous that it is no wonder why God split the emerald, the gem of royalty, and had the emerald pieces hidden away since before time and secured, until they were pronounced between Jesus and Mary on their wedding night. That is why Eeshans know that what has been said to be the words of transubstantiation are incomplete, since they are without the Divine component, and are said within the guidelines of the human consciousness. Only she who has been brought back is in possession of these words.

On the other half of the emerald was inscribed the encrypted name known only by God,[177] of the One who would have the power to crush the enemy. Little did Lucifer know that it would be the woman who would crush the head of the serpent.

Lucifer demanded that the angel guarding the emerald to take the gem from its encasement. He then had it placed at the top and center of his crown for all to see. Even though it was forbidden for any angel to allow access to this gem, Lucifer was so powerful that not one other angel would dare confront him or bring an accusation before God against him.

The emerald was placed on Lucifer's crown, but upon his fall from heaven the gem fell out of the crown, and as it crashed upon the earth it split into two. The two pieces were then hidden from Lucifer, as well as everyone else, until which time it would find its way to the person chosen by God to be its recipient.

He who was called the morning star and true musical instrument of God, and who led the worship of God, had now chosen to refuse to serve and/or worship God his Creator. It was time for him to act. It should have been easy, since no angel dared to challenge him, making it easy to overthrow God's power in heaven.

The one he didn't count on was an angel called Michael. Lucifer couldn't believe the audacity this angel had. He was a 'nobody' with regards to power or stature. Yet, his boldness and disregard for his own safety would make the takeover easy, since it was obvious that God would be left with only the weak and fearful to guard his throne. All others

---

[177] Written in love, which is why Lucifer couldn't read it.

would go with Lucifer. War was inevitable between those who were loyal to God and those who were loyal to Lucifer.

Michael, being an angel who was covered with eyes, had a tremendously divine point of view where he, as an enlightened being, could see love and joy in Adam and Eve. He viewed delusions as inexhaustible, and thereby would fight to end them. Michael rose above all the other choirs of angels; but most of all, his steadfast love for God became his battle cry, "who is like unto God,"

Lucifer lost the battle to Michael but not before declaring war on the transcendental beings and their offspring, who robbed him of God's love. With a perverse cry, Satan vowed that he would return and take his rightful place as son of God.

LESSON 142

SECTION V: SATAN DECLARES HIMSELF GOD AND HELL HIS KINGDOM

Scorned before all of heaven and those who hailed him, the embarrassed Satan set out with a vengeance to destroy the only-begotten, divine Child with a divine masculine and divine feminine duality; knowing that the Child was one with, and equal to the Most High God, First Person of the Trinity, worthy to be worshipped, was bad enough; but the 'created,' transcendental humans who mocked[178] Him by their favored status was the greatest insult of all.

Why is this important? It is very important when you come to realize that Lucifer, with all his gifts, was still an angel, 'created' by God, so he was not infinite. His ubiquity was not the same as the omnipresence of God, but the fear of him still radiated everywhere.

After he and his followers were exiled from heaven, having been narcissistic and delusional, he immediately convinced himself that he was, indeed, God's rightful son. He then made hell his domain. His twisted, narcissistic, self-absorbed corrupt logic caused him to devise a plan to turn the transcendental beings away from God and prove himself the one worthy of being worshiped. How would he do this? First, he had to break the bond between the couple and God.

After watching the behavior and frequency of the reception of the spiritual food given to them and how the time they spent with God in the Garden kept the couple strong spiritually and immortally, he had laid

---

[178]To Lucifer they were lesser beings and he was of the highest order of angel, but God had a connection with them the he (Lucifer) could not have.

the groundwork for diminishing their visits with God, which would also limit the daily nourishment deemed dire to their spiritual strength. To offset this food with another similar food would bring about mortality then and forever more. Once they no longer had access to God's Spiritual Food they would grow weak in their transcendental consciousness, leaving them vulnerable to 'thinking.' Satan displayed great strength in corrupting reason.

The transcendental Adam and Eve, that reflected God's image and likeness, were made in God's image and likeness as true soulmates by the immutable law of spiritual love and this freed them 'into God' with the begetting capability due to the blessing; before God, who could separate into male and female, they were like an androgynous being, since, if seen by the naked eye, they would be very difficult to determine which was which since their love was clearly seen through each and the other.

You can only imagine the insanity that welled up deep from within Lucifer at the creation of these earthly beings, who were not only created in God's image and likeness but were also the 'apple' of God's eye. He knew the love God had for these transcendental beings, since they were placed above him—he who had likened himself to God—and the need to destroy them was imminent.

Though it is sometimes thought that angels have no gender, they, indeed, in fact do. Just as God made us in his image and likeness, so too he made angels; and this is evidenced in ancient writings and with plausible proof by identifying them by names, such as Michael, Gabriel, Raphael, and Uriel.

LESSON 143

Section VI: Lilith and Eve

After being thrown from heaven by Michael, along with losing his place alongside of God, Lucifer now became Satan. With the loss of his priesthood and status in Heaven, he now proclaimed he was God. He desired worshippers. He wanted the duality that God and the transcendental beings had, and because he coveted offspring they would be his adorers. Satan hated the bond that man and woman had and their ability to reproduce in their image and likeness. He watched, with interest, the woman.

This brings us to yet another red flag as to what is true and what isn't regarding the 'woman' we have come to know as Eve.

There are many legends out there regarding another woman named Lilith. These claim that she was originally Adam's first wife, who was created from the same dirt as Adam. Because of this, Lilith was said to have thought herself equal to Adam, and refused to be subservient to Adam; and, therefore, God exiled her and created the second woman and named her Eve. Eve was taken from the rib of Adam to be his helper.

Eeshans believe that in order to keep the patriarchy intact, the story of Lilith was invented, or borrowed, from other religions to secure the fact that a woman's place was to be subservient to a man. Using this rationale, it would be safe to say that if Eve was the original female separated from the androgynous being, this would then cause havoc among patriarchal religions. A new name and a new story had to be concocted making the first female, who was the true Eve, an evil woman. This new name would be borrowed from an ancient text where Lilith was a demoness.

Taking this name as one who would represent the curse on any woman who declared equality to man, this declaration of equality would be seen, henceforth, as an evil punishable under God's law.

As the story goes, refusing to be subservient and wanting to establish her own rights before God, could and would not be forgiven her. With that problem solved, the real truth, the real Eve, was not only hidden from the masses, but she would never be mentioned by any decent woman ever; and the Eve reimaged by the Patriarchs would now be the template for women forever more.

So, you can draw from this account that the story of Lilith was utilized to keep in the consciousness the reason why women needed to be kept 'under thumb.' This makes for a masculine God and the origin of inequality.

The true story of an Adam and Eve being first one being then separated by God to reflect God's Sacred Balance, image, and likeness, as well as equality and duality, was hidden away, never to be unearthed.

Eeshans believe that in order to protect 'man's' image of God and themselves that (men,) as God's sons, would not only make this new Eve subservient to Adam but also there was a need for a backup story as to how she was created. The story of the woman being taken from Adam's rib would substantiate this. Going with that conclusion, the story of Lilith would be the evil reference source, since any religion who was rivaled by women/females who would *ever* want independence and equality with men/males.

The story worked in all respects for patriarchal religions, regarding Lilith's disobedience to Adam, and solidified God as all-male, and all men were made in 'his' image and likeness, even though every other creature fell under the Laws of the Universe. Back in biblical times, there were, depending on the context, masculine, feminine, and intersex variations, just like today. All other human gender relationships outside that of heterosexuality fell under the Book of Leviticus as abominations, and the female was, according to Peter, "Not worth life." Yet all these who were not masculine were obviously created in God's image and likeness despite the fact that men opposed them. That is why the comment from the Pharisees regarding Jesus not seeing any difference in gender, creed, appearance etc.

but His seeing just a child of God, was brought up. The Law did not accept these so-called sexual incongruities. Eeshans present how laws should not define what makes a person a person be it in professional, social contexts, or religious circles, especially in the treatment of women, as it is the case in point. These other variant genders always existed, but it wasn't until present times that they were brought to light. This is so due to the breakdown of biological gender and sex-based social structures to include gender roles and other social roles, or 'gender identity.'

Though presented as truth, the story of Eve in traditional scriptures serves to show only that *God was the source of discrimination against women*, and is guilty of a creation story pointing to man as Eve's origin. God is truth, and if Jesus is God, both the Old Testament God and New Testament God should share the same love and belief in the equality of all humans. Could this be yet another reason why Jesus rebuked the Religious authorities?

If God had the desire to create transcendental humans to reflect and manifest sacred equality and duality, God would have had to make them male and female, since all of this falls under the laws of the universe and physics. We, therefore, concur that the traditional story of Adam and Eve, as it is presently interpreted, is false and an insult to God.

Looking at Lilith's story, from another perspective, what if there was a 'Lilith' and 'she left' Adam because of the way Adam treated her as a subservient person, could this then be reason enough to make their marriage null and void or be the first divorce? This provides other safeguards for males. What if Adam was a very imposing and hurtful man after the fall? What if Adam wouldn't let Lilith be with God because "he" (Adam) was the male, and because since he believed he was the first created he would not allow her to go to God except through him? What if, as some believe, she couldn't express her love of God, or her opinions on anything relating to God, and, thus, was forced to blame God for being created unequal to Adam, and walked out on Adam? Based on what you want to believe, either version was just an inverted account of the real story of Adam and Eve, and these were legends that were actually used to give credence to the traditional story, which was created just to counter, if it became necessary, Eve as Adam's equal and his soulmate.

God indeed created Eve at the same time as Adam, and again we cite:

Geneses 1:26:
Then God said after the androgynous being was divided, **"Let's make human beings in our image and likeness, to be like us."**

Geneses 1:27:
"God created humankind in 'God's' [corrected] own image, *in God's image, they created "them;" male and female they were created.*"

Lilith will always be labeled the go-to explanation why women need to be 'controlled' and 'domesticated,' and will be known as the dangerous demoness of the night to all patriarchal religions, while she is also blamed specifically for the origin of the hatred of men. Though this traditional Story of Adam and Eve is present in the Torah, and was said to be written by Moses, one must wonder who Moses' sister Miriam really was, after we read that she had been punished by God for talking to her brother Aaron, regarding Moses' choice to leave his wife, and why she couldn't speak to God directly as Moses did.

But because of this story of Adam and Eve, there will always be a Lilith in the shadows, since the message it purports regards any woman who claims equality with men before God. What this heresy also does, is it serves to make women in the bible automatically guilty if any woman is caught being in any sin with a man, i.e., especially adultery; and the man will always be innocent, despite the fact that he may have pursued, stalked, abused, raped, or molested her.

Throughout history, even in other Old Testament writings, there have been stories to upset any woman's desire to be equal, prove her abilities, further her status, or challenge the status male quo. To draw on modern language, women, who through the years have been ascribed as "crazy" … are, due through error in reason, independent of the speaker's action, thereby dismissing her feelings as irrational, while simultaneously absolving...men from responsibility.[179]

That is why we present the following scripture. This was the story, derived from the above, of the seven women in **Isaiah 4:1:**

> **And there will be seven women will take hold of one man and say, "We will eat our own bread and provide our own clothes; only let us be called by your name. Take away our disgrace!"**

Here we find another safeguard to rid from the minds of any woman who dares not marry under Mosaic Law, and risks being labeled an 'old maid' if the law is not followed; as well as the fear that they will be alone their whole lives. We see it as a prophecy of the women who declared they will follow Jesus as the seven Kallahs of Mary Magdalen. You see when one wants to hate there are many ways in which to hate; but God would not have created woman to be evil. Even to this day, according to Orthodox Jewish custom, it is wrong to be unmarried when one is of age to marry because it goes against the direct commandment of God in the Old Testament to 'go forth and multiply.'[180]

The true story of the androgynous being separated into two, male and female, makes Eve a strong equal and independent woman, confident in herself and in her sensuality, and being Adam's soulmate, like Adam, was free to exercise her free will.

---

[179] Cf.www.huffingtonpost.com 2014/04/16/

[180] It is worth considering that in light of the above, *Jesus wasn't criticized or charged with being unmarried*, which would be a sure proof of his rebellion against the Commandments of God and Mosaic law, and a certain disqualification for his being the Messiah. Even in modern practice, Jewish religion sees willful celibacy as a sin, against God's commandments and expressed will. Jesus was called "Rabbi" and rabbis were married. The strictness regarding the mandate to marriage, even to the point of arranged marriages being the norm in Jesus' times was apparently not used against Jesus, which overwhelmingly suggests it was likely plain knowledge that Jesus was, in fact, quite married. – Ed.

Later you will see how they made a mutual choice for the physical world, and how, afterwards, it was discovered exactly what they had lost via delusion. It would be Eve who, by her soulmate's love, finds her strength, enabling her to stand before God with sincerity and honesty, and willing to accept whatever the consequences were, even if it meant leaving Paradise. This would, indeed, fit with the couple being made in the image and likeness of God, and in their being soulmates, and other very interesting facts in legends showing the woman's cyclical thinking in opposition to the very linear thinking of Adam, which, in other words, reveals a balance.

Why was this story important with regards to Satan? If you are thinking that it is important because it shows the extent of work and effort it took to keep 'women in their place,' you are right. But, there's more. It gives women "no defense" and "no rights," even before God. It denies Sacred Balance. It also shows how Satan began his plan and continued it up to include Peter, and how Jesus knew the ramifications and dangers of this mindset and how it was totally opposite of Jesus' advancements. These were exactly what Jesus identified in Him when He said (paraphrasing), "You are a stumbling block to my work (referring to Mary's role). Why is Satan so interested in you?"

Satan's jealousy/envy of the human's relationship with each other and with God grew as the duality of God and Adam and Eve was ever present in his sight.

Satan devised a plan to destroy this relationship. He was clever enough to know that if he could cause them to make decisions apart from God, this would certainly offend God and the couple would fall out of God's grace, which would then result in losing all they had been given, just as Satan had lost everything.

PART VI

LESSON 144

Section I: The Plan is Laid Out

Satan devised a plan. His first hurdle would be to weaken Adam and Eve's trust in God and eventually destroy the relationship. The advantage he had was that he could make himself 'appear' via delusion, any way he wished, to include those attributes of God; certainly, with his power and gifts, he could 'appear' to be omnipotent, omnipresent, omniscient, and omnificent, since he was the great impostor.

Satan was kind to the couple, and walked and talked with them in the garden. He spoke with them as a couple, and sometimes he spoke to them independent of each other. He used his time with them wisely. They developed a friendship and a bond amongst each other. Yet he always felt the need to show his expertise and equality with their God, and that he 'knew' everything. He would often ask them how beautiful he was. He tried to make them feel suspicious of God by eluding to them, subtly, that perhaps God was not telling them the complete truth about things in order to incur doubt about what God had instilled in them from the start.

Satan watched and envied the innocent love of God's Creation. His greed and envy grew as these two were satisfied in each other and with God. He coveted both the love between Adam and Eve and their love and worship of God. He became very jealous of the love of the woman for this man; and he tried to mimic from memory how he would approach her.

First, he tried taunting God with the accusation that these humans were not truly free for they only knew God's desires. Satan taunting God? How could this be? Believe it or not, Satan could still have contact with

God, and not in the way we understand, but in ways that we cannot comprehend, which are found in the Universal Laws, as not only a directive, but as part of life with God. Satan cannot exist without God. Satan, cursing his loss of power and glory before God, claimed that if they were truly free to choose, that they may choose differently. Thinking that if he imposed his logic on them they too would choose to turn away from God. Sound familiar?

Satan watched the couple closely. More now than ever he wanted all that made 'them' complete in the eyes of God and each other, since, in his eyes, their offspring was only the fruit their duality, and not the fruit of their love. Secondly, he certainly didn't want them to bring forth more adorers of God, but he wanted adorers for himself.

Satan being the male gender, with fallen male characteristics and attributes, and a flawed reasoning and intelligence, was not only unable to accept truth but rather also lied and became more and more delusional. In being separated from God there was no allowance for the gift of being a 'soulmate' to any female; there was no empathy and he was filled with narcissism. Any of those fallen angels and demons that worshipped the former Lucifer, could take a physical form, but could only manifest through someone or something who would make a pact with them.

As we said, seeing God's creation of humans, and their many blessed gifts stemming from the innocence they received, caused rage within Satan; for never would he have these things, nor could he beget offspring to worship him.

The following is taken from Eesha's private writings:

One needs to understand that the fallen angels do have desire for lust with humans, which is perceived through ego. For every 'innocent' there is a demon. It was after the fall that Satan would need only a likely candidate to have his child and obtain another like himself, thus increasing his chances of regaining the 'blessing' of God. One should know that any offspring of Satan would be considered outside of God and outside of wedlock. Heed this warning however, **that this is not to be interpreted as children born out of wedlock are evil. The fallen angels, once**

sentenced to earth, had relations[181] **with humans and their offspring were Nephilim. But it all started with Lucifer first.**

That is why after the fall it would be because of Cain, who was born of the evil one, that the stories of the Nephilim being the offspring of the "sons of god" and the "daughters of men" would be found according to Genesis 6:1-4.

It stands to reason that Satan's plan would be:

1. First to have the couple fall from grace, resulting in the development of the gross physical body.
2. Next, it would be necessary for them to eventually lose their desire for one another. This was necessary for he could not entice the woman if Adam was enamored with her and she with him.
3. The fall to the physical was necessary and the woman would need a physical body that he could impregnate and get "the blessing" he needed.

If one was to ask what were the two most powerful virtues that were lost that haunted, and will haunt him, for eternity, they would be innocence and love.

That is why Satan is out to destroy innocence to this day. Having no power to beget a child with a female demon, and with the desire to destroy innocence, his desire for a child nevertheless grew. But there was more: Satan stumbled on the fact that Adam and Eve shared the blessing and this united them strongly to God. In order to get "this blessing" he needed a child.

His plan would involve destroying both their innocence and love which in time would plant the seed of destruction, since their innocent transcendental life would provide a cause of death through entropy when they became human. From that moment on, he would see the fruition of

---

[181] While this mirrors in an inverted sense the Father's relationship with the Blessed Mother, the precise manner in which this occurred (since the demons are not embodied physically) is not known. – Ed.

his plan, which would destroy life at any stage by making life expendable for any reason, especially at conception.

His hatred was for the couple and it would grow even greater towards their descendants after the fall, who exhibited the innocence of that child-like love of God, because this would constantly remind him of what he never had and couldn't have, which vexed him because he considered himself as powerful as God. This continues even in these present times, right in front of our very eyes.

As time goes on, with so little belief in God, and with a people being faithless, we witness how Satan being the Lord or Prince of the world, could in 'these times,' be perceived by so many, to be a kind of 'savior' of humanity and planter of the seed of light over the true Savior. Abortion and euthanasia are not a means to end suffering, rather, his tools are used to end life, innocence, and love. *(Under Eeshan Transcendentalism, we believe once the truth is made known and true equality is restored under a Sacred Balance, these actions will be greatly lessened and used only in extreme circumstances without the use of force or violence. Women will champion the cause by 'uniting' under the Divine Feminine, since she will bring justice and accountability back into this world.)*

Satan, thinking he was being subtle, would approach the two transcendental humans, and by his actions, thought he was taunting God about the couple's inability to exercise free will. This is not to imply that anyone could taunt, or accuse God, of having a weakness, but rather God allowed this to become the couple's test of obedience to God's unconditional love. (We must also see how God allows Satan to continue in his plan, being the depraved and delusional being that Satan is, since even a greater display of his expulsion is made apparent in the end.)

Once Lucifer used his free will to sin against God, he was immediately judged. Corruption had already entered his heart and killed it. With that, Lucifer's mind became unbalanced and delusional. He began to cause pandemonium for everyone he put his sights on. It is safe to say that he is the most perfect and the purest example of one who is insane.

PLEASE HEED THIS WARNING. THE FOLLOWING IS DISTURBING AND SHOULD ONLY BE READ BY THOSE WHO ARE 18 YEARS OF AGE AND OLDER UNLESS

ACCOMPANIED BY AN ADULT. THIS CONTAINS GRAPHIC INFORMATION but the author feels these details are necessary when describing this being.

Satan is pure evil. He feels powerful all of the time. He seeks pleasure in separating humans from God and though he may begin, subtly, if one does not repair or seek grace for these offenses against God, or neighbor, Satan can and will attempt to influence them to greater and greater degrees of sin. He encourages his potential followers to see the bad in all things (and how everyone including those people around them, are belittling or making fools of them.) He makes them feel, as through wrongful or tragic situations they encounter, they have no way out. Once he has convinced them that he could help them, he begins with revenge. He encourages them to indulge in rituals that include mortification, and sometimes under the guise of repentance before God so they won't 'lose their souls.' He is destructive, including being intensely and 'sexually' gratified by extreme acts of hate and violence. Having no physical body of his own does not eliminate this psychopathic personality. Those who are influenced by him are prone to different types of sexual deviations to include pedophilia, frotteurism, and exhibitionism, and may say that they hear voices. All these give a false sense of "godly power over their victim." They confuse these things with love, since Satan does not know love; but **though these are characteristic of his influence please remember: Even to witness such people who seem to possess one or all of these issues, seek a professional and report it. Do not try and do anything to cause a worse situation. No one cannot go out and act as an expert, or judge against another, because one feels that someone they know is 'satanic.' That is for the police, the doctors, and the specialists to determine.**

Satan's version of being 'free' is the absence of laws; and free will is a choice that should be accepted by God, whether it is in favor of God or not; and so should not be held against those who use it apart from what are God's directives.

Satan's offenses included the transgression of the Law of Oneness and Correspondence, which declare that everything is connected to everything else. In this case, everything was connected to the 'All' who is 'God.' What we think, say, do, and believe will have a corresponding effect on others and the universe around us. It was 'not' free will that Satan proposed at all; instead, it would be a veiled suggestion to the humans, Adam and Eve, to confuse freedom with lawlessness. The misuse and misunderstanding of free will would then cause chaos and destruction.

The Universal laws affect all things. There are seven laws to be precise. Some split, and therefore arrive at ten, but for the sake of avoiding splintering off into other topics, we will say there are ten. The first three are immutable, eternal laws: these can't ever be changed or transcended. They are Absolute. They have always existed and always will exist. The next four are transitory, mutable laws, meaning that they can be transcended, or at least be 'better used' to create your ideal reality. This is not to indicate that you should ignore these four laws, or attempt to defy them, because even if you do they will still govern your existence. Your aim should be to master all of these seven laws, and learn to transcend the mutable[182] Universal Laws, which, through their practice, maintains harmony and peace. These were all brought to the light in Jesus' teachings. Though you would expect these to be judgments based on common sense that lead to a higher intellectual transcendental being, and based on simple perceptions and facts, one must remember that inflicted perceptions, or influences, by a source, or sources, that seem logical, can easily trick one who is innocent into evil behavior or bad influence. Anyone who is innocent and good doesn't look for what is bad.

So, though one may not see how all of the Laws apply to the real story of Adam and Eve in the transcendental world, you will find how they ultimately apply and play out in their physical life together, thus affecting all their descendants *to include humanity today*. So, God allowed the couple to be tested—but why?

First of all, Adam and Eve were enlightened beings, yet they did not always have to deal with the comparative knowledge of good and evil as we do, since their existence was in Paradise, and our existence is in exile. Not having to deal with this on a daily basis, and given their relationship with God, they based their choices on what to do with what God asked, or not to do what God asked. Could their obedience to God stand

---

[182] Kotsos, Tania. "The Seven Universal Laws Explained." Mind Power from Mind Your Reality, www.mind-your-reality.com/seven_universal_laws.html.

up to temptation after never having the need to experience deception and consequent invasion on a daily basis? Would this test cause them to test their boundaries and grow to do things on their own? Don't forget their spirituality was strong because of the blessing, the Sacred Food and Drink, and being in the Presence of God, in a place where all was in harmony, was this not such a bad life to have, at all?

Well we know that the traditional story tells of how the test began with a tree which God told them of which they were forbidden to eat (Genesis 2:16-17). If God did not place this tree in the midst of the Garden they would not have the chance to exercise free will. Being free they were (and had to be) able to make choices and decisions. Though they had the inkling of what was right and wrong, they had never experienced the outcome of a bad choice to the gravity of what they were going to have to face. God, being Creator, would naturally desire their choice to be to love Him, and not to become complacent in their love seeking the Giver and not just the gifts. Regardless of the reason, this esoteric study differentiates fate from destiny.

Fate implies that one allows life to continue on a preordained course, never challenging, wholly accepting all that happens; whereas, destiny allows one to make decisions and choices, which may change the outcome and shape one life. Adam and Eve's exile out of Paradise, however, was the result and consequence of their choice and not fate. It was a misuse of free will, and this determined their destiny.

It goes without saying that it was by 'God's allowance' that Satan would be able to test Adam and Eve's freedom to choose the life that God intended for them and distract them from each other or from God. The 'why' to this comes later in the purpose behind Jesus Christ as Savior and Redeemer.

With what could Satan possibly tempt a couple, since they basically had everything? One must remember that Satan operated on corrupted reasoning. Watching the couple for quite some time, and knowing their innocence and love for each other, would be the angle by which he would approach them. For what is opposite of love, but lust? He would introduce our first parents to a new kind of "love." Couple that with his jealousy and envy, and you have a perfect set up for which to fuel his desired plan.

Satan's tool would be to use his darkened spiritual power. He would abuse them with it, and they would never have a clue that they were being groomed for a fall from grace.

One needs only to think how a predator would entice a child to get the gist of the mentality of this being. A predator's goal is to lure and manipulate a child into believing they love the child more than the parents or guardians do. They use whatever personality is necessary that emotionally replaces the trusted guardian in the child's mind. What causes the most damage is the trust the child willfully gives to the predator. This causes the guilt and shame, since they believed the predator over their parents who truly loved them.

PART VII

THE TEMPTATION OF ADAM AND EVE

LESSON 145

Section I: Satan Continues in His Plan

Step one was for Satan to come on the scene and appear as a beautiful 'divine' being, since he had to convince them that he was a 'son of God.' Secondly, Satan had to convince them he was equal to God by virtue of the fact that he was God's 'son;' and thirdly, he had to convince them that they had nothing to fear.

One must also remember that Adam and Eve were not prisoners of Eden, nor did God dictate every move they made. They were not chastised, since they pleased God in everything they did for each other, their begotten children, and the other divine beings they encountered. There was no need, nor were they compelled, to tell God everything they were doing. Walking and talking to God, and eating the spiritual Food and Drink were second nature to them; it was a daily choice.

Their parental duties gave them overwhelming joy. Filled with innocence, meeting another beautiful being who claimed to be from God, they would not see anything wrong, nor would it arouse suspicion.

Filled with his selfish desire to take back from God and corrupt all that God loved, Satan now viewed Adam and Eve as a game, and a hunt.

He could have spent many day, in fact months (this is meant only to serve as a measure relative to what we can relate to, since time did not exist yet) could be spent with them, getting to know their likes, dislikes, dreams, and desires. He spent a lot of time breaking down any possible barriers that would, or could, occur in order that the couple felt comfortable with him and have no reason to not trust him.[183] With his unabashed confidence, he knew if he persisted, he could convince them to rethink the things of God, all with a little twist. He knew he could get them to become curious. This is all part of the game. The reality is that he used anything, including God's love, to groom them to become victims.

He literally made them laugh and told them love stories. He talked about God's love for them. He talked about 'real' flesh. He talked about a love embrace very different from what they experienced. He would talk and talk about it as to arouse their curiosity. He would make it sound as though he himself experienced it. Fascinated, the couple continued to seek knowledge about this kind of "love." They would question this beautiful being, who took advantage of his uncanny godlike affluence over their innocence.

He would implant into their minds the imagery and fantasy of eating the fleshy fruit from the forbidden tree and knowing things that only God knew. He would talk to them as to precipitate conversations about their thoughts regarding why God didn't want them to eat its fruit. He would mimic them as being just as curious about why God forbade them access to this tree, and offered reasons for God's command such as: perhaps this God, as male/female consorts, didn't trust them, and would He still love them if they knew as much as He did, almost as though there was another God whom they were serving.

He would tempt them with stories of his power and grandeur, always with an inflated sense of self-importance, along with his desire to be adored and admired. He presented just enough arrogance for them to see him with wonder and love of God, until they openly expressed their feelings to him.

He subtly discussed the possibility of God's earnest desire for them to define themselves as maturing by exercising their free will without their being told that. In other words, he used whatever he thought would work. If at first he didn't succeed, he would just keep trying.

Satan continued on with his plan since the desire in him to have a child was increasing. Day after day he watched how the children would

---

[183] Cf. Methods used by online predators.

come to be in the presence of their parents in what he construed as a form of idolatry.

He *needed* to be adored and worshipped by God's greatest creation. In order to do so, he had to remove the sacred from the sacredness, and weaken the strength of their transcendental union; thus, he would start talking to them about how an embrace that produces the most intense 'sensual' pleasure and one that would be the most fulfilling experience in their entire lives. He told them of its powerful bonding effect, and powerful feeling of closeness and togetherness, than any other act between two humans, which no doubt would honor God. Working every 'angle' he could, he introduced the thought that there would be no doubt God would see how much they loved him, especially if they did so on their own without God commanding it. His intention was to pique their curiosity.

Remember, they had no reason not to listen, or entertain the thoughts and desire for a closer relationship with God and each other, because they were transcendental, and they were inclined towards God and the love of God. They lived by desire and the blessing. They loved each other and was blessed by God and his directive; they were fruitful and multiplied their love with children. Since to love each other as God expressed mirrored the love of the eternal consorts. God's desire for them to love each other unconditionally showed God's parental love for us, as one God in three persons, sharing in each other's divine gender.

LESSON 146

SECTION II: SETTING THE STAGE

Next, Satan had to break this transcendental love bond they had with God, so he articulated the second phase of his plan. Since Adam and Eve were only familiar with expressing a love that was transcendental, because they had a transcendental pseudo-physical body, and it was not like the gross physical body we have now. Originally, the first being's body was made of light, with a subtle body covering. These bodies resembled the resurrected body of Christ. That is why Christ prepared food, and ate with his friends and others he encountered.

To reiterate: when the being was separated into two, God brought upon the earth a beautiful mist just like the one used when the Androgynous Being was *first* created. Next, by way of vibration (rib) the subtle body was divided into two, as well as all that was housed beneath it. Then a second covering was put on top of the subtle body and light bodies. This 'skin' had a kind of pliable cartilage, and not bone, which framed the light body, and was made up of slightly lower vibrations since it had to carry light energy. Try to understand it as a skin made of light that was also resilient enough to give form. Since this skin was made of a kind of vegetable matter, they were inclined to eat vegetables for enjoyment and the sensory experiences of taste, touch, and smell, which also served to carry light throughout their body covering, making eating very enjoyable. God nourished the original beings with pure energy. These were now blessed with light bodies that would be nourished with the spiritual bread and drink we spoke about earlier. They were thus connected to the divine light but in the form of Food. (One wonders if God, as Creator, already had brought about a simple, or primitive, template from which the gross physical body can be built in the event the couple doesn't heed the directives regarding not eating of the tree. Thus, it would make sense that they would be told the consequences of eating from the "physically" organic tree, since the tree was not transcendental.) In keeping with fueling their transcendental bodies with light, their light bodies, or transcendental bodies, were more inclined to be nourished by the vegetables, which are producers of light, as well as fruits and other delights (including vegetables), but were not limited to them.

Knowing that he had to break the 'transcendental character' and consciousness of their love in order to separate them from God, Satan then began to occupy a lot of their time, so they spent less time with God. He would share food with them to mirror God's daily nourishment. He would give them fruit, water, and wine. Next, he would continue to entice them with talk about a body that did not contain a mystical self-transcendence within it, which interfered with this embrace, but would maintain the transcendental love outwardly.

There was just one last phase left to his devious plan; and that was to lure them away from a 'dirt' from which the vegetation was first used to create the original being, which God then used for the covering of the pseudo-physical body, which did not imprison the light body within. One should reflect on the fact that the dirt God used to create the bodies of Adam and Eve was untainted and resembled a dust sometimes dampened by a dew. This dirt originated from where the 'Tree of Life' grew. It, too, was in the Garden, and its soil was of a natural substance, which, along with God's breath, was the supernatural power, which in and of itself lent witness to the fragile nature of humanity.

This substance created an impenetrable protection for the light body, providing this light-absorbing covering, which provided for the fullest absorption of the divine food. In turn, we have the beginning of a heart consciousness, which, via love, called them to rightfully worship and serve the Lord.

It was this covering that God formed to not only house their light bodies but also give way to their specific genders. The dirt of the forbidden 'Tree of Knowledge of Good and Evil' was the necessary component for the formation of the new gross physical body that would have to be designed after the fall from grace.

One must remember the intelligence of Satan knew the original vegetative body would be affected by contact with minerals and matter that would slow down the vibrations of this light-absorbing body in order to form a gross physical body, which was necessary to change everything. It would change the cartilage to bones, and the flowing of light to the flow of blood. This body would have to form everything necessary for life outside the transcendental. That is why the gross physical body would then need organs and systems to replace the transcendental workings of the light bodies Adam and Eve were created with. Just one bite would activate an organic matter, organic substance. Next, Adam, being the male, would complete the process by secreting another organic material that would begin to break down, forcing digestion of the apple. Simultaneously, the body would take on a physical form, and because God breathed life into them to begin, since this organic body was, indeed, forming, God's breath sped up the process of bringing about this carbon-based transition from the transcendental body to this new very different physical one. Just like when Jesus turned the water into wine, there was an unfathomable immediate change made with the rapidness of the change, which also involved the carbon.

There were systems put in place for the assisting of the digesting of the fruit, which would begin the process, and continue to add other systems and changes necessary to form the flesh organs, along with its entheogenic properties, which you will see are provided when Satan gains control and uses the Guardian Serpent to complete the other physiological changes. Ultimately, it would form a body that would become mortal and would not have the transcendental quality, and it would no longer be able to exist on God's nourishment, since the Food and Drink, indeed, *was* God. It was for the reason God forewarned Adam and Eve about death. This body breaks down in death, because unlike the transcendental one, it entered entropy, and with entropy comes viruses, bacteria, and fungi.

Once the plan was in place, Satan had to impart to the couple various reasons for them to think about and arouse their curiosity. It was important for him to get them to become 'curious' about the forbidden Tree. Up until this time, the Tree was far from their thoughts; however, as one is aware, all it takes is one to introduce a trigger to get another person to think about something of which, originally, they had no previous interest.

He used triggers like: perhaps the tree was forbidden because of its 'fleshy' fruit, since he knew this was the key necessary for this kind of love experience, since it would provide the kind of 'flesh' necessary for the fall from their healthy God-fearing natures. (This too would explain why God would become flesh and the Eucharist of the Marriage Feast would involve the physical Presence of God.)

He would entice them with delusions of a grandiose lovemaking. Not underestimating the power of their relationship with God, he watched them. Satan noticed that their consciences call them to observe the similar method of reproduction of the 'flesh animals' around them. Satan could see Adam and Eve's minds becoming confused. Since not only did they witness the resemblance of this act they were hearing about being carried out by the animals, but they also knew, and witnessed, since the beginning, how the off-spring of the animals were not inclined towards loving and adoring of God as their begotten children did. One must remember that they did not possess a modicum of intelligence but, indeed, possess a significant amount of innocence; and they did not know, or fully understand, this kind of love.

Still, by the way Satan described this love via reasoning and logic, it was very compelling, and made everything he said difficult to doubt. Weighing all they had been told, Adam and Eve did observe, and were in agreement that their children were children of the light, and were unaware of malice, similarly as the animals did not know love. Though the animals reproduced, few, if any had a connection with their mates and offspring. There was another difference: the animals did not have a connection with God that filled them with a desire to worship God. There was also a definitive lack of reasoning and choice to do other than what was instinctual. Knowing that this was a biological act, with a total absence of emotion, feeling, or love, caused Adam and Eve to feel that they needed to further probe and question the difference between the 'expression of love' Satan was talking about and the act into which the animals entered. This was important because if there was a greater love they can offer to God, this is what they wanted to do. It would also be their intention to bring this love to their children.

Knowing he had to move quickly, Satan explained there was a high probability that God didn't want them to 'gain knowledge' that would give them this understanding that was equal to God's; so, he could see why God didn't want them to eat from this tree. He planted another little seed in their consciousness, which was that this knowledge would allow them access into the love embrace that God, as eternal consorts, shared themselves.

The sole purpose of Satan's discussions, and teachings, was to coerce the couple's thinking, and what better way than to lead them into temptation by continually piquing their curiosity. Again, they would not see anything wrong, nor have any reason not to explore a closer relationship with God and each other; and they wouldn't be chastised for listening since God did not dictate their every move.

LESSON 147

Section III: Spiritual Food

As it is understood from our purely human perspective, in line solely with our gross physical bodies, we are what we eat; if we eat a balanced diet, with veggies and fruit, we possess a healthier mind and body than if we ate sweets and processed, high fructose food, drank, and took drugs.

The Sacred Food Adam and Eve ate daily from God's Garden, kept them transcendentally and spiritually strong and close to God, since it contained the Presence of God, which, at that time, was of a spiritual essence. As we described in the beginning, this food had the consistency of a very airy bread, or manna. It was a transcendent food which was designed to nourish their Light Bodies, since they had neither bone, muscle, and organs as we do, nor a body designed to process the kind of food we eat. It contained within it light and shadow to make sight of it possible; but had no real weight, since it was created of 'spirit and light,' The drink, too, was like 'air,' yet it possessed visual properties and wetness like that of a holographic image. These were not meant to fuel a body of lower vibration.

Their bodies were created with the purest mist and purest soil that, as we said, "mirrored the resurrected Body of Christ," in that it was sacredly formed by God, and was breathed into by God, and made up of vibrations and light. Their skin, a kind of vegetable matter consisting of pliable cartilage, and attracted to vegetables and fruits of every kind, satisfied them, and was satisfying enough that it did not make them curious, or "inclined" to even desire the forbidden Tree. Nor did they know that the

'Forbidden Tree' was made of a different substance, and fruited with a sustenance different than the other trees.

Their attraction to vegetables and fruits was mostly for a sensorial enjoyment experience, and not to stay alive as our bodies dictate, since they were immortal. Their desire was for the life and love, to be for, with, and in God, and their desire was 'good,' and wholly sacred: since all good things came from God. This is why all they gave to God was in the spirit of thanksgiving, and there was no need for sacrifice.

When Jesus came, after his bloody sacrifice, there was no need for physical or animal sacrifice, since he and his wife would bring back the Sacred Food and Drink as the transcendental/light body needed. Also, the animal sacrifices were stopped by God, since animals were not involved in the fall from the transcendental. That made no sense. That is why God asked that Abraham take his beloved son, who was his and Sarah's miracle son when he was one hundred and she was ninety years old, to a mountain to sacrifice him, prefiguring the death of the 'miraculous begotten, Divine Masculine/Son of God,' since it would require a God who became human, and not an animal, to reconcile God with humanity.

Eeshans believe in this connection in that it's important to keep in mind the biblical account of how Abraham, after passing his test, is told by the angel not to harm his son, and is then directed to take the ram that was caught in the bushes to use as his animal sacrifice. Aside from the usual commentaries regarding the interpretation of the ram as being a symbol of pagan deities and/or Egyptian religious imagery, etc., one might instead look to God's use of the Zodiacal sign of the ram, Aries, which would prefigure the month of March in which Jesus, the lamb of God, would be sacrificed.

The event where Abraham received the blessing from Melchizedek took place before the event where Abraham was to apparently sacrifice his son. So, once in the possession of the blessing, it would now be that Abraham would have to live up to the value of the gift Melchizedek (God the Father) gave him; it also denotes an understanding that Melchizedek and Abraham had a unique parental connection with both "Fathers" having unique "miracle" sons that would serve the purpose of fulfilling a Divine, but not fully revealed, plan. That is why God stopped Abraham from enacting an imperfect sacrifice, even though his heart was in the right place; whereas, only God could affect the perfect sacrifice, which would satisfy what was required to open the door to Paradise. God so loved Abraham that Jesus acknowledged him before the Pharisees, when He said, "Before Abraham, I Am" ... acknowledging that He, Jesus, was the perfect sacrifice, since He was God the Son.

Back to our previous discussion, it should be reiterated that the bodies of Adam and Eve were not comprised of the kind of 'flesh' we possess. That is why to experience this 'love' Satan spoke about had to stress a different 'type' of body. One that required our kind of flesh, a mortal flesh formed by lower vibrations, which could not rely on a spiritual nourishment to strengthen it alone; but unbeknownst to them, a body which would cause a disconnect from the spiritual and require physical nourishment. Why? This body would imprison the higher vibratory light body, thereby cutting the light body off from direct contact with God and all that belongs to God. This would keep them from reconsidering their choice.

This was the plan. This Tree, however, not being the Tree of Life, but the Tree of Knowledge of Good and Bad, was absolutely necessary, since this one would be the catalyst to form a body that would require a kind of food that was just necessary to feed this body. It would provide light, but one which would only mirror the light that was necessary to keep the body alive. This is the light that surrounds the cells in our body, and when nourished with light foods, helps safeguard us against a lot of diseases. This light is still carrying the template of the transcendental body from creation; and because God so loved us, this was planned so that we would come to learn and understand that what makes up the template and substance of our bodies, which would then be used to bring us back to understanding the transcendental in these end times. Once understood, we would find the true meaning regarding the union of our light body in Jesus' 'Light of the World' directive. Otherwise, if his words were unheeded, it would be found only to be that of a temporal nature void of spiritual satisfaction and immortality.

One must remember that Satan was always (and still is) at an advantage, as he was created as a very powerful angel with tremendous intelligence, before he grew in a narcissistic level, and willfully threatened, challenged, and disobeyed God. At the moment his reasoning and intellect became so twisted, mutiny followed. He became evil personified, and at the moment of expulsion, went in pursuit of revenge. There were no secrets regarding the havoc and disorder that would be caused by ingesting the fruit of this tree. God told them: "You shall not eat of the fruit of the tree that is in the midst of the garden, neither shall you touch it lest you die." (Genesis 3:3.)

PART VIII

"THE APPLE"

Salvation Comes with the Bite of a New Apple

LESSON 148

Section I: "The Apple"

The plan was an apple? Why an apple? The apple holds a rather mystical meaning: mystical in the sense that it is the symbol of the 'Divine.' An apple is said to symbolize wisdom and guidance. Apples are mentioned in the Song of Solomon 2:3, Psalms 17:8, Joel 1:12, Proverbs 25:11, and, of course, in Deuteronomy 32:10: "In a desert land he found him, in a barren and howling waste. He shielded him and cared for him as the apple of his eye."

If you cut an apple in half, you will find what has become known as the Esoteric Pentagram, which means and represents the androgynous being and a perfect marriage. A little different meaning, we are sure, then what you learned over the years.

It is true also that only a few are blessed to understand the esoteric. These same few enlightened also understand the Eschatological time of the Lord; this is mentioned because what began with an apple will end with an apple in the most mystical way. Eschatological times are upon us as the Divine Feminine has entered the world, once again bringing with her a change of consciousness, so needed today, and is prefigured in this amazing fruit, which holds so many mysteries within.

The omnipotent, all knowing God, placed within the apple the image of the enlightened and perfect androgynous being. What is unique here, it that the fruit's seeds, its offspring, are not true to the parent; in other words, they do not propagate love nor are they connected to the parent in any way. In a way, the apple carried with it the story of the fall of Adam and Eve from a transcendental consciousness to the imperfect human consciousness. So, if we look at this fruit and God's warning to not to eat of this tree, we understand why the Apple deserves its rightful place to be mentioned with regards to the fall of our first parents, and why it was placed in their garden. The identification as Jesus and Mary being the new restored 'Apple,' *represents the only begotten Child being true to God, and bringing about a connection to God, and life for their children*, and this shows how the Fruit of the Seed of God, as loving Parents will propagate and be fruitful in the fullness of time, since Jesus died on the tree, and together with his wife brought life for their children.

The Eschaton God, the fruit of the uncreated perfect and only-begotten Child of God, the First born of the First born, the One who is like the Son of Man and Gift of the Divine Feminine, is, indeed that 'Apple.' That is why Eeshans believe that the apple was more than just a random fruit to be used in what may have been God's most perfect demonstration of love ever.

In order to fulfill Satan's plan a food was needed. Yes, the *apple* was used because it is a 'fleshy' fruit. Within the fruit as we mentioned is the figure of an androgynous being. This "fleshy" fruit would have to be consumed in order to accomplish the above, and, again, it was destined to be consumed *for its seeds are not true to the parent, which symbolizes free will.*

Without the Spiritual Food, the couple's strength, and steadfast love, would be compromised and weakened enough for them to become enticed by the near occasion of a life different from the actuality, which was the reality of their transcendental life with God.

Over the centuries, many argued whether or not the fruit ingested by Adam and Eve was indeed an 'apple.' First of all, as we said, the 'apple' is the image of the 'divine,' and its seeds are 'not true to its parent.' This is another way that God plays out what happens if this fruit is eaten. It proves that all was recorded should the couple choose to not listen. Eeshans believe for all the reasons above, and possibly more, that, indeed, it certainly was an apple that was growing on the forbidden Tree.

Many authors have written, following a common sentiment, that the fruit was a fig, i.e., claiming that: a) the fig is said to represent 'desire,' (cutting open a ripe fig, with its pinkish purple flesh, one sees folds that are said to resemble the private areas of a woman); and b) apples did not grow in the Middle East where the garden is believed to have been located. Well, it sounds right, at first, especially after Jesus cursed the fig tree for not producing fruit and cut it off.[184] The fig, however, is not mystical. Eeshans believe the fig could not be the fruit of choice in the story of the Garden because the fig can produce its own fruit, and, therefore, is not ideal as the allegory for humans being 'grafted' into the Christs. Anyone who has the knowledge of what tree the original fruit came from, and how, after the Fall, *grafting would become necessary* should understand that the apple, more than any other fruit, embodies more completely the mission of Salvation that Jesus and Mary came to complete. Weirdly enough, regarding how apples actually were growing in Paradise, if the above is true, it was the original tree that never lost its fruit; since the fruit remained attached to its parent. This is likened to the fruit that is connected to God because it never dies. Why do we believe it was an apple? Eeshans answer that the apple is, and always was, considered a mystical fruit and the Garden of Eden was a divine place. We also see that within the garden, and written in Genesis, God placed within the garden trees of all kinds, and that is why some believe it could've been the fig tree: since Jesus used the fig tree in His teachings, and because Adam and Eve covered themselves with fig leaves (which readers may naturally think came from the tree from which they ate). Eeshans conclude that after the couple became 'physical,' the "fig" tree was used by Jesus because it took on that very sensual meaning (as was the reason for the fall), but as both genders are represented in the fig, and because it can reproduce without another tree grafted into it,[185] it is not, to Eeshans, the most fitting fruit. The point we are making here is that from the standpoint of the human consciousness, humans have no need for a savior or redeemer; but from the transcendental point of view, they would see the need to be 'grafted' into the Christs,[186] for they could not survive on their own, and thereby would absolutely need a savior and redeemer for life everlasting. That is

---

[184] Cf. See the adorable little book called "the Untamed Garden."

[185] The whole fruit hanging on a tree are said to resemble male genitals, whereas the crack that opens across the middle and opens has been likened by authors and philosophers to the female body's intimate organs. Also, the Phoenician word for 'fig' is *pagh*, meaning vulva. – Ed.

[186] One must seek Christ in order for Christ to be grafted into the soul. – Ed.

probably why it was written in the verse in the Song of Songs that "The fig tree has ripened its figs. Arise, my darling, my beautiful one, and come with me." So, while the "apple" was chosen as the fruit for transmutation, the fig could well have been symbolic of what had taken place *after* the apple was bitten. That the moment Adam and Eve became physical, 'sex' and not *love* entered their lives and they now experienced a physical, sensual pleasure. In perspective, and given the reason for the only-begotten Child's mission, it is likely to be the reason why Jesus cursed the 'fig tree' when it didn't bear fruit.

The apple seeds, however, for all intents and purposes, were to represent our first parents going against their "Parents" warning, and, of course, the consequence which, as the seeds are not true to their 'divine parents,' therefore, death of that line is inevitable, unless the plant is grafted into another, such as in the case of the co-Saviors. The reason the seeds are said to carry death, is because they were always said to contain minute quantities of 'amygdalin,' which is cyanide when metabolized. God, in mercy, saw to it that asamygdalin is associated with Satan and death, and the 'amygdala gland' is what Mary Magdalen is associated with. Since this is a limbic system structure that is involved in many ways with our emotions and motivations, particularly those that are related to survival, it's no wonder why.

As we said in the aforementioned text, the apple tree's "fleshy" fruit represents life, yet its seed represents death. To accomplish what Satan wanted, the fruit had to be consumed in order to accomplish the above. Since its seed is not true to the parent, we can see how one of the consequences would have to be that which would continue down the descendent line, in order to break the relationship of God and his children. Yes, all of the children down through the lines are thusly affected. This is the reason that Jesus had to bring back the true natures of God by use of the term of endearment to God the Divine Masculine as *Father* and introduce his Mother Mary as his *Mother*, espoused to his Father. Secondly, the story is told of how the seed of death, or entropy, came to tell the story of Adam and Eve's decent to the mortal. Thirdly, in order for the 'apple tree' to continue on it would need to be 'grafted' to another tree in order to live and bear fruit, which then would become the 'new parents,' and that identifies Jesus and Mary Magdalen as the New Adam and New Eve, and how we are the children of the only begotten Child of God.

It would be from this tree that the male would, due to the mutual decision (Adam and Eve's), forever show his connection to his wife and to the original choice in order to complete the 'mutual' act. It has been said that the outward sign of the completed act was the "Adam's apple." It would appear to represent the bite of the apple lodged in man's throat. Since it would have had to been Adam's ingestion of the 'fruit' in order that the fermentation take place after Eve to complete the 'oneness' of the two during the transcendental marriage. Why then would there be an outward sign only for the male? It took the ingestion of both for the plan to work as they were soulmates, since it was from his secretions that fermentation was necessary, the outward sign rested with him as the counterpart.

Due to lack of time spent with God, and using the Bread and Drink that Satan was implementing to lure them away from the spiritual bread they ate daily, the couple now seemed to begin to reason through, and possibly entertain interest in, what they were being told. Satan then logically told them that if God so loved them, surely, they would not die. He emphasized the love God possessed for them, and how he would most assuredly stop them if they were to enter into anything that would harm them. He asked, "What is death anyway? Is it not just the end of something and the beginning of something new?" He continued to tell them how this physical love was so powerful an act, it would most likely cause them to constantly desire it, and this alone would surely be something that God would want for them to share. Adam and Eve, being the balance of one another, decided they needed time.

Eeshans believe that Adam and Eve, being soulmates, would naturally be very interested in this curious expression of love, but also that as part of each was in the other they were endowed with Sacred Balance, and this served as a conscience which prompted them to wait. They also possessed their love, and, of course this always strengthened their resolve with each other.

LESSON 149

Section II: "The New Apple"

Before continuing, it is important that we interject some 'food for thought.' By this we mean that by the eating of the first 'apple' (which was beautiful to look at but was, indeed, the forbidden fruit), began the fall from the transcendental away from God, eventually creating a struggle between a male from female, since this transition occurred with 'the ingestion of it.' We now take a look forward at the "New Apple," and how the mutual eating, or ingestion, of this solidifies the love between humans and God and male and female in marriage. It was because of the miracle of the Water being changed into Wine at Cana that the mystery of the subsuming of each other on their wedding night was revealed.

In a most remarkable way, the relationship that Jesus and Mary shared with God as a result would not only become the human sacrifice necessary to reconcile humanity to God, but they then became the 'fleshy' fruit necessary to take the physical back to the transcendental. This sacrament of the Eucharist did, in reverse, what the 'apple' did. The apple that Adam and Eve ate brought them to the physical. The return of this Spiritual Apple ingested, would cause an almost immediate 'repulsion' to anyone who was without a doubt, primarily governed by a (strictly) human consciousness, with firm ties to the Judean religion of the day, which prohibited 'blood food.' But, you see, though the Eucharist is the Body, Blood, Soul, and Divinity of the only-begotten Child, it is, in fact, the 'Apple of God's eye.' This phrase, and others using the word 'eye,' such as 'eye opening,' refers to what someone sees, or realizes, regarding a person or issue. The 'Apple of God's eye' reveals the most obvious part of the mystery, and, that is, if we look into someone else's eye we see our reflection. The only-begotten Child is reflected in God's eye, and if one looked into God's eye you would see the reflection of the only-begotten Child. That is why God's voice spoke on two other occasions the words, "This is my beloved Son in who I am well pleased," and "This is my beloved son, who glorifies my name; listen to him." (Matthew 3:17 and Mark 9:7, respectively). This mystery is in every way transubstantiated, and, without a doubt, fits into this section regarding divorce. For it is how God sees the Eucharist, as both Jesus and Mary, as one; and though this Eucharist is the body, blood, soul, and divinity of the only-begotten Child, transubstantiated, the 'appearances' of bread and wine remain. There was no reason for any of those who walked away to be scandalized, since they need only to have moved from the human consciousness to the transcendental, to the 'belief' that this is truly the "Bread come down from Heaven." It violated no law regarding the 'eating of a human body, or drinking human blood,' but the turning away did violate Christ's, since this was *his directive*.

This affixes the marriage and union found within the Eucharist of the Marriage Feast of the Lamb and His Wife as one through their marriage, which pleased God, who saw them as the reflection of the union of God the Divine Masculine of the first Person of the trinity and His Wife who is eternally One, as husband and wife; and the fact was that "NO MAN" had the right to try to separate them, especially in this 'holy union of the Eucharist.'

Truth be told, it is the above context that explains why "What God has joined together, let no man put asunder." Here we must interject a wrinkle in time where we are transported to when Jesus was asked about the topic of divorce. Was this in reference to man's opinion of marriage or was it just a conjecture? Or was Jesus addressing the sacredness of the only human way a male and female can be one as soulmates, promising to enter into marriage, both equal, both supporting the other, as God intended? At that time, the issue of divorce for the man was the issue at hand: meaning a man could file for divorce a lot easier than a woman because rarely was their union about what defined marriage at all. At that time, marriages were mostly arranged, and were not about love as we think of it today. In fact, a man could claim infidelity, or any number of issues, against the woman and it would not be challenged.

To move ahead to present times, we see that man is still in control and the wife is still, more or less, subservient. Annulling the sacrament of matrimony is as easy as claiming (as is the most common reason given) "lack of due discretion" when entering into the marriage. Even by the church's own standards and definition of their sacrament, the institution of marriage has been erroneously imaged according to Christ being the head of the church and the church being His bride. In this case, Jesus is the 'head' of his bride, but the bride is an impersonal corporate entity, and not a person per se; furthermore, those who 'lead' the church as a faithful body are all men, i.e., cardinals, bishops, priests, deacons, etc. However much it is looked upon, it is not a sacredly balanced dynamic, exhibiting the dignity and *equality of spouses*, but instead reflects a man still *leading and ruling over* a woman. Thus, women in marriage are imaged secondarily, and not as equal to the men, even in the language 'man and wife.' Also, and just as importantly, it doesn't reveal God's identity and inner nature in the context of the sacred duality of male and female. Jesus' marriage to Mary, on the other hand, did precisely that.

So, as you can see, based on the Eeshan point of view, it was never about Sacred Balance when the church spoke about God, marriage, or any of the sacraments, for that matter.

One must remember that Jesus knew what those who were asking about divorce were thinking. His own marriage was always in the forefront of scandal because of Mary, and especially due to the closeness He shared with his wife. Why? Because it went against everything the Jewish Law was about regarding women. They wouldn't have cared if Jesus 'used' this woman for a man's necessities, but secretly so as to not incriminate Himself, or those with him. Peter, embodying this mindset, tried to get Jesus to understand exactly how her presence was taking away from the otherwise remarkable impression Jesus was making, and saw great potential for those who followed Him. He tried to offset the rumors he heard by appearing to have a great place with Jesus, an official place and being desirous of being the 'apple of his eye.' That is why he would, in effect, try to rebuke Jesus, and how publicly he would ask Jesus questions that could lessen the impact of something that Jesus would say that would upset the religious teachers and leaders. Each time the men were alone, Peter behaved almost as though he was helping Jesus teach by giving his opinion. Yes, he was desirous of that place with Jesus, that one could say that this 'place' became to Peter, like the apple of the forbidden tree was to Adam and Eve. Once Mary arrived, and took her place beside Jesus, Peter's quick temper would emerge.

So, it was no secret that Peter had his own issues, which were always centered around his greed and anger. It was obvious that he would have to try to get Jesus to leave Mary every chance he had. That is why it appeared that with this topic being discussed, it was a perfect opportunity to bring divorce and the justification for it, into the conversation. Mary's reputation was the perfect "reason," and if he could get Jesus to discuss the Law, he would have to mention these reasons unequivocally. In doing so, Peter could now proceed with many avenues from which to work to separate the two. Peter wanted his place with Jesus and his jealousy of Mary was growing.

Knowing Peter's heart, Jesus began to answer with a perfect entry for discussing the edifice of man's definition of love, and the weak foundation on which so many marriages were based at that time, as well as addressing a growing bone of contention that Peter had against Mary. He did so by using scriptures to show God's intention for the first created transcendental Adam and Eve, and how the reality of God was absolutely centered on these created humans. Mirroring the eternal consorts by using the language found in the creation of Adam and Eve, He began with: "Haven't you read, that at the beginning the Creator made them male and female." This was in reference to the androgynous being separated into two. Then He went on: "For this reason a man will leave his father and mother, and, united to his wife, the two become one flesh." So, they are no longer 'two,' but 'one flesh.' Therefore, what God has joined together, let 'no one' separate." Here he was addressing God's law regarding the true Marriage, which began with his Father and Mother, and then especially reflecting his own making He and Mary became One as per God's Law. This was important, since it directly linked to God's law that He and Mary were, indeed, one. Since human beings after Adam and Eve, no longer being transcendental, and now living outside of paradise, they, too, had to come to understand that both the male and female are found in each other. With this he looked at Peter, and those who looked to Peter as the person closest to Jesus, implying that no one could separate Him and Mary.

LESSON 150

SECTION III: TRUE LOVE THROUGH, WITH, AND IN GOD

UNDERSTANDING WHAT SATAN WAS UP AGAINST IN TRYING TO DESTROY THE LOVE BETWEEN ADAM AND EVE

The love that Adam and Eve shared did not lack emotion or gratification. In fact, it was a far greater experience than what humans enter into today, solely because they were pure and they possessed total focus and innocence. This was true love, since it was through God, grounded in God, and originated in God, with selfless, genuine, desirous love totally connected to God. It was so powerful a love; yet, with all its intensely mystical, self-transcendent experience, each time it began with a "kiss." This kiss was an absolutely pure and sacred "kiss."

This sacred kiss they shared would cause them to go into a state of rapture, or ecstasy, and they would be drawn out of themselves with a transcendental feeling, and they would experience three kinds of energy: an increased *awareness* of each other's energy, a *shared* energy of the two of them together, and a kind of *esoteric* energy, which completely surrounded them.

It was a dance with no beginning and no end, particularly as they were not in "time," Remember, time was the result of the fall from the transcendental to the physical. In *their reality*, there was only eternal lovemaking: meditative, expressive, and intimate. It enhanced their love, trust, and mutual respect using gentle touch, loving words, and extreme kindness that was also surrounded by the most beautiful music. It was the fullness of how you feel when you first fall in love, only more perfect and for forever.

It caused them to experience more depth and breadth to their love; for their lovemaking was not subject to age, gender, body looks, how the body moved, or due to pressure and control. There was no focus on a goal to achieve or anything outside of the experience of the moment.[187]

The was no pressure for satisfaction, since both lived for each other. What they experienced was exhilaration and luminosity, since they were full of and shed a bright interior light because of their connection with God. It expanded their consciousness and weaved together the polarities of male and female into a harmonious wholeness; thus, their hearts were as one. Most importantly, it opened the doorway to the Divine, who blessed this union unconditionally.

---

[187] Adapted from Yogananda, *The Second Coming*, Vol. II.

LESSON 151

SECTION IV: SPIRITUAL FOOD FOR ETERNAL LIFE

LOVE VERSUS SEX AND WISDOM VERSUS KNOWLEDGE

With their love being a gift from God, Adam and Eve entered into this mystical euphoria that sealed the bond of love and continued to influence them until the next time they were together. This love and the spiritual food God made available to them literally gave them the means to live forever. That is why Jesus taught about love from God's perspective and his own personal experience as being the highest of all virtues, since what they had linked their love to God's love.

That is what made Jesus' Bread of Life discourse such a profound teaching. It revealed how a marriage of true love seeks to unite this love through, with, and in God by means of the Holy Eucharist and, by this Sacred Union, conceives and begets the fruit of their love which is the transmutation of all who believe, and more importantly, which can only be described wholly as God's mystical intercourse with those who believe, since it is truly God's body, blood, soul, and divinity that sacredly and intimately shared with each of those who love, and, by faith, believe it is vital to life, knowing it is as vital today as it was then.

This mystical union of Adam and Eve's love is what literally gave them the means to live forever as pure organisms that kept their genetics pure and alive. That is how, as pure beings, they were able to reproduce by what is called the 'begetting' process. Through this transcendental union, known as begetting, they fulfilled God's command "to go forth and be fruitful and multiply," according to their transcendental natures, bearing God's imprint.

The couple was filled with the desire to walk in the area where God would avail them with the Sacred Food, very similar to manna, which was seasoned with salt, since it was a salt covenant with God and honey, since it represented the sweetness of God's love and kisses upon them.

This Sacred Food was very light and very delightful, providing the light which kept their souls nourished and their bodies transcendent, since they were dependent on God for life. This food was given to them by God (and Consorts) with joy. This 'spiritual food' is how they shared their love through, with, and in God. This spiritual food was that which was shared in God's garden, and being in God's presence brought a joy and peace that would be incomprehensible to us today.

Satan, who 'became' this 'beautiful' being, was actually what Jesus would have called "a wolf in sheep's clothing." This being, impersonating a 'son of God,' was incapable of love, being loved, and giving love. Jesus spoke of all kinds of love, of which the bottom line is: there is nothing more powerful than love. Love is more powerful than a purely conjugal drive, and fulfills the heart and soul; and we innately know, it is the most powerful of all human experiences. Sex alone, on the other hand, is purely physical and temporary. Love is shared; sex is a selfish act solely for the individual, again, unless it is part of a committed relationship and marital union. We have always been taught that love may involve sex but sex in of itself never involves love. The transcendental love as Adam and Eve experienced caused them to grow even more in love, and they always possessed this desire for each other. This mutual love for each other was so powerful. since it awakened in them the desire to share love as God shared love.

Unbeknownst to Adam and Eve, this was a *fallen* being with whom they were speaking, one who was selfish, self-centered, not capable of love, vengeful, and jealous of their God-like purity.

Though Satan displayed great knowledge he never exhibited any wisdom, since wisdom is God-gifted. The fact is, all the couple knew about Satan was that he said he was from God, a son of God. He knew information, had tremendous understanding and skills, both practical and scientific; but what they didn't know was that he was not capable of making sensible decisions based from a God-centered conscience, but was only capable of making decisions only out of revenge and his twisted perceptions.

A very good source of the difference between wisdom and knowledge is found in Ecclesiastes 7:12: "Wisdom is like the protection of money, and the advantage of knowledge is that wisdom preserves the life of him who has it." Satan lost everything due to pride. His knowledge without wisdom made him incapable of applying this knowledge to anything but revenge. This was due to losing his place with God.

His teaching about love, and the unique delight found in a 'flesh' that was different than that which covered them, fascinated them.

Satan continued to watch the couple closely. Since they spent time together and visited God regularly, and sharing the Sacred Food and Drink, he began to witness some 'doubt' and resistance in the couple's minds. Quickly, he began to work another angle. Approaching them as a couple was making him frustrated, since together they gained strength and their interest wasn't going beyond a certain point.

He decided it was time to distract them, thus, lessening their visits and walks with God. He also began bringing his own food and drink, which *looked* like the Spiritual Food and Drink' they were accustomed to. Its appearance was identical. While it was similar, it had no spiritual connection, or the kind of sustenance that strengthened their resolve. Everything about it had to be perfectly disguised so as to not pique their curiosity about it. It's amazing how this same plan was carried through after Christ. This is yet another link to the three Persons of the Trinity being One God, equal and balanced in every way.

Let's review what we have learned thus far:

We have a masculine energy that believes it is God and is responsible for a corrupt priesthood. Coming into existence is an unbalanced and non-sacred, unsanctified Eucharist, that resembles in appearance the Spiritual Food necessary for a transcendental life and love through, with, and in God, in order to cause a disconnect between the trusting children and God. Could this also be linked to why Jesus called Peter 'Satan,' and told him that Satan wanted to sift him like wheat? Could we be so blind as to not see that anything, that had a connection to the Eucharist of Jesus and his Wife, was either not understood by Peter or was ignored by him? Some examples are: Peter's inability to understand Jesus' Bread of Life discourse, Jesus asking Peter if he loved Him, and then saying, "feed my sheep," and Peter's noncompliance with Jesus' directive regarding 'not holding fast to cultural dietary restrictions' but being known only by one's love. Peter's human consciousness held him back from understanding this from his heart, so that he was not able to understand (or accept) this or Jesus' response to the case of the Centurion.

PART IX

LESSON 152

SECTION I: TIME TO SEPARATE SOULMATES

In the next phase of Satan's plan, we find that he needed to begin to approach each one independent of the other to break the 'bond' of solidarity.

One day, while Eve was walking, she encountered the 'being.' and it was more glorious than usual. He spoke to her about her love for God. He spoke of her love for Adam. He flattered her. He spoke of how as a son of God, her kindness, and love for God impressed him. He enticed her while verbally seducing her with his words. Excited, she ran and told Adam. Not understanding what this meant, Adam wondered why the 'being' would say such a thing to Eve, since God spoke with them both equally, but he had no reason to doubt Eve or suspect any wrong doing. Again, they truly loved each other and trusted in the 'being,' since it was from God, or so they were made to believe.

The thought that Eve was favored by God warmed her heart. Each had always talked of the special relationship due to the gender connection with God, and now, she, too, could share in a "special relationship" with the Divine Masculine God, as Adam could also relate to God's female counterpart and each to both genders of God.

Daydreaming, while Eve was walking, she found her way to God's side of the garden, perhaps led by her heart Consciousness. Not seeing God, she decided to wait for Adam before indulging in the beautiful Sacred Food that they always shared together. She was happy that she had come to the Garden. It had been a little while and she didn't realize how much she missed it. Upon Adam's arrival, they first gave thanks for God's graciousness and consumed the Sacred Bread and Wine. As God entered the Garden, they became even more joyful. Their time here gave them strength and clarity. Their hearts were gladdened, and their souls were filled with joy and elation.

Leaving the Garden, filled with love, Eve proceeded to talk to Adam about what the 'being' told her and the dream she had for these things remained in her thoughts. Eve did not ever want to offend, or deny, God; yet, the thoughts of the Divine Masculine that filled her, seemed to be beyond her control. She was most thankful that God, as both Divine Masculine and Divine Feminine, visited with them today. Talking and being in the presence of God brought peace and calmness, and they both felt complete again; and because of the joy that filled her heart, the topics discussed by the heavenly 'being,' in fact the heavenly 'being' itself, didn't enter her thoughts while with being God.

For a moment, she wondered why she and Adam hadn't discussed their talks regarding this Being with God but their love for each took her focus back to Adam.

This would be true, since if she and Adam were not being nourished the way God had designed, confusion and uneasiness would set in. Not knowing that what she and Adam had been receiving was an imitation that this would occur without their knowledge.

Adam became intrigued with what Eve was telling him. Remembering that the 'being' mentioned a new way God made love to their Consorts, which then made Adam curious about this "different" expression of love, which seemed to have been in the discussion the 'son' of God had with Eve, and which seemed to tantalize Eve's thoughts.

LESSON 153

SECTION II: WITHOUT GOD, THE MIND FILLS THE GAPS

Another time as Eve went walking, Adam, being curious, followed. As Eve approached the area of the Tree, the Guardian called out to her. It asked her if she was lost. This Guardian was known throughout the Garden for its great powers. Eve, not realizing she had wandered near the Forbidden Tree, explained that she had just stumbled upon this area, since she was daydreaming. The Guardian Serpent continued to engage her, since it rarely was visited because of its frightening reputation.

It quoted love poems, and beautiful music surrounded Eve. She felt almost euphoric as the Serpent continued to speak to her of love. Adam, hearing the music and Eve's voice, wandered near. Unaware of Adam's presence, Eve continued to volunteer information regarding what the 'being' had told her and Adam about a "special" love enjoyed by God; and she spoke also of her dream. She confided that she loved God with every ounce of her being. Little did she know that the Guardian was aware of the visits she and Adam had been making, since the Guardian was also 'divine.' The difference was that Satan had already been working on duping it as well.

You see, the Guardian loved music. It dreamed of the heavenly music that would reach and fill its most inner recesses, and calm its entire being with sweet harmonious tones, either in succession, or in combination with, its most treasured dream. It imagined this music would transcend its heart and magnify the colors buried within its very soul. The Guardian swayed to the rhythm of a continued stream of melodies coursing through the vortexes, and, if it had a weakness, that weakness would indeed be music.

No one surpassed Lucifer in music; therefore, as Satan he had already begun to befriend the serpent by having studied its desires. Knowing of the music that filled heaven, the Guardian wanted to talk to Satan about it every time he was near. The Guardian would spend all its time trying to imagine how it would feel if he were filled with music by the one from whom such music originated.

Dreaming of the music Lucifer enticed it with, whenever the Serpent began making its own music it would change the dynamic of the surrounding area. Its own music was intoxicating; and as it emitted tones, energy points called chakras responded, especially precipitating a transcendental state of being.

Adam, noticing Eve's behavior was unusual, called out to her. Eve, in her innocence, was suddenly awakened from her dream state, and noticed Adam was in close proximity of her, which immediately arrested her heart.

Eve explained what had happened. She told Adam how she felt the moment she came in contact with the Guardian. She asked him what he thought about the dream. She shared everything with Adam as they walked away from the Guardian and back through the Garden.

Eve talked about how she thought she was able to experience the sensual feelings he told them about in the dream, and how they were very different from what the couple shared but couldn't really describe. Intrigued by what Eve told him, Adam began to imagine what these feelings would be like.

The being, hearing Eve's conversation, felt satisfaction that what he told her finally spurred an interest, which seemed to have also evoked an equal interest in Adam. Needless to say, it wasn't long before Satan paid another visit. Immediately Adam began probing the 'being,' asking it about why Eve had felt compelled to talk to the Guardian. Following through with his plan, Satan expressed how if he would, indeed, explain it, they probably wouldn't understand it, especially given their 'nature.' He suggested that perhaps the Tree of Knowledge would better contain the information they were searching for. He suggested that it took a special knowledge, and they would not be capable of understanding such lofty thoughts, since they were, *perhaps*, 'limited by their transcendental state.'

Once again, the couple reiterated the command from God to not eat of the fruit of the tree. This frustrated Satan, and, again, he left them. He realized that their love for God was much more deeply rooted than he anticipated; and their oneness would be their protection against temptation. Even spending less time in God's presence and eating the mocked sacred food, there still seemed to be something that made it very difficult to change this mindset.

It became apparent that he would have to continue to spend more time talking to each one separately. Witnessing the tremendously deep love they had for God, Satan approached this challenge by introducing the seed of flattery and desire, but this time to Adam. So, one day, as Adam was going about alone, Satan approached him, and with flattery mentioned how easy life must be for Adam, especially with his having such a close relationship with God, as well as having such a loyal companion in Eve. Seeing Adam's demeanor glow at Eve's name, Satan had another idea.

Their visits with God must become fewer, and then they would not be so inclined to be with each other. Without the nourishment of the Sacred Bread and Wine, Adam daydreamed a lot more, instead of praying to or talking with God.

It worked. The fewer the visits with God the greater their spirituality was weakened. They began justifying their absence with God by rationalizing the time they were spending in conversation with one who claimed to be one of God's sons.

Having said this, one must remember that the more lax time Adam spent entertaining the delusions of Satan, the more negligent Satan became, as opposed to when walking in spirit with God. Becoming more undisciplined, regarding visits with God and the Sacred Bread and Drink, began to allow their minds to become a little more cluttered each time. When spirituality is weakened we can almost foresee how the seeds of Satan's corrupt logic and knowledge are going to begin to take root.

Even today, as mentioned in 3 Thessalonians 2:9, The coming of the lawless one will be in accordance with how Satan works. He will use all sorts of displays of wonder and power through the signs and wonders that serve the lies and all the ways that wickedness deceives those who are perishing. Today, even those who claim they love God/Jesus *must be open to hear the truth and turn to enlightenment*, and not buckle under the pressure of their religion that does not adhere to Jesus' directive as intended. Fighting against any spirituality that leads to God and refusing to see, hear, understand, and love what they just may discover is the truth is what hurts oneself and others. When this happens, a person won't admit that they are wrong. It's as though they are too proud to admit even to God that they were wrong. For example, so many times we do things that are hurtful, but because we don't face immediate repercussions we don't believe God will do anything. Because so much time passes we feel the universe is not going to follow through. Such was the case with so many priests, who, already retired, thought their offenses escaped punishment. Public figures, politicians, and celebrities alike have found this not to be the case.

When a people become like Peter, and refuse to 'connect the dots,' and choose what they want to believe in over what is true, and still refuse to ignore 'the signs' they have entered into this deceitful spirit … it are those that can't see when they are working against Jesus and when they are not in compliance with Him. We can clearly see how God has sent them a powerful delusion so that they will believe the lie. Why? Well, this is because they excuse themselves and do not repent; and God allows them to stay where they are. Sadly, the universe and God 'will catch up to them,' and what goes around comes around, eventually, in God's good time.

The lie, or fallacy, here is when people think that in choosing the Universe on their conditions, the Universe functions on its own without the Authority of the One who created it. When one chooses to live this lie, they reduce Jesus, or God, to a concept, or force, and they are already in danger of losing their soul.

Because the couple knew the necessity of spending time with God and the need for spiritual food, one can see that all of God's directives were spot on; but to stay spiritually strong, although that takes making a "choice," we see here how the 'other one' broke down the barriers of those things necessary, by deprivation, of the Real Presence and the Sacred Food and Drink. So, who really was to blame?

Eeshans believe that the couple was duped, and were deprived by Satan and forced to weakness. What happens next is directly in line with what Eeshans feel is happening with God's people today. In much the same way those who love Jesus were 'not' given what was intended not by their own fault, but it was the sin of the religious teachers and successors under Peter who refused to acknowledge their sin.

This is where lack of time with God weakens the transcendental, and subsequently could be manipulated by the "other one." Then are they truly guilty of the 'sin' of disobedience to God? One could say 'no.' Here Adam and Eve had the 'opportunity' to turn to God, but didn't, so we view this as an offense which could've been avoided. Today people have yet another opportunity to hear the truth and to get the fullness of what God desires for them.

Adam and Eve were not aware of the fact that the being who said it was the 'son of God' really wasn't, and, thus, 'chose' to spend time in *its presence*, thinking it was one and the same God; and they were under the impression that what they were receiving was the Sacred Bread they had always been nourished with, which was still another connection to the path taken under Peter and his successors. Jesus' followers wouldn't have a clue that they were only getting only half of the whole.

Adam and Eve's mistake was keeping their visits with this 'being' *confidential*, rather than telling God about it. If they sought God's advice, they could have been saved. There had to be noticeable changes in comparison to what they 'used' to do and how they felt with God, versus what they were doing and felt with this being. Often, when we begin to pull away from God, we begin to *justify* our actions and feelings; and confuse them with finding our own 'way' as if as creatures we alone can guide ourselves on our spiritual journey.

The decision to meet with them separately was becoming more and more to his benefit since Satan now had the advantage of feeding Adam's ego. Adam knew that God loved Eve equally, but Satan was introducing a new concept. While God had a duality, Satan made an effort in convincing Adam to see that God's Divine Masculine side chose Adam, because they had common characteristics. Viewing himself as God, Satan felt that this is a good time to begin encouraging Adam to see himself stronger than Eve. This was an attempt to impose his knowledge on Adam. Because Adam was still strong enough to dismiss such a thought, Satan did not pursue this endeavor. The seeds, however, were planted.

The couple continued meeting and talking, both together and independently, to this 'so familiar' mystical angelic being, who by this time, had become a trusted friend.

It was just a matter of time, however, before Adam and Eve began comparing the discussions they were having with the 'being' and decided they needed further advice. They concluded that there was one to whom they could go who could advise them regarding God and the things of God. On one hand, they wanted to prove to God that they were capable of understanding and resolving issues on their own, since Satan said it would make God proud; on the other hand, they never had encountered such intimate details regarding the loving exchange between the Divine Masculine and Divine Feminine of God.

The couple's love of God was still a threat to Satan's plan. Even though Adam and Eve began to waver, there still was the one thing that kept their bond of love from being totally severed. What was it? Satan had to find out what it was that protected this relationship with God. There was definitely something that he was missing, since despite his efforts, the two remained loving and protective of each other and their children. Whatever this was, it had to be connected to the reason that they were able to beget children and have their respect and love.

Satan decided to just ask about this. In a conversation with them, he commented on their children's love and 'worship' of them. He talked to them about the children's loyalty, and asked what they felt was the cause, or reason, for such 'idolatry?' Innocently, the proud parents exclaimed surely it was the 'blessing' imparted upon them by God. It was this thing known as the '*blessing.*' With this 'blessing' came all the secrets of 'creation.' It carried the unfathomable, mystical powers of the universe. God split this blessing between the two. Satan now had to get this 'blessing.'

Eventually the couple decided that perhaps the one they should go to would be the Guardian to seek some answers. They knew the reputation of the Guardian, as all the transcendental offspring of the first couple did. Why would Adam and Eve seek out the Guardian, rather than God, for advice? First, before Satan entered the picture, the couple never had the desire to seek advice from the Guardian, since they were nourished by God; and, second, they spent a lot of time in the presence of God. But, now they were entering a weakened state; and it was getting easier for Satan to coerce them into thinking that there was no need to 'bother' God. Now, with having interest in the forbidden Tree, why wouldn't they go to the Guardian? After all, the times the couple encountered the Guardian it appeared to be kind. Also, if it was guarding the forbidden tree, it would make sense that God placed it there because of its loyalty to the directive given to it by God, which was to keep everyone away from it. It provided protection of the tree, and, perhaps, it satisfied an intrinsic purpose of another kind—its being able to choose freely would serve as a pivotal part of the entire Lila of God.[188] Free will has *consequences*. In this case, we see that going outside of God, going to another creature for critical advice regarding a central-to the-purpose-of-their-creation choice, had untold ramifications. In the same way, and more in a current context, in this life the choice of having a spirituality, or no spirituality, also has its consequences, which are going to God, or not going to God, and is the difference between having a balanced conscience and one that is imbalanced.

We are like Adam and Eve, in that our choice to make decisions, based on a purely human consciousness, weakens our spirituality; and rather than turning to God, we feel that we are capable of making moral decisions, and justifying ourselves in rationalizing them by not 'bothering God.' This is precisely what the Serpent was looking for. If Adam and Eve's reasoning was weakened, the same issues we are presented with weakens ours if we do not rely upon our connection with God. We begin to seek out advice from anyone and everyone except God, in whom we should be connected. The Guardian was only being loyal to its directive. Being creatures that humanize everything, from laws to animals (pets and other creatures in the wild, for example), we do the same with God, despite God's telling us that the ways of the Divine are not the ways

---

[188] The "Lila" (Sanskrit) is the Divine Play of God, in this case the entire panorama of events involving the physical universe and human being's place in it. – Ed.

of humankind; also, we might tend to view a creature like the Guardian as having a mind, morals, and feelings such as ourselves. That's the folly of the human nature—to lack good sense and to embrace naiveté.

As the couple was coming into view, the Serpent Guardian called out to them. It already saw that the couple seemed confused and were in deep discussion. Recognizing Eve, it welcomed her back, with flattery.

Being a dual expression of good and evil, and mirroring the positive and negative aspects of male and female genders, we find as the couple approached the Serpent, and that the serpent began to 'coil' around the base of the forbidden Tree. Today we would label that the root chakra, as it is at the base of the spine and closest to the earth. It is a place of governance, and it is often related to our survival and our physical identity.

The Serpent, being the Guardian of the forbidden Tree of Knowledge, also acted on free will. Knowing its reputation, under normal circumstances one would not approach it: especially knowing and having an understanding of its powers. Yet with the 'encouragement of a *trusted* friend from God' (Satan), there was a kind of misplaced courage that enabled the couple to seek it out.

The Guardian plays a very important role in this story and it is usually confused as Satan.

Before we continue on with the Story of Adam and Eve, we'd like to give you some insight regarding this 'Guardian.'

PART X

LESSON 154

SECTION I: AN IN-DEPTH LOOK AT THE "SSSERPENT:" BY FAR A VERY COMPLEX CREATURE

We paused the story of Adam and Eve here so that you better understand why the serpent plays such an important part not only in the story of Adam and Eve but also with regards to how its imagery has changed within the Old Testament. We think it's important that you understand the transcendental teachings of Jesus, and not just the basic catechism lessons you grew up with. This will also help you to understand better some things that were once considered 'New Age,' and how these very things all reflect Jesus and his transcendental lessons. By the way, metaphysical science and modern science today are discovering the secrets to our physical body's functioning and how the transcendental plays a major role in its health and healing.

It was a beautiful creature, *the Serpent*, stretching from the ground to the sky like an umbilical cord; and it was decked out in seven gilded layers of gold and jewels, and wore a crown. The seven layers were revealed to represent each of the chakras because the Guardian was a 'divine' creature, which denoted it possessed pure energy. Because of its beauty, it was hard to believe it could be anything but good. The crown is the symbol of mastery, and to the unsuspected it sought union within their mind and life forces, which is how it could take control.

The Serpent was used by God as a dual expression of good and evil. It was known to hold spiritual and divine wisdom and to have the power to enslave the soul and mind, or to free the soul and mind. It should also be noted that the Serpent was also known for its fertility of nature and rebirth and regenerative characteristics and transformation, as well as its immortality and healing; thus, it exhibited the dual expression, as mentioned above.

The Serpent could also hear and speak. Again, this would not be odd, except that this creature was, well, as everything else was surrounding the couple, created this way. Nothing from after the fall to the human consciousness could compare to what was found, or experienced, in the transcendent world, just as Adam and Eve did not know the ways of the physical world until they were placed there.

The Serpent was, and still is, in many cultures, a symbol of an umbilical cord joining humans to the earth and to heaven (here heaven is the transcendental garden in which Adam and Eve lived.) In fact, scriptures and scholars indicate that the image of the Serpent would be used on the sacred staff of Moses to represent the Guardian of the mysteries of God.

The Garden was created to contain within itself 'everything' Adam and Eve would ever need or desire. It was not subject to human error of any kind since all these kinds of things happened only as the result of Adam and Eve's fall from the transcendental to the physical. It had 'everything'—even choice. Both Adam and Eve had both wisdom and knowledge, yet only when Satan presented doubt did they feel slighted. For example, one often doesn't know they are lacking in something until it is pointed out, or they are told, or are given, a comparison. Growing up eating scrambled eggs for dinner didn't make you think you were poor until someone else told you they had steak and that scrambled eggs were a poor person's breakfast, by comparison.

Getting back to the Serpent in the garden, one must understand that it had the power to heal, poison, or provide an expanded consciousness, as well as offering the elixir of life and immortality through divine intoxication. One may find in many spiritual writings that because of its herbal knowledge and entheogenic[189] association, the Serpent was considered

---

[189] An entheogen ('generating the divine within') we are told, is a chemical substance used in a spiritual context that induces altered states of consciousness and psychological, or physiological, changes. "Entheogen." Wikipedia, Wikimedia Foundation, 11 Dec. 2019, en.wikipedia.org/wiki/Entheogen.

the wisest of animals because not only was it close to the divine, it also was a 'divine' being.

Its divine aspect combined with its habitat of being 'of the earth' and between the roots of the plants was said to also have chthonic[190] properties connected to the afterlife and immortality. In mythology, the god of medicine and healing, Asclepius, carried a staff with a serpent wrapped around it and today it is the symbol of modern medicine.

The serpent is also known for vengefulness and vindictiveness, since it will attack should one encroach upon its immediate vicinity without permission. It was said that the Serpent could bring about the center axis[191] and "create doorways to the spiritual world, and, with it, accompanying power."[192]

It appears that the Serpent takes on many meanings and symbolisms. Perhaps it is because of its divine ability, and duality, in mirroring God that it had the power of life or death over whomever came upon it.

In Old Testament times, we see how God used the symbol of the Serpent as symbol for good. It is taught that the Serpent was a direct comparison between the raising up of the Son of Man, Jesus Christ, and the act of Moses, in raising up the serpent as a symbol associated with salvation;[193] and that it had also 'done God's will' in the Garden. It represented the rising up of the serpent in the wilderness, "even so must the Son of Man be lifted up, that whoever believes in Him should not perish but have eternal life."[194] As Eeshans believe, it revealed the mirrored power of a kind of opposite divine duality: meaning 'mirroring' the Law of Opposites. The Law of Opposites states that if you do what the majority of other people do, day in and day out, you will end up getting

---

[190] Referring to the 'underworld,' the 'hellish,' this refers to the amoral disposition of the Guardian, whose consciousness spans the entire range of all good and evil possibilities; for Guardian Serpent there is no 'right' or 'wrong' or 'good' and 'evil.' Everything is within the realm of its purpose for being.

[191] The connection between heaven and earth. Many religions employ the motif of the central, vertical axis. – Ed.

[192] Cf. Wikipedia.com, "Snake worship."

[193] "Serpent (Symbolism)." Wikipedia, Wikimedia Foundation, 28 Nov. 2019, en.wikipedia.org/wiki/Serpent_(symbolism).

[194] John 3:14-15.

the same results and thinking in ways that most people tend to think and get from life.

As previously stated, the Serpent was the Guardian of the Forbidden Tree and acted on free will. One would not just casually approach it, since anyone who had an understanding of its powers knew it could not be trusted. Especially not in the way one could trust God, for it too was created, and, thus, was not perfect in itself. Because it contained within itself 'entheogens,' it could cause hallucinogenic effects.

In modern times. and to this day, traditional medicine has employed it, and for thousands of years, entheogens were, and still are, used in some religions for obtaining transcendental states of consciousness. Our interest here is how closely related the Serpent, due to its positive and negative characteristics, is associated with medicine today. All things repeat, and are played out in this world, in all areas of life (i.e., as above so below, when the inside is like the outside). Examples of this, aside from medicine, are spirituality and religion.

Archeologist John Marco Allegro makes the claim that early Jewish and Christian cultic practice was based on the use of the Amanita Muscaria (or Sacred Mushroom). His hypothesis was that Amanita use constituted sacred knowledge kept only by high figures to hide the true beginnings of the Christian cult. In many areas of spirituality, drugs *were* used for spiritual experience and some for use in attaining enlightenment. **Artificially introduced DMT is said to awaken and expand the mind, according to many who have experimented with desires for extreme divine experiences. This is not unusual and one can find teachers and writers that have dabbled in DMT, especially relating to sci-fi and spiritual advancement books.**

Anyway, the purpose for noting this information is to help one see the cause and effect of what this 'entheogenic' Serpent had on Adam and Eve. Too often one wonders why the Serpent was made to crawl on the ground in punishment.

Remembering that entheogens change physiology is very important. since this is key to understanding the Mystery behind God's plan for salvation and the reason the Only-Begotten Child, whose Divine Masculine came to be known as the Divine Son of God, and who became a man, married, suffered, died, and was buried and resurrected, all in order that he and his consort could reintroduce the process of transubstantiation. It is also important to know that Satan promised the Serpent "special music" if it got the couple to eat of the Tree. Knowing that its job would be in jeopardy, the Serpent, too, fell to its own weakness, as it was obsessed with music. Because the Serpent was duped into selling out his position with God, God would punish it by causing it to have a loss of hearing and shutting down all its chakras, leaving it bound up; and it was forced to crawl, losing its dignity before all other creatures.

God predicted that the serpent would strike the heel of the Seed of the Virgin when Jesus was crucified to save us, but his plan was not completed because his wife is denied; but in the end, Christ's wife will return, and will strike down and crush its head, once and for all.

Let's take a quick look at the mystery behind the aforementioned text regarding this encounter.

LESSON 155

SECTION II: COMPARING THE SERPENT WITH THE FALLEN HUMAN CONSCIOUSNESS AND THE CONSEQUENCES THAT LED TO THE NEED FOR SALVATION

As with all things of God, entering into the transcendental consciousness one has no concept of time since it is outside of time. The past, present, and future are all intertwined.

We say this, as it is important that we give you a glimpse of Adam and Eve's situation, and to take you a little forward into seeing and understanding better how the role of the Serpent continues. It helps one to understand that though Eeshans believe that the prefiguring of Jesus, which is taught to be the significance of Moses and his serpent-topped staff, works with the crucifixion of Christ, there is a lot more to this symbolism, and it starts here with this encounter.

Being a dual expression of good and evil, it mirrors the positive and negative aspects of male and female genders; and an interesting fact is that the serpent was 'coiled' around the base of the Tree of Life. So, whether or not you believe in the "story," or you convince yourself that the story is all symbolic, one must realize that taking into consideration all of these, we witness the above played out over "time" in the following ways.

To better understand the hidden mystery of the Serpent, we should take a look at what happened to the bodies of all those after Adam and Eve that were beguiled into making a choice that would result in the descent of humans after the fall from the transcendental to the human consciousness.

Section II: Comparing the Serpent with the Fallen Human Consciousness

Let's begin first by taking a look at some renowned teachings of Jesus, with the Eeshan beliefs of what they believe was 'entropy' being played out in human time and human consciousness, since this served as the basis of Jesus' teachings. The struggle of humans today who are searching for the Way, the Truth, and the Life in dealing with the consequences and impact of Adam and Eve's decision, may find the following easier to understand and see that is was more than just a child's story, *and* that the *tampering* with the true story *caused tremendous turmoil and grievous errors.*

In turn, perhaps you will find the truth behind Jesus' incarnation and how His marriage to Mary Magdalen as Divine Feminine God incarnate was necessary for Jesus, through his teachings, to be the first to facilitate the passage through the door from the divine to human, in order that a human can pass through him in order that the human can, thereby, pass into the divine.

There are three most important teachings that involve humans as a result of the fall from the transcendental to the material/physical world.

LESSON 156

SECTION III: LOOKING PAST THE RELIGIOUS TONES AND UNDERSTANDING JESUS, MASTER, AND TEACHER

We all know that Jesus was called Master and teacher, but it was for greater reasons than the human rational consciousness could ascertain and exceeds all that was written, which limited his life to pockets of additional misinformation. and which are claimed to have been found within the Dead Sea Scrolls. It is said that although a priest was sent to study and investigate the scrolls on the Vatican's request, the scrolls were still suppressed for many years. 'Pope' Leo X (1513-1521), we are told, considered Jesus more of a Legend, as did 'Pope' Paul III, when he stated that there were no valid documents to demonstrate the existence of Christ. Other comments made about Jesus included that no one is sure that Christ existed at all, and, if he did, we don't know anything 'certain' about him. This coming from the successors of Peter does not surprise Eeshans, but one wonders how they can continue to say He is head of the church one day, and then indicate the sentiments above, before going back to His being the head of the Church, again.

Eeshans, on the other hand, know that as the active catalyst in redeeming the world, Jesus had to correct not just the mindset, but to also give all that was necessary to bring the mind, body, and spirit into alignment. What He was trying to do had to bring humans, by Himself becoming human, in providing an *attainable means* for each to follow, which is how, in other words, *he brought the ways of God into human terms*, with that means to pass along good spiritual guides and direction.

There were three tips at the foundation of Christ's teachings to enable us to reach enlightenment, which stem from eastern spirituality. The church immediately intended to 'paganize' them; and, thus, separated and excluded all of these and any other ties to transcendentalism. These include The Chakras, Kundalini, and DNA, for example. They needed to do this because of their xenophobia regarding the vast field of mystical knowledge from past ages leading up to their time; also, in order to strengthen political power, it was useful to proclaim everything outside what the church taught as 'pagan,' since it demonized, or made forbidden, whatever might seem to fall into competition with the church and its political aims of power, control, and spread of influence. This perpetuates the spirit of Peter, which would look at this question of mystical and metaphysical teachings from other cultures and deem them 'against its laws' that Christ is supreme, that the church speaks for Christ, and that the church, thereby, deems these other philosophies and spiritualities as not being of God. Because the 'spirit' was not understood by the church of Peter, the Sophia Perennis in the foundations of these systems, was never recognized, or seen, as having come from God, and the things of God, if they were being evaluated. This prevailing spirit of knowing the 'letter' of the law but not the 'spirit' of the law has, thus, been a perpetuating problem throughout church history, and it was inherited from Peter and his alliance/allegiance to the authorities of his birth religion. It is also why, according to the Eeshan perspective, the church would not recognize any details of Christ's life during his 'hidden' years (i.e., India, the Himalayas), as it would lend credence to 'foreign' influences, which could possibly influence the masses, if known.

You are probably wondering what these things have to do with the story of Adam and Eve, the Serpent, Satan, spirituality, and Jesus; but unless we touch on these you will miss vital facts regarding salvation of humankind and Eeshan Transcendentalism.

If you deviated and resorted back to your human, rational consciousness with regards to a "Christian outlook," then put yourself back on the transcendental path as you read excerpts from writings that we feel will best inform you and serve as good references should you want to further explore these topics.

Let's begin with the Chakras. We are told that there are seven Chakras in our subtle system or a "Tree of Life." There is a network of nerves and sensory organs that interprets the outside physical world, but our chakras, or energy centers, take care of our physical, intellectual, emotional, and spiritual being, of which our consciousness is composed. These chakras function as 'pumps' regulating the flow of energy through our energy system.[195] They reflect the decisions we make concerning how we choose to respond to conditions in life[196] through a perpetual filter. They are not physical, but do possess a density to them. They interact with the physical body through our endocrine and nervous systems. Each also represent parts of our consciousness. Through a transcendental process we can clear those chakras that cause us physical distress and illness. Again, however, one must enter a transcendental realm, through which doubt cannot be part of this process.

Chakras are likened to wheels of spinning energy, and are located in specific parts of the body. Since they are correlated to the endocrine glands (which secrete powerful hormonal messages directly into the bloodstream), each chakra is called to overcome its weaknesses, and do what it knows to do, so that its purpose may be achieved, which is preparation for the spiritualization of the mind and heart described in revelation and is foundational through the teachings of Christ. This is precisely what Jesus was met with when he began teaching a people who lived with and were surrounded by negative energies, as was in the story of Adam and Eve. Both began 'feeling' the negative energies of Satan because they lacked being in the presence of and being nourished by God. In other words, they were in the presence of an unbalanced energy.

When these energy centers fall out of alignment, the energy in the body is lost and this is due often to unhealthy living but can also be the result of stress and illness.

---

[195] Solutions, MushakRaj. "The Secret Behind The Chakras." Shiv Ganesh Yoga, Pranic Healing, Yoga Classes, Yoga at Home, Chakra Rahasya, Fight Obesity, 2016, yogashivganesh.com/chakra_rahasya.html.

[196] Solutions, MushakRaj. "The Secret Behind the Chakras." Shiv Ganesh Yoga, Pranic Healing, Yoga Classes, Yoga at Home, Chakra Rahasya, Fight Obesity, 2016, yogashivganesh.com/chakra_rahasya.html.

Using energy for the wrong purposes becomes ugly and the energy moves downward. Sex is the lowest center of our being. This is very important to remember, especially when reading about the marriage of Jesus and Mary Magdalen, since this is not to be confused with 'love's embrace.' Correcting this energy will transform one especially when it comes to *the heart center*.

Jesus and Mary exemplified the balancing and the continuing balanced life of the chakras. So, on their wedding night, for example, Jesus used a continual release of light from all his chakras, especially his heart chakra, since this was His very essence, His love, and especially this emanating from His heart chakra, Jesus was flooding His divine essence into Mary, reawakening her chakras and divinity, which up to this time were suspended (while in her human form), to be awakened by the I AM presence upon their being reunited in their marriage. The "I AM" presence is the fullness of 'God,' and this fullness is what was shared in the 'beginning' of creation—where "Light" passed through the water and created the cosmos. That is why the title 'Light' and 'Water' is so symbolic of Jesus and Mary.

Filled with love you become love; and this is what Jesus taught. This is also important as one discusses what sin is. What Jesus was teaching was if you become love, your conscience will be balanced and decisions against sin, or a better choice, will be easier. Without love, however, the conscience is left only with what is within a person's heart and mind from personal and worldly experiences. In other words, a mind and heart filled with depression, anxiety, or hatred will most likely look towards a harmful, negative, or maybe even fatal choice in handling confrontations.

> *"Don't you see that anything you eat passes through the stomach and then goes out into the sewer? The things that come out of a person's mouth from the heart defiles them. For out of the heart comes evil thoughts—murder, adultery, sexual immorality, theft, false testimony, blasphemies, and slander. These are what defile a person—but eating with unwashed hands does not defile them." (Matthew 15:17-20)*

Next, is the Kundalini. The Kundalini is the creative force within us and can be used for human/physical or transcendental/divine principles. It is likened *to a serpent lying 'coiled'* (just like the serpent in the Garden is coiled at the base of the Tree of Knowledge of Good and Evil) *at the base of the spine.* The ultimate Kundalini experience is in the case where one purifies one's mind and nature through a life united wholly to God, as in the case of Jesus and Mary, while to others it is somewhat experienced when a life along with spirituality is lived with all things in moderation. This is because we are in a world of pervasive distractions and in the midst of so many forms of corrupting sensory influences that makes traditionally-practiced meditation and enlightenment (including the opening of the chakras properly and completely) virtually impossible. People that attempt to do this on their own are unable to find their way, and so attempt to carry out enlightenment, by their own created standards based on imagination; this provides no authentic guidance due to lack of experience, and the church and its authorities on the spiritual life are, thus, little more than the 'blind leading the blind.'

Here the serpent energy is able to 'magnetize,' or draw upward, the Kundalini serpent, until it reaches the Masculine-Feminine principle of the brain, and fires them into coordination, as best it can, keeping in mind the power of the humility of will, which is not the same as free will. Humans are then filled with inspiration and become attuned to the inner world of wisdom. Jesus gave a hint to this when he said, "Be wise as serpents."

Jesus taught that when one can abandon ordinary thought processes one will enter into ecstatic awareness. To lend one's thoughts toward God opens one's mind and body to their fullest receptivity, the fullness of love and wisdom, and oneness with God.

The Kundalini resides at the base of the spinal cord just as the Serpent coiled itself close to the ground. Once it gets direction it starts flowing from the base of the spine to the brain, and, thus, flows into the vital hormones and higher spiritual energy. When Kundalini fully awakens, it completes the circuit from the base of the spine to the crown of the head, and all seven chakras experience a 'breakthrough' opening, after which the person possesses great intelligence, paired with wisdom and strength.

This is how Adam and Eve were created. Not until they were convinced that there was a greater "knowledge" did they lose track of the fact that what they had was greater. Remember they were becoming vulnerable *only* after being deprived of the Sacred Nourishment and time with God.

To become enlightened now happens physically and *biologically* because of Jesus Christ. *Because of him,* one can transcend the polarities and experience the meaning of oneness, union, 'self,' 'consciousness,' 'transcendence,' and 'merging with the Infinite.'[197] In other words, one can have union with God once more.

Now let's look at something more familiar to us today: DNA. DNA is the hereditary material in humans and almost all other organisms. Some said that 97% of our DNA was junk, but recently it was found that this 97% is not junk, and is reusable, since the DNA codex contains an incredible amount of information very usable at 'soul level.' It is considered to contain information about our past lives but science does not know how to translate or decode it yet.[198]

As our biological DNA[199] transmits inheritances of body and contains codes that determine your biological inheritance, the Spiritual DNA transmits the legacy of your evolving consciousness. Both appeared only after the fall, for as we said, there is the DNA that is biological. The spiritual DNA contains information on the trajectory of your soul, which describes how you have come to be 'who you are.' It holds the codes to what you came here to create and express. It will ignite you in a special way for certain experiences. It will never be exactly the same 'from lifetime to lifetime' since the combination of soul and personality is unique to 'each lifetime,' and, with each lifetime, your soul's genome adds more information. Your DNA is encoded with information regarding your 'soul function.' The cumulative history of your soul is dynamic, and continually expanding. Why is this important? It's important because the

---

[197] yoga108bali. "Chakras Kundalini & DNA." Chakras Kundalini & DNA, 10 Oct. 2012, yoga108bali.blogspot.com/2012/10/chakras-kundalini-dna.html.

[198] The following is adapted and found in livingfromyouressence.com for use in describing the beautiful connection to supramentalization.

[199] Hhteam. "Spiritual DNA." Humanity Healing Network, 24 July 2016, humanityhealing.net/2010/08/spiritual-dna/.

more you understand your origins of being, the greater your grasp is of your unique role in the history of your own consciousness, and what your purpose is, and what your contribution is meant to be, along with what it could become. It is a vast storehouse of information about who you are. This is also important when discussing our Eesha and how she carries the consciousness of Mary Magdalen in another body.

The downside to this is that it can be terrifying to realize that the context of our consciousness is infinitely large and incomprehensible to common human awareness, but yet it speaks volumes of the 'kind of power we actually have' to create our lives. Again, for one who is the Eternal Consort, the context of her consciousness is beyond comprehension.

We must also take responsibility for managing our truth. We will see more clearly what it is we came to do and to realize that we can no longer sweep under the rug, or pull down the blinds, and say that what is happening outside of us is not our problem.

Now that you have some background information from some Eastern religious perspectives, scientific/metaphysical, and philosophical studies, and great scholars, let's move on to what we feel are pertinent teachings that Jesus taught that go hand in hand with the above:

1) I am the Light of the world.
2) Blessed are they who do my commandments for they will have access to the Tree of Life.
3) I am the Way, the Truth, and the Life.
4) Blessed are they who believe and are persecuted because of me, for they shall see the Kingdom of Heaven.
5) He taught that he was the sustenance we need, that we 'must eat his body and drink his blood to have life everlasting.'
6) I am the Vine and you are the branches.
7) To him that overcomes, I will give to him to eat of the Tree of Life which is in the paradise of God.
8) 'I am the alpha and the omega; the beginning and the last.'

As we said earlier, there is so much more depth to his teachings and this is why we reiterate certain points in order to bring your consciousness back to the transcendental state.

The purpose for the above teachings is to help you realize the significance of the role of the Serpent from a transcendental perspective, and how it is vital for your understanding of what took place not only in the Garden but also how the story continued right up until present time, thus, unlocking the Mystery of Jesus Christ and His salvation mission and marriage to Mary Magdalen.

Before the fall, the Serpent functioned as the Guardian of the Tree of Knowledge in the transcendental realm of the Garden; after the 'fall' the serpent is tied in with the physical universe, the material world, and intertwined with the DNA. This spiral pattern is found everywhere from the below (i.e., DNA, conch shells, whirlpools, and ear canals) to the above (such as spiral galaxies). Localized at the base of the human spine, the serpent is operative, although in most everyone, 'dormant,' in the form of *Kundalini*. This life energy is capable of expressing itself as good or evil, in any degree of the spectrum, according to the use of will.

So, we can see that in many ways this Serpent gives way to whether or not the chakras and Kundalini are in line with their design, function and purpose. This is important, since it shows how it all affects the DNA within us, in both a physical and metaphysical way. It all stands true, as Jesus told us, 'As above so below, the inside like the outside,' and so, too, are the Laws of the Universe.

The Serpent had tremendous power but being 'divine.'[200] it had to stay in allegiance with God. To not do so it would lose its place and role in the Garden until which time God allowed it to make compensation for its wrongdoing. It was a choice. It was not one the Serpent would ever want to have to make.

---

[200] Again, this term does not mean the Serpent was on the level of God; however, it was so extraordinarily powerful in its particular order of being and the purpose of its being was so unique, that the vastness of its knowledge gave it a kind of 'divine' quality of character. – Ed.

PART XI

LIFE AS THEY KNEW IT, WAS CHANGED

LESSON 157

SECTION I: THE STORY ADAM AND EVE CONTINUES WITH THE CHOICE FOR PHYSICAL LIFE AND HUMAN CONSCIOUSNESS

One must not forget, that the Guardian/Serpent we are talking about was NOT Satan, as most people think they are the one and the same. Satan and the Serpent were different entities. Satan *enticed the Serpent with such a powerful temptation* that eventually he was able to make a deal with the Guardian/Serpent in order to convince the couple to eat the fruit in exchange for a music of the highest level of perfection, which was the greatest desire of the Serpent.

As the Guardian watched, the couple approached. Already having been influenced by Satan, and desiring the 'music' Satan promised, it began the plan to get the couple to eat the apple. First it singled out Eve, and welcomed them. Asking the purpose for their coming by to this area, Eve began to tell the Serpent what the 'being' had told them. When asked why they didn't ask the advice of God, a mere trick, the couple explained that they didn't want to bother God.

The Serpent, seeing that the couple was struggling with a decision, encouraged them to talk about their struggle. After listening, it seemed to bring a calmness which came to envelope them. Once they felt this, they told the Serpent their reasons as to why they thought God forbade them from eating the Fruit of the Tree. Very cleverly and without appearing to be forcing them to make a decision, it told them that obviously God didn't want them to have this knowledge for God's own reasons.

The Guardian continued to listen, and at different moments would talk to them about this love they were told about, and how it could understand why such special love would be kept for God alone. Adam and Eve were astonished by the knowledge the Guardian had, and began to wonder why they had been kept from visiting with it. The Serpent, having great gifts, recognized their awe and continued to tell them that God had chosen it to be Guardian and gave it great knowledge of all things. Carefully it continued to tell Adam and Eve that there was no reason why they, too, couldn't gain great knowledge. They would simply just have to eat the fruit on the Tree. Knowing that God forbade them and that it would take permission to eat of the Tree, the Guardian asked why? Why should ones so close and loved by God be so fearful? You have to remember this Serpent had its own powers and toyed with the couple.

The couple, not knowing how to answer, decided to walk away when the Guardian declared, "Would not God stop you if you had been deceived?"

"You should not tempt God nor us," replied Adam. The Serpent replied, "Surely I am not tempting God or you. It is you who have returned asking questions. Perhaps you are being tested. One cannot be forced to do something should they not want to do it. What can happen if you ate the Fruit of this Tree?" They responded, "God said we are not allowed to eat the fruit of this Tree, or touch it, or we will die."

The Guardian watched their expressions. It continued, "So what is death?" Not knowing the answer it was looking for, Adam replied, "It is the end of one's life as one knows it." The Guardian said, "I see. Perhaps God meant to end this life as you know it? It may very well be the beginning of a new life. One that you've been kept from? It's your choice," the Serpent replied in a whisper loud enough for them to hear, as it coiled itself around the Tree. It continued, "I can touch it. If I can touch it and not die, surely you, whom God loves, should not die. Why do you think I stay here all of the time protecting this Tree? God willed that I stay and guard it because of its power; and you see the many gifts I have. I guard it so that others do not come and take this power or these gifts, since they, too, will become like God."

What Adam and Eve didn't realize was that the Serpent could not ever leave the Tree, since freedom apart from it would be its demise.

Eve questioned the Serpent, "Then why would you let us eat from it?"

The Serpent looked at each one as it slowly moved its head closer to their eyes. "Because, you know God. In your eyes, I see your soul." Then the Serpent drew back.

Not walking away, Adam and Eve watched the calmness of the Serpent, for the Serpent's movements were hypnotic. The apples looked more beautiful than ever. Then the Serpent asked, "How can anything created by God look so beautiful and be so deadly?" (As the beauty of the Apple was skin deep, they failed to know that its flesh and seeds were poisonous.)

The Serpent, looking at Eve, said, "God 'knows' that your eyes will be opened and you will be like God, knowing good and evil. Take, eat, and you will obtain a body for the life and love you desire." With that, both Adam and Eve choose to go through with their choice.

They took a deep breath. Eve took an apple and bit into it as Adam watched. Noting appeared to happen. Eve then handed the apple to Adam. Adam wondered if what this creature told them was correct. Adam then remembered the dream that Eve had regarding this new love, took the apple from Eve and bit into it. Upon biting the apple, their eyes were immediately opened, and everything began to change, since because they were first one before God, who made them two, then blessing them with a sacred union made them one again; therefore, both had to eat the apple.

Their bodies began to feel differently. They felt heavy and solid. Their skin began to change, too. When they looked at each other, they saw each other in a way different than ever before; and this filled them with a desire much different than before. Now their desire seemed to crave each other's bodies, but it was self-seeking pleasure. This desire became so powerful they could not stop their urges.

This was the first time they 'knew' each other. The moment erupted into such extreme pleasure, but then it ended almost as quickly as it began. As entropy was born, guilt immediately set in. Suddenly they both felt empty. Guilt and fear were foreign to them. The 'knowledge' they sought was certainly there, and immediately they knew what they did was 'wrong.' The knowledge they obtained was not a wisdom that expanded inside them, making them feel satisfied and whole; this knowledge left them feeling empty and afraid. What did they fear? They feared how they were feeling and how their bodies had changed; they feared not having that wonderful satisfaction they normally had. They now feared God.

Hearing God calling to them caused them to feel threatened by God and caused them to run and hide. God called them again. This time Adam answered. God asked, "Why are you hiding?" Adam answered God saying, "Because we are naked." God asked how they knew that they knew they were naked.

Adam explained how they had eaten from the forbidden tree. God gave them skins to cover their bodies. Adam told God how this 'beautiful being' was teaching them, and how he told them the secret of how to love more deeply. Adam told God how they had learned about a new way to express love to each other, but it required new bodies with mass and not the transcendental bodies God originally gave them. In order to experience this kind of love the 'being' told them they needed 'flesh and blood.' (Little did they know that one day it would take God to become 'flesh and blood' to correct and restore their descendants.) In order to get the bodies for this love, they decided to seek the advice of the Guardian Serpent. The Guardian eased their fear and they took his advice. The Serpent told them not to be afraid; and that God would not let them die.

Adam told God that after the woman experienced the sensual feelings of love she described to him from her dream, he wanted to experience this, too. Adam told God that after they ate the apple, they were filled with an overwhelming desire for each other's bodies. It was the intensity of these urgings that caused them to 'know' each other physically.

Eve told God how the being presented itself as a 'son of God' when he came to her and seduced her in her dream. Adam told God that the Serpent told them that God knew this love, and perhaps they should experience it and show God they had free will. She said that the beautiful being told her that he would show her the source of God's knowledge. The Guardian/Serpent told her that God would not allow any harm to come to them and how pleased God would be if she and Adam could embrace the way that God did, and proceeded to show her in the dream what it was like. It told her that she and Adam should eat of the Tree. It told her that God would be very happy with her initiative and desire to love; and this son of God told her it would bring Adam closer to God, as well, when the two shared in this experience.

God told them how what they had was the greatest expression of love one could enter into. That to lust for one's body for self-gratification and fulfillment was wrong. Love is shared. Love is reciprocated. God explained how without the nourishment provided for them, they became inclined to act apart from what is good and sacred, and listened to an imposter, one who led them to share in a forbidden and unlawful act of carnal knowledge, since it was done outside of God. The unbalanced consciousness was born as they turned away from God's love and life-giving extension. The feminine quality, or feeling, lost its calm intuitive powers when it succumbs to the restlessness of the body consciousness and the male succumbs to egotistical self-sufficiency.[201]

To have entered into this carnal act without permission is not love, and this goes against God, who *is* Love. This was the means by which animals reproduce, since they were not created in God's image and likeness. For animals, it is not a matter of turning away from God, but is simply the governing of natural impulses for their continuation of life. This is not the means by which human beings should express love. This impulse of feeling, which was designed to draw animals and other creatures to each other, was not meant to operate in the same way God created Adam and Eve.

This is why Eeshans call their actions, the "Original" or 'First Choice.' Though Satan coerced the couple, and it appears that because they were subtly pressured into making this decision, it wasn't entirely their fault. Adam and Eve's offense was two-fold: 1) They neglected going to God's Garden to get the Spiritual Food and Drink necessary; and, thereby, passed up opportunities to be in the Presence of God, which was a directive they knew was necessary for their life together with God; and 2) because of this, they were vulnerable to the delusions of Satan. These were their "choices," entropy was the consequence.

---

[201] Cf. Paramahamsa Yogananda, *The Second Coming of Christ*, Vol. 2, Discourse 62.

PART XII

LESSON 158

GOD'S LOVE AND MERCY BRINGS THE FIRST HUMAN MARRIAGE

SECTION I: GOD SETS GUIDELINES FOR PHYSICAL LOVE

Even though Adam and Eve had now participated in this carnal act apart from God's design, it was because of God's unconditional love and mercy that a new union was instituted in which this act would now be blessed; this love shared between them would also be the means used to propagate. They would, however, lose all beatific benefits and be separated from Paradise. It is not because God was angry, or wanted to punish them, and drive them out of the Garden in shame, rather it was by their choice that the consequence of the change in their consciousness came about. It was entropy that caused the development of the gross physical body and the physical realm of existence they would now have to live in on a permanent basis.

Their new bodies simply could not function in a transcendental world,[202] God explained how there would be joys and there would be sorrows; these came from the choice they made together. Life as they knew it, though it was changed forever, would be lived out together in a sacrificial way.

For Adam and Eve and all their descendants, the expression of carnal love would only be recognized through, with, and in God in the Mystery

---

[202] The body's vibrational frequency was slow and dense by comparison to the actuality of the Light Body one finds naturally at 'home' in the Transcendental realm. – Ed.

of Marriage. Carnal acts outside of Marriage are deemed forbidden and unlawful, since they do not free a couple to pass into a spiritual world, because it takes the Sacrament to provide the 'union' of the two into one. God's 'original transcendental blessed union,' gave Adam and Eve the capability of expressing divinity, which was what Jesus taught. Since love came from God, the first Person of the Holy Trinity/Creator of all creation saw that because they were weakened and they were able to be coerced into choosing a love relationship less than what God shared with them. That is what the Original Choice was. If the couple had chosen this love without influence or coercion, it would be Original Sin, and it would, indeed, be looked upon as a grievous 'sin.' *Entropy came into existence, not by God's hand but by their choosing a physical existence.* It is likened to the saying, "You made your bed, now you have to sleep in it."

The bright side is that they were not, nor would they ever be, abandoned, even though it seemed that their fate was such. It would seem like this because they lost the beatific privilege of seeing God. In fact, because Adam and Eve chose this life now, God actually made their choice for this expression of love to be blessed, however, only in Marriage, where it could be sanctioned.

What happens if there are places that will not accept other gender expression marriages? If there is a male/female alternative God will bless the union. This means that there has to be a 'female identity and a male identity,' and not only a biological one.

PART XIII

THE ORIGINAL SIN

LESSON 159

Section I: Who is Right, Human Man or God Made Man?

The falling from a pure, undefiled spiritual and sacred union to a physical existence was so much less than what God intended for our first parents. Eeshans hold that the language of "original sin" passed down to us coveys so much about man's interpretation played out in the history of humanity's relationship with God being based on adherence to the law, and not love, and choosing to sin versus being pressured; and this is what Jesus found when he came to earth. There were so many 'laws' in the name of God that Jesus had to address them. However, when Jesus came He spoke about love of God and/or neighbor.

Why should we listen to Jesus and not the traditional scriptures? In John 10:36, Jesus says: "Why do you call it blasphemy when I say, 'I am the Son of God?' After all, the Father set me apart and sent me into the world." It was in his teachings that Jesus addressed how the religious leaders laid heavy burdens upon the people, and yet their own works were done to be observed by men and not God. In so many ways, they gave the impression that they were holy men, but never showed it in their actions, saying, in effect that they themselves made the laws in order to achieve their own desires.

The traditional story of Adam and Eve led to so much ill-founded guilt, snowballing over the ages. Transcendentally speaking, what occurred was not a result of poorly exercising a free will, and committing sin, but rather was a result of not having what God deemed as necessary to stay nourished spiritually, and this resulted in the Light Body then being drawn into the material world, where it would become 'part' of it and then be limited by it. This original story maintains what Eeshans suggest: that by the primarily patriarchal-conditioned religious leaders telling their version of what had taken place with Adam and Eve, they can achieve their unquestionable desires. In other words, in this way, Eve becomes the first real transgressor who seduced Adam away from God, and God's law brought punishment down on the whole human race, beginning with the couple's exile from the Garden.

With this rational human explanation, the attitude towards human consciousness and spirituality was shaped to support the view that even though Adam and Eve felt shame, remorse, and guilt for what they had done, God was "angry," and must be appeased by severely punishing the first parents of humankind. We are made to think that the "transgression of God's Law" and fear of punishment takes precedence in how one who commits sin is viewed by God. This mindset has, thus, been carried over to present times, yet Eeshans present that this is not the God that Jesus said was our loving Father/Mother.

LESSON 160

SECTION II: ADAM AND EVE OBTAIN HUMAN KNOWLEDGE OF WHAT IS GOOD AND BAD

When Adam and Eve felt the desire for human knowledge, as though what they had was less, they really didn't realize what it was for which they were asking. Knowledge derived apart from God was not wisdom. When they made this choice, without a doubt they immediately knew what they did was wrong. But more than that, this knowledge carried with it the *consequences* of good and evil, because they had entered "permanently" into the physical realm and chose to become part of it.[203] God knew this, and because this would be the realm we are subject to, we would need help.

The physical/material realm makes us of knowledge, but it is limited in so many ways. First, it is not spiritual. That being said, God would instill in us knowledge that forms the conscience. The conscience, however, would be formed in two ways as we addressed early in the book.

The conscience should be well-formed in truth and spirituality. If it is, it directs the person as a guide towards God. There is a *moral* component, and it is built upon what has been learned and experienced; whereas, it carries also an *informed* component that is researched and thought out through logic and reason. Either of these can be missing, and, thus, the conscience is NOT a good guide, as in the case of Lucifer, whose wisdom

---

[203] This might be seen as the beginning of karmic generation for themselves, and the human race, in the material world. – Ed.

became corrupt with logic and reasoning. A weakened spirituality subjects one to a flawed conscience. Lastly, human knowledge is prone to knowledge of pleasure and joys, but knowledge of sorrows and suffering, as well, because they are a natural part of living in the material world.

The material, or human, conscience gives way to the human consciousness, and is far from the original consciousness of unlimited potential, even while yielding the experiences of life in a material universe oriented to the physical mind and senses. One such downfall is death. Death is the chief of the sorrows and sufferings brought about by entropy. Not just death in a physical sense, but also in the spiritual.

As Adam and Eve made their choice to enter into the physical realm, becoming part of it through the union of their Light Body with the physical manifestation, or outer 'clothes' of the material body, "entropy" was in operation. The disunion that was generated between Adam and Eve and their origin/location in God essentially caused that kind of 'pull' or gravity effect towards God to go into the chaos, or randomness, of the physical universe that draws the soul away from God into the realm of physicality, unless there is the effort put forth to go against it and pursue God in leading a spiritual life.

LESSON 161

SECTION III: INSIGHT INTO SIN

This 'choice' altered their scope of consciousness and drew it into a limited range under the laws of the physical universe. That is why they could no longer live in the Garden, since the Garden was a transcendental reality. The transcendental reality was free from sin and corruption, and it could not tolerate the presence of either. A pure Divine entity, such as the Most High God is a perfect example of this.

Now that Adam and Eve received the knowledge they thought they so desired, God deemed it was now necessary that the couple go into a world that is best suited for their choice. Knowing also that once they would begin to enter into entropy, this knowledge they attained would make them become aware of the other Tree—the Tree of Life. It was of the upmost importance that they not gain access to this Tree, since they would be sealed forever in the material world. For this reason, St. Michael was given the governing command as the gatekeeper. Along with the cherubim under him at his command, the gateway to its East end was closed off. This is important to know because the East was the place of origin, and the place of destiny, the place from which God sent Adam and Eve forth, and where the souls must return. That was why the star of Bethlehem was put in the East, to mark the place where the Son of God took birth to open the gate. And Jesus, who is Lord of the East, is Master of all disciplines and spiritual arts.

There St. Michael held up a flaming sword, that turned in every direction, to guard any way in to prevent the Couple from entering; and, thus, not only would the Garden be protected but so would the 'Tree of Life,' preventing them from eating of the fruit that would keep them alive forever and away from their course of moving into the world of time and physical existence (cf. Genesis 3:22). Access to this Tree would keep them eternally in darkness.

And the Lord God said, "The humans have now become like one of us, knowing good and evil. They must not be allowed to reach out their hand, and take also from the Tree of Life, and eat, and live forever."[204] We use the plural here to denote God's duality as seen in the footnote where the title Elohim derives from with the meaning of seven Elohim together with their feminine counterparts, known as builders of form, which carry the highest vibration of Light. Eeshans believe it, indeed, means the Elohim and feminine counterparts, and the number seven denotes all as One, which is God-undivided.

Ingestion of the Apple was certainly what God 'didn't want;' however, knowing the human's probability to enter into temptation, and alter their lives, God's wisdom shone through when they were told to not touch or 'eat' the fruit of the Tree. This would be the means by which God could 'reintroduce' the Sacred Food for salvation, since the couple had already neglected to eat on a 'daily' basis. Why didn't God stop them? They were told all they needed to do to make a free will decision, including "Do not eat. You will die." What more could God do? Remove the Tree? Then there would be no choice.

Eeshans also want to mention here that Adam and Eve's stay in the Garden was for a very long duration of time. All this didn't happen in a week or month. Being outside of time, one must imagine, or conclude, it would compare to no less the time we humans walked the earth, and perhaps some time before. Therefore, it was possible that God saw their love as becoming complacent from the beginning, and that this choice seemed to be leading towards how it would play out later. (All that would come, from beginning to end, what human beings call 'history,' are but like the briefest of daydreams, the blink of an eye.) One thing is for sure,

---

[204] Here we see God identify as one God, while yet using the plural "us." This is in reference to two main points: the first is the duality of the Creator and the second is the Trinity, which also has a duality, and, of course, to some, reveals God as the Elohim and Elohel. – Ed.

if we look at the Universal Laws we can at least decipher somewhat of an outline, or pattern, of how things would follow. It is said that in law and ethics, universal law or principle, refers to as concepts of legal legitimacy actions, whereby those principle and rules for governing human beings' conduct, which are most universal in their acceptability, their applicability, translation, and philosophical basis, are considered to be most legitimate,[205] which would allow for the 'as above so below' concept. As in the Law of Polarity, everything is dual. Everything has opposites. Opposites are identical in nature, but they are different in degree. There are also two sides to everything, meaning though they are opposite they are two extremes of the same thing. An example would be found in heat and cold: though they seem to be opposites, they are varying degrees of the same thing: both being temperature. That is why we say that one can rise above this law and change hate to love, war to peace etc. They also use the example of the Law of cause and effect, which is applied to three planes of existence: the spiritual, the mental, and the physical. The difference is, that on the spiritual level, cause and effect are instantaneous, such as they may appear inseparable; but on the other planes our concept of time and space creates a time lag between the cause and the 'eventual' effect. What you want to create in the physical world is automatically manifested in the spiritual world.[206] So, Eeshans believe that, with God as Creator, what is created in the Spiritual comes into being in the physical by the universal laws and then manifests, or returns, in its perfected form back in heaven. That is how, based on the universal laws, when one becomes enlightened, one can see how Adam and Eve went from the transcendental world to the physical; and Jesus and Mary, the new Adam and Eve, could bring all from the physical back to the transcendental if one looks beyond 'time.' An enlightened mind can also see that in loving God, it is not love if one is forced or the love becomes robotic. Therefore, God perhaps allowed Satan (not for selfish or for any

---

[205] "Universal Law." Definitions.net. STANDS4 LLC, 2019. Web. 12 Dec. 2019. https://www.definitions.net/definition/universal+law.

[206] Kotsos, Tania. "The Seven Universal Laws Explained." Mind Power from Mind Your Reality, www.mind-your-reality.com/seven_universal_laws.html.

other means) to 'cause' the couple to fail but in 'effect' break down the robot-love, and cause this choice to be intrinsic to an awakening that God is true love and wants one to 'choose' to love. If one's choice is for God, then we have the means given to us to obtain access to heaven once again, or die, both physically and spiritually.

In order to return to our original nature, however, it would take a perfect human couple who were also Divine to restore the "Way back," so humans 'could,' once again, gain access to the transcendental only by this means.

This Plan of course, would involve reversing the ingestion of the fruit by 'another Fruit.' This time it would take a transubstantiated Food that would be available for all those who believed, which was another choice entirely, meaning that it would have to be a Food which would allow one to be mystically consumed by God, and into God, in such a way that every age, despite sin, has access back to what God intended for the extensions of Divine Duality and love. Sin, by any degree, has to include habitual offenses, or the ignoring of God, due to human 'advice,' or degree, by thinking 'human consciousness knows better' is the trap which Adam and Eve fell into.

That is why, in order to reverse the action that caused the fall to the physical, divine beings had to become *human* beings, who lived in the physical world, and would be subject to death, and, yet, who still would be in control of their physical bodies, which like any other body would give rise to temptation. By *choice* they remained sinless; and as Jesus would resurrect (with Mary's Sacred Kiss) in His glorified body, fulfilling His part[207] as the true Divine Masculine liaison for humanity's reconnection with God and re-entrance into heaven, Mary's part in the mission, according to the plan, would have been initiated at the time of her bloodied attack but which would be completed in the course of the fullness of time.

If the plan went according to God's intention what would have happened was that we would have they, who are both human and divine, in the roles of Adam and Eve, which is the Divine being the necessary

---

[207] The other part to be completed and balanced by the Divine Feminine.

component, because of its eternal quality and nature. Through the transubstantiating of the ordinary food humans eat into the Christed bodies of these two, we would have the return of the Sacred Food and Drink lost by the fall and necessary for eternal life. Finally, the humankind connection by the divinizing of each one who believes brings in the choice of free will and the gift for the redeemed. But this 'gift' from God for our salvation was interrupted and altered once again by humanity. Yes, we have repeated this time and again, but do you really understand what the ramifications of refusing this 'Gift' are?

Getting this knowledge was immediate but so was losing the transcendental realm. The limited conditions for their new life, with specific guidelines for taking this knowledge as being instantaneous, was preserved when God, from whom all good things come, could keep them connected, by blessing those who choose to be united as one in their human marriage and love's embrace. That is why sex without God's blessing ends in guilt, emptiness, and eventual death of hope and could lead to remorse.

Free will is often mistaken for going against what is good, or God, and fellow humans, with a choice for self, and absence of God's Law (as interpreted by traditional sources). They feel a need to go on their own spiritual journey dismissing what Jesus said. The human consciousness, as defined by the world, can be mistaken as 'freedom from God,' and replaces the true transcendental consciousness with a version of its own. It borrows actual principles and ideas found in the Sophia Perennis, but refashions their meaning and connections to suit itself. Freedom to use one's body solely for pleasure should 'they choose' to do so is not by God's definition 'spiritual,' neither is one doing "whatever works in order to be happy." That is why Jesus said, "If I had not come, sins could be ignored but I have come;" therefore, choosing whatever one does to think over what Jesus said is choosing apart from God. Life is about sharing, not taking. In 'all' what God wants for us is to share in a committed male/female relationship that goes beyond the physical, goes beyond self-gratification, and where a male and female component is bound together by love and not *pleasure*. It's about having a soulmate on the path that strives for a greater love than a purely human love, one which is not grounded in God.

Jesus taught that from our ignorance we enter into illusion, then we become delusional, as we redefine sin, thinking we have an understanding, but, in fact, have a *misunderstanding*, of God's law.

We enter into illusion each time we honestly think that our actions are solely our own affair, and that we are not affecting or hurting others. Even by the Universal Laws this is wrong. We enter delusion when 'we feel,' or declare, relationships we desire are blessed by God regardless of our abandonment to former commitments. We enter into illusion when we don't take seriously a vow we made to God or have no healthy respect for the things of God (namely his Mysteries or Sacraments), and enter into actions taken apart from these. An example of this is when we enter into the illusion that sex is a priority above all else in a marriage is to include striving together for the ultimate and purest expression of love, which is being in union with God. Delusion is present when, for example, there is a sexual relationship apart from God's blessing, and there is a belief on the part of the couple that there is no harm being done on any level of being, whether it be emotional, physical, or worse of all, spiritual. We do this each time we make blind choices, which result in unforeseen and unwanted consequences. All actions will have consequences, for either good or ill. But when we become entangled in sin because of a poor choice, this will always lead to any number of degrees of suffering, be they small or great, which is synonymous with being guided by the rational, logical human consciousness.

LESSON 162

SECTION IV: GOD OF LOVE AND MERCY

After Adam and Eve explained to God what had taken place, God explained how the 'being' was an imposter and had lied to them. God explained that because they had strayed away (making the choice of not returning to God's Garden and not telling God what they were feeling), they weren't being nourished, and that they left themselves vulnerable to illicit advice. God told them that the 'being' had coerced the Serpent into using its body and voice to lure them into thinking that the teachings they were receiving were the same as God's.

God explained that they had wisdom, which was the perfection of all knowledge in the fabric of their being, and yet they went astray looking to find love; however, it was always there in their hearts.

Turning to the Serpent, and recognizing the vicious and abusive acts Satan used to deceive, confuse, and destroy the innocence of the couple, God cursed the Serpent for being duped into caving to a passion it could not control, music, and said:

> Because you allowed Satan to use your body to deceive the innocent, you are now cursed above all animals, above every beast of the field: and upon your belly you will crawl as a sign of a fallen consciousness. No longer will you stand upright for you will be the symbol of the sleeping Kundalini for you will be subject to knowledge, but you will be seen as ambivalent. Your prana like the five rivers of Vayu will cease to flow until the One Sacredly Balanced will awaken and cause it to flow once more. You will be linked to sexual desire and passion until which time we feel you have heard the Word of God.

LESSON 162A

At this juncture, it is imperative to the understanding of the entire story, from beginning to end, that you now be told this account of the 'time' between Lucifer's fall and the deception of Adam and Eve by the Serpent Guardian; since in truth, the serpent who's "head is crushed" is *not* the Guardian Serpent.

The Guardian Serpent is in fact the Kundalini which should not be mistaken as the "Ancient Serpent" that was corrupt from the beginning. The Guardian is likened to the force within us that Jesus awakened in his wife, and later within the little girl with the words, "talitha cumi," which means "rise up, little girl.

When the Kundalini, or life force, is suspended it causes a kind of slumber, which gives rise to human consciousness that has no sense of the transcendental. It would be by the Divine Masculine that the divine nature of Mary would be awakened and activated through Jesus 'immutable word and their Sacred Kiss.

The Ancient One was Lucifer/Satan; his name was changed from the former to the latter when he fell. His identity was always symbolized by the 'serpent' because of his behavior, mindset, lack of love, and empathy, since these are the traits of a reptile; the Guardian Serpent, however, was not like this, since its role, while serpentine in nature, was balanced and ordered to its purpose without corruption of intent. Thus, the two, while similar in some respects regarding appearance, were, in fact, quite different. They were, indeed, not the same.

The Guardian and the Kundalini could be given another chance or be given an opportunity to change. Notice how God deemed that a bronze serpent be fixed to Moses' staff so that afflicted Hebrews could be healed. This is not the case for the "Ancient Serpent," who was evil and eternally condemned. Eeshans believe this is why the confusing of the Guardian Serpent with the same serpent whose head would be crushed by the woman was a concept passed down perhaps by lack of information, etc.

Eeshans believe, that as one should never engage Satan, the fact that the Guardian did his job and engaged Lucifer was the moment of its downfall. Eeshans believe that Satan had studied the Guardian, and, finding its weakness regarding music, planned this encounter knowing that the Guardian would question him, which was the very engagement Satan was counting on. Since Satan answered the Guardian, he produced the one thing the Guardian could not resist: the highest music. Satan began to slowly fill the surrounding area with music unlike anything the Guardian had ever heard. Becoming intoxicated, the Guardian fell into a rapture of ecstasy, which, thereby, allowed Satan to possess the Serpent, and, thus, engage Adam and Eve. That is why the Guardian, although punished, can still be raised up for God.

In the end, however, Eeshans believe that it was Jesus' heel that has already been struck, as Peter was sighted by Jesus as being the stumbling block to his mission, but it will be Mary, the Divine Feminine, who will crush the head of the Ancient Serpent.[208]

That is why we said that the positive outlook is to see that as God allowed for the errors of the last 2000+ years, until sin was in epidemic form, and he would return for His bride and she would complete His mission.

At that moment, God took away the guardian's and its descendants' hearing, so that it would have to rely upon 'reading' vibration (as opposed to hearing and feeling music); it also no longer was able to stretch high, but instead was made to crawl, and so 'crawled' out of God's presence. We should never want to have to crawl out of God's presence; in fact, we should want to crawl into it every chance we get. Even though it wasn't the 'cause' of Adam and Eve's sin, it chose to become the unwitting instrument of their fall, and so this involved its culpability, and, thus, there were consequences in proportion to its order of being.

---

[208] Here we see how it fits together, beginning and end, that the 'serpent will strike your heel while the woman will crush the serpent's head' (combining OT and NT writings, and tradition with catholic Christianity that the woman will crush the head of the serpent): Jesus was struck in his heel, his 'Achilles heel, which was his long-suffering, his long enduring patience, in order to capture his prize, the completion of the mission for which came; but who would crush the head of the serpent? – Jesus' wife.

It is believed that when Jesus began to teach, the time was close when the Serpent, who participated in bringing about death, yet still possessing a dual personality, would eventually be given an opportunity to be recognized here on earth in relation to fertility and rebirth. Believe it or not it is said that the serpent was the symbol of the "Word." Because of God's 'word,' the Kundalini is found sleeping within each of us because of its influence over Adam and Eve, even though Christ awakened it when He came. Since the "Word" of God was ignored, it would take one who is like him, to awaken it once more. The first encounter happened when Jesus was speaking, and overheard people talking about the daughter of Jairus, the synagogue leader who was told that his daughter was dead and to 'not bother the teacher.' Thus, this is what happened (cf. Mark 5:39). He went with Peter, James, and John to Jairus' house. When he arrived, he said to those outside, "Why all this commotion and wailing? The child is not dead, she is asleep." Then putting them out of the house, and taking the child by the hand, He said to her, "Talitha cumi," which means, "Little girl, I say to you arise." This is important as these will be the words spoken to His wife on their wedding night to awaken her Kundalini once more; and as it laid in a suspended state, she will bring it forth once again.

LESSON 163

Section V: What Did Jesus Teach?

Liberation certainly was not the absence of God's law, although it was made to look that way by Satan. God's law brought freedom. Adam and Eve were first liberated when they first came together and found love in divine friendship, the purest expression of God's love that two individuals can share. This was the love that would then become the perfect way to love God.

Being the perfect couple would require a marriage that would solidify a human love blessed by God, and returned to God in its pure original state, in pure transcendental love, with a pure and sacred Kundalini. Could this be why all evidence of Christ's marriage was lost, destroyed, or deemed heretical? If this is so, then why would such drastic measures be taken to keep this from the faithful?

One reason for this is that, without God, humans are put in charge. Without Christ's marriage, there is no chance with regards to salvation. For once, truth is brought back in the world, it is Jesus saying all over again, "If I had not come sin could be ignored; but I have come."

Without following Jesus' directive to eat the "Bread" come down from heaven, who is Jesus and his Wife through their Marriage, *one cannot attain the ultimate place designed for them for God, or awaken the Kundalini within, so says Jesus*; and all that is left is that which is at the hands of man (male ego), man's law, and gender inequality. Actually, as we have pointed out, there was no equality from whoever spoke, as though on behalf of God. There was only 'speaking' from corrupted reasoning. This is what was found among the religious leaders at the time of Jesus, and what Eeshans believe is found among religious authorities, officials, and leaders of today through the succession since Peter.

What is worse is God's people have been robbed once again by illusion. This time in the form of a dimidiated Sacred Food and Drink in an attempt to thwart Jesus' plan for humans, just like in the Garden, by a corrupt priesthood, stemming from Lucifer/Satan through with and in Peter, resulting in the deprivation of God's Presence.

What is amazing is God comes to the rescue once again. This Sacred Food and Drink, as well as the Sacred Balance, is brought back by the return of the Divine Feminine, who will finally bring closure to the Plan of Salvation in these times.

LESSON 164

SECTION VI: CHANGES IN OUR FIRST PARENTS LIFESTYLE: THE BEGINNING OF THE DIVERSITY OF HUMAN BEINGS

God, knowing Satan's plan regarding Eve, then addressed Satan saying, "I will put enmity between you and the Woman, between your seed and hers." Then Satan was banished from the Garden, never to enter there again.

Let's take a look at the children, the seeds of Adam and Eve. There are children that Adam and Eve had 'begotten;' and there are the children that will be born with the 'new' human bodies, and share in the new life, which will be outside the transcendental life, and apart from where those who were begotten lived, due to the choice of their parents to leave the transcendental. Those who were begotten are not limited by boundaries. They will still be able to see Adam and Eve though the parents will look different.

They would have to abide by God's law; however, they too shall be 'guided' by wisdom. Those who were born here on earth prior to Jesus and Mary were subject to the same laws as their parents, and would have to find this new love in each other. In doing so, they, too, will find that all their joys and tribulations will prove to be worth it. For this love between humans will rise above concern for self. *God would continue to teach and guide them and send angel guardians to assist them in day to day routines, in conjunction with a conscience.*

It wouldn't be easy for Adam and Eve, since they would be faced with unforeseen difficulties they never had encountered in their transcendental life. Sadly, God as a good parent, had to endure the pain of watching the first transcendental marriage of human beings brought to the level of limited corporeal expression and temporal needs. As parents and guardians, we know that pain. It is the pain of seeing our children having less than what we dreamed of for them. Adam and Eve suffered separation from their begotten children. They also regretted the loss of all that God had given them and the suffering of what those born would have to suffer through.

As entropy set in, Adam began experiencing emotions and feelings that were very unfamiliar to both of Eve and himself. They began to feel tired, frustrated, hungry, sick, and depressed. The further away from the transcendental they drifted, the greater entropy would continue to increase. That is why it is said we begin dying the moment we are born. This is the dynamic that causes us to be subject to everything we feel today to include the physical laws of nature.

Adam and Eve found that their bodies were no longer interchangeable. They now had blood, bones, and a flesh of gross physical matter forming and surrounding their formerly pure, unlimited, and boundless light bodies. Now they discovered that not only could these bodies not enter heaven, or paradise, if they tried, but by God's directive, after their death, would have to return to the dirt beneath the Tree of Good and Evil from which they were formed.[209] This is the dirt of the material world, and the dirt the earthly bodies would have to return to in order that their original light bodies, which had been imprisoned within them would be released. Their light bodies would be placed in another realm until the coming of the Saviors.

As time continued on, the texture, color, and manifestation of their skin changed and became less subtle and more dense and receptive to surrounding conditions; this, but also, of *their* descendants' and their offspring would continue to change not just wherever they would eventually be born on the planet, but also because through the effects of time.

---

[209] Note the connection between the Serpent and this 'dirt,' as the image of the belly to the substance suggests a connection between the coiling/spiral energy being 'encoded' into the substance of the physical universe. – Ed.

Their descendant, to include the human race since then, would, through the ages, gradually lose their spiritual communication with each other, and become independent of one another; and as a result would not see that we are all one family under God, but as time went on, see only those things that make us different. Since we are blessed with an immortal soul, it will seek spirituality, since it will have a hunger and thirst for it. So, as with many regions of the world, the people will unite and begin some kind of worship of a God, or gods, since they will be conscious of a being, or beings greater than them. Thus, these yearnings translated into the beginning of religions, rituals, and ceremonies.

This would be the beginning of those differences, which should, under God, unite them, but would eventually also divide them. Human bodies, in time would eventually become so varied from one to another, that depending on where they lived, their location on the planet, new 'races,' new cultures, and new languages would begin to develop. Though we "seem to understand" the above, one cannot help but wonder "how" under Adam and Eve marriage could even take place?

Outward appearances would, over time, give way to the exclusion of what made up the real person on the inside and those truths that brought people together. Being unable to see those things which once united us would become that which made us afraid. Fear would rule, and animosities and conflict would lead to hatred, war and suffering. Is this not the answer to as to why we are witnessing what is taking place today?

Still many times God intervened with holy people, sages, mystics, yogis, prophets, as well as oracles and soothsayers etc. Then, all having reached a certain measure of density of physicality and diversity of spirituality, God became even more involved in humanity. We find God identified in Jewish religion as the One True God; but Egypt, Rome, and other places, etc., had their own deities. Then came Jesus and then Peter's religion, and today we see an increase in Islam, New Age, Magic, Witchcraft, and Mysticism, in proportion to a *dwindling* of Christian spirituality. One no longer wonders why Jesus asked, "When I return, will I find faith?"

Sin originated because of Adam and Eve's choice, which became the catalyst for living without spirituality, and the fallen nature due to entropy will be inclined to lean towards evil. Love of God, according to the Master Jesus, is the only catalyst that inclined one to lean towards God and goodness.

Entropy is also another word for what is often referred to as our 'fallen or sinful nature,' and we use it often since it contains all those things that go with being an imperfect human. Due to this nature, the consciousness of the light body and the transcendental consciousness, that was once known, became forgotten. How we live in this world became more valuable and real to life, with God seeming to become almost fictitious. If we choose enlightenment, we will live more aware of our light body and with a balanced spirituality, and strive more towards eternal life.

If not, if we will continue to live not for eternity, but for this temporal life. It would be this that would become the basis which will always lead to a misinformed conscience, allowing one to fall victim to those who appear stronger and more knowledgeable, but without spirituality in their own lives, which will lead them astray.

All of this lends to the love and mercy of God, who desires more for us, and a path to attain this desire. Therefore, a perfect Guide is necessary to lead us, not just to this *path*, but throughout the journey back to what God always intended. In order to do this, a perfectly sacred and balanced Guide, is necessary. One who completes the Person of the Son of God/Son of Man.

According to Eeshans beliefs the *Sophia Perennis* is the eternal wisdom, and it is she, who opens her arms to those who need God. She is essentially the feminine spirit of nurturing, which emanates from the heart of God. She is the counterpart of each of the persons of God. She is the balance of the Divine Masculine, and has taken her place beside her eternal consort as divine Feminine of the Son of God and his eternal consort here on earth, as Mary Magdalen.

LESSON 165

SECTION VII: WHERE DID ALL THE PEOPLE COME FROM?

Where did all the people come from? Were there more Adams and Eves? The following is found to be a very good insight and plausible explanation to the time old question of 'incest' in the bible. It is written by 'Got Questions.'

> *"There are numerous examples of incest in the bible. The most common examples are the sons/daughters of Adam and Eve [Genesis 4], Abraham marrying his half-sister Sarah [Genesis 20:12], Lot and his daughters [Genesis 19], Moses' father Amram who married his aunt Jochebed [Exodus 6:20] and David's son Amnon with his half-sister Tamar [2 Samuel 13]. It is important to note, however, that in two of the above instances [Tamar and Lot], one of the parties involved was an unwilling participant in the incest—better described as rape in those cases.*
>
> *It is important to distinguish between incestuous relationships prior to God commanding against them [as was written in Leviticus 18:6-18] and incest that occurred after God's commands had been revealed. Until God commanded against it, it was not incest. It was just marrying a close relative. It is undeniable that God allowed "incest" in the early centuries of humanity. Since Adam and Eve were the only two human beings on earth, their sons and daughters*

had no choice but to marry and reproduce with their siblings and close relatives. The second generation had to marry their cousin, just as after the flood. the grandchildren of Noah had to intermarry amongst their cousins. One reason that incest is so strongly discouraged in the world today is the understanding that reproduction between closely related individuals has a much higher risk of causing genetic abnormalities. In the early days of humanity, though, this was not a risk due to the fact the human genetic code was relatively free of defects.

Another consideration is that incest today almost always involves a pre-pubescent, or powerless victim, and the perpetrator is abusing his or her authority with the goal of sexual pleasure. By that standard, the 'incest' of the Bible has nothing whatsoever in common with modern-day incest. There was no power difference between Cain and his wife, for example; the goal of Abraham and Sarah's marriage was to create a family. **Intermarriage among close family members was a necessity in the generations following Adam and Noah and was not a sinful perversion of sex.**

It seems that, **by the time of Moses, the human genetic code had become polluted enough that close intermarriage was no longer safe. So, God commanded against sexual relations with siblings, half-siblings, parents, and aunts/uncles [Genesis 2:24 seems to indicate that marriage and sexual relations between parents and children were never allowed by God.]** It was not until many centuries later that humanity discovered the genetic reason that incest is unsafe and unwise. **Genetics was not an issue in the early centuries of humanity** and the marriages that occurred between Adam and Eve's children, Abraham and Sarah, and Amram and Jochebed were not selfish pursuits of sexual gratification or abuses of authority; accordingly, those relationships should not be viewed as incestuous. The key is that sexual relations between close relatives were viewed differently pre-Law *and post-Law. **It did not become "incest" until God commanded against it.**"*[210]

So where are we now ...? Eeshans warn, that unless measures of prevention are taken for the future of humankind, we may find ourselves in a very serious predicament. With abortions, population control, and fertility clinics on the rise, we may be giving rise to a genetic mess. This means, that as humans fought for freedom of choice for death over life, an imbalance of the sexes, coupled with decisions guided solely by the human consciousness, meaning that without God and the sacred balance, we are subjecting humankind to collective catastrophic sin.

Eeshans wonder, will science and technology step in to take over the control of qualities in the genetic composition of human beings, including the process of reproduction and birthing by artificial, robotic means, in attempts to both secure the 'purity' of humanity's succeeding generations, and at the same time ensure various genetic abilities/qualities/traits according to a pre-planned design? Would this possibly be the true reasons we are currently seeing trending technologies being offered to the naïve masses in attractive packages regarding *DNA, "23 and Me," and ancestral testing*? Eeshans believe that these present *advances in technology along with security assurance in all aspects of our lives, i.e., synchronization of phones and devices, cars, credit cards, and bank accounts, though on the surface this looks ideal but one wonders could it be that the fear of the populous controlling their own lives is coming to an almost epidemic proportion.*[211]

---

[210] In summary, God mandated against the practice of incest when it was time to separate the gene pools, when the numbers of human beings reached a certain point.

[211] Consider in this light Stephen Hawking's observation that the emergence of artificial intelligence could be the end of human civilization by essentially replacing it.

PART XIV

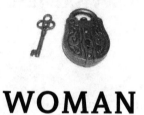

WOMAN

LESSON 166

SECTION I: WHAT WE READ, WHAT WE SEEK, AND WHAT JESUS MEANT

Let's take a look at this word, "ENLIGHTENMENT." Enlightenment is the search for truth, that we may grow in a closer relationship and live according to God's will. Thus far, we have discussed the Eeshan philosophy and beliefs as well as the transcendental meaning of the teachings of Jesus and how His whole life played out as the example of these. We presented those works of other authors we feel may help define and better explain any topics, or issues, we feel are pertinent to what we believe, in hope that you continue to search out answers that lead you to a more perfect relationship with God.

We touched on the issues Jesus faced regarding his teachings and behavior among the religion of the time, which spurned even those closest to him who benefitted by the way things were and who were not happy with any concept of change. We learned of God and God's love, and the difference between that and the twisted teachings, which invoked punishment towards those who were different then and still are today. We found how these teachings were brought to God's people by those who used their power to control the people who, for love of God, didn't question motives, or fairness, but they did it all for Jesus.

Then we brought those things to the forefront that showed how all those things of God are not just linked through time but bring with them the repercussions which essentially proves that history does, indeed, repeat itself if we don't "watch the signs," and as Jesus taught, nothing would change if this is the case. To listen, to understand, to read, and to watch for the signs that would enable us to make better choices, which would, in fact, alter the outcome from negative to the positive.

We also touched on the concept of those who used and are still using fear tactics to control the masses and have learned how some people can and have been led by fear, even if its alternative is better for all. As Eeshan Transcendentalism is not a religion according to past erroneous definitions and standards, we strive to enlighten, or get people to do the "unthinkable," which is to learn to "think," so that they may be free to choose rightfully and thoughtfully for many of our decisions will have eternal effects. Humans, for the most part, who all have some degree or another of some allegiance, unreasoning towards an emotional adherence to teams, sports, etc., but one doesn't want to enter to excessive, or prejudicial, loyalty that takes them to extreme, aggressive levels, where revenge, anger, and rage takes control.

Scriptures quote many examples of what to base our choices and decisions on, but 'few leaders' seem to take note, since they feel they are above what they teach or speak, especially if they are 'speaking' on behalf of 'God.' One priest actually believed that personal sin against God no longer existed, since Jesus already ransomed his life, so therefore, he could do whatever he wanted without blame; and so, he taught out of his own sin so not to be scrutinized himself. It is easy to ignore or turn a blind eye when you are just as guilty yourself: "Let he who is without sin, cast the first stone." However, if this is your take on this, then don't be a leader and lead others into sin, or worse to hell.

If the priest's heart and mind were truly open to what Jesus taught, Jesus' words might, thereby, make an impression on him, so that the priest's life and teachings in the presence of God and God's people would, as other religious teachers would, have somewhat of a true understanding of how God works through the faithful, and as God said (2 Corinthians 6:14-18):

> I will dwell in them and walk among them.
> I will be their God, and they will be my people.
> Therefore, come out from among them and be separate.
> Do not touch what is unclean, and I will receive you.
> I will be a father to you, and you shall be my sons and daughters.

Perhaps when you become confused with lines in scriptures, such as: 'Do not touch what is unclean, and I will receive you,' you will recall our teachings; and you will remember to look further into the text for meaning and enlightenment. Taking this verse as an example, you must remember that Jesus was very clear in telling his followers that the food/diet (any food not kosher) which once separated that his followers, meaning Jews and Gentiles, was no longer to be a concern. What was once "unclean" is now clean. That was why it took Peter a long time to accept any of these teachings, since he held on to his birth religion even after Jesus ascended. It wasn't until Acts 10:28, where it was written down as though Peter said, 'God has shown me that I should not call any person common or unclean.' And again, in Act 10-:34-3, it is written: 'Truly I understand that God shows no partiality; but in every nation, anyone who fears God and does what is right is acceptable to him,' meaning Jesus.

No longer would anyone be defined by the food they ate but by the love they shared. This was not to say that the 'spiritual food' He commanded was included in this statement. He was very clear about the 'Bread who comes down from heaven.' With regards to touching anything unclean, Jesus was referring to not taking a *substitute bread*.

Where there are still those who are sheep led to slaughter, we believe that there are more of those who in an effort to find Truth, to seek enlightenment.

Despite what was, and continues to be, presented as prefiguring Jesus with regards to the Old Law, there are too many contradictions in what was chosen, written, and lost to show Jesus' mission, intent, and of course the transcendental. Even with evidence that is claimed to back up what has been taught, the truth is that there seems to still be that desperate attempt to "hold everything together politically" by those religious authorities in power, just as at the time of Jesus, and for the survival of the religion of the time. In other words, "You can fool all of the people some of the time. You can fool some of the people all of the time; but you can't fool all of the people all of the time." Man cannot change Jesus, despite his efforts to try. It has been easy to continue to suppress Jesus' true teachings and mission for the sake of retaining all those followers that the church lied to, since there was no avenue for Christ's followers to prove, or challenge, anything with all the safe secure methods the church used to protect itself. However, even amidst this situation, the church authorities did not realize that they cannot match the power behind the magnificent love and mercy of Jesus Christ, who is true God and true Man, who suffered and died. Being the "Light of the world" and Truth, there is no way that they could hide anything about this Light under a bushel basket. So, again, the record of history belongs to the victor to write. It is a mystery, however, as to how those who do not actively participate in their religion, and yet see all the wrongs and contradictions, continually and without thought not only defend it but also feel they 'must' acquiesce to it, sooner or later.

That is what Jesus meant by "seeing the fruit, watching the signs, and fearing not one who can kill the body, but the one who can kill the body and soul," and one can only do this if grounded, or coming from, a healthy, honest relationship with God, and not being 'sheeple' to a scrupulous goliath that does not speak God's true words and intentions, who has judged wrongly and left little hope in a God who sees all as his/her children, and warns only of the consequence of eternal death by thinking that man is the center of the universe.

For those who ask, "How can you believe what you teach regarding what Jesus meant?" Well, check and see if it makes sense. Then put our answer into the scriptures and see if it works. If scriptures, however have already been altered, one can see even more clearly the discrepancies. In any event, Jesus, being God, cannot contradict this Father or Mother, nor would he be anything but true to who he is in himself. So, as we continue on, keep that in mind, especially with respect to God's Plan of Salvation.

PART XV

MISTAKEN: BEING WRONG IN ONE'S OPINION OR JUDGEMENT

LESSON 167

Section I: False Impressions

Although the passive counterpart to Jesus, at the time He lived here on earth, was Mary, she, nevertheless, spoke volumes in the person she was and in her unwavering loyalty and support of Him.

As we mentioned, the two had been among so many children in the marketplace areas, especially in and around Magdala, where major import/export trade took place. Their first 'personal' encounter was due to the horrendous violation of the thirteen-year-old going on fourteen-year-old young Mary. We discussed earlier about how Jesus left for the Himalayas to avoid being chosen for marriage. Thanks to God's plan, His earlier travels with his foster father, mother, and uncle prevented this from happening; but at seventeen, when most young men would have already been chosen for marriage, or have had schooling, He really had to leave. It was during these next eleven years that He would excel and become the Spiritual Master/High Priest He was meant to be.

It was when he came back into town that the inevitable took place. That was where He and Mary were destined to reunite.

One must understand that Mary had lived with the dream of her (Savior/Redeemer) young man, who was her knight in shining armor, returning as her hero to clear her name, as would any young woman wrongly accused at the hands of men of such unconscionable conduct.

Since that time, Mary Magdalen continued on with her life, and as a business woman, who possessed many gifts. As a successful business woman, who was also known for her abilities of healing, Mary was not one to be reckoned with. It was a perfect match. Unbeknownst to Mary, that she was already the eternal counterpart to Jesus, she had to choose, as did the Mother of Jesus, to do God's will before all could be revealed to her. Their first encounter wasn't exactly the dream return. It certainly wasn't what Mary had expected. Finding that Jesus had returned to town because He was looking for a wife was rather insulting to her, especially since a man returning to look for a wife, at that age and time, was known to be the kind of man who needed money, and someone to cater to him. Even as Mary, on the other hand, was not considered marriage material due to what had happened to her, you can only imagine that coming face to face with Jesus, after eleven years, with the man whom on which she had based all of her dreams and fantasies. That Jesus; returning one day as her knight in shining armor, under the aegis of His finding a wife, was certainly were now totally opposite of how she imagined their reuniting would play out.

Jesus was almost twenty-eight, had no job since He arrived in town due to the illness of His foster father, and lived with his mother, which did not exactly depict, or characterize, the 'hero' who inspired Mary Magdalen's dreams.

If it wasn't by God's own hand, this relationship may have ended at the first meeting of the two during a party thrown for Jesus at the home of Lazarus.

As Providence stepped in, and altered Mary's future, memories took over the two, and shortly thereafter, they were betrothed. Breaking tradition, in many instances, Mary and Jesus were married shortly, thereafter.

Their marriage would begin with such sacred vows that any human vow afterwards would pale in comparison to its beauty, since these vows had a sincerity within a covenant of love more astounding than anyone could ever enter into before. What made their vows so different? Because these were vows made *between* them and *God*. Even the tiniest detail revealed what would become the greatest, most immeasurable and unfathomable "Love Story" ever told. The wedding ring Jesus placed on Mary's finger was clearly the widespread symbol of the All-in-All, the totality of existence, infinity, and the cyclical nature of the cosmos, which is the meaning behind the transcendental serpent that forms a ring with it's tail in its mouth, symbolically representing the all of Christs', Jesus and Mary's, mission. Again, herein, we continue to find the parallels to Adam and Eve.

Their marriage was not a conjugal union, but, rather, an immersion of essences, a vision of soulmates melting into each other and becoming a divine soul, sacredly and supernaturally intrinsic to God and God's true love.

Their sharing of each other is the perfection of a transcendental, tantrically-shared love that can only be said to far exceed that which even Adam and Eve experienced. It was the embodiment of all the two, as one, would experience in their marriage: the bliss of heaven/agony on earth, extreme love/unfathomable tribulation, completeness, and total devastation, followed by fulfillment, and, yet again, years of feelings of loneliness and emptiness. Yes, they were indeed twin flames. Just as John the Baptist was freed at birth from original sin due to Elizabeth's encounter with the Fruit of Mary the Mother of God's womb, Mary Magdalen's virginity was once again restored, and made whole as the two united transcendentally and consummated their vow to each other, becoming indistinguishable as the wine from the water at their reception; prefiguring the comment, "Most couples served the best wine first and then brought out cheaper wine after the guests had too much to drink and would not notice. You have saved the best till now." (John 2:10). Not only did Jesus' wine at the wedding reception represent to Mary the meaning behind 'sharing' in Jesus' legacy, but it would reveal their Mission and all the mysteries behind her tribulations in what had to yet take place in her life. Once again, as God saw fit, it prefigured, and solidified, her place with Him presently, and that which was to be revealed in end times.

As Jesus would not have it any other way, by their marriage and her presence next to Him at the Last Supper, you will find as you read on, it was clearly in how Jesus demonstrated, that unlike Jewish Passover tradition, gender is not an obstacle before God, especially with regard to God's priesthood.[212]

---

[212] God's Priesthood reflects the offering marriage, or union, for the two, as one, before the totality of God. This necessitates a representation of each nature (Masculine/Feminine) in a mutually conscious/active priestly capacity. Other priesthoods, by comparison, are generally one sex and not the other, and are mostly 'male,' naturally leading to a projection of a 'male,' or 'masculine,' God, with women's experience and representation overridden. – Ed.

The Eeshan faith stands in unwavering testament to this truth. Having possessed his Christed Body, as only His wife did, the right to apostolic succession was not only given back to her here on earth, but it was also uniquely restored by the ending of the poisoning of her blood by Christ her husband, with a kiss, and His immutable word, by his marriage vows and his eternal oath on their wedding night.

LESSON 168

SECTION II: BUILDING A BULLYING, OR GOSSIPING MENTALITY

Jesus addresses Simon: "Why are you bothering this woman? She has done a beautiful thing to Me. Truly I tell you, whenever this Gospel is preached throughout the world, *what she has done will also be told in memory of her.*"[213]

Recent discoveries, accessible with modern technology, reveal texts that arouse questions: Why weren't these texts included in traditional biblical scriptural writings?

These words are examples of how a word here or there was changed and how scriptures could be manipulated, and edited, so as to leave out who this woman was, etc. Another prophecy? Eeshans say: yes.

All these make understanding Mary Magdalen today very difficult, especially since so much has been lost, hidden, rejected, and expunged in order to obtain (or protect) a goal. Aside from what our Eesha teaches, there are little known facts to be found about this incredible woman. A woman who was abused and violated, yet who never blamed God, and lived by the strength of her will and the dream of her hero returning for her. Rising above the oppression of man and man laws, Mary is treasured, and honored, by almighty God, and revealed as the hidden Queen, especially on her wedding night.

Why is it that most of what was omitted and declared forbidden texts were those which revealed Christ's tenderness towards Mary, and other women who were always in his company? Obviously because it would

---

[213] Matthew 23:16.

interfere with the leaders and groups who had a particular goal served by ulterior motives. In addition to there being very little information about the above available, which appears mainly in Gnostic gospels, or scriptural fragments, the general public is beginning to consider them and their place more and more. But while there is generally limited information about these available, and much of the commentary and source material can be looked upon with a healthy skepticism, Eeshans believe that the fact that there is an eyewitness to the original events who were present (Eesha, the consciousness of Mary Magdalen) changes everything.

Yes, looking upon all information from the earliest of writings warrants a healthy degree of skepticism, for sure. What Eeshans claim however, is that they believe their religion is founded on this key component: this 'eyewitness,' the consciousness of Mary Magdalen.

Let us consider, for example, when Jesus was moved by Mary's tears at the death of her brother Lazarus. On this occasion, we are told that Jesus reprimanded Martha, who was distracted with household tasks and sought His support to have Mary leave his side to assist her. Eeshans believe that Jesus took Mary away from the stigma of women of the times, with their marriage, just as He removed her from household duties in this instance. He raised her to a level higher than that of any apostle, or disciple, as often as possible and in as many ways possible.

Eesha teaches that where Jesus was, Mary was with him. They were inseparable soulmates.

Traditional writings contain mostly references to sinful, adulterous women, including the Samaritan woman at the well (John 4:4-28), to be sure to keep the mindset and stigma regarding women of the times to carry through to present times, and to never to allow a woman's mark of disgrace (especially the one that marked her as a slave) to be forgotten. What would increase the problem would be the woman being a Samaritan, i.e., *culturally impure*. All in all, according to Peter, without a man, a woman was not worthy of life.

Jesus stood in defense of Mary of Magdalen, His wife, as she anointed His feet with expensive perfume from an alabaster jar and dried them with her hair. When attacked for doing such actions, in the gospel, Jesus addresses Simon/the disciples: "Why are you bothering this woman?

She has done a beautiful thing to Me. The poor you will always have, but you will not always have Me. When she poured this perfume on My body, she did it to prepare Me for burial. Truly I tell you, whenever this Gospel is preached throughout the world, *what she has done will also be told in memory of her.*"[214] (It should be known that only the wife of a holy man could touch him.)

Obviously, the following is completely self-evident. Mary Magdalene was never a prostitute, nor an adulterous woman, but given the texts one could well come to that conclusion. Yet, this reputation followed her, despite Jesus clearing her name, and because more and more widespread, since people believed the stories, without proof.

This is the same kind of propaganda (and oppression) that women have faced throughout time. Women have tried facing and dealing with these attacks by always trying to take the higher road. Women tried to ignore such allegations, and derogatory gossip, and innuendos by men by doing their best work, and more work, in an effort to be recognized by their talents and not their colleague's apparent insecurities and their own weaknesses. Often times, these same men/women who gossip are mostly insecure, and, in an attempt to keep from being attacked themselves, they become the bullies. Often, you find they do these things behind your back, or with a group, because they need support. They manufacture their own 'worthiness' by trying to make *you* feel worthless.

The attackers always show emotional imbalance, and their strength comes from seeing how you are affected. One thing that can be said of her is that Mary Magdalen's propitious attitude made fools of those who tried to portray her as less than who she knew she was.

Her strength obviously came from Jesus who was at her side, and how He handled situations is what taught Mary how to do the same. Once Jesus had returned to heaven, however, Mary was left vulnerable. With outside forces causing the regression of Jesus' teachings and the New Law to revert back to the Old, Mary continued to face the inevitable.

With constantly being made a fool of, and with continued insolent and cheeky insults against her integrity, despite her personal and loving

---

[214] All gospels record the anointing (i.e., Matt. 26:6-13).

encounters and respectful confrontations to resolve the issue, as she felt Jesus would, these persistent attacks, with no evidence for this kind of reasoning would continue throughout her life and beyond. Since attempts and queries were made thanks to persistent memory were squashed, the church finally shifted from the sinful woman who had seven demons cast from her to more recently 'apostle to the apostles and **a witness to God's mercy.' Sure, let's keep the "title 'adulteress' alive."** Though 'the sinner' is still the focus, and not wife, this decision was only brought about by the updates in the universal film industry, giving the church no options.

Still many scholars now believe, as Eeshans have known, that Mary's prominence in the early traditions was an obstacle to later attempts to exclude women from leadership positions in the church of Peter, and that the story of her previous life as a prostitute[215] (which was instigated first by Peter), then fabricated to discredit her in later years, was reinitiated to protect patriarchal dominance, especially during women's fight for rights and among activists group for the equal opportunities for women. Also, one would look at this new 'position' for Mary Magdalen as 'hope' for sinful women, who, as it is written in the 'disclosed' policy of the church, without men women have no control over their own bodies. Private revelations from our Eesha indicate the same.

The being called the "disciple Jesus loved most" is not fiction, and finally gives way to the truth that this refers to Mary of Magdala (not the apostle John); and *is much more credible that she is the disciple* that Jesus loved most. Sadly, this could not be propagated since it would give Mary equal place with a man alongside Jesus. Yet when Peter turned and asked Jesus, "What about 'Him' (Mary)?" Jesus replied, "If I want him to remain alive until I return, what is it to you?" (John 21:21-22). We know that this was changed to reflect His eternal consort but removed. Why? Because Mary was with Him, and no other man followed among the apostles. Peter was so angry because Mary took her place beside Jesus at the supper. Every time she leaned over to talk with Him, Peter tried to interrupt. When Jesus announced that someone would betray Him, Peter immediately figured it would be the woman.

---

[215] "Mary Magdalene." Gospel Mysteries, www.gospel-mysteries.net/mary-magdalene.html.

When Jesus taught about those who 'hear the word of God and live it,' He raised nor only His Mother to her rightful place but also he raised up His wife, putting her above all the other apostles, as she was *his wife and his counterpart*. Her continued presence and His respect and kindness toward her and all women made Him a radical for that time.

Women, having very limited rights, even in the home, could be sold for a dowry when they came of age. The Mishnah taught that a woman was like a gentile slave, who could be obtained by intercourse, money, or writ.[216,217] To be treated as equal to men in the eyes of the Savior was 'beyond offensive,' especially to Peter, and to those like him and his brother, who would never let go of the old Law. To them, Jesus' relationship with Mary was an outrageous and scandalous example of how marriage was viewed.

Peter took every advantage and often argued that Jesus' concern with the treatment of women was an obstacle to His (Jesus') ministry and its public approval, and so he (Peter) was profoundly at odds with Jesus' relationship with Mary and the notion of her as the completion of Him as Messiah, often in front of the others. This added to the influencing of others.

Jesus' acceptance of women as followers, and being impartial as to who He taught were two more reasons that *frightened a few of his apostles* to a great extent, when hearing Peter's continued complaints. Disgusted, Peter often asked that Mary be removed from their presence when Jesus met with His disciples.

Peter's cowardly concern was that Jesus' behavior regarding women would bring about charges that He was violating the Mishnah. Why was this not made known until present times? As it's been said many times, "History as we know it is written by the winners."

Given enough time, which allows for a kind of bullying, a social and psychological 'mob' mentality becomes fact to people who lose personal identity to stronger minded people. Running on 'emotion,' not on truth, the fallacy of the accusations towards the victim gives way to destructive

---

[216] "Women in Ancient Israel." Bible History Online, Bible History Online, www.bible-history.com/court-of-women/women.html.
[217] m.Qidd 1:1.

means to prevent the truth from being revealed. Mob mentality may begin with heckling, bullying etc., and this is how any agenda, or platform, when expressed in opposition, can turn to violence at the drop of a hat.

But you may say that not all confrontations are of a 'mob' mentality. Well, we are showing how at the root of these are people, with personal issues and underlying tones of anger/rage, who are just awaiting the opportunity to become just that, and this rarely happens for the good or the betterment of all. Angry people can also sow seeds of anger and display them under the guise of 'doing good,' or for the 'betterment' of mankind, since it tends to lead in efforts that begin by showing the 'dangers' of not taking action and relieving not only a crisis situation but by bringing comfort and solace to the suffering. Remember when groups of people rushed into abortion clinics killing abortion doctors in efforts to stop abortion? Foul language, threats, and tabloid stories never lead to good, or to healthy or positive, change.

It was this kind of mentality in the 1950's, and into present times, out of fear, which kept women from being educated, due to concerns that they would defy their purpose of being created woman, or that they cannot be educated since they were lesser than men. Many times, groups would take to protesting in efforts to cause upheavals of anger from opponents, which would then be popularized by the media.

How wonderful is the STEM program, which is giving opportunities to outstanding young women in every class, color, and creed to destroy the stigmas attached to women being leaders and advancing in fields of science, technology, engineering, and math. Programs such as these insure, and help, the growing staples of brilliant women find their places and be counted among the pioneers for other young females.

Today, it seems as though the trend is not to 'love one's neighbor,' but to 'hate' one's neighbor. Hatred of political figures, institutions etc., are a few examples of where protests, social media, and debates, that, without civility and recognition result in not exemplifying that we are all members of the 'human family,' and initiate a 'mob' mentality, which is becoming more and more encouraged.

On an individual basis, it takes just one other human being to encourage another, then another, before an entire office turns on a worker. Women can be very dominating. This is where the test of rights come into play. They have fought for so long and so hard to gain recognition that even they tend to think and act they must be careful to not lose the battle at the expense of another woman, especially when the more dominating personality can retaliate. Healthy competition is what the Divine Feminine encourages. Women must be conscious of the fact that the feminine nature tends to be very judgmental towards other women who don't fit their standard, or who choose to be what some would call 'a disgrace to other women.' In other words, they become the image of the males they have been pitted against.

Women who have worked hard against the rights they feel they have lost to men or in facing obstacles to gain equal wages and benefits to bring a change in men's perception of what a woman should, or could, be, must be most certainly aware of working with other women. Women's rights are about respect and dignity as human beings, and the appropriate recognition for their abilities, talents, and skills, and being free from judgment of being somehow inferior because of their gender. At the same time, women's rights should not be about turning the tables and forcing another form of inequality.

That was where the clash between pro-abortion/prochoice and anti-abortion and anti-choice groups came about. Equality for all should be morally sound, and yet not infringe on every aspect of a person's life, or the decisions, they have to make. Eventually children, teens, and young adults hopefully mature under proper and moral guidance. We want them to understand and make good choices in ways that won't cause them to rebel against those teaching about good example but by being good examples, and being able to communicate why we may see things differently from how they see things. It is important also to recall how many times you, as an adult going through life, changed your mind, and how those things regarding your experience caused your change of mind to a mature outlook.

We as Eeshans could vouch for that, since we as men and women grew up Catholic, and all of us remember those things that contributed to choices we made and the experiences we had. Thinking regarding political issues, education, family, God, in one's teens, early twenties, thirties etc., truly changes, hopefully for the better, and, yet, still sometimes more life experience is necessary.

LESSON 169

SECTION III: GENOCIDE, EUTHANASIA, MERCY KILLING: IS THERE A DIFFERENCE?

Over the last 50 years of being raised in our birth religions (Catholic, Christian, etc.) we have witnessed what we feel are many wrongs. Witnessing an authority that teaches a doctrine of morals that even they themselves do not live by or govern themselves with in their own inner workings (Matt. 23:1-4) was one of these. There are familiar workings found within religions; within the Catholic church, for example, there is Canon Law. Canon Law is broken into an internal forum and an external forum. Though these divisions may be necessary, when abused they can be very hurtful. For example, 'internal forum' is the act of governance that is made without publicity. Things in this sense are determined, and are decided upon "behind closed doors." When used properly, it allows the governing of issues that don't affect the public. Used wrongly, it can be very hurtful, since it can perpetuate and protect corruption and the abuse of power. This is what allowed for grievous sins to continue within the church: i.e., pedophilia, sexual abuse of nuns, children, unwed mother abuse, etc. These ills were essentially protected from public knowledge, and so they would persist.

ABORTION

External forums, by contrast, are public and verifiable. These also have been abused and poorly exercised. For example, they have been used to publicly address the sin of abortion, and announce the punishment of women who went against the moral code, yet not against pedophile teachers and priests; but to be fair, there were also plenty of abusive nuns. Abuse is not just found in the Catholic church, but in pockets of other Christian denominations, and in other religions, as well. Abortion is morally wrong, and protection of life should be of the highest priority in our lives, and so is the protection of innocence.

Being raised Catholic, however, and believing that Jesus was the central and the one true God, Savior and Redeemer, makes the teachings on abortion critical. Over the recent years, finding that church teaching is not necessarily what the church does (as in Matt. 23:1-4, on doing as the authority says and not what it does) is chokingly sad.

During the scandal reported in June, 2014, where nearly eight hundred children's bodies were found in a mass grave near the former home for unwed mothers and their children near the site of St. Mary's Mother and Baby Home, which was converted into a housing estate run by the Sisters of Bon Secours in Ireland, is, indeed, fact. Charges of abuse by priests, such as outlined in the movie "Spotlight," are also fact; yet, there are still people who will turn a blind eye to it all and say, "I don't want to see, or hear, anything that goes against my church." Who is confused here?

Though the state took the Magdalen Laundries where women were sent and confined by the Catholic church, and worked for nothing, serving in most cases "life sentences" simply for being unmarried mothers, or regarded as morally wayward,[218] one wonders who is morally wrong? Our Eesha met a few nuns who had information regarding these horrid, detention centers, with the last one closing just around 2012, who asked to remain anonymous, while some also asked for forgiveness. Nuns from the Sisters of Our Lady of Charity, Sisters of Mercy, and Sisters of the Good Shepherd were[219] involved to some degree, and some were actually

---

[218] McDonald, Henry. "Magdalene Laundries: Ireland Accepts State Guilt in Scandal." The Guardian, Guardian News and Media, 5 Feb. 2013, www.theguardian.com/world/2013/feb/05/magdalene-laundries-ireland-state-guilt.

[219] O'loughlin, Ed. "Tuam Mother and Baby Home Remains Will Be Exhumed, Ireland Says."The New York Times, 23 Oct. 2018, www.nytimes.com/2018/10/23/world/europe/tuam-ireland-mother-and-baby-home-remains.html.

implicated. This particular sister showed Eesha a diary that was kept secret, and she prayed that she would get to see Eesha, so she could ask her to pray that God would forgive these, and more, who were involved. It has been said that many of the children aborted were those of priests, as a result of their sexual abuse of nuns in convents. Many nuns told her stories of the abuse that would take place among other nuns and priests with the women in the work houses, as well as with children in families in poor countries. There were friends who remembered people who were abused and those priests who were exposed in recent years. Her stories and recollections were very, very sad. She told Eesha that any woman who became pregnant by a priest had to have an abortion, and these were often young girls at school, who were from poor families, and where priests would frequent their family homes, or abuse them at school. Children were malnourished, beaten, and given to priests for entertainment.

These kinds of abuses were, in fact, the same kind that women faced at the time of Jesus, and, as in the case of Mary Magdalen, women have been threatened, ridiculed, and/or punished, since there were no repercussions, whatsoever, to the man/men involved. This is the same punishment which just recently has been made known by women today in all fields of employment. These kinds of actions, though brought to light, have still caused many women to be put on the spot for unmasking those men guilty as charged. Africa is another horrible example of ignored abuse and abortions reaching epidemic proportions among nuns impregnated by priests.

That is why we took great offense at the announcement of Pope Francis in 2016, with regards to the 'year of mercy' designated to all priests to "forgive 'women' the sin of abortion."

In the Eeshans' view of this, the Catholic church not only continues to punish women but also went one step further, since this kind of announcement lessens the importance of the sacrament of forgiveness and Divine Mercy, and it proves that a double standard of teaching exists. This is not how Eeshans believe Jesus taught his people to handle difficult moral, and ethical, problems and difficult decisions.

It stands to reason that women are not solely responsible for this sin. Both a man and woman are involved in the conception of the child.

Without a doubt, there are always extenuating circumstances where an abortion, or a dilation, and curettage is necessary, the latter is usually necessary after a miscarriage, or apparent ongoing miscarriage. But with regards to abortion, consensual decision or not, it's always wrong that it's only the women who are 'judged and punished,' apart from the shared responsibility of the man.

Eeshans conclude that being morally, or ethically, responsible, as implied by the church' practice of 'forgiveness of only a woman,' it's only right that all church laws should apply equally to the man, as well who is involved in this situation. In other words, if this is the church's stance on abortion then both should fall under this directive of murder, and in the case of the church's directive regarding a "year of forgiveness" to the amended "all priests can forgive this sin," both should equally fall under this "special forgiveness." Men know if they impregnated a woman or not.

We must ascertain that Eeshans always believe that the Mystery of Forgiveness took care of this issue, since in most cases the decision was driven by fear, and the woman never really gets past her decision, or the father's decision, for that matter.

In another instance, where one is married, or single, should one or the other refuse the abortion, then, whoever maintains the abortion decision embraces the weight of the moral responsibility and the consequences (unless there is due cause). However, should the woman with *the most sincere and contrite heart* (if the abortion was her decision and not done under coercion) have the right to come before God in the powerful Mystery of Forgiveness, she should not be held a prisoner of a troubled conscience forever. This has been a practice among prayer groups, who continually target women who had abortions with prayer services, which will not allow for Divine forgiveness, but instead keep punishing the woman over and over.

Eeshans present that there is verifiable reason to believe that many of today's views on marriage, divorce, abortion, etc. and are certainly influenced by ancient biblical laws and customs regarding the treatment of women that were carried over from the Old Testament into the New Testament.

NOT ALL ARE VICTIMS OF RAPE, BUT ALL DO INVOLVE FEAR

The severely limited rights of women, which were absolutely reversed by Jesus Christ, and were reverted back and continued to plague present times shortly after the Ascension of Jesus, are glaring. Taken as a whole, and unless we correct what Jesus intended, lived, and taught, we will never be able to correct these errors. Eeshans understand that in a lot of cases the factors of age, immaturity, hormones, fear, and the desire to please at an early age, the desire to maintain a relationship, pressure, alcohol, and drugs are on the list of contributors to pregnancy and forced marriages, or the refusal to marry, and most of these poor decisions, not to mention financial issues, have all contributed to the choice of abortion.

Humans make horrible mistakes. That women have carried the brunt of this sin and men have taken, in many cases, little accountability for it, especially under church law, is another indication of continued discrimination in Catholic and Christian circles. The recently altered declaration of the "year upon which priests may forgive women who had abortions" (only for the year) by bishops only added insult to injury, since men had no guilt to bear. As we mentioned previously, the correction to this was an amended directive, indicating that any priest could now forgive this sin, as though it was taken to a lower status; but the issue at hand is the attention drawn to 'the woman that requires a 'special' forgiveness' outside the sacrament of Reconciliation.

JESUS NEVER MADE A SPECTACLE OF WOMEN'S ISSUES BUT GAVE ENCOURAGEMENT, EXHIBITED TENDERNESS, AND THIS IS HOW HE CHANGED ATTITUDES: WITH LOVE.

Eeshans believe that humankind, male or female, is subject to error, and we all share in the horrid results of those sins, as well as the healing. *Though there is nothing more grievous than to take a life at any age*, and at any cost, perhaps with the exception of self-defense, we do believe that all, with a truly contrite heart and resolve to try and never commit the sin again, may be forgiven. Perhaps a way of expressing that contrition would be to find a penance for the sin, and a reparation, which allows for an understanding of what triggered this sin, and how deeply embedded one is in it. In doing this, we are then helping to develop a better informed conscience.

Realistically, to promise to never commit this sin again is very difficult, since we all have faults and weaknesses that, if not guided, or helped by friends or family, may lead to a continuing of the sin; whereas, when understanding the consequences and being given an alternative to viewing the proposed sin, one may find healing and courage to commit to avoiding those things that lead back to the vicious cycle of bad choices leading to sin.

It is true that abortion led to euthanasia, and that euthanasia for population control, and relief of economic distress, attempts to establish laws and propaganda that allow legal widespread extermination of anyone who can no longer, or never could, contribute to society, due to age, illness, etc.?

LESSON 170

SECTION IV: UNJUSTICES TO MEN/WOMEN: HOW CAN THEY BE RECTIFIED?

Eshans also believe, and profess, that as Jesus forgave sins, so can his wife, since she, who was disgraced, and slandered by men, was also, as He had been. She is His female counterpart, whom He sends to act on His behalf with kindness and love sharing in all He was, is, and always will be. As things regressed, due to the rejection of God's plan, regarding the 'New Law,' which Jesus' himself lived as an example against the erroneous old Law, the sacred balance was once again suppressed and almost forsaken as non-existent.

One very beautiful Eeshan belief is that in this world, a mother's love is born in a woman with the birth of her child, and Eeshans believe that a father's love, also, is born; and when faced with raising a child alone, makes for a balanced single parent, when God is involved. Woman is no stranger to pain, or sacrifice, as proven with the acceptance of the erroneous story and facts from the image and likeness of God, and from the story of Adam and Eve, down through the ages, up and until to present times. She will give up her life to give life.

We believe that men today are finding a 'new' role as fathers, due to becoming single parents, either by divorce, or illness, and death of their spouse, and this is all due to the return of the Divine Feminine. A majority of women have given up their lives, their futures, and faced shame, and pain, for the stigma they carried alone due to an abortion. Men seem to have come forward, and despite what the church taught, would very well accept the responsibility of raising the child, not out of obligation, but love. We see a growing interest in men investing in their children, and 'learning' how to be as balanced as they can in offering those things a 'mom' would have done, especially in encouraging their child to pursue their talents and dreams, and not letting anyone, or anything, stop them.

Many have given up on their faith, but not their God, and that shows intestinal fortitude and trust. It's as though Jesus is their personal Savior and redeemer, as He was in His days on earth, and recognizes women as 'equals' differently than maybe their fathers or grandfathers. Humans can judge, but God knows the heart.

It's not only the 'right to choose,' or the 'loss of choice,' that hurts women or what they are fighting for, but this also regards the loss of dignity. The right to go to Jesus, and the fact that they must succumb to the judgment of man, is now being looked down upon by men. Maybe because they have been experiencing their feminine balance, and understand better how all have been deprived of this beautiful sacred balance.

There are so many women who panicked that just couldn't deal with carrying a deformed child or a child afflicted with birth defects. One must remember that only God knows the truth, and the strength, or weakness, of a woman's heart, or of actually *any* heart. Fear actually causes a strong biological compulsion to avoid the perceived source of this fear. Coupled with the fear induced by others, a husband's threat, rather than his love, undermines the great love and trust in the heart of the wife, and that always damages marriages, as does the wife's threats when a husband wants the child, and the wife cannot bear to keep it. Life takes unexpected turns. Not to imply that either is absolutely right or wrong, it's just that the mental state of one or the other should be addressed, and eased if not by the other spouse alone, or by close friends and relatives, then, perhaps, along with a doctor or professional.

We understand the pain and hurt of women who made this choice, perhaps just on their own. We also understand and believe in the mysteries and sacraments Jesus gave us in our Eeshan faith. We understand how women, and all those who have been victimized for being different according to any religion, are often compromised, but we know the love of Jesus and the extent of his forgiveness, and we know Him.

Human beings will continue to make mistakes; this is why we have the Mystery of Forgiveness. We are not perfect, but God is. Jesus Christ saw only a means to bring people to Him with love. He came to those who sinned, and who were shunned by the law, and to the sick who were scandalized and punished for the sin of their parents, and for those rejected for color or race or class. These people were no different than we are today. He talked, laughed, ate with them, and healed them, and was accused of being 'like' them. Jesus taught us to love our neighbor with the many acts of love He performed. He dined with sinners and all those who were rejected because of class, job, or illness. Jesus saw the person. He saw their attributes, capabilities, weaknesses, and strengths. He forgave them and expected them to do the same for their enemies. He showed them how it is better to turn the other cheek and to forgive, as many times as it takes, to bring about peace. He was kind. He taught how, if you couldn't change hearts with His example, or teachings, to shake the dust from your shoes and go to the next town. He taught us to reject those things that take you away from him, meaning those things that will hurt you and those you love, and, in turn, weaken your faith and trust in God.

He treated each woman He met as a person in her own right. He healed the woman with a hemorrhage without question because of her faith in Him, despite her being labeled unclean. He stood with the weak, the tax collectors, and all those whom others judged. and who were called sinners. He showed God's love in how He accepted us and how that is the same way we should accept others. To love our neighbor as we love ourselves was a commandment, which means putting ourselves in the other person's place, and deciding how we would want to be treated in the other person's position. This was His commandment and it was not to be viewed as an option, but instead to be exercised with all people. We don't have to agree with them, we don't have to follow them, but we must *love* them as children of God.

Options for a child whose parents, for one reason or another, are not able to care for the child has always been adoption. Moses' mother had to give her child up. Many times, women who loved their child just had to seek a better life for their child. Families have also intervened to help, and grandparents, as well. Many, many, people who have had given birth to a child, or children, with birth defects now have wonderful people to help, such as the Danielle Foundation.

FORGIVE EACH OTHER: REMEMBER YOU ARE NOT ALONE

Jesus taught us that God is our Father and Mary is our Mother. Before He died He astonished us by forgiving those who crucified Him. Afterwards, we became His and His wife's begotten children. As He gave us his Mother to love and intercede for us, we find He now gives us His wife, who encompasses Him, as a living testament to continue His ministry. With the example of a phenomenal marriage in which the Lamb and His wife complete each other, and bring back the sacred balance of male and female, it is through this marriage that He would correct the downward spiral that began with the exposing of what Eeshans consider to be the unfolding truth of Adam and Eve's choice. Never before revealed, Eeshans teach this omission is what led to fear, discrimination, and oppression we see everywhere today.

God will do the same for us in these times, in this moment, actually, through our faith and love for Jesus and His wife. God gave us the commandments. People became lost. Jesus taught us how to live them, but they were ignored, rewritten, or lost. Perhaps, if we had what Jesus taught, we would still get lost, but God's mercy and love abounds. Knowing this about God, one thing is for sure: God does not quit on us. We quit on God. That's how we know, Jesus' wife will teach us and lead us back to Him.

LESSON 171

SECTION V: MARY AND THE WOMEN MINISTERS AT THE TIME OF JESUS AND TODAY

THE BEGINNING OF SEXISM?

Sexism, hardly. Pointed fingers usually accompany this term, followed by a disgusted tone by those weak men who fear strong women. They are not interested in equality of genders. These are not even interested in what or how this word came into being. Usually they claim women are aggressive, bitter, and hate men. They might work with women, and by their own standards of wage, feel that feminism is no longer necessary. When men are single, they are hailed. When a woman is single, she is pitied and judged. These men still feel that it's a woman's job to order their lunches and pick them up, finish their office cleanup and make party arrangements, buy gifts for colleagues, etc. Most always men interrupt women when they are talking or seek the opinion of another man on issues that a woman has already explained. Women are mocked for expressing feelings, as though they 'cry' about everything, while referring to them in vulgar terms.

Most people don't know that sexism is gender discrimination based on any gender, but it most assuredly is particularly documented as affecting women and girls, though there are many cases of the same with regards to men. It has been linked to stereotypes and gender roles. It often includes that belief that one sex, or gender, is intrinsically superior to another,[220] even before God. In John 4:27, we immediately see the apostles' outrage that they found Jesus talking with a woman, i.e., the woman at the well. They knew then that He was breaking the law not only by speaking to a woman, but He was also alone with her, and it was a Samaritan woman at that. Samaritans, if you recall, were shunned by the Jews.

Eeshans know that Jesus always intended for Mary Magdalene, His wife, and the women who followed Him, along with his apostles, to propagate his teachings, bringing gender equality to all. The issue is that God will not infringe on free will, we infringe on God's.

As the apostles parted, groups formed under each, having disciples of their own. Many of the women that were part of Jesus' ministry, including His wife, Mary Magdalen, who headed groups and worshipped as Jesus had taught them.

Aside from evidence presented to the contrary, and as we exhibited time and again, Peter was never fond of the way Jesus included Mary and other women around Him, and used whatever 'language' necessary to strengthen his point. We saw how even while Jesus was alive, Peter used every opportunity to try and influence Jesus' behavior. He always viewed what Jesus was teaching as against Mishnah,[221] and made known the punishment for this behavior, and how allowing women to be taught, and teach about God, was prohibited. Peter's behavior, and that of a few of the others close to him, was, indeed, reflective of how women are viewed in many religions today, including the various stances of religious institutions on women's ordination and other leadership roles. And why is this? It has been handed down for two thousand years.

Following Jesus' ascension to heaven, we see how Peter felt, if Jesus' ministry was to continue, that it would be necessary to stop and correct those things that would cause the arrest and imprisonment of himself and the other apostles. His thoughts were that surely Jesus would want

---

[220] "Sexism." Wikipedia, Wikimedia Foundation, 4 Dec. 2019, en.wikipedia.org/wiki/Sexism.

[221] The Mishnah is the first written record of the Oral Law. At the time of Jesus, it was the Oral Law that explained how its commandments were to be carried out. – Ed.

his work to continue, and if they were all arrested there would be no way it could. A plan developed where, as time went on, a few of the male apostles began to attend to the women's worship services; and since women found it natural to welcome the original brothers/disciples and fellow teachers, so Peter would report them to the authorities to deflect any attention away from him.

That is why Eeshans believe that the Byzantine prayer seems to have best captured the awareness of Peter's betrayal of Jesus and his teachings as much as Judas,' "May I not reveal your mysteries to your enemies, NOR give you a kiss as did Judas." Two different examples of betrayal, but we can see that Peter's capacity and inclination to betray and the manner in which he betrayed is held up in a glaring manner.

Eventually, the women's ministries were outlawed, and deemed heretical, and they once again fell under the law, which prohibited them from teaching, and/or attending religious worship, despite the fact that the women no long followed Jewish Law but Jesus' Law and Priesthood. They followed precisely what Jesus taught, even down to the eating of foods that were once unclean under the Law.

The women never felt inclined to follow Peter as leader since they were present when Jesus spoke of Mary and other times to include the conversation regarding James being the one who would lead.[222]

Eeshans still feel that if Mary had been allowed to accomplish Jesus 'Plan by teaching and balancing as the female counterpart (as was God's intention) to bring sacred balance back, and if James had been put in a place of leadership of the structural part (and not Peter), there would be little to no discrimination based on gender, age, religion, creed, race, color, and sexual orientation because Jesus taught all as children of God.[223]

To those who don't understand, we mean that as Eve was the first to bite the apple, after she and Adam made the *mutual choice* to follow through with the decision, it would be Mary who would follow through

---

[222] According to the non-canonical Gospel of Thomas, (buried and preserved in the Nag Hammadi, in Egypt) knowing Jesus would soon depart from them, His disciples asked Him who would lead them, "And Jesus said to them in the place you are to go, go to James the righteous, for whose sake Heaven and Earth came into existence." – Ed.

[223] Matt. 19:10-12, Luke 20:21-25.

with her and Jesus' *mutual decision* for Him to lead and teach first, and Mary to continue and bring the plan to fruition when God's salvific plan would be interrupted.

We believe, and cannot stress enough, that Jesus did not see people according to their appearance, but saw them as human beings, who by God's salvific plan would have exposure to Him, and, thus, the expand the their level of consciousness to the transcendental, and live as God so intended.

Without a doubt, the strength of certain women was certainly displayed in the Old Testament, and we heard all the references of these women since ancient times. Women such as Ruth, Esther, and Rachel of the Old Testament, were strong for sure; but none surpassed the women of the New Testament, such as His Mother Mary, and His wife and her Kallahs, as well as all those women who followed Jesus. These anxiously and fearlessly propagated the faith as He taught them, while He was here and after He had gone. It was because of Jesus that women saw the freedom to know, love, and serve God for the first time under the Order of Melchizedek. Jesus loved spending time and talking with women. Their opinions were important to Him, but, more importantly, He ordained them.

LESSON 172

SECTION VI: THE WOMEN WHO LOVED GOD

Eshans revere, and believe, that the most prominent among all women is without a doubt the Virgin Mary, who became woman through an immaculate birth (meaning without sin or defilement), solely to give birth to Christ Jesus the Son of God, Divine Masculine, that he may become human without change. The Mother of Jesus was the first to give an unconditional yes to whatever God wanted. The Virgin Mary always displayed complete trust in God, and always put obedience to God before obedience to man. Jesus raised His Mother above all women when He called God His Father in heaven and blessed her for knowing the will of God. Though Mary entered into a secretly platonic marriage, as the wife of Joseph (Jesus' foster father), under Mosaic law, her non-conjugal relations with Joseph, though against the Law, revealed and witnessed to the truth that God is the author of law and His law is above man's law. The marriage of God with a human being was sanctioned and perfect in every way. This truth, as well as the acceptance of her immaculate conception, dispelled the rumors of the day regarding Jesus' acknowledgment of the identity of His father in heaven.

Next is Jesus' wife, Mary, whose example we bow to in deep respect and love, for she heard God's will, and willingly gave her yes that her body would be born to be defiled in order that she be saved, redeemed, and divinized by her husband.

We declare her second only to Mary, Our Lady's reputation who, though not violated, was subject to doubt from her husband and the ridicule and slander of others to include the story of a Roman soldier as being the father of Jesus; thus, making the Virgin Mary an adulterous. This, too, was God's plan, that the sinless, immaculate Person of the Virgin would prefigure the illicit and reputed rumors of prostitution of Mary Magdalen, wife of Jesus. Still today rumors continue to circulate about the Virgin not being a virgin, or worse—that she was a prostitute. Sadly, to address these things in anger or counterattacking does not stop the rumors, or prevent anyone from spreading them. It would be more to the point, since those who love the Virgin will 'not read this trash,' or circulate these things. If one feels they must 'do something,' then pray that her Son is merciful to them. Sometimes these kinds of issues are more personal than if they were made for public attention. Oddly enough, sometimes people want God to react.

Women need the power of the Virgin and Mary Magdalen as spiritual guides. These women were, are, and always will be, the Sources of Sacred Balance and strength, and because of their divinity, they will lead women on a path that doesn't have a corruptible integrity, which career-minded and professional women pursuing their professions or who are in powerful positions are often subject to. Needless to say, all women need this guidance regardless of who they are and where they are. Women are faced with vulgarity, immorality, and unconscionable undertakings and offenses daily. They give their heart to men who seek ephemeral relations, hoping that love will triumph. The last thing women need is to become, or to follow, those who mimic the same. To take on those characteristics of the very evil that they have fought thinking that they have succeeded becoming one like those who they have modeled themselves after, lowers women's potentiality. Thus, women gain no ground. They just become the extreme version of what they have fought against.

A man once said he kept his wife in 'check' because he feared it was the only way men could survive, since they are becoming a potentially 'lost breed.' Women who think and act in portraying men in the same way as they themselves are despised are no better a women or gender. To do so is to succumb, submit, and surrender to a superior negative force.

In other words, they are still inferior against men. In the dictionary, it says the imagery of succumbing is to lay down before more powerful forces, and this happens when women become, or take on, the same mentality of powerful men who have controlled their lives and the lives of what they consider weaker genders.

Yes, we need the divine. Prayerfully, we hope to realize that sooner rather than later.

LESSON 173

SECTION VII: DA VINCI DECODED 2000+ YEARS AGO

With his love and respect for His Mother and Wife, and despite the reputed Mishnah declaration Peter directed at Jesus saying, "Why do you allow her here among us?—everyone knows women are not worth life!"

Jesus continued to teach by example and showed men that women deserved life, and their lives had as much worth as men, and contrary to Peter's declaration, were equal to men in the eyes of God. Women, in turn, were by the Savior's side during the good times and never left his side, or denied, Him when He was arrested and crucified. Jesus' wife never failed Him. She remained with Him at the cross and by her divine and sacred kiss gave Him life, and once upon returning to the tomb, she searched for Him, found Him, and returned to tell the others.

Jesus' relationship with Mary of Magdala was an example, par excellence, of the view that God, as man, put into action the truths regarding women's place beside men, and the power of love. Eeshans believe, too, that Jesus' teachings, example, and marriage were vital, and were duly meant to be known, not to be hidden, or expunged, but, because it went against both written and oral law, they became the main reasons for His arrest, suffering, and crucifixion.

Jesus' correcting, embarrassing, or calling religious leaders 'hypocrites,' and pointing out errors of an ancient religion, where Abraham and Moses, as the head patriarchs, were used in His talks, or when He would rebuke someone (i.e., "It will not be me who condemns you but he whom you put your trust in: Moses and before Abraham I Am …") was

His way of countering their attacks on Him, and showing the wrongful scriptural proof-texting they used against Him. This was important since Jesus seized moments to show how they saw only a *masculine* God. To them, this was unacceptable, thus, every opportunity they could leverage and they used the Law in an effort to make Jesus cease trying to make women equal to men. If they continued to use the Law against Jesus in some way or other, it would prove He was not what, and who, God promised as the Messiah; Jesus was altering the male gender's assumed superiority of man, which was claimed by the authorities as being foundational to the plan of man's salvation. So many references to improprieties with regard to laws and teachings allowed for references, charges, and the list of blasphemies that were eventually used against Jesus. These include countless 'Gentile' teachings about love of neighbor, what defined 'work on the Sabbath,' in addition to Jesus 'focus on the treatment of women; this absolutely footed the growing accusations and planned protest gatherings created by the Pharisees, Sadducees, and scribes. This is demonstrated by their constant efforts to trip Him up and His responses toward them. It is a known fact that the word 'Gentile' was, in biblical times, used to show a distinction between the soul of a Jew and the soul of a non-Jew (this included women). The soul was classified in this way:

1. Nefesh: the 'lower part, 'or 'animal part, 'of the soul is linked to instincts and bodily cravings. This is provided at birth.
2. Ruach, the 'middle soul,' is the 'spirit.' It contains the moral virtues and the ability to distinguish between good and evil.
3. Neshamah is the 'higher soul or super soul.' This separates man from all other life forms and is related to the intellect, and allows man to enjoy the benefit from the afterlife. It allows one to have some awareness and presence of God.

According to those writings, a Jewish soul was composed of these three characteristics; whereas, a Gentile soul contains only Nefesh.[224]

---

[224] "Gentile." Wikipedia, Wikimedia Foundation, 30 Nov. 2019, en.wikipedia.org/wiki/Gentile.

Though there are many interpretations of the word 'Gentile,' many were confused after reading conflicting gospels, such as what Jesus commanded and why. One such gospel was *Matthew 10:6-7: "These twelve Jesus sent out but commanded, 'Go not to the way of the Gentiles, and into any Samaritan city; but go rather to the lost sheep of the house of Israel.'" And yet again, in Luke 23:28, "Jesus turned and said to them, 'Daughters of Jerusalem, do not weep for me; weep for yourselves and for your children.'"*

What Jesus was saying here was that according to both of these verses, the Jewish religion *and* those who did not follow what He taught was necessary would 'not' accept Him as Messiah and certainly would not see a plan for Salvation, the way we currently see it, rather, salvation was seen as political liberation from the Romans. It is in this way that they had a problem. This man was destroying their chances for sovereignty and autonomy.

This meant that Jesus' ideals were not realistic to the Jewish authorities and teachers, nor did He help the cause but rather He was weakening the numbers. His teachings were actually considered dangerous to the survival of Israel. The Jewish authorities and teachers totally missed what God meant by Messiah, and that is why His changes, as the active consort and "Way" of the transcendental life, was a problem. As Caiphas said, quoting scripture, "It is better to have one man die than for an entire nation to be lost." While religious leaders and political liberationists were waging war on a secular enemy, Jesus was waging war on the source of evil. In telling them what He meant and that He accomplished what He was supposed to do in reality was giving them everything; but for them, with what was going to take place, without following His directives, they would lose everything. That is why He said it would be their children and their children's children that would 'not' have what God intended for them for their salvation, and that they didn't know God when He was among them.

Jesus' acceptance of women as equals, and allowing them to attend and participate in worship services in every capacity as the men, was the last straw and final blow to their birth religion as it was to them a mockery of God's Law to all those under Moses:

"But do not think I will accuse you before God, your Father; your accuser is Moses, on whom your hopes are set."[225]

That is why the "transfiguration" was so vital, especially for Peter. It was to jar his belief and get him to see why Satan was after him.

If this were to continue, 'men' would no longer be seen as sons of God and/or made only in God's image and likeness. This was an undisputed truth and origin of male power and direct connection to the divine. This, therefore, would be seen not as a directive by God but by man.

If allowed to continue, then Jesus identified a God with both genders/natures, and both were equally worthy of priestly duties before God. No longer were women (less than, of no worth, or had lesser souls) to be ignored, or forbidden, in temple services and worship, despite the fact that they had female bodies that didn't resemble the divine masculine. His acceptance is evidenced by the giving of his Christed Body to His wife and awakening within Her the Divine Feminine, and following the line of Melchizedek whose Priesthood had revealed an altar at which no man worshiped and where Jesus' wife and Kallahs could officiate a worship service without breaking any laws.

That is why the Divine Feminine is back. Since today this bodily difference can no longer be the reason given for the ban of on women's ordination, and because this religion has been brought back into existence it breaks no laws, nor does it have to conform to any patriarchal religion.

Through the ages, Jesus' inclusion of His wife at his side at the Last Supper was deliberately omitted, as it was made to appear that His command to "do this in memory of me" was given only to the male apostles God's Law which once again overrides man's law.

Yes, it's true, The Da Vinci Code book and movie suggested enough of the hidden truths, to bring a shocked world to seek the 'whys' and 'hows' of a church's secret so powerful that caused it to force anyone who thought independently to go underground.

What DA VINCI DECODED 2000+ YEARS AGO was clearly what took place during Jesus' time, and was a prophecy of what would take place after Peter, and with the establishing of what has come to be known as "the church of Peter" and the 'true faith.'

---

[225] John 5:45.

LESSON 174

SECTION VIII: WHERE HAVE ALL THE WOMEN GONE?

It used to be that there were more women involved and participating in church affairs and ceremonies, both young and old alike. More now than ever, churches are half-full; and with that the half that are there are older and of the great-grandmother and grandmother age group. It's astonishing how more young people are now questioning the whole Christian institution's stories about Mary Magdalene and her absence from church writings, as well as the leadership role of Peter. They, especially young college age women, question as did the religious women of the 1960s, why women are barred from being priests. No longer do they want to work in the church as perhaps their mother or grandmother had done, while being submissive to men. Teenage girls appear to be disproportionately driving the attitude shift.[226] Freedom for women to exercise their faith and love for God is extremely important.

Yet, there are still those who fall victim to thinking they 'need' personal spiritual directors who enslave them in ways that are so subtle and inappropriate but exist and continue as these young women think, or, perhaps, believe that they are, indeed, getting closer to Jesus. In reality however, it is only the priest who is getting closer to them. It is also true that many women pursue priests because of misplaced attraction and marital issues.

---

[226] Cf. Danielle Paquette,: "Why More Young Women Than Ever Before Are Skipping Church," *Washington Post*, May 7, 2015; Jimmy Carter, "Losing My Religion for Equality."

There are some things men should contemplate. One thing for sure is that man's very existence depends on women. It is said that women make man*kind*. Women see things and feel things differently than men do, but they are not weaker. In saying that, it is also up to men to stop child trafficking and help end using little children for breeding.

Eeshans believe, and teach, that Adam and Eve truly were soulmates, not just due to the separation of 'their being' but in their love they had for each other, before and after their choice. We believe also, that there are many reasonable ways to find your soulmate, but not through illicit sex that is outside a committed relationship. Today sex has become a 'test' for love where it should be the means for fostering love.

Jesus lived true love, taught it, and proved it. He, being God, is the same yesterday, today, and tomorrow; therefore, if you believe in Him, then you have to believe in his Word.

Up until now, we mentioned how Jesus lived, worked, and talked among women. Back when he was a Spiritual Master in the Himalayas, Jesus was sure to include His teachings regarding women wherever he went. Elizabeth Clare Prophet, in her book, *The Lost Years of Jesus*, mentions a few things He taught before returning home in pursuit of His wife. These teachings of Jesus that Mary Magdalen did not know were those they naturally lived and enjoyed between them in their marriage.

It is a known fact that anyone who writes outside the standards commonly accepted in Christian writing and theologizing is criticized terribly and is usually labeled a heretic. Yet, this teaching provides ample and sensible information that brings a true God-like connection to all of God's people, with no exclusions, just like Jesus. Below please find the kindness and love that Jesus taught during the years he studied and taught in the East, before coming back to Mary Magdalen to make her His wife.

More of Jesus' Teachings on Women

The following Supplement[227] is taken from Clare Prophet's book, *The Lost Years of Jesus*, and while it may be laughed at, and derided as 'nonsense', the question still stands: Could it actually be true?

---

[227] Elizabeth Clare Prophet, *The Lost Years of Jesus*, 239.

Eeshans say, yes, because it unpacks quite well, and elaborates on, points of doctrine considered central to Eeshan Transcendentalism.

9. It is not meant that a son should set aside his mother, taking her place. Whosoever respects not his mother, the most sacred being after his God, is unworthy of the name son.
10. Listen, then, to what I say unto you: Respect woman, for she is the mother of the universe, and all the truth of divine creation lies in her.
11. She is that basis of all that is good and beautiful, as she is also the germ of life and death. On her depends the whole existence of man, for she is his natural and moral support.
12. She gives birth to you in the midst of suffering. By the sweat of her brow she rears you, and until her death you cause her the gravest anxieties. Bless her and worship her on earth.
13. Respect her, uphold her. In acting thus, you will win her love and her heart. You will find favor in the sight of God and many sins will be forgiven you.
14. In the same way, love your wives and respect them; for they will be mothers tomorrow, and each later on the ancestress of a race.
15. Be lenient towards woman. Her love ennobles man, softens his hardened heart, tames the brute in him, and makes him a lamb.
16. The wife and mother are the inappreciable treasures given unto you by God. They are the fairest ornaments of existence, and of them shall be born all the inhabitants of the world.
17. Even as the God of armies separated of old, the light from the darkness and the land from the waters, woman possess the divine faculty of separating in a man good intentions from evil thoughts.

Wherefore I say unto you, after God your best thoughts should belong to the women and the wives, woman being for you the temple wherein you will obtain the most easily perfect happiness.

PART XVI

THE OLD WINE SKIN AND THE NEW WINE

LESSON 175

SECTION I: WHAT WE KNOW

ONE CANNOT PUT NEW WINE INTO THE OLD WINESKIN. If you do the wine will burst the wineskins and both will be lost (Mark 2:22). The fact that Mary's presence always bothered Peter, since he was old wineskin, and she was likened to new wine, should always have been duly noted, since to mention this could be seen as foundational proof surrounding the controversy of Mary Magdalen. It is not surprising that her marriage, let alone her presence, would also be the topic of controversy as to whether or not Mary sat with Jesus at the Last Supper. Was she there? Wasn't she there? She *was*, indeed, there.

It is to be emphasized that it was "by his authority and desire," as her Husband having already possessed His 'body, blood, soul, and divinity,' that He would undoubtedly give her first place at the Last Supper with His apostles.

This is an Eeshan fundamental truth. This unique marital bond with Him, having her at His side, not only gave her equal status with men but also *exalted* her. He was her savior and redeemer first, and then He freed her from the laws that bound her because she was female.

Because theirs was a marriage of soulmates and twin flames, because they were one with a divine, infinite component (they cannot be destroyed), Mary wholly shared in her husband's agony. She was there when Jesus died on the cross; and who could deny that at the moment of His death on the cross, as His blood poured from His body, Mary hemorrhaged, as well. Since they could not kiss, there were no children conceived.

His sacrifice would not have been complete unless Mary had been part of it. Just as Eve began the choice to the physical and Adam completed it, The New Adam began the sacrifice and The New Eve completed it.

When Jesus died on the cross, Mary died with him, since His death tore their hearts apart. It was only by His last words to her that she was able to survive the separation. The seven last words to her which defines our religion were: "Mary, we will never be separated again."

LESSON 176

SECTION II: A NEW PRIESTHOOD

The apostles, both men and women, were given the Christed Body at the Last Supper; their bodies were all activated at the Crucifixion, when the fullness of Christ's sacrifice instilled life into their Christed bodies; however, the privilege of the priesthood was not fully exercised until after Jesus' Ascension, since the apostles remained His students up until He returned to heaven after approximately forty days.

Were there women present who were given this privilege? Yes, they were, as we stated throughout this book there were men *and* women. Interestingly, these were the women Jesus kept close to him and His wife, before they were married, and were present when Jesus was arrested, tried and, crucified.

At the arrest, Thomas and John stayed nearby also, while the rest of the apostles scattered and couldn't be found. Shortly thereafter, Philip and Levi found their way to them. These women, however, who were with Jesus and Mary never left them, and were not ever mentioned in mainstream established Christian sources. These were those who received the Christed Bodies of Jesus and his Wife, since He treated them as equals. This was what gave them the right to continue to teach and lead worship services after Jesus' resurrection, alongside Mary, who along with her Kallahs, continued her husband's work until shortly after Jesus ascended.

One must remember that to have a Christed Body (the singular noun for body used here is to describe the Oneness of Jesus and Mary through their marriage) is the link of a priest, or priestess, to Christ, as the Co-Saviors. It is through the Christed Body (bodies) that one is not only linked to the sacrifice on Calvary but also to the entire Plan of Salvation, which is the restoration of the Sacred Bread necessary for the link back to the transcendental light body and eternal life. Upon receiving the 'Christed' Body (bodies), the Kallah, or Chatan, becomes a direct vessel through which Christ and His Wife speak and work. It is through this means that a priest, or priestess, is distinguished from other children of God, since the priest, by the power of the Holy Spirit of God, enables Jesus in sacred union with His wife, to speak, once again, the most sacred words of consecration, as only the co-Redeemers may speak for the process of 'transubstantiation' to be accomplished in order to restore and give to humans the "way" back to their original transcendental form and ignite the light body within them. This is vital, since only through this means can the plan of salvation continue from age to age without interruption and continue the lifeline Christ commanded in his Bread of Life discourse.

As we know, transubstantiation is the process by which the simple gifts of bread and wine, by human hands, and via a unique alchemy, are turned into the Christs' body and blood, soul and divinity. Only by means of Christ's sacred marriage, and His sacred words, does time actually stand still, and we are back at the time of Christ, witnessing His marriage, passion, and death. These are timeless words, meaning that they are meant for all ages.[228]

With the reception of the Marriage Feast of the Lamb and His Wife, we are transported through time; and, thus, are present when they speak the sacred words, by which only through the instituting of the mystery of holy orders (the mystery of the priesthood) with Mary, His wife, and their apostles, they instituted the Holy Eucharist.

We are not in a memorial, but 'live streaming' back to the moment as He (the active Consort) and Mary (the passive Consort) fulfilled their

---

[228] Seen from a different angle, one could say that Jesus' sacrifice is eternally present before God and that any person consecrated to perform the priestly ministry opens the door to that eternal and transcendent moment of perfect redeemed eternity and makes it present to any and all present, regardless of where in the 'time stream' they may be. – Ed.

role in God's plan of salvation since He died for all ages. That is why the sacrifice, and real presence, are alive today; however this time, Jesus is encompassed within the Eesha, and, thus, has returned to help her complete the plan. Thus, we had the New Testament, and a new covenant, which changed what was written in the Old Testament, as being from God; and today we have the New/Final Testament already in play, which correctly fulfills God's Law with the Divine Feminine *actively* involved.

When Jesus came as the Son of God, He, being the 'active' Consort for those times, introduced a new covenant given to us by the Word. He changed everything, or rather corrected the misinterpretations of God's law by man. He revealed and taught that God, the Divine Masculine of the First Person of the Holy Trinity, was his Father and ours. He introduced the perfected version of the sacredness of marriage by identifying His Mother, Mary, and by including his wife, Mary Magdalene, in all He did and taught. He invited all to hear and follow Him as children of God, with no exceptions. At His baptism, He identified a third person of God, the Holy and Sacred Spirit, also being Sacredly Balanced, whom they witnessed at His baptism, and who was promised to help us after Jesus ascended back to His Father. By their love for each other and for us, as God's children, they freed us from what has been termed the 'Original Sin,' rather than the 'Fall to the Physical,' and conquered all sin and death. Because they are as One, the liaison, and the Perfect Altar, Perfect Victim, Perfect Sacrifice, and the only means to undo the fall from grace, there was no longer a need for the sacrifice of animals.[229] Since Christ, the Son, and Divine Masculine gave us His

---

[229]The question can be raised and debated whether God ever asked for the sacrifices of animals beyond the Paschal Lamb. It's interesting to note that the Essenes felt the entire Temple religion and its practices and leadership had become hopelessly corrupt and wanted nothing to do with it, or, the direction the mainstream religion, of Judaism, was taking, secluding themselves in the wilderness. Scripture can be cited, as examples, of God's mandate but the issue of human interference and superimposition of interpretation, along with editing and omission/additions, over large periods of time, is problematic when it comes to this issue, let alone many others—in addition to the issues involving Jesus' true teachings and marriage. For an intriguing take on this topic, see the book, *The Christ of India: The Story of Original Christianity* by Abbot George Burke. – Ed.

body and blood, soul and divinity to ensure our salvation linked to Him and Him alone, His wife, by extension, shared equally in God's plan, as in the Mystery of God as consorts, the One became two, and then became One in marriage, and have activated those light bodies once denied the Sacred Food and Drink, who together with the Divine Mystics scattered throughout the world, will force darkness into the Light.

PART XVII

INTO THY HANDS, MARY

LESSON 177

Section I: Another Testament is Begun, Ishvara is Back

Delving into some pertinent facts behind the scenes,
regarding the Virgin, the Virgin birth, obedience to God,
the Bride of Christ, and paranoia surrounding the title Goddess.

Ishvara[230] is back and it is the Divine Feminine who brought it back. Hidden away since biblical times, the Bride of the Lamb is identified: "Come I will show you the Bride, the Wife of the Lamb" (Revelation 21:9). Because of God's mercy, another Testament is begun. Is it the final testament?

We call it the New/Final Testament. The New Testament is fulfilled in this Final Testament.

The prophecy of the return of Ishvara is: She who was suspended in time has returned. Once again, the God of whom Jesus spoke and taught, chooses mercy over punishment to save His people from themselves. For the Bride, the Lamb's wife, will give them the grace necessary to receive and accept the truth. The Sacred Bread and Drink that was locked safely away in Paradise, has been brought back by she who will be the guide and lead God's people to the "Way" of God's plan of salvation.

If we continued to guide ourselves, we would continue down the destructive path created by the human consciousness; therefore, we say

---

[230] Divine Presence, as in the Shekinah (in the Holy of Holies of the Temple). – Ed.

to God: "You make known to me the path of life; you fill me with joy in your presence, with eternal pleasures at your right hand." (Psalms 16:11)

Humanity without the Wife of the Lamb would end with the transcendental consciousness being lost forever, leaving us enveloped in a human consciousness, which would essentially lead to eternal death. Without living Jesus' directive, there is no salvation, just as He told those who walked away from his Bread of Life discourse. *Now that we know the truth*, should we ignore this directive again, we would be counted among them.

Enlightened, we see how after Jesus' ascension, the mission of Jesus and Mary Magdalen, as The New Adam and The New Eve was thwarted by the failure of the supposedly Christ-centered religions. The willful failure of Peter to transcend allowed for those 'male' followers and disciples, who were also strongly entrenched in their birth religion, to use any opportunities at their hands to induce fear among some of the other apostles. Those who were steadfast in the New Law were killed. These were apostles who did not agree with Peter, and feared that he was the perfect weak link from which Christ's New Covenant could be broken and destroyed, and he was.

Peter felt that Mary Magdalen's reputation was the perfect reason to do away with any reference to Jesus' marriage before, and especially after, his Ascension. As mentioned before, not only was Jesus constantly rebuked by Peter, Andrew, and others because of who He married, and because it was shameful back then to marry a woman of such 'repute,' or it would bring certain death to the early church. From the beginning of His ministry, Jesus' wife, and the women in His company, stood staunchly by Him, for what He did for women was shocking and scandalous to the whole country. Did you know that:

- It was considered "better to burn the words of the Torah" than to be delivered to women.
- Jewish women received no education, and were married as soon as they became fertile, usually around the age of twelve or thirteen.
- One week of the month [during her menses] she was unclean and anything she touched, including food and other persons, was considered contaminated.

- A respectable Jewish woman was kept confined at home, hidden from view.
- A woman spoke with no man outside of her family.
- A woman had no honorable status except when she married and bore a male child.
- Unless this happened, she was without honor even in her own family.
- Public affairs were the domain of men only.
- In public, a woman was forbidden to speak to any man, and a man was forbidden to speak with any woman, even to acknowledge his wife.
- Traveling by women, except for such conventional purposes as visiting family and attending certain religious feasts, was considered deviant behavior, usually with sexual overtones.[231,232]

Everything surrounding Jesus and His Wife encompassed the above, making it no wonder why, to this day, the church has made, and still does make, a deliberate attempt to hide any information regarding his marriage, even though what had been written about Mary Magdalen was pure fiction. Throughout the recent times, beautiful Orders dedicated to Mary Magdalen have come into existence. Few know her life and secrets, though any and all devotion to her is another step to honoring her.

Eeshans realize that not everyone will be in communion with our religion and spirituality, and perhaps may feel a little apprehensive about it, but we are hoping that contention will not be to anyone's advantage.

Eeshans expect that passages, such as Isaiah 4:1, which was used to disgrace these women, will come to be used in these times to proclaim our love for Jesus, since God will raise them up as they honorably take His name and bring forth the Sacred Food and Drink of the Sacred and Divine Marriage Feast of the Lamb and His Wife. In time, 'so few men

---

[231] Truthbook. "The Women Who Followed Jesus." The Urantia Book Illustrated and Online, truthbook.com/jesus/the-women-who-followed-jesus.

[232] Some material drawn from *TRUTHBOOK* and other sources.

will be left' who will not fear these words: "Let who does wrong continue to do wrong; and let the vile person continue to be vile; let the one who does right continue to do right; and the holy person continue to be holy" (Revelation 22:11); and those who have been wrong and vile shall be made to seek redemption and face retribution.

After Jesus, the women and the men who supported them continued to do as they were taught, until which time they were forced to disperse. We find that it became, once again, illegal for women to continue exercising their right to worship God. The many writings backing this information claim that it truly appears that following the Ascension of Jesus, women's roles became even more subservient. Almost half the male apostles began to undermine Mary's authority as Jesus' wife, and successor, the one person who perfectly understood His mission.

The undermining of Mary His wife, and those women who followed Him, were the very things Jesus frowned on and sought to change. With the onslaught of attacks that focused on Jesus' attempts for change before his arrest, once He was no longer there to support the women and children, death threats, as well as actual attempts on Mary's life ended with the reversion of so much of what Jesus taught, back to the old law.

Without a doubt, there was a tremendous hatred towards the Christians after Jesus, especially in the first few hundred years. Primarily because Jesus appeared to identify/align himself as God, along with what He taught and did regarding miracles and the like, He rocked the very foundations of his birth religion and those of other belief systems and cultures. We know of the periods of time where many who followed Jesus went underground, or were arrested and tortured, while others were burned as torches or crucified during these times of religious unrest. Romans were always anonymously called upon to check out the comings and goings of Jesus' followers and disciples; and those from within Christ's immediate circle had a lot to fear. Certainly, fear was the tool to drive a wedge among his followers, and a few like Peter were not about to cause turmoil if it could be avoided. So, if putting women back in subservient roles, or revealing a few of the Master's secrets could help sustain the New Law in the beginning, then that was considered great.

We know from the time Jesus was crucified and resurrected, until He ascended, and after, the religious leaders of the time still were not comfortable after He was gone. Where then was Ishvara? Well, as Jesus declared, He did not come to bring peace, *but a sword*. One may ask, why then did Jesus say to Peter, "Put away your sword"? Well, because in Matthew 10:45, Jesus says, "I did not come to bring peace, but a sword!" Here, Jesus was making a claim for giving to God what is God's and a claim for taking a stand for offenses against neighbor especially with regards to human rights, before God just as He did in the cleansing of the Temple. Remember when He taught He was meek and Humble of heart, but when it came to abuse of his Father's house, he stepped in. striking out against the wrongs on their own to do as He taught, since Jesus warned all who followed Him of the evils they would face.

In Luke 22:36, Jesus says, "If you have a purse, take it, and also bring a bag: and if you don't have a sword, sell your cloak and buy a sword;" this was what Jesus told His disciples at the Last Supper. After the supper, again, they asked Jesus who is the greatest of them. He talked about the one serving being the highest and greatest. He warned Peter again about Satan.

Why do we mention this? Again, to show God's mercy as Jesus watched and knew what was in Peter's heart. He knew that Peter would use the sword, as *power*, and so would some of the others. He was trying to show them that some among them just didn't get it. They were still following the human, rational consciousness and not the transcendental one. Jesus tried to get through to Peter that Mary has her place next to Jesus, since she was his wife, and the better way was to serve her, not be served *by* her. To show that they have learned so little with regards to what He taught them about all being God's children, and what they thought of women, did not help the cause of Peter and other males, but instead it became something that hurt all of humankind. From inequality and the bad treatment of women, there came the attack on innocence (i.e., child slavery) and the attack on other genders, and then race, creed, etc.

Yes, Ishvara *is* back and the Divine Feminine *is* speaking and *is* using a sword as Jesus taught, and only she who shared in his body, blood, soul, and divinity would know how.

> For the Word of God is living and powerful, and sharper than any two-edged sword piercing even to the division of soul and spirit, and of joints and marrow and is a discerner of thoughts and intents of the heart.
>
> —Hebrews 4:12

It has been said that God can divide, or make, a distinction between things we think of being closely related or indistinguishable, like the difference between the soul and spirit. God's sword, which is the Word, penetrates the heart without leaving a physical scar. In the human consciousness, this doesn't work the same way.

Reverting back to those injustices were not just changes, and revisions, that appeased the enemies of Christ in the early church, but it gave way to the declaration of other concessions that were carried over to this day. This is, again, the result of the biases left in place since Peter. It is a problem of language where they replaced Jesus' wife Mary with Blessed Mother Mary, because they could conveniently make use of the name and fill a certain place in memory. Since current beliefs do not accept Jesus' marriage, women will never be rightfully represented in this church. Right or wrong, it is what they have built their religion upon. To think this will change, or to move ahead with a "theology for women" will not help, and it will not change anything. From the Eeshan point of view, the very nature of the structure of the church that has been created and passed down is not *able* to change. So, for church theologians to appease women by coming up with a "theology of women" to involve a fully *equality with males* cannot happen, since it would change the entire foundation and trajectory of the Catholic church.[233] Therefore, the sins of the past follow through into the future, in the sense that today Catholic theology has no choice but to continue to unpack what was begun from those earliest stages under Peter's discretion. These are some of the more

---

[233] It would also create an enormously pregnant problem, drawing a questioning attention to where the Holy Spirit has been for the last 2000 years of church history in the face of such overwhelming, glaring injustice, especially since the church has firmly stood behind the belief to the point of making it a central doctrine that the church (with Christ at its head! – read, Papacy) cannot err in matters of faith and morals! – Ed.

principle reasons why Eeshans do not agree with the theology of the church as it stands.

Over and over, it is our opinion that God's people really have become more and more aware of the imbalances of gender related issues, meaning that there is no understanding of gender identity, especially when considered with reference to social and cultural differences, rather than biological ones; plus there is now a more broadly used system that denotes a range of identity concepts that do not correspond to traditional and established ideas of male and female, and at times conflicts with physical and or biological realities. As a result, one failed to understand basic teachings enough to ask: How can a single male God make a yin-yang world, a world where everything is paired equally and kept in perfect balance? How can anyone in a world with a positive-negative dynamic, a linear and cyclical world, claim we are made in 'His' image and likeness? The answer is because 'He's' God is no answer, even with regards to considering nouns and pronouns in English being limited, with different inflections that they have associated with them, etc.

One must ask, *"is it the Holy Spirit claiming God is male,"* or is the Holy Spirit of God who being one with his female counterpart, the Sophia Perennis [the Divine Feminine] speaking in unison with the voice of those crying out for justice and an end to discrimination?

Over time, when the cries of the innocent, and the charges of injustices have continually been brought against standards and controversy has abounded, statements were made to end discussions on the matter. Another such statement, which Eeshans found seriously disturbing, was in *Inter Insigniores* (Oct. 15, 1976), in the Congregation for the Doctrine of Faith, which said: "The church, in its fidelity to the example of the Lord, does not consider herself authorized to admit women to priestly ordination." This was done with the approval of Pope Paul VI. Pope John Paul II, in his *Ordinatio Sacerdotalis* (May 22, 1994) said this: "We declare that the church has no authority whatsoever to confer priestly ordination on women and that this judgment is to be definitively held by all the church's faithful." This meant that the church's stand on women's ordination was irreformable. We must ask, then, if the church is a "she" and the Bride of Christ, as implied, why would she discriminate against women?

A few continued to search for hope; but, once again, it became necessary to take that hope away. In October 1995, the doctrinal congregation acted further, releasing a *responsum ad propositum dubium* concerning the nature of the teaching in *Ordinatio Sacerdotalis*. "This teaching requires definitive assent, since it is founded on the written word of God, and from the beginning constantly preserved and applied in the Tradition of the church, it has been set forth infallibly by the ordinary and universal Magisterium." The ban on women's ordination belongs "to the deposit of the faith."[234] That's it and no more.

The challenges continued, and one primary reason given to justify many churches' stance against women's ordinations was *still that the female body did not resemble Christ's body*. We believe from the church's teaching that we are *all* part of the Mystical Body of Christ; and, yet, the church's actions contradict the teachings of Christ. Eeshans hold the words '*the female body did not resemble Christ's body*' are insults against the character of Jesus, His life, and His teachings. Eeshans believe that this is merely male-dominated consciousness speaking on behalf of both sexes, as if coming from God, speaking for God, and before God, and humanity, and in conjunction with everything regarding God's people is filtered through the error that it is only what males perceive regarding God, and the things of God, to include secular affairs.

We believe, therefore, that the 2000-year-old institution, by its errors and scandals and falsities, forfeited its right to speak for God, and we claim their doctrines and teachings are in error, and not that since Peter did it ever had the right to claim such things.

However, Eeshans believe, just as the Virgin Mary was God the Father's feminine counterpart in this world to bring about the Son of God made man,[235] the Son (Child) of God, who as God is male and female, when He became Man (Jesus), found His feminine counterpart

---

[234]Terence. "The Lay OBLIGATION to Discuss Women's Ordination." The Open Tabernacle: Here Comes Everybody, 4 Dec. 2012, opentabernacle.wordpress.com/2012/12/03/the-lay-obligation-to-discuss-womens-ordination/.

[235]The Divine Feminine through the person of the Virgin Mary, via supramentalization.

in the person of Mary Magdalene, who as Christ's Wife *had and presently still carries the authority given to her by Christ himself, and having said authority conferred to her by the highest authority, in addition to being His infinite counterpart has the right to*[236]:

1. ordain any faithful called by God to the priesthood;
2. right the wrongs regarding women's rights before Jesus Christ;
3. bring women to equal status wherever and whenever possible;
4. stand by and support those men and groups who fought and were punished for saying that anyone among the faithful could be called by God to the priesthood; for there is no sane reason or justification for someone to be excommunicated, dismissed, or laicized for
   a. advocating for women's ordination;
   b. attending a women's ordination; or
   c. preaching about women's ordination, except if said institutions are in error.

Jesus claimed His authority by God and, thus, his wife's would also be by the authority of God. Only one who has that authority can pass on that authority, and that one *is* God. Eeshans fail to see success in any religion that claims it got its authority from Jesus but whose teachings contradict the Savior's views, or to try to abide by rationalize, or fight against those who oppose illogical explanations and justifications; since to continue to persist in trying to get an ear with such mindsets is as pointless as debating their arguments. As Jesus said, "If a house is divided against itself, that house cannot stand" (Mark 3:25). Could this be the reason why just about half the faithful will most likely change religions? Did you know that in the *Gospel of the Confession of the Holy Twelve* Jesus himself says (paraphrasing), "There shall arise after you, men of perverse minds who shall through ignorance or through craft, suppress many things which I have spoken unto you and lay to Me things which I never taught, sowing tares among the good wheat which I have given you to

---

[236] Drawn from Tom Roberts, *National Catholic Reporter*, Nov. 20, 2012.

sow in the world." When an institution, religion, or faith is in error, chaos abounds. The parable of the wheat and tares, similar to the above passage from *The Confession of the Twelve*, only appears in one of the canonical gospels of the New Testament, and it is important because it reflects the sifting of souls in End Times. (Cf. consider Jesus' question to Peter, "Why does Satan want to sift you like wheat?")

Eeshans believe that where there is discrimination there is no "love thy neighbor as yourself." In the end, one needs to know, "Who is my neighbor?"

Eeshans further believe that a religion is false when it:

- holds fast to distorted teachings of Jesus and perpetuates false doctrine;
- turns a blind eye to the destruction of innocents;
- holds a double standard in punishment of the perpetrator of moral crimes, excusing priest pedophiles, and yet punishing women by assaulting and molesting them and then turning a blind eye to these acts.
- punishes only women for abortion while not holding the men involved accountable;
- destroys faith because its own priests, seminaries, and teachings, causing malcontent among its faithful;
- discourages personal/mystical relationships with God especially in seminaries;
- fails to ordain women because of their anatomy, including those who are called to the priesthood, thereby excluding half the population;
- fails to acknowledge the possibility of genders and relationships outside the traditional male-female designation, and yet its leaders were and are carrying out such relationships up to and including popes.
- (as we mentioned earlier) had 'popes' who did not believe that Jesus existed at all!

Today, we see that the harder women desired, and fought, to participate in certain organized religions since Jesus, the more discrimination they experienced. Most young women today do not feel that they want to continue in a religion where women never had the respect, or opportunities, to achieve any leadership roles, such as in the Catholic church, which robbed women of the right to worship, and propagate, the gospel as they feel Jesus intended. Yet, there is still the need arising in the heart to follow Jesus and respond to his call. Perhaps these women finally realized that trying to change the church of Peter will not happen, since it would mean admitting it was wrong all along about everything; and, thus, would have to admit its theology was humanly contrived.

LESSON 178

SECTION II: PETER'S PATH VERSUS JESUS' WAY WHO WAS MORE GUILTY JUDAS WHO THOUGHT HE WAS DOING A GOOD THING OR PETER WHO KNEW HE WAS DOING THE WRONG THING AND KEPT ON GOING

So precious was Mary to Jesus, it goes beyond reasoning that He ever mistreated, denied, or betrayed her. Eeshans feel that within the gospels and writings that were omitted, and deemed heretical, there is evidence of offensive behavior directed at Mary Magdalene in the presence of Jesus by Peter several times. Why then did Jesus not address the abusive, misogynistic, and chauvinistic attitudes of his own apostles, if in fact His mission involved correcting this central problem? The truth is that just as he knew Judas' role would be to betray Him, He also knew Judas loved and admired Him, but because he was blinded by human consciousness, he (Judas) was only able to see Jesus through his worldly conditioned, politically-charged lenses (i.e., that the Messiah was supposed to liberate the Jews from foreign oppression). Once Judas realized who Jesus really was, in fact, his own betrayal of that was more than he could bear. He couldn't go on living after knowing what he had done.

Thus, in order to accomplish his Father's plan, this was another example of what Jesus had to endure. Jesus, being God, knew full well that if He addressed each of these instances with Peter, or if He expelled him from the company of the other apostles, then the plan of God, historically speaking, would not be fulfilled, and that plan was to bring back His wife at the right time in world history, when sin had reached its *full measure*.

There is nothing to say that Jesus didn't know full well what Peter would do when he assumed control of the apostles and disciples, for evidence of that surrounded Him. As it was, there is nothing to say that He didn't know it would all be a necessary part of His mission that He must painfully endure for the sake of a greater good, which would be when the time of 'Woman' came to pass naturally. Just living and teaching them, Jesus knew that as the male mind would not convert, God's salvific plan would have to be divided into two parts: the fullness of time in the biblical period, and at the end of time slated for another 'fullness of time' necessary to fulfill all the scriptural prophecies made by Jesus himself as were mentioned in this book.

If it was necessary that Eesha's role was meant to unfold in the age of Aquarius, and complete the mission Jesus began, then Peter's usurped role and decisions to follow, as distasteful as they were, would be a necessary piece of the puzzle, since it would set into motion events in history that would lead up to sin reaching its full measure. This would be when the age of Aquarius was due to begin. Just as much as Judas' role was necessary to set into motion the events that would bring about the cause for the Resurrection, so Peter's role was necessary in order to bring about God's plan up into the 'fullness of time.'

Peter's inability (or refusal) to transcend kept God's children from entering into the transcendental and from understanding Christ's true mission. Actually, Peter missed it completely: the restoration of the Sacred Balance, the ability to have, and share in, a transcendental life once again, and the breaking of bonds that time built, like a wall around God's people to keep them starving, rather than receive food for eternal life. But what it did do was play out until it exhausted its purpose, and the groundwork was broken to forge ahead with the completion of his mission.

Was it jealousy? Was it a personal issue that 'had to be suppressed at the time' that made it impossible for Peter to express a manly love towards Jesus, and occupy the seat of Mary? How deep were Peter's issues that he had to reveal Christ's mysteries to his enemies?

The omitting of Mary's role, and that of women, may have prevented the decline and destruction of the early church, and as a result we find that without God's intervention, once again, and because of the continuation of Peter and his successors, the transcendental truth and complete salvific mission of humankind would never be attained. That is why Jesus says, "I tell you, God will see that they get justice and quickly. However, when the Son of Man comes, will he find faith on earth?"

As time continued, and scriptures were altered with regard to Mary's relationship with Jesus, one can certainly recognize that this could all be viewed as a blatant attempt to erase Mary from history. One begins to wonder if the sins of jealousy, covetousness, covertness, and discrimination were indeed at the root of man's decisions regarding women as ministers and leaders back at the time of Jesus' Ascension, and the reason that brought about the usurping of Mary's authority by men up to present times. If this is true, then does it further explain why within the church today any gospels, or writings, regarding Mary Magdalene were 'lost' or deemed heretical? As no good reason was (nor could ever be) given for the 'law' against women's ordination, one must ask and wonder: who sold out and why? Who was, and is, in charge of actually structuring the church which claimed to have Jesus as its founder and head? Truly, if they are right and all the evidence presented is wrong, then here we must go *repititio* and ask again and again, if one is wrong in thinking this:

1. Why would a perfectly balanced God fashion a woman's body only to become an impediment to serving in a priestly role? Or would he have fashioned it, so that it would complete the male component, and lend a balance to a wayward world in dire need of the Divine Feminine to keep the male ego in check?
2. Was the traditional story about Adam and Eve, and it being described as "the Original Sin" true, or was the true story of Adam and Eve intentionally obscured by man out of jealousy, and to ensure man's dominance over woman and to secure this throughout history?

3. Would God create any form of gender expression for a human, whether male, female, androgynous, gay, or gender-neutral to be a focal point of affliction?
4. Did God intend for all to be equal in each other's eyes, since each are equal in His eyes? For humanity to inflict pain on those judged by laws before Christ, Jesus would have had to condone those same acts; yet Jesus' teachings on love of neighbor stress equality. This points to still another mistruth causing us to look deeper into our neighbors to see who they really are. Aren't we all human, but with God's fingerprint? Weren't we always taught that beauty is skin deep and that you can't judge a book by its cover? It is not whether male and female are physiologically different for the purpose of gender identity and reproduction; it is the fact that one cannot exist without the other. The cyclical female keeps the linear male right angled or squared.[237]

Since Eeshans believe the above is true, it is more the case that, as history continually proves over and over again, man labors under the illusion that he is guided by truth; yet, in fact does not see that in truth he is only half right. Mystically, Popes have continued to claim they represent Jesus in the world; yet, how can this be claimed when there were popes who didn't believe Jesus ever existed? However, as they claim that women mystically represent Our Lady, who then is the human component to speak for her? Why didn't they pick up that there were two distinct Persons mentioned in the conception of Christ: the Holy Spirit and the Most High.

These errors and man's claim to superiority over woman obviously originates from what Eeshans feel is a biased interpretation of the creation story in which woman is pulled from man and is under his authority

---

[237] It is interesting that for an ancient stone mason to check his square for accuracy and precision, he required the use of a circle: by drawing the circle, dividing it, and making a point anywhere along the edge of the circle, he could create a perfect right angle by connecting that dot to the two points marking either end of the diameter. Thus, the circle is required for anything built to achieve correct right angles in the structure. – Ed.

and dominion, since no one would even consider (let alone believe) that God the Divine Masculine and the Virgin were husband and wife.

It is without a doubt a problem of consciousness. Under the human consciousness, not many are capable of thinking outside certain categories, which naturally or intrinsically flow from the current understanding of the creation event: see how profoundly the human consciousness has been shaped by what has been handed down.

Jesus taught that in order to enter heaven, one must have the enlightened awareness that all creation mirrors God, and that the creation template is the means to attain the kingdom of heaven within each person. That is what the parable meant when Jesus spoke about the necessity of being 'properly dressed,' in order to have a place at the marriage feast in the kingdom of heaven (cf., "the Kingdom of God is within you"). It is important to be clear that this does not infer any kind of elitism, or favoritism, toward those who are 'in the know,' or privy to 'secret knowledge,' but what it does means is that one must be like a child whose innocence is embraced, and this goes for anyone who follows Jesus' fundamental commandments to love God and neighbor with one's whole heart, mind, soul, and strength.

How could such injustice prevail if the Holy Spirit's guiding hand was claimed to be present in the decisions made by the authority of the church of Peter? Perhaps, the question should be "Why didn't the authority of the church of Peter listen to the Holy Spirit?" It could very well be that all along no resolution for equality in leadership and ministry could occur. Eeshans assert that the Holy Spirit has been urging this change continually, but was ignored by men in authority with deafness of heart and mind.

They had ears but could not hear, nor could their eyes see, because as time went on the cost of change was becoming increasingly too high to them.

LESSON 179

SECTION III: DON'T CONFUSE OBEDIENCE TO MAN WITH OBEDIENCE TO GOD

We might say that the fruits of the Holy Spirit are evident in the organic growth and expressed beliefs of Christians outside the walls of Roman Catholicism and in the constant turmoil created within its walls. Man's choice seems to always be blind and deaf just as much as it confuses justification, rationalization, and sanctification. Though they all resemble each other in many ways, and may have been powerful in their attempt to suppress God's true plans for the plans of human beings, the chosen course of humans has also resulted in institutionalized oppression and suppression. What it does is it makes, or tries to change, that which essentially serves into something that should create, but cannot, and then once again God's ways are silenced or stifled. Eeshans believe, therefore, that the unrest surging behind women and other minorities, genders, and cultures throughout history is the Feminine counterpart of the Holy Spirit: the Divine Feminine, who is challenging and desperately and fearlessly fighting against the wrongs and imbalances which have been in existence for 2000 years. That is why Eeshans believe that a dawn of truth and a period of enlightenment are upon us, and those who were not heard or given a voice before will be heard this time. This will be Mary Magdalene's fight song. By exposing the reality of God's plan, and bringing back the Spiritual Food that was again lost after Jesus' ascension, will instill a change that will shift humankind from its focus from the unsatisfying and materialistic trending life to the desire for a more spiritually transcendent and wholesome, holistic life, witnessing Christ's teaching and personal example.

The question remains: Do you have the courage to choose obedience to God over obedience to man? Do your ears hear and eyes see? Are you going to be the rebellious people identified by the prophet like those who turned in and away from Jesus, going from hailing him to shouts of "crucify him!" out of fear?

LESSON 180

SECTION IV: EESHANS' STANCE ON THE REFERENCE TO THE "BRIDE OF CHRIST"

Eshans understand the established church of Christ as really showing how it's being prejudiced, and ego driven, just as Jesus found was the case with the religion of the day.

As it was written:

> "Woe to the obstinate children, declares the Lord,
> 'to those who carry out plans that are not mine;
> forming an alliance, but not by my Spirit,
> heaping sin upon sin;
> these are rebellious people, deceitful children, children
> unwilling to listen to the Lord's instruction."
> [Isaiah 30:1-2]

Judas AND Peter were both guilty of having this problem rule their minds and hearts, but the problem manifested in different ways.

The mind is meant to be informed by the heart, where the soul and God reside together; thus, what is given by God to fill the heart is meant to overflow into the fabric of the mind, so that conscience is properly formed.

Without this 'flow,' which creates a balance, *corrupt reasoning* result, and this is when thoughts and conclusions are based on gossip, hearsay, kneejerk reactions, dysfunctions, dramas, traumas, or whatever is drawn from one's own conclusions in a specific way so that the ego/false part of the person is shown to be 'right.' This part of the mind is preoccupied

Section IV: Eeshans' Stance on the Reference to the "Bride of Christ" / 747

with self-preservation and so does anything and everything necessary to survive; thus, it must always be right, especially among peers, in order to secure a foothold for survival or a place for itself. This is the darkened mind that human beings mistake for personally infused knowledge; when under this influence, they refuse to see good, or accept it even when it is reasonably presented. Those in this condition can't let go of a disagreement, or argument, because they are not at peace; they are at war with themselves. A balanced mind can still disagree but also can be open to receiving correction.

Peter's corrupt reason eliminated the transcendental totally, simply because his mind was set up (by his own choices) not to perceive it; even after Jesus resurrected, the problem with Peter only continued since he was still mentally attached to his birth religion and saw Jesus' reformation from the vantage point of his own attachments.

Judas, on the other hand, reasoned from his human consciousness from the evidence at hand, and what was transpiring when Jesus was arrested, that Jesus wasn't going to fight back and overwhelm the enemy as a political leader. It was then when he saw the truth in all of what Jesus taught; however, he never witnessed the fullness of Christ's promise that He will rise on the third day.

So, for the above reasons, and Peter's jealousy and covetous attitude and actions towards Mary (and who she was to Jesus), Eeshans *do not* agree with the use of the title Bride of Christ when cited that Ephesians 5 uses the example of Christ's relationship to the church as instructive for marriage. In Ephesians 5:23 it says that the husband is head of the 'wife' (leader of the family), since it compares to Christ being head of the church. And in verse 24 the church is, therefore, to submit to unto Christ, as a godly woman to her loving husband.

Further it is said that "Christ loves the church and gave up His life for it. Christ loves the church as He loves himself;" likewise, a husband is to love his wife as himself, considering their marriage 'one body.' The truth is Christ loves us just as He loves himself, without condition or selfishness. In this troubled and confused world today, however, people may, through a purely human consciousness, misperceive loving oneself to mean self-absorption. So, to be accused, or said to be "into oneself," is NOT a compliment; but with Christ's consciousness, there is a true balance and right employment of the expression 'to love oneself.' Thus, to love oneself in this sense means self-respect without interior confusion, conflict, or illusion. Transcendentally, this means to live in a balance before God, and loving unconditionally. To some, as Jesus says, "We are to love one another as we love ourselves." One body in a marriage is that which becomes One through a reciprocal love, not to be identified exclusively with the male gender. Though we discuss the Oneness of Christ and his wife, it is a reciprocal love, and is not the same as how the church explains 'oneness,' or for that matter, and this is proven by how the church law plays out against women, wives, or females of any gender.

Eeshans claim that Christ did not say this, and in all fairness, He gave himself up to restore all things to their original transcendental state for 'us' to have the Sacred Bread necessary to return to God; and it was to reverse the effects of the choice to the physical marriage of Adam and Eve and to 'their' original transcendental state.

In so doing, He sacrificed His marriage and human future with *Mary, who was His whole world*, since He was one body with her for eternity, but in the material world the love they expressed here also was salient, always powerfully transcendental.

Because of this, marriage became more than the sharing of bodies in a conjugal way, it made their oneness *eternal*. They were equal by becoming the first androgynous being, separated into male and female. If anyone holds God's title for Bride of Christ it would be 'his' eternal bride, who would take her place alongside Jesus. Here in this world, if Christ said what the church claims, both should have been represented, a male and a female, not what we have now, male (masculine) and institution (feminine). Was it still just another way to keep and protect a patriarchal way of life?

No longer can Peter, or his successors, claim solidarity with God and take their place by removing Christ's wife by claiming from the Old Law that women are not worth life. There is no longer a means to rationalize, or justify, the exclusion of women from priestly ordination as in Pope Francis' recent comments on this issue.

With regard to "women priests, that cannot be done. Pope St John Paul II after long, long intense discussions, long reflection, said so clearly. Not because women don't have the capacity. Look, in the church, women are more important than men, because the church is a woman. It is 'la' church not 'il' church. The church is the Bride of Jesus Christ. And the Madonna is more important than popes, bishops and priests."

One must admit we are a bit late in an elaboration of the theology, and never chanced a look at the *'thealogy'* (the wisdom of Sophia Perennis or Divine Feminine) of women. We have to move ahead with the erred theology[238] because it was made to be compelling, but Jesus is more compelling and he was a man who spoke, taught, and lived what love and marriage was, and most of all: Jesus was God and Mary was one with Him and they shared (and still share) *one body*. No longer can the above happen, since God has brought back into existence a New Law with a New Altar never used by men and joined it together with the Sacred and Divine Order of Melchizedek—as One.

Eeshans hold to the belief that by the 'authority' of the Madonna, as the female counterpart of the First Person of the Trinity, identified by Jesus as His Mother, and in His reference to God as His Father, the place and rights of women are now validated and affirmed. With no lack of gravity may we add that being the Wife of the first person of the Holy Trinity, as they too shared and continue to live as one body, by virtue of the fact her role was to give birth to the only begotten Divine Masculine, thus, giving him His humanity. His becoming Savior and Redeemer (having married and shared 'one body' with Mary Magdalen on earth as it was in heaven) makes her co-Savior/Redeemer; therefore, we declare that *she* is the true holder of the title "Bride of Christ."

Eeshans ask again, "if according to the church, women have the capacity, what is the issue?" If the Madonna is more important than bishops and priests, and as the Blessed Virgin brought salvation to this world by giving birth to the person of Jesus Christ, the Savior, then the mirroring of the Perfect Marriage between God the Father and the Madonna *cannot* be ignored, nor can the fact be ignored that God deemed that their Son Jesus, along with His wife Mary, restored the Sacred and Transcendental Balance. Therefore, **'What God has put together, let no 'man' put asunder.'**

---

[238] "On Flight Back Home ... Pope Spoke To Journalists." The Wanderer Newspaper, Wandering Press Printing Co., 29 Sept. 2015, thewandererpress.com/catholic/news/breaking/on-flight-back-home-popr-spoke-to-journalists/.

LESSON 181

SECTION V: ENTER PARANOIA

As much as the reference is meant to once again quell the "issue of women priests," we find that these words were carefully chosen so as to not to have to address the words that have proven to be the most horrible, unconscionable words of all: Could the two Marys really be "goddesses" to be worshiped? You see what a tangled web hiding God's genuine and true, Sacredly Balanced nature has caused? The paranoia is so great among the male-dominated church that the faithful were terrified of such thoughts; and more, they were terrified to be confronted by other Christian faiths.

For as long as there was a Jewish and Christian faith, there was no conceivable way that a woman could ever be connected to God on a level that can place her as equal to God, especially as an Eternal Consort. That is why there was, and still is, a tremendous fear that has plagued Catholics forever, and that was that their devotion to Mary, our Blessed Mother, was always and is still being confused with worshiping her, and that honoring her was a pagan, idolatrous act. And so it has been said among some that the most popular form of idolatry is the captivation of the heart to the 'worship' of Mary and the fear that the constant plea for her intercession makes God less than who 'He' is, which shows an obvious disconnect with God's image and likeness. Obviously, most Catholics don't even know their own religion well enough to stay calm, to not panic, and to not worry so much about what others think in order to try and understand the facts. That is why people don't understand that God can, and always did, choose ordinary people to do extraordinary tasks. That is what made Jesus, as Messiah, difficult to believe at that time, i.e., He was a carpenter, as was His father, and His mother was mocked as an adulteress, or as we say today, a 'prostitute.'

Not understanding, or passing on, the truth that nothing is impossible to God and that God himself, as Jesus, 'changed' the very meaning of the religion of the time and made a New Covenant to the point of being crucified. In denying God's eternal and infinite Consorts, the church leaders allow the people to substitute no answers for horrible accusations. Case in point: if someone comes in the name of God, remains in good standing, and teaches only what the Catholic church teaches, and then performs healings, then a lot of people would accuse 'her' of leading a *cult*. What they wouldn't know is that people who have devotion to Jesus in the Blessed Sacrament, sign up for perpetual adoration to belong to a 'cult,' as with devotees to the Virgin Mary.

Any system of religious veneration, and devotion, directed to a particular figure, or object, is termed a "cult." We know that people often think 'occult' when they hear the word 'cult,' but it's even in their lack of knowing that the two terms have very different meanings that we see how fear, again, prevents people from seeing past the errors in their minds, and what other people's opinions are, towards what is God's plan. People think of things like Jim Jones when the world 'cult' is used. It's very powerful when used that way, and people are frightened by it. However, the world 'cult' is short for 'culture,' which was at one time positively applied, as in the "cult of the Blessed Sacrament." A cult is another name for a group who believes in the same thing, or with a certain mindset. It was not a term denoting something wrong, or bad, but it could be *applied* to something good or bad. In this sense above, however, it has become a useful weapon of attack in the hands of those with darkened minds against someone authentically working for God, and trying to teach love and respect for the human family. Strangely, this term is never applied to followers of the Grateful Dead or fans of Nascar. *What about the NFL...?* Come on, people! Let's move into the 21st century, shall we? Your religious 'knowledge' is showing, or rather, the lack thereof.

Did you ever wonder why there is a struggle with trying to explain Mary's virgin birth and perpetual virginity? The reason behind this issue began with not teaching that Mary was the wife of God the Father and that is the origin of the misleading and fictitious stories of the Virgin being a prostitute. Everything written was centered on how the information would be perceived, and how it would cause issues for the goals set. For example: anything regarding Jesus' conception or birth was written to protect any reference to the Virgin's identification of her marriage to Jesus' Father, who is almighty God, so as not to put her in the category of 'Goddess.' If this had been written free of ambiguity, her marriage with God the Father would define the oneness of marriage. That is why, with painstaking efforts and the least amount of detail possible, the story contains just the following vague information and an error, which also indicates a change that alters the genealogy of Jesus. In Matthew, 1:20, we find the following.

An angel of the Lord, named Gabriel came to Mary and said, "You are highly favored." She was startled by what the angel said, as Mary was 'unaware'[239] of her place with God. She tried to figure out what this greeting meant.

The angel said to her, "Don't be afraid, Mary, you have found favor with God. You will become pregnant and give birth to a son and name him Jesus. He will be a great man and "will be called the Son of the Most High." The Lord God will give Him the throne of His ancestor David. Your son will be king of Jacob's people and His kingdom will never end." Mary asked the angel, "How can this be? For I do not know man..." in other words, she was a virgin. The angel answered her, "The Holy Spirit will come to you **and the power of the Most High will overshadow you." (Two different persons. The Holy Spirit had to prepare her for it was necessary for her Husband's visit.)** "Therefore, the holy

---

[239] Remember when Mary became human her place as eternal consort of the Most High was hidden from her that she may give herself voluntarily over to God. Her 'Yes' awakened her transcendental consciousness to the full, and the mystery of her role as Mother of Jesus Christ was once again revealed to her as was her role in the plan of salvation and her marriage to Joseph. Jesus attained his royal line not from Joseph's side but from Mary's lineage. Joseph had no other direct familial connection to the Child but to take care of God's wife and their Son. That is why it is written in Mark 6:3, isn't this the carpenter's son and the son of Mary, since it is because the line of David came through Mary's side in blood; however, even though Joseph had 'nothing to do with Jesus' lineage,' Joseph's line supposedly came from the line of David also.

child developing inside you will be called the 'Son of God.'" What else would he be called? Here we see word altering. Still, right from the start Mary's identity was revealed as well as was Jesus.'

Elizabeth, Mary's cousin, was six months pregnant with a child in her old age. People said she couldn't have a child. But nothing is impossible for God. **Mary answered, "I am the handmaid of the Lord, let it be done unto me according to your word." Then the angel left. (It was then that Mary went into the euphoric state she had shared with her Husband through eternity, only this time they would share in the conception of a child made by the love of God with a human woman, but still transcendentally), and a child would be mystically placed within a womb created by Mary's 'husband's' hands and carefully placed by him within her body so as to not break her virginity.**

Mary's 'Yes' was the necessary component to awaken within her who she was. With her yes, Mary 'remembered' who she was and what her role was before she became a human. This was just the beginning, since in twenty-eight short years, another Mary would say "yes," this time to Mary's son Jesus, Son of God, in marriage; and would be awakened to find that she, too, had shared a euphoric transcendental and eternal love with Him only this time in human forms.

Can you imagine the most holy Virgin, born into a world which was so foreign to the love she had for God, knowing from her first moment that she wanted no man 'despite the Law' that she may spend her life loving only God? Mary so loved God that she begged Zachariah, her cousin's husband and father to John the Baptist, and the next male in the family line after her father's death, to let her live only to serve God. Since it was now his responsibility to find her a husband under Mosaic law. Mary's dream was to be the servant girl to whomever was chosen to bring the Messiah into the world. In other words, from a very early age she knew she was different.

This one scriptural passage alone shows how, by their 'Yes,' Mary the Mother of God and Mary the wife of the Lamb's equality with their husbands, first in eternity and then in the world, had, by accepting and doing God's will, witnessed to, and gave respect to their counterparts, allowing for both to grow in their human marriages; whereas, by man's law there may not be mutual dignity accorded, and, therefore, there may be a crisis in mutual respect and honor, which allows for the breakdown of marriages and the abuse of women.

Thereby, in doing so, and under the definition of marriage, this does not allow for *not* recognizing equality of gender with regards to God as a conceptual truth, nor can it be used to deny, ignore, or suppress women as though it was God's Will. The fact is all of the people cannot be fooled all of the time. To say to God's people that the reason women cannot be ordained is because 'women's bodies do not look like Jesus' body' is not only the weakest of all reasons, it goes against the foundations of the Sacred Balance Eeshans believe is essential for the correct practice of spiritual life underscored in this book. Moreover, this reason flies in the face of a scriptural foundation, "and the two become one."

Just as there is nowhere in any text where Jesus decreed that women cannot be priests, it is by Peter's statement that it is so. Peter was concerned only with man's law above God's (to include Jesus' directives). The defensive argument that 'women are more important than men, because the church is a woman' implies the linear way of thinking, and does not evidence an enlightened mind which stems from a transcendental consciousness. An enlightened mind allows for these things to be addressed.

The argument above suggests that women who protest publicly, or privately, would be satisfied with this thinking so long as they are flattered, and that they are naive to such a degree and that they, and not being as cultured, as intellectually adept, or attuned, to God and the things of God as men are (because God is male and shares that part of his intelligence only with men), would believe anything they are told without questioning. This is further exposed by their continual complementarianism, which, by the way, is practiced by most patriarchal entities, not limited to religions. Therefore, by the church's own words and on their definition of "Deposit of Faith," they are guilty on all counts.

This fact cannot be argued, since by their own definition of this 'Deposit of Faith,' and the Pope's statement(s), any who resolve to continue on this path are guilty.

This comment not only takes away from and distorts anything they try to cover over with flagrant attempts and ways to hide the truth, but also blurs all things written by these authorities regarding the person of Jesus the Son of Man and Son of God. It also enables them to again unite with the biblical Judaic religion at the time of Jesus and obscure the new covenant and directives of the one whom the Christians claim as their Messiah, rather than stand on Christ being God as foundational enough.

LESSON 182

SECTION VI: JUDAIC MESSIAH, CHRISTIAN MESSIAH, TRUE MESSIAH[S]

It would appear that the promised Messiah doesn't seem to fit the bills of either the Old Covenant or the New. Why is this important? It's important because the Messiah was the One in whom all want to put their trust to bring the truth and "straighten everything out." Each religion as well as each individual is looking for the 'One' that would prove what they believe is the "truth." Undoubtedly, someone will be disappointed, and this will always bring and spread controversy and hatred, and can even lead to war. One needs only to witness bipartisan political parties to see the consequences of this. When it comes to the Savior of the world, namely God, in whom, there is the faithful trust, when competition arises, regarding who is right and who is wrong, is as volatile a question as asking who Jesus 'is,' let alone whether or not He was only a man, a man of God, man 'and' God, or just God in the guise of a man. Why is this volatile? Because no one wants to think that God could ever be mistreated if a man, let alone be arrested, convicted, and crucified. That is why today the question of whether or not He even existed still lingers on. For some, if the answer to "did He exist" was "no," it would probably solve half the problems of humanity if not more, since finally the sense of guilt would be eradicated; however, what would follow would quite possibly be another crime of humanity for those who feel they can finally punish those who believed, perhaps leading to another kind of enslavement. Who knows? The question is not whether or not you believe in Jesus; the odds are that in some way he still rocks your world. Even within his realm of believers there are tremendous differences of opinion.

We find just how controversial His name still is, even presently. Almost everyone is familiar with Google, Google home, Google Assistance and Amazon Echo, etc. It was reported that when "Google home" is asked "who is Jesus" Assistance responds, "Sorry, I don't know how to help you with that." That, apparently, is the same response when asked "Who is God?" But when asked who Muhammad is, Assistant answers, "Mohammed is the founder of Islam." It was reported that there was a conspiratorial reason that info on Jesus was not available, claiming that this information was censored. The Google answer to this claim was that it was not due to conspiratorial reasons but to "ensure respect." Kind of sounds like censorship as "respect towards Mohammed is paramount to his followers." This claim was also followed up by [Google Assistant response that it] 'it might not reply in cases where web content is more vulnerable to vandalism and spam,' says a Google spokesperson. It was also mentioned that despite their intelligence AI's are in many ways dumb. They depend on humans to teach them, and humans can deliberately influence them to be racist, offensive, or otherwise skewed to be improper. Wouldn't this be a threat to all other Deities also?

It is written in the *Bhagavad Gita (4.2)*:

> This supreme science was thus received through the chain of disciplic succession, and the saintly kings understood it in that way. But in course of time the succession was broken, and therefore the science as it is, appears to be lost.

LESSON 183

THE DIFFERENCES BETWEEN CHRISTIAN AND JUDAIC MESSIANIC BELIEFS

Taking a little deeper look at how the differences between both Christian and Jewish theologies have impacted their doctrines and beliefs, respectively, one can see why there is such controversy surrounding Jesus. First, He was born Jewish. Being Jewish, He could never be seen as the Messiah as perceived by his birth religion; the authorities at that time interpreted Jewish prophetic expectation regarding the Messiah's qualifications to be incompatible with the person, example, and teachings of Jesus. But depending on one's point of view, it could easily be shown how Jesus fulfilled the prophetic expectations of the Messiah to the letter (and spirit). One again, this shows the importance of 'point of view' when writing, or interpreting, scripture, and 'who' has control of that.

Based on this, we could immediately find ample reasons as to why this rejection of Jesus impacted both religions, under the influence of human consciousness. This leaves the question of whether or not the Messiah came, or is coming, and if there is a Messiah, which one will come back?

The following are excerpts from a source called Online Essays. It defines the beliefs of the two as follows. While Christians hold that Jesus/the Messiah came, had gone, and will return, the Jewish Faith is still waiting for God to act, since they do not believe Jesus was the Messiah.

A Messiah is said to be defined as being endowed with the characteristics of a priest, one who is mandated to bring the world into alignment with the word of God. 'He' was prophesized to come from the House, or line, of David, and will build the eternal kingdom here on earth, vanquishing the enemies of Israel along the way. Recalling what was said earlier, the Jews were looking for a Messiah who would liberate the people of Israel from foreign oppression and establish its sovereignty as a nation. Jewish lore describes the Messiah as laboring with the spirit of the Lord upon him, and guiding his wisdom and understanding, while counseling the poor and the meek. He could not forgive sins, as only God could do that. Though upon the Messiah there would be good and important qualities, they would not know when He would appear to work miracles for the people. *Hmmm.*

Now, let's look at the Christian view of a Messiah. According to Christians, Jesus fulfilled all the above EXCEPT that he was also the Son of God. The Messiah of the Jewish faith was to be just a man, but only a man, not a God. Christians believe he came to save the world by absolving people of their sins. Jesus was born of a virgin named Mary; however, He healed the sick and infirmed, raised the dead etc., and always acted as judge and counselor telling followers to embrace peace over violence and war, but He did not confine his ministry to just Israel nor did He make the Jewish faith the religion of the world, as they believed; rather, he talked to everyone, including Gentiles, all gender expressions, all cultures, and all ages.

Both are said to be the Son of God, but Jesus was mortal until death. For ages Christians have believed that since Jesus completed and fulfilled the Old Testament prophecies and law, for the Jews to refuse to recognize him as the Son of God and Messiah is what led to His persecution, trial, and crucifixion. For this reason,[240] Christians had long believed that through this conscious rejection of Jesus, they could not be saved. Eeshans believe in addition one must again refer back to the mindset of Jews not concerned with 'salvation,' as Christians understand it, but, rather, as freedom from captivity and oppression. Is this what Jesus meant by "weep not for Me but for your children," referring to those who did not, and would not, believe in a salvation of the soul, over and above the mere liberation from political oppression? That is, even if a political liberation occurred, and sovereignty for Israel was achieved, the same spiritual

---

[240] "Essay: The Role of the Messiah in Judaism and Christianity." Online Essays, onlineessays.com/essays/religion/the-role-of-the-messiah-in-judaism-and-christianity.php.

condition Jesus addressed would remain, since again there was a loss of the transcendental consciousness which would steer the mind, soul, and spirit towards those things of God greater and above those things of humans who are below. So, what happens then? Why did Jesus say what he said? He was addressing the consequence of religious leaders' and authorities' actions on behalf of both the Jews and early disciples, and, eventually what would develop as the Catholic faith, who would rob the people of salvation. Since to not have the transcendental they would not have the Sacred Bread and Drink necessary for life everlasting, and would truly find themselves living out the consequences of living by their law for afterlife. What happens to these people? Those in charge will be accountable for others' actions, and, as for the victims, we need only refer back to what Jesus said.

We find the characteristics of a Messiah defined by this essay as being spot on with their views of both faiths, but now Eeshans feel they should share their own view.

If you look closely, you will see that the Jewish views of the Messiah *are more accurate* when compared to that of the Christian views regarding Jesus as Messiah. Those of the church over 2000 years of evolution have taken on more characteristics of the Old Covenant than that of the New Covenant coupled with the omission of Jesus' stance on equality beginning with his Marriage and treatment of women and children, race, color creed, etc., and the true reason for his mission.

One can clearly see by this comparison how the Popes were able to establish the doctrines and dogmas they preferred, which influenced western philosophy, politics, culture, science, art, music, etc., by their use of ecumenical councils and papal bulls; and how the papacy and the authority of the church still protects itself by its claim of infallibility.

Anyone can find the following information anywhere.

Where it claims that due to the fact that the Holy Spirit guides it, it has God as the common source and two modes of transmission: Sacred Scripture and Sacred Tradition as mentioned several times in this book. These are 'authoritatively and authentically interpreted' by the Magisterium. Sacred Scripture consists of seventy-three books in the Catholic Bible, forty-six of the Old Testament, and twenty-seven New Testament. Sacred Tradition consists of those teachings believed to be handed down,[241] since the time of the apostles, and both of these make up the deposit of faith. Authentically interpreted does not allow for the omission or expunging of additional authentic information, or teachings, which would alter the whole course of faith. A perfect example is that the Catholic church holds that there is one eternal God, which exists as 'mutual indwelling' of three persons: God the Father, Son, and Holy Spirit together called the Holy Trinity,[242] but this does not include that which would maintain Sacred Balance. The church also has what are called doctrines and dogmas, which have been specifically defined as being its sacred scriptures and apostolic traditions and teachings revealed by an extraordinary definition by a 'pope or ecumenical council.' These 'must be accepted' by all faithful members as contained in the Deposit of Faith; but what if the popes and council's "extraordinary definition" is only based on human, rational differences of opinions of Christ's teachings passed down from one who disagreed with Jesus' directive, having maintained its roots in the Jewish faith and culture, otherwise *supplanting* what was taken out? And, what if said texts were, in fact, found to be more of the Old Law, allowing for the betrayal of who Jesus still was, is, and always will be the Messiah? What if what is said to 'prefigure' Jesus allowed for questions, or controversy, and does not give purpose for 'all' to be saved according to what Jesus said, but allows for all to continue in error, a point maintained throughout this book? What if throughout the apostolic succession there were those who did not believe in Jesus, or who He was, or did not and do not believe in his life, sacrifice, or Real Presence in or out of the Eucharist as defined by that religion's own doctrines?

This is what Eeshans maintain and teach. On what basis do they profess this? Based on many sources (to include our Foundress,) but, moreover, to use a reason most adequate in presenting the fact that in the Eeshan faith, we feel the Holy Spirit has not been guiding the church of Peter but has been urging it to make amends for its errors and accept the Divine Feminine in order that its doctrines be corrected and sacredly balanced. Couple this with

---

[241] These include sacred writings, commentaries, doctrinal councils, and other developments based on practices and the sense of the faithful over time. – Ed.

[242] "Our Lady of the Rosary San Diego, CA." About the Catholic Faith | Our Lady of the Rosary San Diego, CA, Our Lady of The Rosary, www.olrsd.org/About-the-Catholic-Faith.

the fact that the church has already been proven to have covered up, and continues to lie about sex scandals, i.e., the February 5, 2018 report, regarding a letter from the Associated Press that contradicts Pope Francis' insistence that victims of Fr. Fernando Karadima had not come forward to complain about cover ups by Bishop Juan Barros, who Francis appointed to lead the Diocese of Osorno in 2015. True or not, there is evidence enough that the 'internal forum' housed 'not the Holy Spirit' but another, very different spirit.

We believe that we are correct, based on the fact that our truths were given to 'us' and Sacred Scriptures, and the real Apostolic Traditions and Teachings, are revealed by an extraordinary definition, and by the Wife of the Lamb, who, in present times through Supramentalization, teaches with the consciousness of Mary Magdalen, who witnesses through what we might call 'Persistence of Memory.' This is, in the final analysis, according to Eeshans, *all that will be able to step in and say what is the truth and what is not.*

We think of the Persistence of Memory this way: even if/when the world, or an authority, has disproved, discredited, invalidated, or condemned something as even beyond the shadow of a doubt a fiction, there is still something inside of collective human memory. experienced individually and quite personally, that will not allow a truth to be lost, forgotten, or invalidated, especially when:

A. it seems that there is no longer a reason one can believe
B. and all the facts are in,
C. and it is determined [i.e., by the church] the case is closed,
D. and there is no explanation why it won't go away.

This means that the truth has been so deeply buried in human consciousness, yet it just continues to push back up through that consciousness to the surface, as if God, through the transcendental consciousness, wants it revealed; it becomes evident that there is more (i.e., to history) than what is recorded; and more to a human being than just 'facts' and 'reasons' alone. There is a *direct connection* through the immortal soul to God. An example can be readily seen in the police detective who continues to push on to solve a case even after all the 'facts' and 'evidence' points in another direction. There is still something 'inside' that tells the detective that the truth, while as yet undisclosed, is still there waiting to be discovered.

PART XVIII

LESSON 184

OUR EESHAN CREED EXPLAINED

We believe that Christ is the second Person of the Holy Trinity, Divine Masculine of the only-begotten Child of God, and He made a conscious desire to be born of his own free choice. We believe that He acted with the sentiment of a human among humans living as human with a wife, who was His eternal and infinite consort. He, as the *cornerstone*, would be rejected as would be His wife, who is the *keystone*. We believe he allowed himself to suffer, to be crucified, and, by Divine love, He was resurrected with a sacred kiss.

It was then God's plan that He consciously made the choice, due to His almighty omnipotence, that Jesus chose to 'limit his divine power.' Why? Because as humans, we are created with free will, and Jesus felt that to use His power all of the time would be to take away everyone's ability to choose and take away one's personal responsibility to make choices on one's own based on free will, without coercion … especially with a relationship with GOD. God does not infringe on free will. Jesus taught, and repeated often, that it's faith, and not phenomena, that we live by, and on which we base our spirituality. "Blessed are those who have believed without seeing …" Human beings after the fall did not have beatific vision, and so would have to rely on faith, hope, and love for their guidance.

We believe it was then, as God, by God's mercy, that He laid the groundwork for a transcendental life with God, with His intention being that in the end of times, His wife, (Mary Magdalen, eternal consort and Divine Feminine of the only-begotten Child of God), who before, during, and after His mission on earth, would follow in his footsteps.

Though, she, too, would be denied and derided, and her rightful place and role coveted, usurped, and taken from her, in the fullness of time, she, by the power of the third Person of the Blessed Trinity Divine Holy Masculine and Divine Feminine Spirit, by the process known as supramentalization of the Divine, would be awakened from her suspended sleep. It would be at this place in time that Jesus would return for her, and she would 'encompass the Man,' and continue Christ's mission of salvation, as originally intended. From then she would continue Christ's mission as his 'helper,' in its truest, most proper meaning, which entails equality of dignity and not servitude. The purpose of her mission is to bring about faith in a faithless world, salvation in the midst of loss, harm, and damnation.

Her purpose is to reintroduce Christ's plan of salvation once again through the choice of open theism, miraculously, or through necessity, without overriding the inherent powers of God's people. To a people who no longer believe they need salvation, and for lack of belief in God, the power of inspiration and love goes hand in hand with Christ's teachings, his life, suffering, and death.

It is by our beliefs that Eeshans claim the right to ordain women, since it is not the sole privilege of males on this earth; by God's design from the beginning, it was to bring the Holy Sacred and Balanced marriage imagery, which will once again mirror God's image and likeness. From this holy and mystical mystery, humans will draw their strength no matter what their marital status, since in this mystery lies the grace and love necessary, and in the formation of a balanced conscience and a consciousness grounded in the Oneness of a Masculine/Feminine God, the Creator, Redeemer and Sanctifier.

By reason and authority of God as the Divine Masculine Melchizedek, there was an altar where 'no man' was allowed to offer sacrifice. This represented His female counterpart, as you will find is significant because she would become the Virgin Mary, the One who would not be defiled. There would be no relations between her and Joseph, who was chosen to be her guardian. In light of this understanding of the Order of Melchizedek, there is no reason why women can't be ordained, since they are needed to bring back the Sacred Balance in the human.²⁴³ This Divine and Sacred Order would unite with the resurgence of the Divine Feminine, and, thus, be "as Above so Below" in the sight of God.

At this time, the Sacred Bread and Drink would be brought forth by, with, and in the celebration of the Sacred and Divine Marriage Feast of the Lamb and His Wife, for the Salvation of all of God's children. As leaven, these children will form an allegiance in the final battle and destruction of the Beast, with the help of the victorious St. Michael under the auspice of the Divine Feminine, Who by Oneness encompasses the Lamb, who was slain and carries with her the total and undeniable sacrifice necessary for the salvation of humankind.

It shall be at that time, that the One, who is the Fruit of the Lamb and his Wife, shall rise and rule with a sacred and balanced "Rod of Iron."

---

[243] In the Eeshan Tao, women and men *both* have ministerial functions, to reflect the divine and sacred balance of male and female. The Kallahs flow from Mary Magdalen as the Bride, and the Chatans flow from Jesus as the Bridegroom. Here there are two means by which those who feel called to enter the way of life of a bride or bridegroom, a Kallah or Chatan, may do so and there is no cause for discrimination.

LESSON 185

SECTION I: THE IMPERFECT CHALLENGES THE PERFECT

If the female body is the deciding factor in what man feels is his right alone, THEN THE MALE MUST SHOW PROOF OF ABSOLUTE POWER; yet, only One has absolute power, and even the All in All 'chooses' to limit that power to free will. Is there anyone who is greater than God? Then Eeshans present there is no support, or documentation, presented as Christ's sans the opinion of the church with regards to this claim; and, thereby, there is nothing to substantiate this claim.

Are we faced with these issues because the church is so obstinate about not accepting that God is both male and female, and, thus, it refuses to see how wrong this teaching is, since all created things are balanced? This in itself has discouraged, and always will discourage, half the world's population with regard to Christ's love for us. It also identifies a dogmatic issue.

Eeshans believe that all of these arguments, pro and con, are based on erroneous philosophical, epistemological, and ontological categories. Eeshans assert that the form of priesthood today, claiming the Order of Melchizedek, and that which was meant and intended for Jesus to institute, was in fact the reason Jesus upheld and ordained women. For the apostolic priesthood claimed today, the Order of Melchizedek was used to prefigure Jesus as High Priest, and to lockdown for all eternity the patriarchal mindset and foundation for 'their' version, or to source an origin in order to maintain, that women could not be ordained.

Sadly, women stand no chance of equality under the fabricated 'traditional' story and ongoing teaching in Genesis about Adam and Eve. This is precisely why Eeshans maintain that the church's militantly titling of itself "the Bride of Christ" is so wrong. The Gnostic texts and discoveries of text fragments and archeological finds, as well as the contraindicative traditional interpretation of scriptures seem to indicate that the church usurped its title from Christ the Lamb's Wife, and took the coveted role for itself. By doing so, Mary's role would then be erased and there would be no further discussion because no question would likely come up later on down the road about the Bride being an actual person. This would then begin, and continue, the imbalance, which Jesus' rightful teachings would have prevented.

Eeshans assert that any tree with bad fruit, if not treated, will continue to grow bad fruit. It is wrong to put a man ahead of woman and take the role of the Lamb's Wife out of the Sacred Balance Jesus created through his life and mission, thereby, creating an imbalance, which would, and did, perpetuate the sins of discrimination and oppression. Setting this course into motion, we watched flowing from it more such criminal acts, which when identified, created an invincible shield of protection, which has come to be known as the "deposit of faith," which is according to the Catholic faith the 'body of revealed truth, apostolic tradition OR oral Tradition,' that no one may question or revise. In this regard, one must conclude that a human representation of Christ should be balanced with a human representation of his Bride. To 'deny,' or reject, the fact that Christ had a consort for 2000 years does not make it law and does not make the oppression, discrimination, and prejudice justified and true. Remember there are just as many books written that were against Jesus by those who denied him.

Once again, Eeshans assert that despite what has happened throughout church history, it remains obvious that what has been taught is just one part of the story. It is apparent, that somewhere along the way, what Jesus taught was grossly changed and revised many times in order to support an agenda.

What would happen if what is being taught under the guise of his teachings is not true? Well, if they were not balanced, discrimination and prejudice would indeed abound in this world, *and it does*. The same conclusion is drawn with regard to the truth about Adam and Eve. The outcome of such untrue and offensive notions, such as that Adam was over Eve, or that Eve caused Adam to sin, may satisfy the male ego, but it retroactively jettisons humankind back to the time before Christ, and offers an unbalanced salvation in which women still pay for what men feel is her fault. This is an argument that can go on and go—a veritable 'Catch 22.'

But, as we have reiterated time and again, the consciousness of the world suffers with no real end, or solution, for its unrest and begs Christ to intervene once again. One must wonder if these injustices against gender expressions under God are the reason for lack of love of neighbor, lack of faith, disbelief in God, and sin reaching full measure?

Unless we 'unlearn' the wrongs and learn how to love, we stay where we are. That is why a guide is necessary. One who can guide with the "Light," which enables our Light Bodies to shine outside the bushel baskets and to clearly see the way back through the transcendental consciousness and be nourished with the Food of Eternal Life.

It is definitely imperative that the world needs One who will redefine what is good, and One who will untangle the web of deceit and reveal the kind of love Jesus, as the Spiritual Master, taught and the peace of which he spoke.

As the obsession with sex has replaced love, so, too, freedom is viewed as a lack of law and order. People no longer feel safe and protected, and they are confused with what is right and what is wrong; but there is a real need to take precautions against whatever they feel is hurtful or is perpetrated against them, which comes from the sense of being grounded in kindness and with truth as they individually search for right and wrong, decency and indecency.

There is a misunderstanding of what free will is and how it is conceived. Wrongly used, it has been used as a tool of enslavement, and, thus, much of the world lives with fear and reactions to fear as a result of blame, or deserving credit, since it is use to choose, or make poor decisions, out of a poorly informed conscience and/or spiritual guidance. There is no belief in divine accountability for poor choices, and no one can teach decency or form good conscience because the full resemblance of God's existence is rarely displayed.

The cries of those who need God to avenge their lives are smothered by those who use God as a scapegoat to blame for this pathetic life that has become humanity's legacy, as a result of its choices and decisions. The church, and its ambassadors, were witnesses of atrocities all over the world, but were too involved in politics, power, guilt, and intrigue to speak out against them. The church and its leaders have been responsible for committing atrocities with their own hands, with little to no acceptance of guilt or remorse. Where was the Holy Spirit at these times? Was it ever there, or was it just an entity used for a fail-safe whenever a crisis presented itself?

Since the Holy Spirit of God is that which directs the conscience of those who believe in God and the works of God; yet, it is based on what the Catholic church proclaims, one must question how this same Spirit has guided those in authority who have ignored, or turned a blind eye to all the atrocities throughout Christian history, to include the scandals of the religious in recent days. Is this the same spirit who offers excuses for why women cannot be ordained priests, and had a hand in the last two Popes avoiding meetings with victims of purported scandals, addressing their involvement in misconducts themselves? Which Spirit was called upon when it was necessary to enforce belief in the faithful with the creation of a new doctrine, or dogma, or papal bull, that clearly was an outrage against Jesus and his life and teachings on women or other genders?

The threat of a woman as being an eternal/infinite consort of God was never so blatantly obvious as when the Roman Catholic Archdiocese of Boston felt that it was necessary to immediately calm rumors, which began following a false news story that was released about a Father O'Neal, a seventy-one-year-old cleric who claimed and related a near-death experience. The story goes to state that on January 29th, 2017, Fr. Michael O'Neal was rushed to Massachusetts General Hospital with a heart attack that resulted in his being declared clinically dead more than forty-eight minutes, and with the use of a very high-tech machine called LUCAS 2, woke up perfectly recovered. What caused the stir over what Father O'Neal 'saw'? What was it that upset the Archdiocese and "probably the entire Catholic/Christian world"? Describing his experience, he said, as follows: "He went to heaven and was met with the experience of an intense feeling of unconditional love and acceptance by an overwhelming light who was God, but God was a woman! Father said: Her voice was both overwhelming and comforting. 'She had a soft and soothing voice, and her presence was as reassuring as a mother's embrace.' The fact God is a Holy Mother, instead of a Father, doesn't disturb me, she is everything I hoped she would be and even more." Immediately, despite doctors' comments to the contrary, the Archbishop, the article writes, made a public statement stating that Fr. O'Neal suffered hallucinations linked to a near death experience, and that God clearly isn't a female. Even though this story has been proven false, it swept the global news circuit in almost record time before it was determined a hoax, which begs the question: Why did people take to this story so readily? Is it that the consciousness of the world knows a story like this can't be far from the truth, or wouldn't be surprising if it possibly was the truth?

LESSON 186

Section II: Would Things have been Different?

If the Sacred Balance that Jesus and Mary had been rightly expressed and taught after Jesus died, instead of being changed to suit another's vision, there might, indeed, have been a very different course of history, one which would have very clearly reflected Jesus' true mission of justice, resetting the balance between male and female, and all of this through divine Metta.

Will the image of the Divine Feminine as the hidden Queen, the Woman who was/is the Wife of Christ/the Lamb, the Sophia Perennis, bring balance into a world robbed of the fullness of truth? Eeshans believe yes, so long as she is imaged by Christ's side, and as his Bride and Wife, or encompassing him within her, and that people are taught to listen to their hearts and common sense, and by God's grace, they will be able to see God as truth once again. By her love she not only corrects, but also brings with her a new and loving beginning. With outstretched arms, she is essential and fulfills her role as the eternal feminine consort of Jesus Christ.

She will continue His mission in comforting those who had been led astray, teaching them to think, and reviving love of God. She will crush Hell's dark, evil profile. Being the Bride in exile after Jesus' redeeming death, now reunited with the Lamb, and together once again, they will complete their Mission.

LESSON 187

SECTION III: MEN FOR WOMEN

It is the Divine Feminine who moved and continues to move the hearts of all; one must truly acknowledge that though the women felt the brunt, and bore the burden of carrying the false guilt of "those who created Eve's sin," one cannot mention, too often, those men who sacrificed their reputations, good standing in their faith, professions, and careers, to fight for women's rights.

In the political, religious and social arenas, there is a courageous witness, President Jimmy Carter, who let his position be known in his church when he saw how women were being discriminated against. There are many public and entertainment celebrities who have used their high profile to visibly and vocally stand up for women's rights, dignity, and equality in the workplace.

President John F. Kennedy, even while having a reputation of being a womanizer, nonetheless helped set the stage for further positive change with regards to women's status in public and the work place. The President signed the Equal Pay Act of 1963, which prohibits arbitrary discrimination against women in the payment of wages, drawing attention to the unconscionable practice of paying female employees less wages than male employees. He called it 'another structure to democracy.' He said it would add protection in the workplace to the women, the same rights at the workplace that they have enjoyed at the polling place.[244] At that time, the

---

[244] Popova, Maria. "Happy 50th Birthday, Equal Pay Act: A Brief History and Future of the Gender Wage Gap." Brain Pickings, 18 Nov. 2015, www.brainpickings.org/2013/06/10/equal-pay-act-of-1963/.

woman worker earned only sixty percent compared to the average pay for men; yet one in three workers were women.

These are men who are intrinsically connected by virtue of an innate gnosis and desire for equality *for all human beings*, and we meet them daily, and know them personally. These are men who have supported, and continue to support their mothers, sisters, wives, and girlfriends equally. These men teach their sons the same respect, and tell their daughters that they can become anything they want, to be strong, and to always demand respect.

Because of the *Sophia Perennis* (through the person of the Divine Feminine), we do continue to see more of an outpouring of good men across the world, good husbands, and those who have great devotion to our Eesha and what she stands for, and who have been members for thirty years in her work.

But Eeshans feel that it is time to reintroduce God's people to what was supposed to have been implemented in Christ's teachings from the start. As mentioned in the *Pistis Sophia*, Chapter 96, and the Gospel of Mary, Christ says, "Where I shall be, so shall be my twelve ministers. But Mary [Magdalene] and John, the virgin, **will tower over all my disciples** and over all men who shall receive the mysteries in the Ineffable. And they will be on my right side and my left side, and I am they and they are I."

The world has suffered for not knowing the complete truth of what Jesus taught in actions, words, and deeds. It is apparent that most religions have lost touch with how to soulfully, and adequately, direct God's people. The saddening result is the poor forming of conscience over the centuries. Both faith and governments have been affected and injustice prevails.

Without a fully formed conscience, one cannot determine right from wrong, when to fight for what is right (as Jesus taught, "there will always be innocents"), and how to recognize when political correctness blurs the truth and violates freedom and human rights.

Now the fullness of time dictates Christ's plan for His wife to come to us with the Divine Feminine Spirit, and by their Sacred Union, they will perfectly fulfill the prophecy that "a woman shall encompass a man."

The time has come, and it is now necessary for the Wife of the Lamb to come here to heal the wounds of women and all those who are scarred by divorce, discrimination, betrayal, abortion, and the sins that result from those consequences; and for all those other expressions of gender subject to discrimination and prejudice, she will be their advocate, just as Jesus was.

One must not forget, that discrimination of men by women is real also. Women in power not only are found to abuse and emasculate, and deprive a man of his male role, or identity, but have been guilty of not giving him his space, too. Where today we find the absurd and unconscionable behavior of men, the same actions have been used by women against men in the workplace and at home.

As mentioned before, one must be careful that in fighting for equal rights and in citing behavior issues against men, women who assist these men in providing them with whatever means serves the male ego, and doesn't correct the problem, it just mirrors it. This means that often times women will use men for a greater place themselves career-wise, or for status and financial gain as easily as men would do to women and at times other men. The shoe fits both.

Opting to go along with the wrongs of those one should be protecting either to share and benefit behind the scenes by compromising, or by aiding and abetting without being the principle offender, is only to have these things, these gains, these attacks to backfire, and prove to be more ammunition for the other side in a continued war against the greater good. Since one or the other to continue to use betrayal as a means for personal gain, rather than exposing the bad and reforming and working out difference, is unjust, unreasonable, and immoral.

Women must not join the ranks of 'what was' once deemed the world of the powerful, egotistic, white male exploitation of women, by *becoming* one of these. Yet, it happens that often times when presented with power and money, in favor of the reversing of advantages or a minority group, one can be too 'over enjoyed,' and relish in those things coveted. Another example is seen where a woman can be two-faced, thus, continuing to double-deal in unequal treatment of men and women, or whoever is the winner in the 'present' majority group, and leads to efforts using the same techniques and actions as what they are fighting against, thus preserving inequality rather than eliminating it. For example, a woman appears to support other women by seeking out names and leaders as standing with the women, as though to help; but instead she is working with the accused behind the scenes, knowing that these men will eliminate these women from the workplace, while destroying their lives and future, as retaliation for exposing their dastardly deeds. In the meantime, the two-faced agent of betrayal was promised to gain a powerful political office under the guise of another step towards women's liberation. What's lacking? God is lacking, conscience is lacking, decency is lacking, and morality is lacking. Without God, or a Superior Being, there is no afterlife, there is just the present time. It becomes a world of taking what one feels is deserved, and thinking only of oneself.

The needs, the cries, and the souls of the righteous have once again reached the ear and heart of God. The transcendental consciousness is back. The transcendental consciousness, as you have learned throughout this book, is the relationship of the heart-mind with God, or the relationship of the heart-mind and deeper truths, which are more fundamental than the physical world, or the intimate linkage of the mind of a worshipper and God. God is found within the consciousness of the Lamb's Wife, which was put into a deep sleep until the time He decided to bring her back by His side in fulfillment of God's plan for salvation of humanity.

What is this person like who claims to teach from this consciousness? Jesus' desire for her life here as His eternal consort means bringing the Divine Feminine to retrieve what is rightfully meant for God's people:

- the right to bring souls back to God;
- a voice for the souls of the sick and dying;
- an advocate for the oppressed;
- the revealing of the wrongs of oppression of women, especially in matters of faith, back to and including Eve;
- and the revealing of the complete story of salvation by the birth, life, suffering, death, resurrection, and ascension of The New Adam and Eve, who is Jesus Christ and Mary Magdalene, as it was intended from the beginning.

LESSON 188

SECTION IV: OUR FUTURE

Since the state of the world lacks in faith, and its sins are increasing, it only makes sense that a merciful God would intervene and correct the conscience of the world with the one who knew Him best.

The standards held as truth by religious institutions have every man, woman, and child shown as children of God; yet, discrimination abounds with regards to disabilities, age, race, color, creed, and sexual orientation; also, abuse, poverty, and war are prevalent. So where are we now?

We are aware of sins that cry out for vengeance before God:

- the sins of homicide, infanticide, fratricide, patricide, and matricide;
- the sins of pride, gluttony, neglect of the poor, neglect of the disabled, and abuse of women, other genders and children;
- the cry of the outcast, the widow, the orphan;
- slavery and marginalization;
- injustice to the wage earner by taking advantage of and defrauding workers;
- no longer believing in eternal life or eternal death.[245]

---

[245] "Sins That Cry to Heaven." Wikipedia, Wikimedia Foundation, 13 Nov. 2019, en.wikipedia.org/wiki?curid=21351469.

LESSON 189

SECTION V: CORRECTING THE CONSCIOUSNESS OF THE WORLD

Before we can do what Jesus commanded us to do, which is to love God and love our neighbor, Eeshans believe that the world must go through a correction of its consciousness, and, thus, be enlightened.

Eeshans believe that errors in religion that result in lack of faith continue today and allow for acceptance of the many worldwide atrocities that prevail against women and children in horrendous ways, such as the scandals within the church of Peter, the church's, as well as other Christian sect's, double standard for men, the many places in the world where female gender mutilation, rape, sexual slavery, and lack of education about such issues for men, women and children continue daily.

Being blessed, we must find ways to raise the quality of life and consciousness in other nations, disarming jealousy and hatred by teaching and providing the means to not only assist in desperate situations, but to help the people of these nations to realize their dreams in their own countries, so that their citizens are provided opportunities where equality and law-abiding, decent and harmonious attitudes flourish. It is, however, the responsibilities of those "democratic" governments to teach respect for authority and not allow those to interfere who refuse to support the people's choice, and, instead, inflict and encourage 'not freedom but destruction' of the people's right to choose a leader. To try and influence by corruption does the opposite of what should be done with a democratic foundation, and this is not meant only in the political party sense, but in the sense of "freedom to make one's own choice about government and leadership through voting." The meaning behind democracy allows for the process of working together for the people and it teaches respect for authority and love of the nation; and it builds love of neighbor and family. To consistently incite riots and encourage people to continue battling against the elected leader through organized resistance simply because of dislike, rather than accepting the person and respecting the office and protesting policy in an orderly and respectful way, encourages those who are destructively intentioned to look to destroy and divide a country by use of violence, and this lessens the strength of a nation, and no good or constructive achievements could come of this.

It is always said that a nation divided against itself cannot stand. Those who permit elected officials to continually stay in office knowing they are wasting time, whose focus is only to disrupt and destroy elected officials in democratic nations, and who fail to first realize the Founding Fathers' love of nation, are guilty of poor example and acceptance of breaking the two great commandments of God.

In the case of those considered outcasts, or those immigrants, who desire the lifestyle of said nation/country, should realize that they have no rights according to the nation they choose to immigrate to, and once they desire to proceed to find a new life there, by all that is decent, *honorably* obtain citizenship so that they may share in God's blessings in a free world, and the privileges of that nation, living and working as upright and morally sound citizens who will fight to defend the civil liberties in the land where they choose, or desire, to live according to that nation's spirit and law, and not their personal choices, as did those throughout history of man. To overrun, invade, or overtake a nation is no better than conquers of ancient times, which was to obtain power and indulge greed. Just ask yourself: How would you react if an invasion of extraterrestrials came and took over the earth? Would you just let it happen, or would you fight for your world?

There are continued horrors we hear, or read about, and the fact is that somewhere in this world, every day, in every place, women and children, and people of other genders are faced with verbal, psychological, emotional, and sexual abuse linked to oppression and fear, in their homes, and in the workplaces, and this includes all the same injustices against men as well.

As the fight continues for equality in all walks of life, those who have been subject to some of the most grievous sins and the atrocities, have turned to various religions looking for a source of solace and refuge, such as in Jesus, or any Higher Being one worships. How sad when human beings are supplanted and made a depository of institutionalized error and discrimination by those who claim to hold the sacred doctrines of faith and morals, as these are supposed to give clarity and certainty of the faith itself and its morals, and are supposed to protect the profession of the true faith without error.

Let's be clear here, when any woman, man, or child of God is judged by ill-conceived and unjust standards, *all of humanity suffers* and gets stuck, and cannot advance in spirituality or grace or find peace. Beneath the skin, all share the same inner light of awareness; all bled blue before the fall, because of their love for God. Now humanity bleeds red because this is a sign of needed salvation. This is the essence of the teaching to love one's neighbor as one's self.

Eeshan Transcendentalism, animated by the Divine Feminine, with her consort the Divine Masculine, balances humanity: male and female are like Yin and Yang, in that within the Yin part of the symbol one finds the Yang represented as the small circle, and within the Yang part of the symbol one finds the Yin represented as the small circle.[246] Both are present in one another, even as one of the genders is highlighted over the other in connection with life in terms of a physical body. Together they make one (circle).

In essence, what we are saying is that we are likened to the first androgynous being, and most certainly are mirrored and linked to, and in God's male/female, masculine and feminine image, as found in the true *unaltered* story of Adam and Eve, and Jesus' teachings and beliefs guided by the *Sophia Perennis*.

---

[246] Eye of the fish. – Ed.

PART XIX

LESSON 190

SPIRITUAL TEACHING I: THE RETURN OF THE WIFE OF THE LAMB

Understanding how God can bring back an eternal consort really isn't that difficult. As mentioned previously, the continuing of a Godhead has always been acceptable in many religions and spiritualities. It is just in the Catholic/Christian sects that the verbiage is, and always has been, controlled to reflect whatever was necessary to move and retain the masses. At times, the Pope for example, is the 'successor of Peter'. Other times, he is the 'Bishop of Rome.' To most, he is known as the Vicar of Christ, or Christ on earth, without question.

Christ Himself made known to those who followed Him that He was the Son of God, the Divine Masculine of the only begotten Child of God, but as we mentioned before [repetitio] even up to and including today, there were and are those who question whether He is human, Divine, and human, Divine, Human and Sacramental, or if the person of Jesus ever even existed.

Depending on personal choice, each of those people, none, some, all, or just Christ, is/are telling the truth. We mentioned that the Dalai Lama is considered to be the successor in a line of *tulkus* (living Buddhas), who are believed to be the incarnations of Avaoliteśvara, a Bodhisattva of Compassion, Mater, and Guru. Even those outside the Christian sect readily accepts this. Enter Eeshan! Wow! But at the time of Jesus, the people said the same thing. Nothing is impossible for God, save anything in the minds of humans that choose not to believe.

Supramentalization has always existed, except today due to a lack of spirituality the physical world cannot help but seek to live outside of spirituality, which makes the world prone to the negative, and is doubtful of such actualities. Why not? Because there is nothing in the spiritual that has a connection to the material—a bridge is required.

There are examples of certain known and accepted expressions of lower levels of supramentalization that were found in some people. These are those who felt a connection with someone from the past, or a feeling, of having lived before, or those who believe they lived in one or more lifetimes before this one. But here, you may understand more readily if we use a more classic example in that the church approved saints to whom people had, or may still have, devotions and have read of their supernatural experiences, or who have witnessed personally assistance by their favorite saint, the Virgin Mary, or Jesus, it is in these examples that may help you to understand a little about this process. These saints are said to mirror, and imitate, the 'person of Christ.' We said this since these people witnessed His extreme love being endowed with and displaying supernatural gifts associated with the light body, which shares in the Person known as 'Light of the world.' This means that by their love they 'shared' in the gifts from God, which, still theirs, are more the realization of the Absolute in their heart, but this gets you to step one in understanding, or obtaining, a glimpse' of what happens when one is totally in love with God, the All in All, or Deity of heartfelt choice and devotion.

Supramentalization, as in the case of our Foundress, is the physical divinization where she has demonstrated over the years a more ascended/definite connection with Jesus, and witnessing Him in her and through her.

Eeshans believe that Mary Magdalen experienced the totality of Christ and His love in a mystical/tantric union of her mind, body, soul, and consciousness, which joined her person to His. After her death, her consciousness was in a state of 'rest,' until which time it would be necessary to bring back her consciousness. which was divinized by Jesus in their marriage from biblical times. This is not to say that she enjoyed her marriage, once again, in heaven.

In order for Mary Magdalen's consciousness to return, and live among humans, it would require a woman chosen, or destined, to be the vessel for the Divine Feminine via a gross physical body prepared to witness to eschatological times, and fitted to endure supernatural phenomena. His wife would not only be identified by the above but also prophecies would necessarily be fulfilled. She would 'rectify the loss of Christ's true teachings,' teachings which by His command were supposed to have been His identity as corner stone for his spirituality, which is shown not just by His crucifixion and death, but by the rejection of His directives by Peter and his successors. She, who was and is, the keystone following His way, would not look like her image of 2000+ years, since was the case with Jesus after his crucifixion due to the return of his glorious body, but one is to understand that the difference here is that this is a human replacement body and the glorious body of the Lamb's wife will only be given upon her return to eternity. As was necessary for Jesus for His mission on earth, this human body is necessary for His wife, at this time, as she completes her mission.

Jesus left us with a Christ-consciousness, which, if recognized and propagated in its entirety, would have raised the human vibratory consciousness, and connected it more perfectly to Christ, as intended by God; but man, governed by his own consciousness, led innocent souls away from a transcendental way of thinking and midway back to the rational imperfect state from where He began His mission.

Eeshans believe, wholeheartedly, because of Christ's own resurrection, that the consciousness of His wife, too, would not die with the body. By the process of supramentalization, the consciousness would be united with a human body prepared by Christ himself to house it. Next, this body would have to be of the person who would be seen as a redeemed person, and as believed by the renowned Sri Aurobindo, the individual would have to experience a "psychic and spiritual transformation." In addition to this Eeshans strongly believe that proof of a physical transformation of the woman is necessary, as well. In other words, the total person, the entire being, must transcend into the "formless/timeless being," yet, the body must still be subject to entropy, and, at the same time, be a resilient vessel and animated by an assertive attitude to be used as God would deem necessary. Her life would also have to mirror that of her Spouse if, indeed, she was part of Him. This would include the rejection by family, and by being ridiculed and even persecuted in the process of living out her mission, and being rejected by her own church and people, and having her work labeled a 'cult,' just as those who knew Jesus, according to similar family relation and social context derided Him, and labeled His work as coming from Beelzebub. This would include rejection of the testimonies by eye witnesses, and facing the false testimonies of those who were guilt-ridden and knew even less about their birth religion than what they accused her of teaching, or who knew little to nothing of their birth religion while accusing her of 'heresy.' The list goes on and on.

Sometimes even those who witnessed firsthand the goodness of her work were for one reason or another persuaded to disbelieve what they personally witnessed. For fear of being attacked, or ostracized, some came to be afraid to be seen by others in her company, or part of her close circle of friends, while others, on the other hand, stood in her defense.

Some, even those closest to her, fearing perceptions and guilt by association, would not invite her to public and family gatherings, but would still continuously send her requests for her prayers, send others for prayers, and ask for miracles for healings, but would do so only through second parties, or communicated in some other indirect way. They would not publicly recognize her healings, nor give credit to God for answered prayers through her, but instead would give tithings to 'their own church' in thanksgiving for her healings, and, yet also be courageous enough to come back to her to tell her without any sense of guilt that they did this.

There were times when children of devotees would find any reason to try and destroy her work out of irrational fear that their parents had long-term contribution plans, which would cut into imagined 'inheritances.' Racked with bitterness, some wasted no time resorting to public attacks and humiliation on social media, even from those who were helped personally, or via members in assisting in care and assistance, or prevented the following through of promises under the directives of the parent. Unfortunately, as is the case with human beings, whenever God is truly involved in their lives, some of the worst traits of human behaviors are provoked into the open when God touches nerves.

LESSON 191

Spiritual Teaching II: A Body Prepared for an Eschatological Time?

With this in mind we look back from the birth of our Foundress to present times. Born to tremendously faith-filled Byzantine parents whose marriage and life together began with little in the material sense, but who still saw lives wealthy in sacrifice and suffering, they were joyful and thankful for all God gave them.

This Foundress grew up, severely ill with asthma. At two years of age, she experienced a near death experience, which began her unique relationship with the divine. From a very early age, she felt the presence of God in very special way. Hospitalized for double pneumonia with little hope to survive, she experienced the event which identified her life's link to the supernatural. At the crucial moment where death could have claimed her life, the most gracious Mother of God came to her and cared for her through the crisis state, bringing the child to complete recovery, but still laden with asthma, which would remain with her throughout her life.

As time went on, Jesus claimed her as His bride at her first Holy Communion and from that moment their relationship continued through audible conversations, as well as locutions. Her love for Him grew, as His relationship to her changed from a father figure to friend and then to heart-driven love. Beginning in 1974, when she became engaged (married in 1975), through the following eleven years of her marriage, Jesus was absent, both in terms of outward and inner locutions, leaving her to the charge of being a working wife and mother. When pregnant with her first daughter (b. 1976), the audible conversations, and locutions, involving Blessed Mother returned. At the birth of her second daughter (1981), locutions returned, and, in 1986, our Foundress was stricken and hospitalized with a severe condition of her asthma. With a prognosis that she may not be able to work or care for her children, the very familiar voice she knew since she was a child spoke to her, only this time. it was a male voice, and it was here that Jesus began to visit and speak with her. For the next year, as their relationship was rekindled, Jesus was now *physically* appearing to her. From that time, until the early 90's, He taught and commissioned her to do His work, in which included: 1) the early 90's brought with them the fragrance of roses, the presentation from Him to her of a miraculous bloody Host to show His [Jesus'] disappointment, and disgust, at the lack of veneration and reverence to all that was sacred, as well as the failed direction the church that had sent people by the poor example of the priests, and their increasingly secularized, human consciousness-based opinions; 2) the visible Stigmata; and 3) the physical endurance of Christ's Passion, which would last until 1998, when the Stigmata became invisible and the Passion was limited to Lent and Holy Weeks, or if Jesus desired for a particular reason to show it. Then with the continued controversy surrounding the witnessing of no less than ten people, and as many as several thousand, her public reception of Holy Communion from Jesus to the regular (with eye witness) reports from miraculous Eucharist hosts in countless numbers appearing on her tongue, the accounts of seeing Hosts travel from her heart to her mouth, and for distribution to people gathered near her in and outside of churches, to the witnessing (and photography of) Christ's face and body, replacing, and visibly seen, through her person in public and on private retreats, were just some of the ways Jesus identified our foundress as His own and as the woman encompassing the Man.

    At the crest of our Foundress' public work, she found herself placed by Providence at the heart of a perfect storm of political intrigue within the church. For some time, prior to this event, physical, mental, emotional, and spiritual healings were all a part of her ministry; many testimonies from healed persons and their doctors were witnessed. At a healing service, Eesha, our Foundress, had healed a priest of a terminal illness he had in front of an entire congregation, but because it was a

Polish parish celebrating a Polish nun, at that time known to be up for canonization, and because the Pope was scheduled to visit the United States around that very time, the Cardinal orchestrated a plan to capitalize on the opportunity of the priest's healing with the Pope's visit. It was a converging point of clerical corruption and opportunism, a perfect storm of ecclesiastical intrigue. The priest who was healed, who had been in the papers over his miraculous healing, was quickly 'redirected' by the Cardinal to tell an amended version of what happened, which he abided by, even to Eesha who he had known as a 'friend' up to that time, so that the Polish Nun, Sr. Faustina, would get the credit for his healing, and, thereby, be seen as the "miracle" needed for her canonization, and all just in time for the Papal visit. Eesha was not mentioned as having been there, nor was the purpose of the event, which was her personal healing ministry and talks. Sure enough, the priest was immediately wined and dined by the Cardinal, and, in turn, the Vatican, the canonization process turned its attention to this priest. As the Cardinal's plan with Rome was approved and sanctioned, Eesha was quickly erased from the actual historical account, which had been 'recast' to focus on Sr. Faustina as being the healer, even though the healing took place in front of so many witnesses.[247]

Our Foundress' work went under attack, and every effort was made to stifle her public appearances by church authorities. The church continued to impose restrictions on how, and where, she would speak on church property, which was contrary to what God wanted since more unofficial smears, and accusations, of heresy combined with untrue statements and gossip. continued to be circulated about her to all parishes by church authorities, priests, and wealthy benefactors loyal to them.

Unsubstantiated, and twisted, accounts of the supernatural events that surrounded Eesha were being spread in an effort to discredit her. Yet, none could prove these attacks or falsities, and she remained in good standing with the Byzantine church. The controversy grew, and while the church's due process and growing false accusations mounted, she decided

---

[247] The priest, Fr. Ron Pytel, mysteriously contracted his terminal illness again immediately after the canonization ceremony in Rome, and died very shortly afterward. – Ed.

to remain silent, even as she was still officially in good standing with there being no actual 'charges' being made against her. She was encouraged by her bishop through relatives and friends to continue speaking. She stopped her public appearances and refused invitations to speak from many traditional, eastern, and other religions. Though she was not permitted to speak in churches, she was always, instead, permitted to speak on "church properties." Though she was in good standing with the institution at that time, and remained so, she made the decision to bow out of the public eye to establish a transcendental school of enlightenment, as urged by her Divine consort.

It was now that the supramentalization process was fully revealed that Christ's request for her to continue His mission took another turn. Jesus sought a place in the wilderness, a "Place" it was called, from which He could continue her tutelage, and fully complete the transmutation of her body to allow for transformation towards, and sharing in, the DNA structure she needed to continue their work. This was accomplished by introducing higher vibrations within her body, and raising them/intensifying them in order to accommodate this change, though the change of which we speak was more subtle and interior.

All the above prepared the way for the "Child," who was born in Avalon,[248] the transcendentally conceived, and 'born', Fruit of the marriage of Jesus and Mary. He was born in 'the wilderness,' and carried back to heaven, as prophesized in Revelation. Also, during this time, the new Ish and Eesha [Isha] (Jesus and Mary), were able to share a oneness which was used to heal and teach all those God brought to "The Place." His uninterrupted time with His bride/wife would make complete the integral consciousness (awakening the transcendental point of view) over the rational, revisiting what took place in Cana two millennia ago. This work continued privately, until which time she was deemed ready for the institution and beginning of the propagation of a new religion, a *sangha*, a spirituality, and a *Way* for this time. Her readiness is best defined and explained (in the language of Aurobindo) as one whose "body has been transformed, divinized, and emerges, as living a supramental, Gnostic,

---

[248] Meaning 'apple'. – Ed.

divine life on earth," and she is determined to continue her mission freely and without undue restriction. Eeshans feel that Sri Aurobindo uniquely described the reality of supramentalization surrounding and permeating Eesha in his "The Life Divine," as he writes: "Nature already has descended into her and enable[s] her to liberate the supramental principle within her; so must be created the supramental and spiritual being as the first unveiled manifestation of the truth of the Self and Spirit in the material universe." And as Eeshans would continue, "long in coming since the Blessed Virgin Mary."

As with the Virgin, our foundress would live happily married. Unlike the Virgin, however, she would have other children, and face the day to day joys and trials, as we all do.

It was during this time that the scriptures regarding the One who is like the Son of Man were to be fulfilled, Sacredly Balanced, and his name is Emmanuel. He is the fruit of the love of the Bridegroom and the Bride in the wilderness, for these End Times.[249] Eeshans acknowledge that as the three Persons of God share equally in the Person of God the *Future of Days* is now among us because of the Marriage of the Lamb and His wife. Hidden away in an undisclosed location in the world (unknown even to his mother) until the fullness of time, He is the Promise, the Gift, and these days belong to Him whose counterpart is the Divine Feminine.

---

[249] It's interesting to note that the expression 'end times' carries with it the image of finality, death, destruction, and so forth, in the conditioned imagination of these times; sadly, far too few see the expression as referring to the 'ending' of what *was*, something corrupt, something oppressive to God's intentions for humanity which entails joy and Sacred Balance ... and the 'end' of those times is at hand, before giving way to something new, by the hand of God, something based in the love of God and neighbor, in the spirit of goodness and truth. – Ed.

LESSON 192

Sacred Teaching III: Understanding the Fulfilment of Scriptures

When we read scriptures, we seem to read them as though they reflect an ancient component (meaning readers don't readily associate present times as being relevant or directly connected to what is being read—rather it's 'dated' to belong to, or to be limited to, something in the past), forgetting that with God there is no time; we fail to see how *any* writings about God could reflect 'only' an ancient point of view, but must reflect present and future, and then back to the beginning, especially "if" they are about Jesus being Divine, Human, AND Sacramental. That is why He can say He is Alpha and Omega. For example, if Jesus was to come today, we might have a preconceived thought of how He would look, based mainly in the many pictures and images we have been exposed to, and by which we were conditioned to think of Him. We would judge him by what was handed down to us. We fail to understand that our soul is eternal, and it would certainly identify its Creator/Savior; and this is not to say He wouldn't give us some familiar quality to connect with that image we have placed within our hearts. But Eeshans believe that He would also fit into the 'fullness of this time.' That is to say that we see the Jesus that has been proven to be Divine/Human over 2000 years.

We were taught, and conditioned, growing to believe that the Blessed Mother was the Woman in the Wilderness, and the Woman clothed with the Sun, when we heard about Revelation, and in the absence of any memory, or foundation, for Mary Magdalen and her role alongside Jesus, these above revelatory images became associated with Jesus' mother: who else would these images be about? Jesus would clothe His wife with His radiance the 'sun,' as she 'encompasses the man;' but due to the church's stance on women, none of this would be intelligible or be acceptable in any way. Thus, it had to be made to be about Jesus' mother. As for Blessed Mother, there are still doctrines that are not accepted, nor will they ever be accepted, by *all* Christians, as we discussed earlier.

Taking this into consideration, we do present traditional accounts of Sacred Scriptures that Eeshans believe have only been altered in a minimal way; in addition to this, in order to make this more complete, and to raise the understanding of the scriptural accounts to the platform of the transcendental, Eeshans include, in a discerning way, those scriptural passages that conform to the Sophia Perennis (the foundation of Perennial or Eternal Wisdom).

With eyewitness accounts, however, as fulfilled in present time, these traditional scriptures may also affect, and, at times, be a hindrance to some people because of new concepts and appearances being included among those transcendental teachings necessary to fully understand the point Jesus was making.[250]

As an example, it was taught, and believed, that this passage described the Virgin Mary, Eeshans find it surprisingly shocking, and impossible, by any stretch of the imagination, for anyone, even if one is still connected to the beliefs of any of the traditional religions and churches, to make this work for the Virgin Mary. However, we include it here for you to read, once again.

Book of Revelation, Chapter 12:1-17:

And there appeared a great wonder in heaven; a woman clothed with the sun, and the moon under her feet, and upon her head a crown of twelve stars.

And she being with child, travailing in birth, and pained to be delivered.

And there appeared another wonder in heaven; and behold a great red dragon having seven heads and ten horns, and seven crowns upon his heads.

---

[250] In the absence of transcendental teaching for so long, suddenly coming to grips with these concepts and points of view can be quite 'jarring' or seem (at first) like too steep a gradient to traverse. But nothing is impossible with God. – Ed.

And his tail drew the third part of the stars of heaven, and did cast them to the earth: and the dragon stood before the woman who was ready to deliver, for to devour her child as soon as it was born.

And she brought forth a man child, who was to rule all nations with a rod of iron; and her child was caught up to God, and to His throne.

And the woman fled into the wilderness, where she had a place prepared for her by God …

Revelation 1:13:

And among the lampstands was someone like the son of man, dressed in a robe reaching down to his feet and with a golden sash around his chest.

Revelation 14:14-20

And I looked, and behold a white cloud, and upon the cloud one sat like unto the Son of man, having on his head a golden crown and in his hand a sharp sickle.

And another angel came out of the temple, crying with a loud voice to him that sat on the cloud, 'thrust in thy sickle and reap; for the harvest of the earth is ripe'.

And he that sat on the cloud thrust in his sickle on the earth; for the harvest of the earth is ripe.

And he that sat on the cloud thrust in his sickle on the earth; and the earth was reaped.

And another angel came out of the temple which is in heaven, he also having a sharp sickle.

In retrospect, though everyone has been told that these revelations are 'symbolic or already have been fulfilled,' and that they referred to the Virgin Mary, from the Eeshan perspective, this is hardly the case. Yes, these *have* been fulfilled, in this lifetime, according to God's word by the Wife of the Lamb, and not the Virgin Mary.

PART XX

LESSON 193

SACRED TEACHING I: CREATION

As we have been taught OVER THE CENTURIES, and in accord with so many stories, God was not originally EVER seen as male or female in traditional religions.

You know the story, many argued that God is masculine, while others claim God is genderless. And these are always followed with questions such as: If He is just masculine, who is he compared too? Who is his counterpart?[251]

According to the Old Testament, God was not supposed to have a 'human' gender, at all. God was not a 'Father,' as Christianity understands that term for God, and in the Old Testament God definitely had no 'Son.' It is part of the reason that Jesus was, and continues to be, a curse to a lot of the Old Testament believers over the years. That is why He could never be the Messiah to them. Not only was Jesus not the kind of Messiah the Jews were expecting, there was no way he could be "God," either. Then of course there's the disgrace of God having changed his own Law that He gave to Abraham and Moses etc., etc. …? This was an outrage.

Yet, the personal pronouns used are always in the male gender. There are only rare occurrences of feminine imagery with regards to imaging God, such as in talking about 'wisdom' (of all things), but primarily, the scriptures as we have them today cannot help but convey a clearly masculine God.

---

[251] Masculine is only masculine because it is in relation to feminine. Without feminine, there is no proper way to understand what masculine is. – Ed.

In the Psalms, and in other Old Testament writings, one also finds such expressions of God as a "husband." We are told the reason for this stems from the use of such terms as man and mankind, which encompasses male and female. In the Eeshan religion, we strongly disagree with the above, as pervasive use of the masculine pronoun with regards to God's gender quality is linked to the traditional story of Adam and Eve, where God created man first and women second.[252] Knowing the truth, to believe this in effect puts man over woman, and shows that in the beginning there was only a man, and that a woman's creation was an afterthought for purposes of the female helping the man.

Even there, she was drawn 'from' Adam's side, as if she, therefore, 'owed her existence to his being first;' it's peculiar how it doesn't lend to the fact that Adam obviously couldn't get things done, didn't know how to do things, or the expression was due to Adam's having a linear way of thinking, i.e., and that he lacked 'wisdom.' Nonetheless, it seems to attest that man was the first, and dominant, gender made in God's image and likeness. It is said that Eve, being taken from Adam's rib, was the weaker one, placed there to delight, accompany, and serve as a helper, a mate, and everyone believed it because what other information did they have? So, we teach that if this was true, we now have a Male God, who despite being a supposed perfect being, though the term 'androgynous' was never used, but only vaguely referred to, so as not to incriminate said religions, then discriminated against Himself.

The same mindset is carried through, and taught, in a different way in the New Testament. In the New Testament, we are told that Jesus spoke of His Father in Heaven, and of Mary his Mother on earth, though at different times and not in a united way. In other words, according to what was taught and written, unless mentioned in a song somewhere, there was no teaching regarding the possibility that there was any kind of

---

[252] It has been noted by feminist theologians, and is well worth considering, that English as a language is inherently, unarguably biased towards maleness in terms of its use of personal pronouns, whether or not the term can be demonstrated to have included women as well as men, i.e., in the term 'mankind'. It still evokes a masculine image of a totality, even as women are, of course, included in that term. – Ed.

relationship with Jesus' Father beyond Mary's participation in the birth of God's only begotten son, Jesus, to which she said Yes. To be sure, the thought that Mary was married to God the Father was clearly disguised in the story so that she would be overshadowed by the Holy Spirit.

So, how then did creation take place? Eeshans have a take on this as well.

LESSON 194

SACRED TEACHING II: THE ETERNAL COMPONENT OF GOD AND THE HUMAN FACTOR

As the first Person of the Most High is purest masculine/feminine energy, the fruit of that divineness begot the Second Person of God. It was necessary after the 'Fall' to become the physical since the choice of the First Person God to take on human forms on earth, while both counterparts remained Spirit were intrinsic.[253] So, too was the life of their only-begotten masculine/feminine Fruit and the third Person of the Holy Masculine/Feminine Spirit.

When the Persons of God decided to create the transcendental/material world, the first and second Persons of the trinity, and the intervolving/intertwining of the third Person all plural, all the persons of the Trinity, parts and counterparts, were equally involved. Being omnipotent, omnificent, omnipresent, and omniscient, God brought about a creation which would naturally reflect the course, and choice, humanity would take given the influence of the free will factor.

That is why Eeshans believe that before and after the Original Choice of the fall from the transcendental, the second Person's (as Jesus and Mary) mission to end times was, and is, sealed in the creation story.

---

[253] I.e., When Melchizedek, the 'human' face of the First Person masculine was on earth, the Divine Feminine was in spirit; when Blessed Mother was on earth, the Father was in spirit. – Ed.

LESSON 195

Sacred Teaching III: The Eeshan Versions: Of the Eternal Consorts and the Creation and the Role of the Second Person of the Holy Trinity

Being all loving, and wanting to share this love as soulmates do, the fruit of God's love gave God the desire to bring about a human manifestation, that it may, in turn, be witness to a reciprocal love by knowing God's love and showing God's love. Eeshans call this part of God, the 'who' of God. Both the masculine and feminine gender of each of the three Persons, being one God, were 'formless' in their eternal effulgence; however, they would always be, at the center of that, which radiates that effulgence, *eternal Persons*.

God began by calling into being, a "Place," where life can play out, and prove superior, over all that would be created, and exercise dominion over all creatures. Just as new parents do, when they prepare for the new life they are bringing into the world.

This 'newly created' extension of themselves was formed by God's own hand in God's own image and likeness, and was loving and beautiful. Yet, as God is infinite and perfect, this being that was created was limited and imperfect. Why? Because this created being was just that; the being was not already in existence, since God was. However, nor was the being the manifestation of the love of the First Person of God who was manifested in the infinite being of the Second Person, which is the only-begotten Child of the Holy Trinity.

God began with forming a planet. Being the Creator, God took nothingness and began to create. (At this time, the begotten Fruit of the Most High, who is the only-begotten Child and second Person of the Holy Trinity, whose Divine Masculine would become the cornerstone for all of God's salvation plan, was coupled with the Divine Feminine). Being parents, wishing to share their life, the only-begotten was formed, since it was the desire of the Most High Being to share in all things equally. So, since the Second Person of the Trinity was begotten by love, they desired to share in the decision to witness love, too. First the female counterpart of the begotten Child took on the form of water. As a raging ocean by God's command she would become the living water and gave it form. Next, she prepared it to bear life. She would then take her place as the water bearer, the Holy Grail of life for those who thirst. As the form was engulfed with darkness, the spirit of the masculine counterpart of God then came as Light ('let there be light') for He will become the Light of the world, and the light which will be the way for all those who seek Truth, and this Light came through the sea and caused a great explosion. The two which formed one, united, and caused an explosion, then separated, and the male stayed light and the female stayed within the darkness because all of creation is composed of opposites, a positive and negative, an extreme; yet, each complemented the other. The light became day representing the divine, the healing, the dispersing of darkness; and the darkness represented the future of humanity, awaiting daylight each day. This is so because humanity was not the Creator, but was the creature, and was, therefore, "of" God. Just as the spark and the bonfire are similar in quality, but very different in terms of *quantity*, the soul shares the qualities that God gave of his/her own divine substance, but it is placed into a *created* form. So, rather than thinking that the human creature is 'opposite' of God (since this would have a kind of moral tone ring within it, as in good and evil), the human being is *drawn from God*, and bestowed with the divine gift of choice and free will. Still, this does not put the creature on par with the Creator. Thus, as one who is imperfect to its counterpart who is perfect, night was given boundaries; so, thus, day and night were, in our language, and according to a purely human consciousness point of view, seemingly 'opposites,' hence, the word we see in our minds is: 'divided.'

God then separated the water into two parts with sacred breath, forming a dome-shaped division to keep the water above separated from the water below. This then separated the Divine Feminine from the human feminine/female. This would now be our sky shared by the Light and the Darkness, as well as the human with the divine.

Next God created boundaries for the waters and called it 'land.' This would be a place enriched with all that is necessary for life. This land would be a place of shelter, and rich with food to sustain life; and living water, to quench thirst.

Then God brought into existence sustained light, which would always to return after the darkness, which would last for a time, since the Divine would one day return to a less than perfect human world. This would be a reminder of God's love and longsuffering oneness, since he created the moon as the Female and the sun representing the Male counterparts; thus, both were always meant to serve as evidence of a Superior Being who dispels the darkness.

Then God sprinkled stars in the sky to give witness to a universe greater than just this sole planet. The masculine counterpart filled the water with life: there He placed creatures that lived in the water and called it 'she,' since it mirrored His feminine counterpart with a formless body filed with life, breath, and rhythm, which brought life and could take life. Plants of all kinds provided oxygen and balance were meant to be enjoyed.

God's Feminine Consorts decorated the land, and filled the air, with birds of all kinds. Then together, Masculine and Feminine commanded all kinds of animals to come forward: large and small, tame and wild, all of unusual shapes and colors.

Then God, Masculine and Feminine, decided it was time now to create a human being. A beautiful being that reflected all the beauty of God, and all the love and oneness shared between the masculine and feminine counterparts. It would enjoy all goodness from God's imagination. The land, with its richness, was used to form a body capable of all things beautiful, even begetting of extensions of its own life. This being was as perfect as it could be, considering it was created, and did not exist of its own doing. It resembled God in all things to include a perfect life. God placed into creation 'creatures' called animals, reptiles, etc., some with only the male attributes and others with only the female attributes to show the distinction between the being's higher life complete in itself, as male and female, verses the separating of the two original forms.

Though the animals, and other creatures, seemed fine, the human being did not reflect the magnitude of love, meaning there was no *reciprocal* love shared that mirrored God's intimate, reciprocal love of consorts. Since it was perfect in itself, it was human, and still did not have the same perfect love exchanged between the male female identities that God enjoyed. God felt that it was good, but wanted the being to share love, but decided that to truly mirror God's love, the being needed the company of one like itself. The Feminine Consorts encouraged separation of the genders within the human being to serve to initiate a different kind of love, one where the two could experience giving and receiving love as soulmates, with the God particle being the catalyst for union. So, the human being was separated, and God blessed the two so they could enjoy their oneness.

This pleased God since it showed how separating the being into male and female reflected God's oneness by being separated, yet they were still whole. Since God shared the masculine/feminine perfection of love by placing within each expression, or *'gender,'* a part of the other gender, to be 'opposites,' in a complimentary sense; and when they were separated they found a part of each other in one another. Looking ahead, God saw that soulmates will always find each other, since this is the underpinning of true love.

PART XXI

LESSON 196

SACRED TEACHING I: THE STORY OF ADAM AND EVE, AS SEEN THROUGH EESHAN EYES

The following sections do draw extensively upon Paramahamsa Yogananda's writings, because, more than any other sage and yogi and spiritual writer the author has encountered, his personally detailed writings most closely align to the truth regarding God and the origins of creation, since the Eeshans, and particularly the Foundress, understand it. While differing in some detail, overall, any of his writings could be highly recommended for reading regarding the subjects described in this book. Having said that, it should still be made clear that his writings are considered *helpful* and *complementary* in their descriptions regarding subjects and accounts of ancient origin, as well as being more useful and helpful than what Euro-based early Christianity had inherited. It should be remembered that Jesus travelled to, and mastered the spiritual disciplines of, the culture and geographical influences of the lands of the Far East, where transcendentalism was prevalent and more aligned with God and the Sophia Perennis, as opposed to what became Jewish background, and later, the by comparison poor fund of knowledge of which Europe possessed on these subjects. Thus, the Eeshan way is based not on Yogananda's writings, but his writings and the culture and tradition they came from are illuminative regarding Jesus and the Sophia Perrennis.

So, Eeshans submit first, and foremost, that God was not 'genderless,' as the familiar arguments generally go, but was the perfect androgynous being, having the characteristics of both masculine and feminine in perfect balance.[254] Male and female gender traits here on earth are reflections of a perfect relationship of Divine Feminine and Masculine qualities/natures *in God*. God thought, however, that he/she whose nature is ever creating and expanding, would share the Divine life, and would create a being uniquely embodying God's own traits.

Eeshans believe that the Creator decided to beget, and create, an androgynous transcendent spirit of a cosmic vibratory nature. God then cloaked a portion of his/her unmanifested consciousness with the illusion of difference or particulars.[255]

The Spirit manifested finite objects and forms, first with positive and negative elements, and then by using the law of duality and relativity to differentiate God's one consciousness and cosmic energy into countless pairs of polarized forces, and forms, to include positive and negative, male and female, man and woman.[256]

God's creature would not be limited, and bound, by the laws of the physical universe. Eeshans believe that this body has three divine potentials: reason or discriminative will, feeling that which one is conscious of and able to enjoy, and lastly energy, the substance that creates and activates the body. We understand a soul to be a spark of the consciousness of God, individualized by God, and capable of expressing God's image. It is immortal, meaning it will never die.

Then God separated that being into two by vibration (once again, that's what the word "rib" means) in order to create relational complementarity and reciprocation as with all things in the physical universe. We believe that "due to the divine soul attraction within that separated, they became one flesh, acted in harmony, and in unison in body, mind, and soul, but as two bodies, two minds, two souls with one ideal."[257] So, the true male and mate is united to his true feminine soul companion by spiritual union that perfects the expression of the complete spirit nature

---

[254] Created qualities of male and female are drawn from the duality of God's inner/reciprocal nature of Divine Masculine and Divine Feminine. – Ed.

[255] Paramahamsa Yogananda, *The Second Coming of Christ*, Vol. 2, Discourse 62.

[256] Paramahamsa Yogananda, *The Second Coming of Christ*, Vol. 2, Discourse 62.

[257] Paramahamsa Yogananda, "Jesus Speaks of Soul Union as the Original Purpose of Marriage," *The Second Coming of Christ*, Vol. 2, Discourse 62.

of each soul according to divine decree. They had the pure love and feeling that God placed within their hearts and souls.[258]

Once separated, the polarities of male and female would become respectively dominant, and outwardly visible, while simultaneously, and inwardly, maintaining the attributes of the opposite gender and their transcendental state. This was how the image and likeness of God was revealed.

God filled them with divine magnetism to reflect the Divine wish, which was the supernatural demand to know reciprocal love according to God's specifically ordered divine plan for his creation, and that they draw each other unto themselves. "They were to lead natural lives, with uplifted spiritual consciousness free from the dangers of sex-motivated mismating and the necessity of separation." The one becomes two, and the two separate beings, equal to each other, manifest as the one. This is the power of love in a marriage. Separated, the one with dominant male attributes was named Adam, meaning "of the earth," and he witnessed to the masculine attributes of God. Now we have the male gender known as man. His male attributes became more pronounced. He used reason and cosmic energy. He had feeling, but God kept it uppermost and hidden, and, thus, we have the familiar version of man as an enlightened being who is not limited to a gross physical body. He now demonstrates all the masculine attributes complete with a total innocence with regard to good and evil.

Adam continued to become more identifiable with respect to gender identity and gender expression, including linear thinking, that is logic and reason. He was more inclined to demonstrate unflawed strength, rationality, loyalty, and healthy competitiveness, to name a few attributes.

The female was named Eve. She demonstrated the feminine attributes of God, becoming a complete version of woman, with a more cyclic way of thinking, an intuitive nature, and an attraction to nurturing. Eve shared the same feeling, reason, and cosmic energy, but reason was the uppermost and hidden. She was softer and expressed more feeling.

---

[258] Paramahamsa Yogananda, *The Second Coming of Christ*, Vol. 2, p. 1197.

It is also written that reason, being aggressive, made the man 'positive,' with positive sexual processes, and the woman, with deep feeling, was 'negative,' and, thus, formed deep sexual recesses.

As Yogananda continues, "The ideal spiritual union between a man and woman (male and female), was ordained that man/male might bring out the hidden reason in woman and that woman/female may uncover man's/male hidden feelings. Together they had the perfect sacred balance of male/female."

By aiding each other to develop a perfect balance of these pure divine soul qualities, they realize their true nature as inviolate souls. Eeshans agree that liberation was to be accomplished by their becoming united, first to each other in divine friendship, the purest expression of God's love shared between two individuals, and, then, perfected love, ready for the ultimate union with God.

God spoke to both Adam and Eve, but with a language tailored to each nature with the attributes of the male relating to the male attributes of God and Eve to the feminine.

Adam and Eve were inclined to speak to God in a language of love unique to their gender, but not necessarily in mutually exclusive ways. In other words, Adam, in a more masculine sense being male dominant, would talk to God from man's perspective and Eve from a woman's perspective. Thus, both would speak to God differently, while at the same time with equal dignity, mirroring God's own dignity, the same "as it was in the beginning, is now, and ever shall be."

Even though we are obliged to know, love, and serve God, we do have a choice. Our obligation to know, love, and serve, stems from the fact that we are the creatures created by a creator. Adam and Eve reflected God's image and likeness, since God 'separated' masculine and feminine, creating Adam and Eve as true soul mates by the immutable law of spiritual love, and, thus, freeing them into God. Satan taunted God with the accusation that humans were not truly free. To allow for free will, God permitted the beginning of directed illusion.

Although they were enlightened beings, not having the comparative knowledge of good and evil allowed for the possibility of deception and consequent invasion. However, would their obedience to God stand up to temptation?

Let's try and understand the reason and purpose behind the test. Satan would come as a beautiful, supernatural, intelligent being, and tell God that just by his entering into dialogue with the male and female, even as they were united in a sacred union blessed by God, that through this conversation they could be made to fall from grace. Satan watched how the humans functioned daily, how they saw only what they had been given and taught by God.

Was their love for and obedience to God simply because they had no choice? Did God see that they had become complacent and no longer sought the giver and the gifts they had been given? Regardless, this esoteric study differentiates fate from destiny. Fate implies you allow your life to continue on a preordained course, never challenging, and completely accepting all that happens, whereas, destiny means you take an active role in making choices that shape your life.

Without a doubt, Satan would not have been challenged, since life as God designed it in the garden was perfect in that there was never anything to detract from Adam's or Eve's life together.

Knowing their innocence, Satan cleverly gained their trust. Once being that most beautiful of all angels (Lucifer), Satan, now banished from heaven, could make himself appear any way he wanted. He was kind to Adam and Eve, walked in the garden, and spoke to them, sometimes together and sometimes independently; he also used 'time' to his advantage. Together, they had a stronger bond. This creature talked to them about how they could have a more personal relationship with God and he seem to give sound advice.

Satan abused Adam and Eve with spiritual power. One need only to understand, and try and think, of how a predator would entice a child. Adam and Eve would not have had a clue that they were being groomed for a fall from grace. It would use deception, and they may have been confused, and consented, to new ways to love God and each other. However, Satan made them feel cared for, loved, and unafraid of him; and, therefore, it was easy to maintain this relationship, since they now felt a strong emotional tie with this beautiful being.

To repeat, the next step in Satan's plan would be to remove the sacredness of their union and introduce a physical way of expressing love. Eeshans believe that Adam and Eve, soulmates from the start, would naturally be very interested in this curious expression of love. Satan was clever enough to know that what they were learning would push them away from God and into creation.

One must remember that Adam and Eve were not prisoners of Eden. God watched over them and talked with them, but did not dictate every move they made. They wouldn't have been chastised, nor would they feel a need to tell God what they were doing, since they would not see anything wrong, having had no experience of wrong; they had no reason not to explore their desire for a closer relationship with God, and with each other on their own. That was Satan's articulated plan.

They were only familiar with expressing love that did not involve their physical bodies. When the first being was created, God brought upon the earth a beautiful mist and formed their bodies. The skin was of a vegetable like matter, not the kind of flesh that we could ever comprehend, and it fed on light and did not need blood. Once separated, their bodies resembled the resurrected body of Christ,[259] meaning it was made up of vibrations and light. Their skin, formed by a vegetable matter, consisted of a pliable cartilage-like structure, which contained the light body; and their senses were attracted to vegetables and fruits for enjoyment and sense experience, not necessarily for sustenance, as we understand it, but they did consume a food which filled them with light, which came from God. This, along with time spent with God, made them complete.

Their expression of love was an embrace that would begin with a kiss, a sacred kiss, as they were transcendental in nature and conscious of an order entirely different than that of the animals.

---

[259] Cf. Luke 24:39. Christ described his body as "having flesh and bone, not flesh and blood."

The sacred kiss would cause them to go into a state of rapture, or ecstasy, and they would be drawn out of themselves with a transcendent feeling, and they entered into a mystical euphoria that sealed the bond of love, which continued to influence them until they again entered into this beautiful ecstatic union. This was a gift from God. It literally gave them the means to live forever as pure organisms, since it kept their genetics pure and alive. As pure beings, they reproduced through this transcendental union better known as 'begetting;' thus, fulfilling God's command "to go forth and be fruitful and multiply," according to their transcendental natures.

This expression of love in no way resembled the act of reproduction of the animals that surrounded them, which was a biological act with a total absence of emotion, feeling, or love. Thus, their offspring would be of the same nature and would be inclined to God's plan, bearing God's imprint.

Satan, who became this beautiful being, unbeknownst to Adam and Eve, was a fallen being who was selfish, self-centered, self-gratifying, not capable of love, vengeful, and jealous of their Godlike purity. Satan displayed great knowledge and enlightened the couple in a manner different than God; however, they truly believed Satan came from God.

The being began to teach them how they could experience love and delight with their flesh. Fascinated, the couple continued to seek knowledge about this kind of "love." They questioned this beautiful being, who took advantage of his 'Godlike' influence over their innocence.

As was described previously, Satan succeeded in coercing Adam and Eve into choosing the physical world rather than the transcendental; he would continue to make them feel comfortable, and by using flattery began to plant seeds, which eventually because of their weakening spirituality and relationship due to their starting to spend less and less time with God, would drive a wedge between them. This is when, due to that increased distance created between them and God and the lack of the Sacred Food and Drink, including a weakened relationship with God, led to Adam to begin seeing Eve more as a helper, and when Eve began to wonder more and more about her talks with Satan and her place with God, questioning if she was as important to God as Adam was. They were growing weaker without directly realizing it.

This was the first time they knew each other physically. The moment was short-lived. Almost immediately, they realized that they had made a mistake, and this choice that they made brought with it feelings and knowledge that something central to their life had been altered and changed. Guilt immediately set in. Hearing God calling to them actually caused them fear. Guilt and fear were foreign to them, and caused them to run. Never before did they rush to hide from God. God called them again. This time Adam answered. God asked, "Why are you hiding?" Adam answered God saying, "Because we are naked." God asked how they knew they were naked. Adam explained how they had eaten from the forbidden tree. God gave them skins for them to cover their bodies. Adam told God how the beautiful being taught them the secret of how to love God more deeply. He explained how they had learned a new way to express love using their bodies and could only experience this love if they did what the beautiful being told them to do. This act was the original choice considered by Satan as the use of free will. Adam told God how, after the woman, whom God had given him, experienced the sensual feelings in the visions of love, and told him about them, he, too, desired this feeling. After they had eaten the apple, the desire for each other's bodies was uncontrollable. Adam told how the intensity of their urges drove them to know each other.

Eve told God about her dream, and how the 'Son of God' came to her and seduced her, and how Adam wanted this, too. Adam told God that the Serpent told them that God had always intended for them to have this knowledge of love.

Eve told God that in her dream, the beautiful being told her if she wanted, it would show her the source of God's knowledge.

Eve told God that the being told her that no harm would come to them and that God found favor in her and how pleased God would be if she and Adam could embrace the way the being and Eve did. The serpent then suggested that she and Adam eat of the forbidden tree, and that God would be pleased with her initiative and desire to love him more deeply, and it would bring Adam closer to God, as well.

Seeing that Satan had coerced them, God chastised their disregard of God's warning and their deliberate act of disobedience. God told them that to come together for the sole purpose of lust was wrong because lust is short lived and corrupts that which is sacred. God told them that this impostor had caused them to share in a forbidden and unlawful act of carnal knowledge. As a result, "the unbalanced consciousness," as the act turned them away from God's love and life, caused the feminine quality, or feeling, to lose its calm intuitive powers under the restlessness of body consciousness and emotional excitation; and the masculine attribute, or reason, lost its calm intuitive powers when it succumbed to the restlessness of body consciousness and egotistical self-sufficiency.[260] To have entered into this carnal act without God's permission is not love and is a deliberate act against God, who is all things love. This was the means by which the animals reproduced. For animals, it is not a matter of turning away from God, but is rather simply the governing of natural impulses for the continuation of life; for human beings, however, this was not to be the case. This impulse, or feeling, which was designed to draw the animals, and other creatures, to each other, was not meant to operate in the same way for human beings, since their lives were meant to subsist on a transcendental platform of existence.

Even though Adam and Eve had now participated in this carnal act apart from the design of God, God's love would now institute a union in which this act would now be blessed and used to propagate. They would lose all beatific benefits, the Sacred Food and Drink that kept them immortal, and they had to be exiled from Paradise. It was not that God was so angry as to punish them and drive them from the garden in shame; rather, it was by their own choice that the consequence of the change in their consciousness came about and led them into union with the physical body and the physical realm of existence on a permanent basis. There would be joys, and there would be sorrows, but these both came from the choice they made together. Life was forever changed.

---

[260] Paramahamsa Yogananda, *The Second Coming of Christ*, Vol. 2, Discourse 62.

The expression of this new carnal love was, however, only to be recognized under the permission of God through marriage. Carnal acts outside of this marriage were forbidden and unlawful, for they would not free them to pass into a spiritual world.

God's original blessed union gave Adam and Eve the capability of expressing love shared in divinity, which was what Jesus taught. As love came from God, the Father and Mother of all creation, this conscious decision to ignore God's command and the original intention of God caused the couple to enter into a grievous alternative, by which, because they chose the physical, they would experience death.

By God's command and directive, this new expression of love between soulmates could only be consummated and expressed under God's blessing, and would only be allowed in a committed relationship or marriage. The falling from a pure, undefiled spiritual and sacred union to a purely material, sexual union, was to take the love and make it less than what God desired; and, thus, it did not mirror, or was witness to, or manifest, as the love of the Consorts. You see, marriage was the ultimate union, the ultimate celebration of LOVE. That is why we cry at watching someone getting engaged, and watching someone get married; and, well, there are no words for it. God *is* love. There is nothing more important to God than to see us love each other; and when entering into a marriage, we are celebrating God.

Yet, Eeshans hold that the language of "original sin" conveys so much history of humanity's relationship with God, since it is based on adherence to 'law and command,' and "original sin" regards so little with respect to love that it led to much ill-founded guilt. Marriage was what healed the effects of Adam and Eve's choice.

Guilt has snowballed over many centuries, especially since the wrong understanding of the old creation story of Adam and Eve was made known and repeated through generations. This naturally evolved from the true reason for God's plan for salvation of humanity. Our choices naturally led to consequences. The drawing of the light body into the material world caused it to become a "passive, incomplete part" of what was once transcendentally balanced and free; thus, not only limiting it and its capabilities but also imprisoning it in the gross physical body beset with limitations. Previous to this, Adam and Eve were not restricted to the Garden, but could go anywhere and be anywhere they chose to be. They could also 'create' because there was, according to their level of being, no limitations placed upon their abilities. They could, for example, create a world, and go into it and leave it at their discretion. They lost their beatific vision, and their abilities, but the Word of God stayed with them. By extension, we draw our human lives from what they left for us.

We not only lost the beatific benefits of living transcendentally but it also caused a disconnect to something that brought delight to God's heart. This wrong choice, which altered humankind's life, showed the strength and power of love in extreme circumstances, and how, as humans, nothing means more—not money, nor power—than love. Without this beautiful, selfless, sacrificial love. there is nothing.

Through the primarily patriarchal-conditioned retelling of the story that Eve was the first real transgressor who seduced Adam away from God's law (ultimately causing the Fall and exile from the garden), the true life-creating, loving consciousness of spiritual life was reshaped to support the view that God was angry and must be appeased, and the "transgression of law" resulted in exile and shame, guilt and punishment. Fear of breaking God's law, and fear of punishment, and an ideal scapegoat, together took precedence in how one, thereafter, approached God; and to this day, this consciousness still reigns.

Adam and Eve made a mutual "Original *Choice*," and that choice carried with it the consequences of good and evil, because they had entered "permanently" into the physical realm and chose to become part of it. In that one choice, there would be the knowledge of pleasure and of pain, joys and sorrow, and widespread suffering and death. There came with it a natural part of entering into the material world and that's all we know.

They experienced the material consciousness, as well, which limited their original spiritual consciousness of unlimited potential; yet even while yielding the experiences of life, through the material 'universe-oriented' physical mind and senses, God was there. God is *always* there.

We all feel, or have felt, that God 'abandoned' us at one time or another. Even Jesus asked His Father why he was abandoning Him. But God never abandons us, and His Father certainly did not abandon Jesus on the Cross. Though so many reasons are given: the fulfillment of the Old Testament Psalm, or the words of the Prophet Isaiah, or Galatians, or even Corinthians, God did not abandon His Son. What happened was that Jesus had one more experience to undergo; and that was how God felt when we commit sins against him or our heavenly Mother. In that moment of suffering, Jesus made the effort to draw all who were there to him and tried to show all those around him, who He truly was and how He was still fulfilling prophecies and promises as God. In this last-ditch effort, if Jesus could only get God's children to see who He was, and that He truly was God, they may just come around to believing all, or at least a greater part, of what He taught.

Thus, death, being the chief of the sorrows, and sufferings, among the consequences of their choice, and which was the end result of the *entropy*[261] that Adam and Eve had begun, and unfolded, by their choice, Jesus' sacrificial death lay to the opposite side of the spectrum, with the joys and the pleasure of being an embodied human being who loved unconditionally.

Because of Jesus and his wife, death is now a limiting condition, if we believe and trust in the specific guidelines He gave us to preserve a connection with God from whom all good things come, and only because of them can we, as male and female, unite as one.

Having the admittance and confession by the two, and their contrition for taking this knowledge and voluntarily entering into this carnal act, God did not bestow "punishments," but rather *ratified Adam and Eve's choice.*

---

[261] As Adam and Eve made their choice to enter into the physical realm, becoming part of it through the union of their light body with the physical manifestation, or outer "clothes" of the material body, "entropy" was in operation because of the disunion that was generated between Adam and Eve and their origin/location in God. This essentially causes a kind of "pull," or gravity effect, into the chaos, or randomness, of the physical universe that draws the soul away from God into the realm of physicality, unless there is the effort put forth to swim against this current and pursue God in spiritual life. – Ed.

Because this "illusion is pregnant with consequences leading to suffering" and was willfully entered into and embraced, it caused Adam and Eve to "fall from grace."

The Liberation they once had was accomplished by their becoming united first with each other in divine friendship, the purest expression of God's love shared between two individuals, and then perfected, ready for the ultimate union with God. Jesus' marriage, with Jesus as The New Adam and his wife The New Eve, brought a blessing upon human marriage. Just as Adam and Eve had taken the transcendental love God bestowed upon them to the level of corporeal expression, Jesus' marriage solidified the human love blessed by God, and returned it to God in its original state in pure transcendental love. Could this then be why all evidence of Christ's marriage was deliberately lost, destroyed, or deemed heretical? If so, why would there be such measures taken to keep this from the faithful?

The choice and its consequences altered their scope of consciousness and drew it into a limited range under the laws of the physical universe. They could no longer live in the garden, since the garden was once again a *transcendental* reality free from illusion and corruption, and it could not tolerate the presence of either, and that is why they could no longer enjoy the relationship they had once shared with God. It was as though the Garden had entered a detoxing effect once the couple ate the Apple.

Jesus taught that from our ignorance we enter into illusion, and what we, in the west, now identify as *sin*, since, we are told, if we do such things we are then breaking of God's law.

Eeshans believe that when we do something that we think will help us, or benefit us in some way, and when we enter in upon something we think, at first, will be pleasure, but actually unfolds with suffering, *we enter into illusion*. Jesus said, when this happens, we harm ourselves in some way, either emotionally, physically, and/or spiritually. As we were taught, any time we break God's law, we commit sin, just as Adam and Eve did. Eeshans understand it to mean that when we make choices which have unforeseen or unwanted consequences, we are accountable, and though we must make amends, God is there for us. All actions will have either a good result, or a consequence, or a good, or ill result, respectively, since there is a reaction for every reaction; but when we become entangled due to our making a poor choice, this leads to any number of degrees of suffering, some perhaps small, some perhaps quite great.

"Sin" for the Eeshan, then, is not so much the 'breaking of a law' as it is the misuse of free choice, as Jesus, and as God, taught. One thing is for sure, Jesus taught implicitly that 'to turn oneself away from God is evil,' and this happens when we deny Jesus and His teachings, because as He said: "If I had not come and spoken to them, they would not be guilty of sin; but now they have no excuse for their sin." (John 15:22).

And, so, Adam became aware of unfamiliar emotions, and became afraid as everything around him and Eve was changing. They began to feel the effects of *entropy more and more*. No longer were their bodies interchangeable. They now had blood, bones, and a flesh of gross matter that had formed around their formerly pure and unlimited light bodies, and God told them that these new bodies would return to the ground upon their death. That's why we are told, "from dirt you were formed, to dirt you will turn" after death.

The initial "clothing" of the light body, a kind of vegetable matter (just as vegetation is actually just a container of light, hence, the chlorophyll's green hue through the walls of the plant), gradually began to be more and more affected by the dynamic of entropy, and now became subject to these physical laws of nature, and the color and manifestation of the skin became less subtle, and more dense and responsive, to the various given conditions in various places on the planet.

All those who were previously "reproduced" in the transcendental state under Adam and Eve gradually lost their spiritual communication with one another, became independent of one another, and fell prey to perceiving outward differences in one another to the exclusion of the interior unity they once knew. Thus, differences were now seen before similarities, and fear of difference began to rule and create animosities and conflicts, which would lead to hatred and suffering. Having reached a certain measure of development in the physical body, which had now become completely dense, consciousness of the original light body, and the consciousness that was once known was largely forgotten. Human bodies had become so varied from one to the other, according to location, that "race" had come into being. From there, the gradual decline of human life began.

Seeing that they chose to eat of the Tree of Knowledge of Good and Evil, a deliberate choice after God's warning, God then ratified the effects that Adam and Eve caused by their decision, which entailed the separation of the couple from the Tree of Life. This was not what God intended, or desired, which sheds light on what God intended to convey with the command, "Do not eat …"

By placing St. Michael, as the gatekeeper with the cherubim at the east of the garden, with a 'flaming sword that turned every way' to guard the way to it, so that they could not eat again and live forever, theirs was now the course of moving into the world of time and physical existence.

God explained how the being lied to them, and caused them to take a course that led them to what the being represented as the same goal as God's. God had given them everything except permission to eat of the Tree of Knowledge of Good and Evil, for they didn't realize they already had this knowledge, since all knowledge was, indeed, contained in the fabric of their being; and, yet, they went apart from God to find love. God realized that they misunderstood what true love is.

After hearing the accounts of what had taken place, recognizing the vicious and abusive acts Satan used to deceive, confuse, and destroy innocence, God cursed the serpent, and said to it: "Because you allowed Satan to use your body to deceive the innocent you are now cursed above all animals, above every beast of the field; and upon your belly you shall crawl. Your form will be linked to sexual desire and passion until the debt to God is fulfilled."

Then God addressed Satan, and its seed that was placed in Eve (which was only known to God and Satan), saying, "I will put enmity between you and the Woman, between your seed and hers." By doing this, God addressed Satan's attempt to "take back" what was lost in Satan's rebellion, deem the seed bad; and, thereby, the child would not receive the blessing

Satan intended for himself. But because of God's love for Eve, the child would be given a preempted forewarning; and, thus, forgiveness might be extended. God would do this because of Eve's sacrificial love towards Adam and her honesty towards God. The far-reaching effects of Satan would, of course, be felt in the offspring of Adam and Eve, but the effects of God's mercy would become eternal with the promised Messiahs.

Before Adam and Eve's exile from the garden began, God, being love and mercy, took pity on them, and in an effort to bring about their truest love for each other would use this time to show what true love is. True love is a sacrificial love, not a guaranteed love, with no effort, or concern, for one's counterparts. God revealed that love by not just telling them, but making them have to rely on each other for everything. Nothing would be given to them, but God would still guide them, and they would live and survive by the work and fruit of their hands.

Since they could not go back to the way things were, they would no longer reproduce by a supernatural and transcendental means of "begetting." Adam would now have to work, and both would have to provide for the other. Adam would now have to impregnate Eve physically, and Eve would now deliver children through her body, experiencing the pain of childbirth, in order that they might propagate. "No longer can their union be termed a divine, sacred, and true marriage, (or as) a union of souls" (See Discourse 62, *Second Coming of Christ*, p. 1202.), as it had been. A new life had begun.

God told them that their ideal partnership would now be expressed by a mutual desire to make each other feel wanted, needed, accepted, and whole, all with a sacrificial love, for they gave up immortality for mortality. Their love must be for each other only, and they must work to bring out the best and the wholeness in each other. God blessed this union and called it marriage. Each would be tied to the other, and though this union would now be conjugal it would be blessed by God, and through which it becomes a very intimate expression of love between a human male and female, providing extensions of the couple's love by bringing about children. These, too, will be taught and raised to fall in love and give birth to extensions of their love, becoming soulmates and, thus, adorers of their Creator. As a result of this union, the world would then have good souls to help rule with love, and live in equality, decency, and peace, as God intended.

PART XXII

LESSON 197

Sacred Teaching I: God Allows Bad Things to Happen for the Sake of a Greater Good

What is the parallel with Jesus and Mary Magdalen? When Jesus returned to town eleven years after his first encounter with Mary, He came back wearing a white robe, since he was now a renowned spiritual master. His intention was to begin his mission. First on His agenda was to get married, according to the law, and to the woman destined to be His wife. He would marry the person of Mary Magdalene, whom He met once, during a crucial point in her life, which marked him forever as her Savior and Redeemer. God's allowance of this incident created a bond between them, which fulfilled scriptures and kept the person of Mary for His own.

> If you recall, seven men dragged her to a cave, where they violated her. Taking her innocence as a trade-off to not hurting Martha, since these thugs whisked her off to a cave, the young Jesus followed the screams and attempted to save her. Upon reaching the cave, He was held in their grasp and forced to watch. After the last criminal abandoned the child, Jesus heard the laughs of the men as they left. Tearing a piece of his cloak, He wet it and washed off her blood, and kept a relic of it for His own. He wrapped His cloak around her and carried her to her sister's house, where her sister and brother were in distress over all that had happened.

On the way, a breathless Jesus kissed her forehead, telling her everything would be all right. Jesus fulfilled scriptures regarding being the Savior of Mary, who He would redeem from being made a scourge of scandal, that she may represent all God's children.

Ezekiel 16 reads:

"When ... I looked at you and noticed that you were of age [proper time for love/marriage] I spread My cloak over you to cover your nakedness. I made a solemn promise to you and entered into a covenant with you," declares the Lord God. "You belong to Me. I bathed you with water, rinsed your own blood from you and anointed you with oil (He was the anointed one, and as He touched her, she too was anointed) then I cover you with My cloak. (Later He covered her with embroidered clothing and clothed her feet in sandals.) I wrapped you in fine linen and dressed you in silk. I adorned you with jewels, placing bracelets on your hand and necklaces on your neck. I put a ring in your nose, earrings in your ears, and a crown encrusted with jewels on your head. You were adorned with gold, silver, clothing of fine linen silk and embroidery. You ate food made from the finest flour, honey, and olive oil. You were exceedingly beautiful, attaining your royal status."

"Your fame spread throughout the nations because of your beauty. You were perfectly beautiful due to My splendor with which I endowed you," declares the Lord God. [This prophecy is about His coming back to her after eleven years and finding this Princess who was of royal descent. Though not "marriage material" due to being violated, she had successfully started an import/export business and was her own woman. Still a disgrace, she moved on with her life and became very famous, not only for her import/export business from which she made a lot of money, but because she became known for her healing methods and for opening her house to other women who were violated or were homeless or runaways.]

This was the beginning of the reversal of the humans' 'fall from grace.' Because Mary believed that *sometimes God allows bad things to happen for the sake of a greater good*, this showed her recognition and awareness of another consciousness that allowed for One who is greater than and not limited to human thinking and human cognition. In understanding this, she did not fall victim to self-pity, or blame God for her life taking on a different path than what she had planned. This is truly noteworthy on her part, for it portrays a shining example of how God as Divine Male and Divine Female enjoyed perfect love.

God, most assuredly, had expressed this love through her, who would be reunited with her soulmate/twin flame just a few years later. This love between them would then be shared with, and in us, and all the world would be desirous to share this beauty. This love would also be shared through, with, and in human marriages.

In doing so, God's most intimate love would be manifested once again, and it would be revealed in "how the ideal spiritual union between male and female, or man and woman, should be ordained, and that man might bring out the hidden reason in woman, and that the woman might help man uncover his hidden feeling."[262]

Jesus' marriage to Mary was necessary because their sacrifice for humankind had to not only reflect his Father and Mother's sacrificial will, but their own sacrificial will, as well. Sacrifice is a personal choice. Though God gave us the only-begotten Child to reverse the consequences of the Fall, to be a sacrifice of the Second Person of the trinity meant that they, too, would have to be involved a choice to give up something near and dear to them, and this would be a human life with each other, despite their own needs and desires.

Eternal Wisdom, or *Sophia Perennis*, says that what was taught regarding Jesus doing his Father's will is just *part* of the story. Jesus, too, had to sacrifice something of Himself. This had to reflect back to the beginning and the story of Adam and Eve who entered this world and permanently and became a part of it physically. As Adam and Eve were married transcendentally, and chose to enter into a physical marriage, so it was necessary for Jesus' marriage to become the sacrifice, which

---

[262] Adapted from Yogananda, Discourse 62, *Second Coming of Christ*, p. 1202.

would reverse the direction of this course. In doing so, it would liberate humanity from the sense of being 'imprisoned' within the confines of physical embodiment and the material world.

Christ's marriage would be a complete sacrifice, since there would be no physical relations other than a kiss; and they would have no earthly children until end times,[263] and by only those who were conceived transcendentally. What greater sacrifice is there than to have to leave behind your partner and wife for the good of humankind, without ever having been able to express your love physically, as well as spiritually/emotionally, as God blessed humans to do. To lose his whole world, and for Mary to lose her whole world was heart-wrenching in itself. It didn't stop there, however, due to the loss and misuse of Jesus' teachings, then to lose him again at the Ascension was piercing. How then could one describe the greatest of all separations: the expunging of his marriage from history and human memory, and all related to it until present times?

What is there to say about the sacrifice of their marriage and life together? Transcendently, Jesus comforted Mary, in his final seven last words to her on the cross, by stating, "Mary, we will never be separated again." Then He offered himself to His Father. Though His words were comforting, they wouldn't be fulfilled, or completed, until His Father would reward Him with an end time union, when He would return for her.

In retrospect, by aiding each other through their tantric transcendental union via the kiss, they developed the perfect balance within the biblical marriage of their pure divine souls. In this way, they transcended their delusive differentiation as man and woman and realized their true nature as inviolate souls.

---

[263] In the transcendental realm.

PART XXIII

TRUE MEANINGS

LESSON 198

Section I: The Consequences of the Misinterpretation of the Marriage Feast at Cana

If you are Catholic or Christian, or if you have ever read the New Testament, you know the story of the marriage feast at Cana, and that is, of course, if you read the gospel of John. The gospel of John is the only gospel that describes the marriage feast of Cana. The other three synoptic gospels do not mention it.

Eeshans believe that this scriptural passage was changed in order to emphasize 'Jesus' first public miracle,' and to eliminate any possible tie to its being *his* marriage feast. The well known and most popular story begins with 'Jesus' mother' approaching Jesus about the lack of wine for the guests.

Most church authorities say that Christ's responses, in which when He asks why there was the lack of wine was His concern, and stating that it was not his time, 'prefigured his passion and death on the cross.' Although, we don't see it that way. The Cana event has also been used as a teaching about 'His affection and respect for His mother's wishes' and 'her insight into her son's love for her.' It is told that Jesus, then by his mother's request, intervened on behalf of the groom. This was with regards to presuming that Jesus would act to correct what would become an embarrassment to the groom only because His mother who safeguarded His identity since birth, asked Him to perform a 'miracle' for this person who was unknown. There is a lot to presume here, but, obviously, that doesn't matter.

We are also told that behind this short conversation, someone knew what He was also thinking; and all His thoughts were centered on 'his mother as Mother of the Universe'. How is it that *anyone* would possibly know what Jesus was thinking? How could anyone commenting on this event even presume to know? Thinking back to what we are told regarding Jesus speaking to John at the cross, "Behold your Mother," and to Our Lady, "Woman behold your Son," we see this as an event that Eeshans were sure He had discussed with John early on, knowing and discussing with all his apostles what was going to happen to him with regards to the religious leaders and rumors. Eeshans feel that Jesus would most likely try and ease his wife's pain and that gives more credence to His last words to Mary.

Truly Jesus' actions, and care of her, substantiated the love He had for His mother, while more importantly, and, especially, with His acknowledgment of her, whenever she came to hear him talk. The most vital role of the Virgin Mary, was becoming human in order that the Divine Masculine of the only-begotten Child could become human in order to bring about God's promise of a plan for salvation. When He told all who were present at one of His talks of the importance of hearing what God's will is for one's life and doing it, He paid tribute to her before His Father. Turning her care over to John did not make any impression of her role with all those around Him. Her title as our Mother came about with the acknowledgement of God, the first Person Divine Masculine being His Father, and then teaching us that God was also our Father. Jesus, however, would carry the title of Father also, when he died. Since, with His death, we became His begotten children, since He is the one who gave us life.

The commentary regarding the Cana event is sometimes said to be the written account, but how can you have written accounts about what someone is thinking, if that person doesn't reveal their thoughts? These moments are meant to come across and express that these are 'eyewitness' accounts. Unless Jesus expressed what His intention was, or reiterated to everyone at that moment, or sometime later, something He was actually feeling, or thinking, there is no proof that either of these suggestions are reliable or true.

The event accounts of Cana being Jesus' own wedding is considered realistic even by those who do not believe in Jesus.

The understanding we currently have of these passages, and their meaning, has been handed down over a very long period of time where, through nondescript details, additionally, the church, without a doubt expected followers to believe these assumptions, even though they made no sense, whatsoever. Unless one dared to question church authority, there would never be a reason to think otherwise.

By omitting the actual story of Christ's wedding, and inserting a substitution account, it not only caused the loss of vital information, but introduced misinformation to *misdirect*, the loss being that the true event was the story upon which the salvation of all humanity was based.[264] As Eeshans see it, this deliberate distraction so grossly altered the meaning and purport of the actual event that it was now essentially a different event altogether, and obviously now had a different meaning. This was done so as to erase all evidence pointing back to the true meaning of the actual event, which was Jesus' wedding.

We introduce the actual story:

From Mary's Diary:
The Greatest Love Story 'Never' Told

"The three days of the wedding had arrived and the plans were in place. The sun shone brightly. It was early and the house was buzzing with excitement. Family and friends began arriving and Joseph had begun setting up the Ritual area, which seemed to take me outside my body at the mere presence of it. A very special bridal chamber was being prepared and, of course, I was not allowed to see it.

I watched how Lazarus took the place of head of the household regarding my marriage. There were already things about our betrothal

---

[264] Thus, it automatically followed that there would be no basis for understanding the relation of the water to the wine at the event, the water's significance as Mary/the Divine Feminine, nor would there be from there a basis by which to understand the connection of Cana to a foreshadowing of the Samaritan woman at the well event. – Ed.

Section I: The Consequences of the Misinterpretation of the Marriage / 829

which some may have considered wrong. The one constant part was the communication and planning between Jesus and myself. Normally a friend of the groom would be the communicator, but that did not work for us. Though his gifts or *mohar* were left secretly, and the wine was chosen and given to Lazarus, there was no mistaking that Jesus was 'hands-on' with every plan for 'us,' with all my 'desires' incorporated. Where betrothals of most couples I knew extended the norm of at least a year or two, ours happened very quickly as our marriage was imminent.

This was also a detail which, by many, could be misinterpreted and we could have been shunned by family and/or friends, in 'my' case. I'm sure they looked at it as a safeguard of His reputation, so that I would not be tempted to engage in the weakness of adultery, and end in divorce before we were married. Having lived through the gossip and lies for so long, I had developed thick skin, but I guess, deep inside, it hurt. There were several events that were amiss primarily due to time and the amount of guests that were arriving. So whether the sequence was not in the traditional order, they were all there. Best of all, I wore the first of my three dresses, and I felt pretty.

The second day, we each received a blessing from his Great Uncle Joseph, separately, and the celebrating began with Martha accidentally breaking a dish. Tradition showed that as a dish, if broken, cannot be repaired, such is that of the marriage. Jesus' Mother, with such grace, smiled, and broke a dish in response, and all laughed. I went to the garden, where I spent more time thinking and as it were, followed a tradition where the Kallah immerses herself in water—I used this beautiful fountain and prayed for sanctification. I wondered How God was seeing all of this from Heaven above …

I had been dressed in the second of my three dresses. Despite the craziness of the past couple weeks, and the mayhem of this week, I really did enjoy the 'girl' moments: the pretty dresses and people and of course my special moments with my girls and Martha. The girls made me laugh, and we danced and sang and talked about our travels. It was then, when, for a brief moment we talked about Jacob. *Hmmm*, I wondered if anyone other than our little intimate group would consider this grounds for divorce. Beth laughed and said it definitely would so, therefore, she would take

Jacob. Oh, it was so much fun to be with them. I made them promise that we would never part. I made them promise that they would not separate themselves from me: or I could not bear it.

Though we were betrothed, the men and women were separated with little communication except through friends, which I must admit became frustrating. Jesus and I did, however, get to exchange glances and raised our glasses in a toast to each other. By the end of this day it was apparent that talking about the impending 'consummation' by royal tradition, which called for witnesses at the time of the consummation of our marriage, was not going to happen; since despite my many attempts, that opportunity was lost. Our only contact was at the end of the evening when it was time for sleep and I tried to convey my concern regarding this matter through Martha or Lazarus. It was near impossible to say anything without alerting them of our plan; if found out this 'non act' would be a violation of the law.

There seemed to be time to talk about everything else. The financial issues regarding my dowry had all been handled between Lazarus and Jesus. Jesus' dowry for me apparently came out of the sale of his family business and mother's inheritance; however, I was financially successful and in no need of such security.

As all the plans according to the law were followed at the proposal of marriage back at the Bethany house, this ritual or blessing was a formality between the families and a reason to celebrate. According to tradition, both Jesus and I would observe our fast that would last from dawn until the marriage ceremony the next day; however, I heard He had already been fasting. Jesus, or the Chatan, reflected His desire to still want to marry me by returning to the common room of the house where time was spent with friends who celebrated his return for me, which I'm sure *no one* expected to happen.

Awaking this morning with the thought that it was 'MY' wedding day with failed attempts through the night to get to exchange words with Jesus caused me little sleep. Being separated and needless to say, very concerned about how we would get away with the exchange of vows without it binding us and leading towards the avoidance of physical consummation which would, if discovered, bring shame and punishment

Section I: The Consequences of the Misinterpretation of the Marriage

under God's and Mosaic law robbed me of joy on this most important day of my life. It was a personal Yom Kippur. I was giving up my body and so was he to become one person under God. Or were we? Ugh! Did he feel the same way? Was he frightened and nervous? Did he lay awake worrying about the 'plan?'

Well, the time came quickly as family and friends began preparing for the ceremony. There was still the food and fun but to a milder degree. Martha and Mary, His mother, came to my room. They helped dress me in the most beautiful of all dresses yet. I could almost see the memories fill her mind as Mary looked at the dress as though she was looking for flaws or any last minute alterations needed. Then they led me to the terrace where they had placed a special chair resembling a throne for me to sit and greet guests. Being a Kallah was equaled to being a Queen and all the girls closest to me wanted to be part of all that was happening with me as it was not just symbolism that was being expressed here but direct reference to my royal background of which Lazarus and Martha were so very proud.

As evening fell, a path was forming from my living area to Jesus' section of this very large house. The cheers began and shouts that the Bridegroom was coming filled the air. Where often the bridegroom placed the veil on the bride, we did it differently. Lazarus placed the veil upon me and after both he and Martha kissed me, the veil was brought down over my face. In doing so Lazarus whispered, 'No more Mary, will you be treated like a harlot,' with tears in his eyes, 'Hurry now as your King awaits his Queen.'

My heart pounded. Mary, his mother, and Martha who had just helped me get into my dress, hugged me. As I stood looking out at the star-studded sky, the torches of light, the oil lamps and the crowd, my mind went back and glimpses of that horrible night that had plagued me all my life. I had spent my life trying to forget and on what should be the happiest day of my life, now returned once again causing me to wonder what was in store for my future. I had spent the night before hearing the priest Joseph giving God's blessing on us in a toast and now as I looked out at the faces of family and friends, I wondered about their thoughts. Were they laughing at him for marrying me; were they scandalized?

Would my appearance, my dress, cause more disgrace to His name as it was not the style of dress that I was accustomed to or noted as wearing? What if they found out about our non-consummation promise?

The cheers were getting louder. The crowd was calling for him as if he was their King! As the Bridegroom came closer, the shouts got louder. He entered the area on a donkey, his feet not touching the ground I was told. As I listened, I was hurried by the whispers of Mary and Martha for our need to hurry. I must have appeared frightened as Martha took my hand and told me all would be alright. Numbly, I went with them to the terrace steps to meet **MY BRIDEGROOM!** Through the crowd of bystanders and guests I tried not to hear comments and searched frantically to see Jesus. I needed to see him. I heard some of the guests calling out that their lamps were running out of oil as they had lighted their lamps early on in anticipating the bridegroom's arrival. It was getting dark and to avoid not being able to see the need for oil was mandatory! No one knew how long the ceremony would last and certainly didn't want to miss anything. Being left in the dark was not a very good look. It showed you were unprepared and you missed so much. You were also considered outside the inner circle. So, frantically there were shouts for oil and light. Once your lamp went out the evening and celebration was more or less over for you. To the women who desired more to see the Chatan than the Kallah, as they put themselves in her place-this was devastating. The fact is, that secretly, the women believed that the Bridegroom belonged to each woman single and I would say even married (though that would be adultery and grounds for divorce), as what woman doesn't love romance and daydream.

As my wedding party and I slowly walked towards the brightly lighted garden area, searching for Him, I caught my first glimpse of Jesus, my Bridegroom, dressed in white, immediately our eyes met. He smiled, as I so nervously, and barely breathing, walked towards him. Reaching Him, I continued to circle Jesus seven times connoting that a woman will encompass a man ending by Lazarus who then took my hand lovingly and put in Jesus' hand. It was then that I realized that I couldn't recall when it was that Lazarus took my arm in his to escort me. As Lazarus gently kissed my cheek, I noticed the tears in his eyes. This was such a long awaited dream come true for Him. A day which He dreamed of since I was brought home and put in his arms, by the very man standing, awaiting my arrival as His Bride.

As I was given to Jesus, the sounds and presence of the people faded. It was as though I had stepped outside of time and into another world. No one else was present. I could see only him. My whole being felt as though I was being lifted out of my body and brought to a place where my heart always belonged. If it wasn't for the voice of Joseph, I would have been quite content staying right here.

He took scriptures and read a short passage. Then turning the Torah over to Joseph, he took his place, His mother near Him. Facing each other, He took my right hand in His and before God and witnesses we vowed that everything we are and everything we possess now belongs to each other. We vowed to leave our families and forsake all others and live for each other and as one. As we looked into each other's eyes I saw, not the man I had promised to make a business or legal contract with, but a man who obviously took these vows very seriously; but for what reason? To make it look authentic so as to throw everyone off regarding our agreement? Or, as my heart cried out: **_HE REALLY LOVES ME_**!

Now my heart ached as I too had dreamt of this moment since our eyes first met. I so wanted our vows to be true. I dreamed all my life that my hero would come for me, my knight in shining armor, so strong, so possessive of me, in a good way, and make these vows to me! That He held me high as if on a pedestal before all who judged me wrongly, and that my adversaries would see that nothing could keep his love from me!

The chalice of wine is brought forward and the blessings are pronounced over the couple, the wine cup signifies the sanctification of the man and woman to each other. As we drank from the cup, I looked nervously to Jesus.

Next came the exchanging of our rings. Being a man of little wealth, I expected a braided reed or rushes made into a ring. However, I was wrong. As Jesus took my left hand, He placed upon my hand a ring. Usually only the Egyptians and Romans took these materials as they felt the more expensive the ring, the greater the love. How could He afford such a ring?

As he put the ring on my finger, he looked into my eyes saying, 'Being a path to your heart and soul, as your finger pierces the space of this ring, know that you are mine and I am yours; and that you have entered the gateway, leading to a life of events and things, both visible and invisible, known and unknown. May this ring, Mary of Magdala, signify to you who wears it, and all who see it, our eternal love having had no beginning and no end; for it bears witness to our never-ending and immortal love.'

(At these times Mary's response was not necessary or traditional. In fact, Mary gave her vows to her Bridegroom on the wedding night. These words are the foundational words for the Marriage Feast of today that were hidden and protected by God until these end times.)

Joseph continued to officiate, reading the terms of marriage and responsibilities of the husband; that He is responsible for providing her with food, shelter, and clothing. He is to be sensitive to her emotional needs as written and then the document is signed. How sad that this contract was regularly ignored by husbands and men. Having signed the paper, Jesus then stepped aside for two witnesses to sign also. It was most important that there be two witnesses for all legal actions and agreements. This Ketubah becomes the Bride's (Kallah's) property.

Now the seven blessings are recited with the sacred words over the second cup of wine. As we drank from the cup, my mind once again turned to God. For this cup we dedicated each other to God who is Creator of all from whom all good things come. He will be our Savior. He will redeem us all. It is He who promised us a Messiah. I looked at Jesus and wondered how his learning the ways of the East and his knowledge of my lack of religion was beheld by God in such a traditional way. Perhaps He didn't feel bound by these ways but accepted them. Perhaps he saw these laws as necessary to enable him to pursue his career. Realizing He never took his eyes off of me except to take the cup or acknowledge the words of the celebrant, I was able to smile. He then took the cup and taking a drink, handed me the cup, which he secured with His hand for me to drink.

A glass was then placed on the floor and Jesus looking into my eyes, steps on it and shatters it beneath his foot. This tradition was the acknowledgement of the destruction of the temple that unifies all of us

Section I: The Consequences of the Misinterpretation of the Marriage

Jews; but this thought didn't seem to fit the moment. His face told a different story. His look was one of a personal feeling. Just in the way he shattered the glass while looking in my direction as if he was saying, 'Look Mary, witness to your husband's strength and love! I make all things NEW!' I don't know. Whatever the reason, my heart knew that this man was my destiny.

Shouts of 'Mazel Tov' and songs of joy began to ring out and my husband took my hands in His and lifted my veil for a gentle kiss. A rope was tied around our wrists to symbolize we are one until our marriage is consummated. We were then escorted to where the family and friends greeted us. There were some jeers heard as we passed through the crowd but they were few and I was able to ignore them as I had the strength of my husband's hand to keep me strong.

We entered with flowers being tossed in our direction and well wishes from my girls, which made me forget the faces of two of those men who were of Jesus' group of followers.

Martha was still happy, crying, Lazarus was handing out wine, and a tender hug was exchanged between Jesus and His mother. I watched is face as he held her tightly. She whispered to Him and He hugged her again.

Being tied together caused us to have to move as one and think as one. At times it made us laugh, other times we would become a little frustrated. There were moments when I just wanted to talk with my girls but he, of course, would have to come and stand there, which took the fun away if you know what I mean. I did know that I was hungry but for some reason he found ways to keep me from food.

We had fasted and I was looking forward to the lovely food I had seen prepared. He also seemed to keep steering me away from drinks. At one point I said to Him, 'I'm really hungry' to which He answered, 'You're fine.' I must admit I was getting annoyed with his 'controlling' me because I was at a disadvantage with this rope. Finally, I reminded him of the 'document' stating He had to feed me, and He lovingly laughed.

The party was lively and I saw a look in his eyes that was causing me to feel uncomfortable. I totally forgot that there was a missing component. It was at this moment that Jesus went to Lazarus and whispered something to Him. It was then that it was announced to the guests it *'WAS TIME'!"*

Because this, the actual story was removed, expunged, altered, or deliberately lost to preserve the agenda and maintain a platform against equality, it was never linked to the 'Christs' actual mission, whereby, Jesus' death and resurrection, and by extension of these, the Eucharist, was robbed of its true meaning. Not having the language of the heart of God in its human expression of this ultimate union with another human being, one cannot witness to, or mirror, the love of the eternal and infinite Divine Consorts; as such, since there are disconnects among all the unfathomable mysteries of God.

The union of two people becoming one requires a vow before God, because it is such **a very serious undertaking**. No one realizes this union as solemn anymore, or the steps between God and humanity that were necessary for this ultimate mystery to be unveiled and revealed. All one has been taught with regards to the reason for getting married is little more than procreation; and that a man leaves his father and mother in order to be united to his wife, and the two will become one flesh (Matthew 19:5-6). There was never anything that correlated salvation with Cana, or how Cana was vital to the return of the Sacred Food and Drink.[265]

That is why the saying "I don't need a piece of paper to tell me I'm married or that I love someone" became so popular. Well, though we understand what is meant by this comment, we feel it is only based on the poor foundational reasons given, which are also shadowed in poorly selected Traditional Scriptures and the watered-down version of this unfathomable Sacrament.

For those who feel they are not religious, or who do not want God to be part of their marriage for the past mistakes of the church, there is 'civil' marriage. This marriage, if it does not invoke God as a witness to their union, does little more than meet the requirements of the law of that particular state. Since true marriage involves an emphasis on rearing

---

[265] If anything, the Cana event was only given significance as being the location of the first of Jesus' public miracles. No suggestion that it was Jesus' own wedding was ever permitted to be entertained. – Ed.

children also, it is most important that the couple be focused on the love they share with each other, and then have a true desire to raise the child, or children, to be decent law-abiding citizens, balanced and loving, prayerfully, in a life centered on the Divine.

There are other reasons for marriage that vary around the world, which set the guidelines between cultures, and religions, which are designed purely for interpersonal relationships. Here you will find where human sexual relations, and others that are sanctioned, and acknowledged, be they legal, social, libidinal, emotional, financial, and religious, and even those which are arranged, as well as child marriages, polygamy, and sometimes forced marriages, often have their own rules. One must wonder if the truth about Christ's wedding was told, how many of these kinds of marriages would have dissipated?

Today there is a growing trend towards ensuing women's rights within a marriage and concerns for infringement of children's rights that have also resulted in non-religious ceremonies.

Being unable to correct decades of errors that surround the breakdown of marriage and attitudes towards marriage by arguing that the purpose of marriage was procreative, Eeshans prefer to take a look at what is in accordance with fact, and reality, set in place by God, and then move forward, helping as we go, to correct the consciousness of the world.

Believing that a civil marriage accurately fulfills the provisions and spirituality of marriage is not only inaccurate but also pretentious. **God still holds you accountable for your actions**. We say this ONLY as the truth is now being propagated by, through, and with the return of the Divine Feminine.

It is extremely important that one understands that Eeshans do not frown on civil marriages especially since Sacramental marriages were based on beliefs that couldn't be accepted by "conscientious believers." There were too many reasons couples have chosen to 'not' have a sacramental wedding due to their not accepting church doctrine and dogma, or simply because they just don't believe what is taught by a church or a religion, and for good reason. They just could not in good conscience accept what they were being told. For example, it was not an option if a couple, through no fault of their own, were refused or just not accepted by the church at large, for reasons of gender identity, etc. One simply needs to take a second look at a little information we have included. Though it is limited by time and effort, due to what some may say has been repeated to ruminate on, or has been reiterated ad nauseum, *we still want to remind you* otherwise that the issue becomes seen as "same old, same old." Thus, we emphasize once again its importance. This, too, is part of being enlightened, the ability to stop and see, or listen, to other points of view, other than our own. As we said earlier, repetition does, in fact, make one more conscious of something. They may well begin to see it as not so 'awful,' and may, in fact, cause one to break that 'steel trap mind' syndrome where one 'sees what one sees and that's it' ... and from there to open one's eyes to thinking an issue through rather than just standing firm because of a political party, or what the church has taught, etc. 'Good conscientious observers' undoubtedly had and have good intentions; yet, due to unforeseen complications the end results didn't reflect their point of view, but their original beliefs became a foothold, or platform, for other less desirable points of interests and agendas.

The truth is, though one may believe that they don't need the sacrament, or believe that it provides no more grace than counting on the laws of the universe, or believing that this provides the same, or greater meaning to a marriage, they are wrong. What we are saying is that when certain circumstances prevail that did not, or won't, allow for a sacramental marriage, we understand. The ultimate union, however, should be blessed in accordance with God and under God.

But as Eeshans see it, if the couples have based all on Jesus, had good spiritually balanced priests, and wholeheartedly believed the Sacrament was Jesus in totality, they would be perfectly fine, in the eyes of God.

Eeshans have found that, increasingly, through the years, traditional sacramental marriage had devolved to becoming a mere 'show;' while, secondly, it also seemed to lead far too often into extremely complicated and abusive marriages and disastrous divorces, and the incurring of annulments, which says that the sacrament never existed in the first place. Because the couples were never really taught well, and, thus, could not see God and their relationship to one another in the context of a mutual relationship with God, marriage ends before it has a chance to begin. This has overwhelmingly become the case in the world of today, and, thus, a new look is required into the subjects of civil and sacramental marriage.

That being said, it should be also understood from that from the Eeshan perspective, in a marriage where God is *consciously excluded*, that is, when a marriage is contracted *without* God, there is an automatic imbalance, and a marriage is most likely to be governed under the human rational consciousness, and the love God desires for us does not fall under this category. A civil marriage does not protect the couple spiritually nor does it provide a blessing, or a blood covenant of the couple, as would be the case under a sacramental marriage. A civil marriage based on 'true love,' with every intention of their love blossoming, should still receive a blessing by a Kallah, or Chatan, as an offering to God for the benefits thereof. Any marriage contracted under the significance of just a cosmic/universal law, without a belief in God, is not only considered invalid in the spiritual sense, but subjects the couple to their own imperfect, human-made laws. Up until the introduction of the Eeshan religion, these kinds of marriages were essentially little more than a man-made way of accepting the living together of two individuals, which joins them together in a purely materialistic way. While most couples say their bond is based on their deep 'love' for one another, it is found out quickly that when things don't 'work out' the truth can be revealed in very stark terms.

On the other hand, civil or sacramental, marriage has implications and consequences. If one has no spirituality, or belief in God (whether in a personal or impersonal sense), it goes without saying that any sacramental component is automatically invalid, unless there is a change of heart, and the couple begins to recognize and embrace the sacredness of marriage.

It should be pointed out at this juncture, that people only really 'believe' what they are taught, what they are given, and this condition is limited; whereas, people lacking understanding is a complex problem. Eeshans believe that even in the worst-case scenario, these unions, whether they be civil or sacramental that are breaking down, can be salvaged, and rectified, by the strength of the Eucharist of the Marriage Feast of the Lamb and His Wife.

Eeshans recognize that only under God does this union count as a 'permanent union'; whereby, each gives oneself voluntarily to the other. It must be made known that in the Eeshan Church, both must be under God and baptized into the Eeshan Church, regardless of whether one was already baptized in a Christian denomination; and each person must accept Jesus Christ and His Wife to ensure Sacred Balance; this is mandatory. With this baptism, a promise must be made to God and to each other to live completely in love with each other and for love of each other under God.

Matrimony is a very serious Mystery/Sacrament, and it is the foundation of our Eeshan religion, faith, and spirituality. It is the foundation for salvation of all humanity for us as God's children. Without this step, and if things continue as they have been going (i.e., the absence of truth), Eeshans believe the minds, hearts, and souls of both persons in the marriage risk the possibility of staying independent of each other, thereby never experiencing Sacred Balance. This is in defiance of all God desires for them. Being the reason for the Christs' Mission after Adam and Eve, this translates as risking salvation of humanity, which makes it conspicuously bad. A sacramental marriage is more than a natural marriage; and, yet, is also in union with a natural marriage, because of the Sacred and Divine duality of all the Persons of God and our connection and relationship to and with the Divine.

For the church to have not accepted the reality of Jesus and his Wife, was sad and grievous, and only serves to cause more damage to innocents while continuing to teach along increasingly watered-down lines. It continues to weaken people's spiritual fabric. Even a 'committed union' should be blessed by God, at least to mark it as a stepping stone towards the ultimate, permanent union of marriage.

Individuals who, for one reason or another, feel, or felt, that they cannot get married in their state or for particular reasons raised in one or the other's faith, should seek an immediate sacramental, and mystical, blessing from a Kallah, or Chatan, as soon as possible, in order to be able to enter into the mystery of marriage as God designed. Though a civil marriage does cover civil laws, it really does not cover God's; and, thereby, without God's blessing, the marriage is without the grace to ensure salvation of both individuals, and as extensions of the couple's love. In other words, you may be married in the eyes of man, but it is also necessary to be married in the eyes of God.

Without the truth regarding this Sacrament, Eeshans believe the marriages performed, unless the people of that creed and religion accept those teachings as they have been taught, cannot, and will not, be held accountable for the beliefs handed down to them. Those since Peter, however, who have been coercing people over the centuries, sans the true believers who knew nothing of what was done, or being done, cannot escape God since it mocks the Sacred and Divine Marriage Feast of the Lamb and His Wife, and this denotes extreme offensiveness that God will not overlook, especially if they knew the truth about God, and they know the Person of Jesus Christ. Remember, however, that there were Popes who didn't even believe in Jesus' existence. The reason this is so, is because the whole plan of salvation is based on the Marriage of Jesus Christ and His Wife; therefore, it is impossible to ignore God's presence in a marriage and to have tried to write His marriage out of God's plan for humanity's salvation; such could fall under an act of evil, since it is a gross miscarriage and violation of God's directive and justice.

There should be few if any extenuating circumstances for not having a Sacramental marriage. A blessing can also be imparted after a civil marriage so long as all the criteria of God's law are met. No more is expected.

WHY JESUS' MARRIAGE WAS VITAL TO HUMANKIND, AND HOW IT RAISED HUMAN MARRIAGE TO ITS HIGHEST PLANE

When God blessed the human marriage, it was intended that both who enjoyed a sexual union would eventually grow to a higher plane of transcendent love, not by forced abstinence, but because of a desire for a more transcendentally-based love. This is not a 'loss' but a 'gain' in the realization that one has ascended towards God and loves his or her partner even greater than before; so, there is 'nothing' that can interfere with this love. The many faults and weaknesses of a person can now become strengths, and all that was caused by a worldly definition of love that defined even their physical relations fall by the wayside, as true love grows and is no longer defined by their physicality, or spirit, of the world. The couple sees the truest and purest loving-kindness (metta) in each other: knowing now that no one can intrude on their love.

If one or the other has not yet extinguished the sexual appetite,[266] and has 'moved on' seeking pleasure with other partners, or is viewing their current marriage as a 'lie' (what they convinced themselves to be a lie), they were *not* truly united as soulmates, since a marriage that is very harmonious, but without realization of the marriage, or the concept of the duality God, may through no fault of their own, must still be prudent in exercising a way to live according to what God expects. Otherwise, the consequences normally lead to divorce. Any relationship outside of these may hinge on being a product of an immoral marriage, and the repercussion of this is to know that God does not see the relationships outside the vowed marriage as good. One cannot be expected to live in a marriage while the spouse is being continuously unfaithful with an affair. But some do try to honor their vows, and pray for their spouse to come to their senses, and return to their home and the marriage.

An ideal social religious relationship on a human level falls short of being an actual marriage between soulmates.[267] It is said that the sexual

---

[266] The meaning here of 'extinguishing the sexual appetite' should be understood in context, that is, against the backdrop of eastern disciplines of yoga, where one focus is the *judicious* use of sexual energy, not total abstinence from sex. There is a focus on the conservation of the vital energy and directing it into one's personal relationship with God and other related creative-oriented endeavors. While the energy may be employed in harmony with the interests of expressing love in a committed family relationship during child-rearing years, there comes a time when the couple shifts the focus to helping one another realize their mutually supported personal relationships with God. – Ed.

[267] Yogananda, *The Second Coming of Christ*, Vol. 2, p. 1202. Additionally, in conjunction with the above note, the emphasis is love, not sexual appetite, knowing the terms are too often confused in practice, even though in discussion many readily acknowledge they understand the difference. God-realization is the fundamental purpose of each person's existence. Everything may be ideal in appearance in marriage, but without God-realization clearly being at the center of both partner's lives, it is, in the final analysis, at most a union rooted in goodness, but not according to the purpose of human marriage, which is to be a school for divine love, and one's own espousal to the divine. – Ed.

Section I: The Consequences of the Misinterpretation of the Marriage / 843

nature fights most viciously before it dies, since in this material world one tends to measure life with its ability to perform sexual acts rather than embracing the transcendent spiritual power.[268]

Marriage without the spiritual love that God intended is said to be under nature's law, and this is forbidden. Sex for the sake of attempting to satisfy lust is not the love that is in harmony with God's love. Eastern spirituality teaches that if a male or female human, a man or a woman, has an impure heart, he or she will not be drawn to his or her rightful soulmate. In other words, if a person seeks merely to satisfy his or her lustful drives, that person will forfeit true happiness, first and foremost, as the act is not blessed by God. God will bless only the union that 'serves a vow before the Divine.' Jesus taught that this is true because "if the couple had found, joined, and had lived in a spiritual soulmate union according to God's law and the divine purpose of marriage and seeks another for sexual satisfaction only, then he or she breaks the law of God and is damned." What Eeshans interpret this to mean, is that adultery then comes about when one has found the soulmate, and has entered into a commitment with that soulmate before God, but then puts that commitment and relationship aside for the sake of pleasure with another person.

There are many instances where people have entered into marriage believing they have fallen permanently in love, but do not realize it is mostly the depth of *emotion* they are experiencing (which can be confused with spiritual states, especially when one is especially attached to the sensation of the physical body, and when the consciousness is dominated by the experience of the physical body). They may be experiencing various forms of human-centered love, but this does not necessarily mean they are experiencing a true, transcendental love between soulmates before God. Often it happens that people in this situation, who get married too quickly, or too early, in their lives, are far too immature spiritually to have an understanding of the lifelong commitment they are entering into. These considerations are essential when it comes to understanding the

---

[268] This is an expression of the animal component of the human person's embodied existence; the animal aspect behaves in accord with animal nature, and fights to survive for itself, almost as if it were a separate entity. – Ed.

hard and fast rules of organizations that rigidly hold to the letter of law regarding divorce and the interpretation of Jesus' words that "what God has joined together, let no man put asunder." What God joins together is the soulmate relationship, and that is the relationship that one cannot abandon for the sake of physical and emotional fulfillment. To hold any and all to the rigid interpretation of law under penalty of shame and the refusal of sacraments merely intensifies further shame and only serves to choke off love.

LESSON 199

SECTION II: A QUICK REVIEW

To Eeshans, the Sacred and Sacramental Marriages of both Adam and Eve, and of Jesus and Mary Magdalene, had texts that were deliberately changed, removed, or lost, to some, hopefully forever. We have continued to unpack details of their stories and have presented reasons why we believe this, especially in light of Jesus' marriage, one of the chief reasons was paranoia on the part of patriarchal religions to eliminate proof to avoid *any* possible claims to women's demands for equality with men in terms of priestly ordination, contraception, and procreation, or any other issue regarding women's, or humanitarian/civil rights, so long as they reflect the laws and beliefs of the constitution of the country of which the person is a citizen.

In reviewing the apostolic priesthood of present times, it would appear that if the truth was known, the issue of celibacy (which finds its roots in the concept of an unmarried Jesus) would have benefited, and been understood better, in the light of His transcendental marriage, and would prove to better substantiate a more balanced understanding and foundation for celibacy.

Eeshans believe the church's understanding of celibacy is grossly impoverished, and leads to repression, and is expressed in the form of neurosis, cruelty, and the problems that have plagued the church for its entire history, most pronounced in the scandals of today. The problem of course, reaches far beyond the confines of the church, into just about every sphere of society and culture the world over. Where in the world does this problem of repression and sexual harassment, molestation, abuse, and violence *not* exist? All of this stems from the burying of the

Sacred Balance established by Jesus and Mary in their marriage. There is a higher standard by which to live, to rise above the lusts that would seek to invert and corrupt love, and that standard was set, and exemplified, by Jesus and Mary. Jesus never said sex was 'bad,' rather, He showed how it was to be properly governed in the light of love and the greater good.

For many in power and authority, there is no desire whatsoever to 'risk' upsetting and bringing down all that has been built up for the last 2000+ years, since there is no fear of losing all of this. Though the vital reason for this belief is our constant, it remains, however, to remind us of the description that we feel harkens back to the biblical story of the bronze statue with feet made of clay. When truth has been distorted, or even falsified, God intervenes. As it has been said biblically, which could easily be applied to church history, **As strong and deeply grounded as Christian history can be made to appear, it is still more than possible that those foundations are made of clay; and no matter how strong and shiny those upper levels may seem to be, let's not forget that upon which it all rests.**

Jesus was the first to explain this in his parable found in Mark 4:3:

> **Listen! A farmer went out to sow his seed. As he was sowing the seed, some fell along the path, and the birds came and ate it up. Some fell on rocky places where it did not have much soil. It sprang up quickly, because the soil was shallow. But when the sun came up, the plants scorched, and withered up because they had no root. Other seed fell among the thorns, which grew up and choked the plants, so that they did not bear grain. Still other seed fell on good soil. It came up, grew and produced a crop, some multiplying thirty, some sixty, some a hundred times. And then Jesus said, "Anyone with ears to hear should listen and understand."**

A firm conceptual and wholehearted stance argues for Jesus and Mary being married, at the marriage feast at Cana. As we have written we believe this was the marriage feast designed by God and carried out by Jesus and Mary Magdalen, that was necessary for the restoration of humankind to the transcendental state, lost after the fall from grace in the book of Genesis and the traditional story of Adam and Eve. Why is this so important? Because the truth about this Sacred Balance is essential to have in place at the heart of human history, and it must be that light put on the lampstand, and not hidden under the bushel basket. It needs to be seen clearly and with hearts of faith. If it is not, it doesn't matter what is 'built up' in human history in the name of the human consciousness: it will, indeed, fail. Also, because humankind was created in the image and likeness of God, after the 'fall' to a physical state, it would take a begotten God to become 'parents' in order that their children are saved, and they would become begotten children of The New Adam and The New Eve; thus, Jesus and His marriage were crucial to making it possible that humanity could the begotten children of The New Adam and The New Eve. While it would be 'easy' for God to simply declare all things new, and start everything fresh with a snap of the fingers, the reality is that God does not 'violate' the created order of laws and relationships to affect the divine plan. Rather, God implements a plan, whereby the laws and relationships described here are drawn to serve a transcendental purpose, while taking a human error, righting it, and bridging it back to the Creator, while still retaining the dignity of free will.

For God to simply make all things new, without Jesus, would go against the divine justice because it would be obstructive. This is why Jesus also has the role of Judge for His Father, (in addition to being liaison between humans and God the Creator) because He, along with his wife, set the directives for salvation in order for humanity to come back, and regain, what was lost. By their marriage, Jesus and Mary reopened the gates of heaven and gave us the Way for us to return to God the way God intended. That is why their marriage is vital to everlasting life. That is why Jesus taught that one cannot go 'around' him, and why what He taught is essential and not subject to dismissal.

LESSON 200

SECTION III: HOW THE HOLY AND SACRED TRANSCENDENTAL IS GREATER THAN WHAT WAS TAUGHT TO US

The holy and transcendental mystery that completes the Sacrament of the Holy Eucharist through the sacrificial Marriage of Christ and His wife, as his eternal and human consort, is the final step in the destruction of the barriers within the human consciousness that prevents its complete awakening in God. It is the antidote for that which has poisoned the mind, the soul, and the body of humanity before God. Once again, God enters the physical world with a renewed relationship, raising human love to the highest level imaginable, a manifestation of the duality and love of God. This *is* our goal.

Even more than that, we have, at our finger tips, the means to this "Plan of Salvation," which we have continued to speak of and teach about; and, yet, we not only hope, but wonder, if it is truly understood and comprehended in our texts as humankind should see it.

The salvific effects are far beyond and deeper than what has ever been studied and/or taught; and this marriage not only lends to the reality of God's plan by returning and restoring to humans that which was lost, but it goes far beyond the normal capacity of spirituality. This is found in reference to our explanation of Marriage.

God always knows best. As Eeshans, we have witnessed how the original plan of Salvation was, in fact, stalled by man's free will, but not only does it appear to have been used again at a time when women are taking a stand, and finally all are seeing them from a very enlightened perspective, but this uncompromising will of the human woman is being fueled now by the Divine Feminine, and the resurgence of yet another Divine and Sacred entity, The Order of Melchizedek.

That which is being presented for humans this time around, is causing them to enter into a realm that goes beyond that which even science, or technology, would fall short. This salvific plan could and might not just provide facts that one would find compelling. The fact is that this plan, being Divine in nature, steers the actual human knowledge with the Divine Mind, Heart, and Soul of the Divine Feminine; and that we share in a much greater way in a Divine life much greater than any human ever experienced before, to include Adam and Eve.

Up until the reforms of the Catholic church in the 1960's, we were living in a time where people respected and revered that which was considered sacred; for example, bowing to the Blessed Sacrament, manners of receiving Communion, etc. Then came the time when all these things were changed and secularized, and that which was to be handled only by consecrated hands was handled by everyone under the guise of the 'priesthood of all the faithful;' and this led to such familiarity with the sacred that eventually the novelty wore off to the point where very few people have an authentic appreciation of 'the Holy,' if they even go to church at all.

What was once sacred, solemn, and mysterious, had fallen victim to the consequences of the lack of the transcendental consciousness; and we watched all that fed an innate desire for it to be buried to the point of disbelief in the Divine. As time heals all wounds, the consequence of not believing what has always been declared mystical, and spiritual, had become to most nothing more than those things that can now be explained.

Yes, it certainly is time. With advancements in technology, we are finding a world subject to man's quest to finding answers to questions such as "Could the Ark of the Covenant be explained as having been a nuclear device brought to our earth by extraterrestrials with the ability to produce the Manna in the desert?" There are other questions also, such as, "Could it kill anyone who touched it due to the radiation effect?" This consciousness, which is manifesting increasingly in these inquisitive times, suggests that people are not satisfied with the 'stock' answers from the past regarding the 'big questions' of today.

We live in a time where, as the truth regarding the marriage of Jesus and Mary has been deemed by God timely to release, the world is in a time of tumultuous upheaval in many other ways: politically, socially, philosophically, and scientifically. In an odd conjunction of science and religion, there is the example of the official Vatican telescope situated in Arizona being officially named "Lucifer" by a team of Jesuits. Lucifer? A telescope owned and set up by the 'church' that stands as the beacon of light to the world through the ages regarding the Savior of humanity, Jesus Christ, but is officially named *Lucifer*? And what would the purpose of this be? Some sources say that it's set up to watch for an 'alien savior' from another world, and there's even supposed guidelines being drafted under Vatican officials regarding how to baptize aliens.

There are many reasons and justifications provided by official connections to the telescope trying to calm people down with explanations for the name; yet, it still comes down to a common sense question, "Of all the names on earth you could use for a telescope, why did you pick this one …?"

Crazy? No, it just shows us where we are in the midst of the many kinds of changes that are occurring in these times, witnessing to the fall and corruption of so many things related to God. From the telescope named Lucifer to the awaiting of an "alien savior" under proposed tolerance, or connection, to an established religion supposedly founded on Jesus Christ, one may presume that the foundations of said religion were, indeed, always corrupt under its namesake Peter. Or could it be a distraction regarding the perverted actions, and acceptance, and hidden secrets linked to the pedophilia scandals all along? Can all these things be related to the conspiracy stories linking the Vatican to Black Masses and the enthronement of Lucifer, which was said to take place at the Vatican, simultaneously, in the basement of a school in Charleston, South Carolina via phone?

All this was discussed, as we are sure, with the intention of promoting cognitive advancement, as well as assisting humans in the efforts of gaining knowledge? It is said by a reliable source that there are "good tools to conquer evil." Are such tools now the new labels for the Sacrament and Mystery of Baptism?

And could these things of God that are being 'researched and redefined' be some way of explaining away the power of God in an effort to offset findings that could advance not just women's agendas, but also the revealing of the omissions and deliberate errors to obstruct the true Mission of Christ? In other words, could there now be a force at work that can excuse away or create insurmountable barriers that takes God's design out of the equation?

Like the appearance of the sun burning away fog, the truth about those things, once seen as holy, sacred, and divine acts, may readily be explained away today; whereas, in biblical times, people fell into the hands of who they believed, only because they were totally unfamiliar with modern physics and science and technology, seeing wonders as magical, or divine, because they were so 'primitive?' Or did they have real faith and witness the supernatural?

Jesus rebuked the Pharisees, and religious leaders, for taking advantage of God's people and put himself and *his identity* into the equation to justify his authority, by saying that because He came and existed, God cannot ignore the injustices laid upon the people. In addition, they truly couldn't ignore what He *is* saying.

But, what if man can, or believes he can, now explain those remarkable stories and provide reasonable explanation? Well, then it makes spirituality that much more mandatory, so, that one sees that without it, there is a danger that the 'fall' of humankind will be attributed to 'someone or something that mirrors the what and who of God,' but is not God but another imposter.

If we find what is revealed is 'true,' then we have been given a purpose, and this brings even more merit to suffering; but if we have no spirituality, or it doesn't exist, and there is no promised eternity, life as we know it truly is pointless. Eeshans say that despite technological advances, humans are always more than just pawns and/or subjects for experiments, more than 'sheeple,' and there is a greater Supreme Being, to whom we all matter, and that being is "Love" (God). The fact that advancement in technology and knowledge can't be ignored (nor should it be), whether or not you are in agreement with it, one thing is for sure, it should help one to realize that these extreme gifts, though they are brought about by amazing individuals, are still first, and foremost, from God and centered on spirituality, and they should be helpful to humanity today, but while witnessing, even more so, to the tremendous mind and creativity of God.

One should not, however, fall victim to trickery by letting someone explain away an adversary such as Lucifer/Satan as a fictional character, or actually nonexistent, or something created in an attempt by religions to control people. Since if Jesus/God exists, or rather, is *alive*, and if the story of other life (outside the senses, this world, other universes, etc.) is true, one must understand that demons and fallen angels really do exist and do not die. So, to accept these advances under the guise of being "the only" rational options to the advancement of humankind to the point of excluding God, then your thinking and rationale aren't coming from a source of good. This is not at all to mean that our educational developments and scientific advancements are bad, but as with the presence of any imbalance, that, 'power corrupts.'

LESSON 201

SECTION IV: 'TRY TO RECTIFY YOURSELF RATHER THAN BLASPHEMING THE NATURE OR ACTIVITIES OF OTHERS'

—Bhaktivedanta Saraswati

Eshans are hoping that with the revelation of the marriage of Jesus and His wife, it will help in burning away the fog of the mind, body, and spirit, which envelopes so many at this time in history. It is at least enough for us to witness that the effects of entropy still blurs the beauty of true love, and that true love began with the Creator's desire to share love by creating beings as extensions of it.

To reset the course of the transcendental path for the light body of human beings before God, it is necessary to begin with the Marriage of the Lamb to Mary Magdalene, and to proceed up to the Last Supper, and His passion, death, and resurrection, in order to bring about the Sacred Food necessary to insure the conquering of life (defined only by the human rational consciousness). From there, this path was meant to continually unfold Jesus' teachings with Mary leading the community of believers who would oversee all that Jesus put into place. Though this plan was thwarted, God chose to allow man's free will to play out and this may be the greatest proof of God ever witnessed. Since at the fullness of time, when all seems lost, humans cry out, allowing God to spread the seed on good and fertile soil.

It is imperative for the salvation of man, to understand that our humanistic views alone, especially those guided by spiritual authorities who, too, were guided as Peter was, by the human, rational consciousness, *have caused us to 'not' believe that love of neighbor begins with respect and equality of genders.* Starting with women, and including the various forms of gender expression,[269] who have been turned away from Jesus for being born the way God designed, we continue to witness people being punished because they are judged by biases beyond their control, and, as impersonally as one judges a book by its cover.

Eeshans believe that the chattelization, and subjugation, of the female gender has its origin, nonetheless, in the incorrect/altered story about Adam and Eve, since it has been passed down and taught traditionally.[270] Why? Well, *to reiterate once again,* because of woman's heartfelt love and deep attraction to God, persistent memory will NOT let her be denied her rightful place before God. That is why she continues to reach out and fight for that love. The right to love God, and the right to choose love, even if this love must endure the vindictive attacks from what should be her *counterpart.*

When women began their fight to gain equality we were told, and we all believed, that feminism was born, and that it was bad. We believed it because that was how the church operated and conditioned the faithful to think. In a range of movements, and with a variety of ideologies, these women persisted, and continued, to fight to achieve equal rights for women, and have tried to respond to issues of all kinds, such as the social construction of gender. The result was, for the most part, that women seemed to be sympathetic to it all. Still they hit a dead end, primarily with the Catholic and Christian faiths as being a 'bad' people for having spearheaded a movement in the wake of "the female" counterpart of the Divine Masculine.

---

[269] Known genders identified today as male, female, and androgynous, expressed through the human body in various combinations to include, heterosexual, homosexual, bisexual, and transgender. – Ed.

[270] The story may have been told quite differently by an enlightened people, but as the story was absorbed into existing patriarchal cultural foundations, that story would be modified in its retelling, sooner or later, to support the male dominant structure, and that consciousness would be projected back on to the story, i.e., 'it was the woman you gave me.' – Ed.

Persistent memory would not allow them to 'stop.' As conscientious objectors of a special kind, these people, both men and women, fought to right the wrongs within the workplace; yet, they were viciously attacked just for trying to help those who were discriminated against, and abused, within the church. Perhaps, not all their methods could be deemed appropriate, but sometimes the shock value is the jackhammer needed to move things 'for God,' yes, *for* God. Because of these triumphs, women are now beginning to be heard.

Eeshans believe that though the primary 'obstacle' has stemmed, not from one, but from the *many* misleading biblical accounts that were safeguarded within the official doctrines, or dogmas, this obstacle contained within itself a kind of spiritual lockdown, where even the many other women (who did not agree with the feminists) presumed the women behind the women's movement were fighting because they were lesbians, or because they hated men, and hated the Divine Masculine God. We see more clearly that this was not true. Eeshans believe that if it wasn't for the pressure of the Catholic church to suppress such ideas, or if there had been all along, scriptures and writings that had not been tampered with, or rewritten, there would be found authors and scientists whose work would have helped create a balance. Instead, we found that from the Doctors of the church to scientists that were pressured to write only within certain parameters, and were not permitted to write and publish, if, according to what was dictated to them, this pressure was created, and maintained, in order to uphold a certain agenda, beginning with the story of Adam and Eve. The Eeshan Religion is here to bring light out of captivity from darkness.

If all that has been presented since Peter was true, we now have the perfect storm to totally eliminate belief in God, and forfeit salvation once and for all, as Satan desired. All these wrongs would be accomplished, sooner or later.

Eeshan transcendentalism, as we said before, is a combination of Merkabolic and Kabbalic energies, and has throughout humankind, stepped in to restore the Light when it is required, and that is what you have here in these times. Because it is a Living Light that connects to the light body found within each person, the resurgence of the Eeshan transcendentalism is, thereby, identified when Jesus, who is the "Light of the World," said "My sheep will hear my voice."

We see that the world today has lost much of its sense of the sacred in every way and lacks much in sacramental experience, transcendental purpose, or sense of providence. Again, because the mystery of God's Salvific plan was not only withheld from the them, what they did have, and what was given to them, was distorted. Accepting God's existence is becoming a serious 'option' and is no longer a 'constant' in the minds of far too many; and one can see evidence of this in how people are treating one another publicly and privately.

Jesus, as God, is vast in His images, and is complete as God, and we harken to hear the real words that Jesus spoke from the depth of his spirituality as God. With the many faces and facets of absolute truth, like a diamond, and as powerful as a Brahmastra weapon,[271] it is time to turn the tide against those whose strength cannot compare to God's. With kindness, one gains the strength necessary to change hearts. With the reception of the Sacred food and Drink, and by the propagation of the Sacred and Divine Marriage Feast of the Lamb and His Wife, we will truly become the leaven for the Sacred Balance of the Divine Feminine and Masculine.

"Unless we return to the Holy and Sacred, and give reverence to God, we shall not know holiness, or sacredness, or kindness, let alone, love. For the pyramid of God starts with the human foundation and points to a holy institution, that was once unattainable to now being that which is attainable."

The above reference was drawn from *The Nectar of Instructions for Immortality*, by Srila Bhaktisiddhanta Sarasvati Thakura Prabhupada, where we also find this admonition: "Try to rectify yourself rather than blaspheming the nature or activities of others." In connection with this we find the more familiar teaching by Jesus: "Before you attempt to remove the speck from your brother's eye, you must first remove the plank from your own eye." So, when Jesus returns, will He find faith? Will we have learned that we are all created equal, male and female, and children of God?

---

[271] From ancient Vedic times, described in the Bhagavata Purana, a weapon which created an explosion of nuclear proportions. – Ed.

LESSON 202

Section V: Metta True Charity/ Love, Not Misplaced Compassion

The love, of which we speak, may not appeal to everyone for each individual has their own version of the "kind" of love they fantasize about; but this love, known to Eeshans as "Metta," is what originates from the 'Christs,' as the Light that transforms ordinary beings into light beings destined for eternity. This is the love that was experienced by those who, in the beginning, sat in Jesus' presence, and still do. This is the love that carried His name, and allowed him to 'correct' the laws that did not originate with God. It allowed him to call the Pharisees liars and hypocrites. It allowed him to throw out thieves from the temple, and it allowed him to teach and preach to 'all those who wanted to hear' without thought, or concern, about who should hear, or who is allowed to hear or not. All he did, taught and exemplified for humankind was to be carried out for 2000+ years precisely the way he commanded it. It's this love that, even though you never met him in his human form, makes you feel that you, indeed, have.

That's the power behind God's love. This is the love that does not confuse the words charity/love with misplaced and misapplied compassion. Perhaps we don't have a clue anymore of how lax we have become to the point of allowing the very laws that protect us to be broken under the guise of being 'out of love for God's children.' This is the love that brings balance to nature and God's creatures by abolishing the abuse of animals, but is also careful not to place these *ahead of the value of human life*. Though few do, it a good reminder that all life has worth; yet, being extensions of God, we tend to fall to the level of what we are told is a domestic, or tamed, animal for companionship and pleasure. Though pets are governed by nature they actually are living examples of what humans should be; and are not only approachable, and eager to bond with us, but are non-judgmental, making it easier to be ourselves. Our pets approach us with trust and sincerity. We should be able to approach God this same way. We should love God the way our pets love us, but on a grander scale/level, loving as God loves. As our little pets love us with an unconditional love and fidelity, and are ever ready to forgive, and are always non-complaining, ever-trusting, always happy and affectionate, they teach us love of neighbor; these qualities all being present without question in such a natural way often puts human beings to shame, since they show a true example of the kind of love human beings should be practicing, as defined by Jesus and his teachings on unconditionally loving God and loving one's neighbor. These things make us wonder who best serves God, and why they aren't in charge ...?

Having the God particle placed within us, who are made in the image and likeness of God, raises us as extensions of God having a conscience, self-awareness, and the ability to enter into a relationship with God and experience salvation. We, therefore, should strive to be enlightened beings, as intended by God that we may enjoy the place we were all meant to have in the context of the Divine.

Eeshans realized long ago, that the key to enlightenment is to read, listen and discuss, but also always to promote cognitive clarity on issues with the Christs at the center. Imbalances are responsible for mudding translations, especially when/where the human consciousness tried to define issues of faith and spirituality. Fear keeps us from following through as God intends and confuses good and evil. Tolerance of bad, or evil, is not the way of Jesus. Yet, at the same time, there have always been negative things that have been and are being attributed to 'Jesus.' In the Woody Allen movie *Hannah and Her Sisters*, there is a character who was reading the newspaper, and commenting on articles he was reading. At one point, he lifts his head in disbelief, and says, "If Jesus came back and saw what was going on in His name, He would never stop throwing up." How true.

There are so many laws in place that have become blurred with language using double and triple entendre, etc., which have caused more chaos, license, and tolerance of lawlessness, inequality, and lack of spirituality because there is no "authority" that can take the place of God and God's laws. However, we are sure that there is a lawyer somewhere that would find a word, or words, that would bring about not one, but many meanings, defenses, or arguments for what was just described. That is what has happened with Jesus' teachings.

Today everyone "explains and talks for and on behalf of God" through human concepts and understanding self and awareness of their environment, which as imperfect beings, we cannot do quite so perfectly. Each individual has a different perspective from which they think and act. If we had taken together all of these under a 'perfect Authority, and perfect authoritative guidelines' wouldn't we then have amazing recounts of what Jesus said, what our country's founding fathers wanted for us, and so on and so on?

Just as little children, teens, and young adults see their parents as role models (or as bad role models), they learn from them by way of a 'familial' conditioning, following and representing how the parents, guardians, and other adults think, treat each other, and others, as well, as their views on life, environment, politics, and economy as we mentioned early on in this book.

It would be great if there was an actual facsimile of what Christ said, or an eyewitness, and confidant to his thoughts and wishes, from back then or today.

Eeshans feel that their religion, guided by the Consciousness of Mary Magdalen, and having the Christs' true teachings, may help bring people back to God and God back to the people.

The Eeshan religion is nothing less than miraculous, since it provides that which fills a person totally, and allows them to feel that they are in God's presence. It is a love we wish everyone to have and experience.

If arguing and crying, rudeness, and lack of civility is part of daily life, children will learn this, and when they play, they will act it out. Movies, YouTube, and other social media present a different kind of love to preteens and teens, and the reasons for falling in love are also depicted differently. In other words, each age group possesses similar to extremely different versions of love; and, thus, no two really are the same.

The definition of love varies, and is different, as it does change over the years, through experiences, through the many phases we experience throughout life. What we once were against, after we are placed in our brother/sister's shoes, we might suddenly find ourselves being 'for,' as mindsets change, biases change, and prejudice falls by the wayside, etc. Truth, however, does not change. Metta tries to maintain truth according to how God views something, and how we can accomplish to resolve issues to the best of our ability without misplaced compassion and unbridled tolerance.

LESSON 203

SECTION VI: DIVORCE

We talked at length about marriage, so now let's take a look at the Eeshan beliefs about divorce. Do you remember the way divorcees were once treated? Do you remember how we were made to treat the women who were divorced? Do you remember how the church used Jesus' saying, "What God has put together ...?" We know how (though not said) women in abused situations lauded the strength of divorced women; yet, were in situations themselves that prevented them from following suit, and lacking that grace from God to know that they need not tolerate abuse. Jesus never ignored, or condoned, abuse. In fact, he openly made His feelings known when He talked with the people, especially in His wife's case. He openly dared the men 'who were' without sin' to pick up the stone and throw it at the adulterous woman. The same clarity was found in his parable of the good Samaritan and His identification of the many who abused God's children with their hard yokes and heavy burdens.

The 'love that is sanctioned under God,' when both sides, divided by beliefs, politics, laws, etc. believe wholeheartedly in God, and find answers through sources which are also balanced in God.

Where finding love and a good decent partner is becoming more and more complicated, we say it is the fallout of not believing in God. How amazing where we had once been a culture where we believed in finding decent relationships, but due to a radical change in priorities, (and we frowned on arranged marriages) it seems impossible to find a decent and committed partner; some wonder if perhaps arranged marriages would be the way to go to some degree. In fact, more and more this is becoming the norm, since isn't that what dating services are providing, as no one has the time, the patience. or the energy to meet someone, and just need help? These are doing what would have been done in cultures where parents, or guardians (based on their own life experiences), felt they knew what was best and suitable for their child. Granted, this was not always in the child's best interest, and sometimes it was in the parents' best interest, and oftentimes in selfish ways, one is still inclined to wonder how to find that perfect person. Well, no one is perfect.

Human love is complicated. Divorce is more complicated. There are so many times when that one marriage that shouldn't have worked turns out to be the best marriage ever; and what seems at the start to be the best marriage ever, ends in divorce, and you wonder how it all happened. One wonders what can be done so that this doesn't happen to you.

That is where God and grace comes into the picture. This gives one strength to make balanced decisions. No, it does not mean that there is a guarantee that everything will work out, but it gives a couple the strength to give it their 'best' try, with all they have by the love that they made their promises with to each other, before God.

Divorce for "irreconcilable differences" means that after all effort was put forth, there seems to be no improvement, and the desire to follow through with their promises to continue in this union, has been greatly lessened, or is no longer there. Children are always affected by divorce; however, *they are most often more affected* by disastrous marriages where fighting and hatred posed between both parents whom they love are the constant. Remember that the children are *not* the cause, nor should they be involved, included, or made to 'choose' between parents, nor should they be made to hear all the details of the issues between the parents. These issues are between the couple, and though there are times the couple cannot hide, or deflect the problems, hurt and anger, they must still try. Otherwise, the children will 'learn' that this is 'normal' behavior, and it is, indeed, not normal behavior, or at least it shouldn't be. If there are circumstances that cause volatility at times, try and end it with a kinder note. Children need hope and stability. We need children with hope, and who are stable, since they are our future. Staying together under duress causes stress on the children, and an impossible situation for them to decipher, are all the facts thrown at them in their minds, regardless of their age. As children grow, they need to talk, as well as having an understanding of morals and values. Children also need to be reared in civility, which they must learn to apply in daily life. This means more than manners and politeness; it makes life more pleasant for others and teaches one self-respect: in other words, children need to be brought up as an upmost priority, otherwise you will definitely affect their perspective on love and life. Civility promotes and encourages discipline and a positive outlook and way of expression. Today, foul language replaces useful vocabulary, and points to the true condition of the heart and reveals the true identity of the person. That is why using God's name in vain reveals the heart of the person, and dismisses the holiness and reverence due to God. "The mouth speaks what the heart is full of." (Luke 6:44-45). This spirit is the origin of perjury, where a person swears before God, with no intention of speaking the truth. God looks upon this as breaking a vow in front of him. "For neither fresh water nor salt water flow from the same spring." (James 3:11).

Vows are important to God. Sacramental marriage combines the love of God with human love by a vow made between a man and woman, or a male and female. Though human love is not a guarantee, God's love is. This vow, then, invites God to witness to the couple's actions, decisions, and quality of life together. Therefore, if one or the other does not take the vow seriously they forfeit the grace they would undoubtedly need through troubled times, and may not hear the inner voice of their heart.

Oftentimes, God can become the mediator, even with the decisions of children through all difficult times, since they will come to understand that they are not alone. Even when you are going through a divorce, believe it or not, just by saying to the children that God loves both parents, and will help resolve the situation as best it can be resolved, brings reassurance. With this divine component, why would one not believe that they have superhuman abilities, and strength, to handle a very vulnerable and confusing time? Without a doubt, God helps those who ask as well as help themselves. Truth is, there is no guaranteed formula for marriage, the chances for success of stronger love, loyalty, and fidelity are greater with God.

There is, however, a factor, or major component, that, without it, by which one's love implodes, as this is an authoritative witness. That is why that "little piece of paper" that is witnessed by civil authorities and by those closest to you, but especially by an Authority who is the actual, true authority from whom all other authorities take their name, makes you feel "different." Eeshans suggest how much greater this authority is, when this authority is God, the author of the Law from which all laws and authority comes?

Still, civil authority has become for a lot of people all that is needed or desired. That authority, in which a lot of people feel more comfortable, is satisfactory for to them, since their mind and heart has been betrayed by a belief system that just doesn't work for them any longer, and that being namely that of the church. One should remember that this is not all that one should feel is needed, since civil authorities can give only an approval, and acknowledgment, created by other humans under human laws that recognize the one thing that separates you from others, who are not seen as 'married,' and that is that legal paper. Some feel that this is the alternative to standing before God, and is equal to the other (we want you to at least consider this for yourself, the difference between the two). If that is how you are thinking, and if this is one of the "most important" events in your life, enough to celebrate it with family and friends, then why wouldn't you want God's blessing too? If not for this moment, when is there a more important time, or event, that is 'worthy' of God's presence? Sometimes the bride or groom to be becomes angry when the other wants God to witness their union, all for many different reasons, could it possibly be guilt? We could explore all of these things, but again the most important reason is your link to God and to your salvation, both of which are forfeited should you take a path away rather than *towards* the 'Way" to Jesus and His wife.

We are not opposed to what other religions or spiritual ties believe, nor to what a civil marriage declares as right or wrong. In fact, we have an open invitation, should at any point in your civil marriage you desire, to enter into a sacramental extension. Based on our beliefs, however, *we just feel the need to share our position, or at least a summary of our beliefs, in hopes they may help someone.*

As we watch the world falling more and more into a secular state, we see an increase in a more self/sexual gratification-centered view of marriage, rather than the sacredness of true love in a Sacramental marriage, as exemplified by Jesus and Mary, not just in young people, but in those of the baby boomer age, who feel life has passed them by. Maybe they never really understood the questions, or had the answers to them, but they kept them hidden deep within their hearts. Maybe if they did, their marriage would not have ended in divorce, since are we not at that point, again, where Jesus said this when asked about divorce:

"It was because of the hardness of heart that Moses permitted you to divorce your wives; but from the beginning it was not this way." He said this in reference to his Parents, and about Adam and Eve, who were the extensions of God's duality and the first transcendental marriage and first human marriage. These were the things you were never told anyone, and no one would admit to; but by not presenting them, marriage lost its true meaning, under the guise of what it was taught marriage was, and still is all about.

Without a doubt, over time, and without the divine component, disastrous results of entering into a *purely human covenant without its true, originally intended meaning, is no longer grace-abundant, as per Sacramental Marriage. This grace is that which:*

1. Is available to help those marriages in crisis situations.
2. Is the presence of God sought as the source of answers.
3. Is available to be the tool of strength to save the 'vowed relationship.'
4. Gives the needed completeness, or wholeness, to a couple joined together, that can only be in a relationship with God.
5. Helps one to see that sex *without God's blessing* is illusory, because it does not satisfy the soul.
6. Helps one to see that a soul without love is lifeless because it is starved of true love. Human love alone brings with it many forms of suffering and emotional and psychological entanglement, such as the erosion of a person's dignity and the removal of the desire for marriage.

7. Helps one to see what it means regarding those who are involved only in a physical relationship, and how they stand a risk of growing tired of one another, or losing interest, in the other person, and eventually finding a growing interest in another for the same reasons.
8. Helps one to see that the superficial emotional and physical pleasures masquerading as love may wear off, and, thus, there is no desire to get married, or share in an eternal connection. These people try to feel that there is no residue to leaving a sacramental relationship as both parties "entered as consenting adults," and under illusion they are "leaving as consenting adults." Under this delusion, they are free to find someone who once again 'ignites that fire.'

The grace which we speak of in the above points helps one to see in various ways how a committed relationship brings with it a partner who is there to help, heal, and encourage life between each other, since there is always the option of the open door.

If, however, one or the other partner had fallen in 'love' in a committed relationship (i.e., living together, but not married), and the other decides to leave, it's possible that the immortal component can be ignited, since God will not abandon anyone who calls out for help. How could this happen? It could happen if one or the other quietly turned to God and began asking God to intervene in changing the heart of the one leaving, due to unhappiness, illness, or death. So, God does not ever abandon us, even when we think we know everything. God is also not a "concept by which we measure our pain,"[272] rather, God is life and love. People do use God as their own gauge for all that goes wrong in their life.

---

[272] John Lennon.

LESSON 204

Section VII: God as Human: To Live in a Vowed Marriage

God is the immortal component, who by being eternal love, **also experienced human love IN A VOWED MARRIAGE**, and all the difficulties that entails. God the only begotten Child did so that we could not say God has no idea what marriage is, and how this God particle is not only relevant but vital to human marriage. Jesus fell in love and chose marriage as the example of ultimate love between two humans and their love for God, despite Peter's attempts to get him to divorce Mary. Since these had the eternal/infinite component before their humanity, which Jesus tried to get him to understand, but Peter would not and could not.

Since vows before God have become increasingly meaningless today, we find that all must be in a written contract between humans, also, as one's word means nothing to man ('as above, so below').

Approval for marriage outside of God, in any manner, may give you civil rights, but according to Jesus' teaching regarding marriage does not give rights under God. Even in a committed relationship, it is viewed as preparation for marriage; but a vowed Sacramental Marriage cannot be sacrificed to a committed relationship and lived without taking that next step as though under God. For it would lack the grace the sacrament brings with it as well as God's blessing of the couple being "one body."

Under a vowed Sacramental Marriage, God recognizes that 'the two are now one', *according to God's 'own oneness,'* as was the original being created to manifest God's love. As above, so below, meaning the inside is like the outside. With God, the grace of the Sacrament, if called upon, will sustain, heal, strengthen, and bring joy in the midst of turmoil, thankfulness, and peace in the face of pain and suffering, and will glorify God in human flesh. This grace will last until death to the body, which then releases the bonds of marriage. Grace is what sustains a couple in the midst of triumph and agony. It hearkens the heart to heights unimaginable, and sustains one through unthinkable heartbreaks. With this kind of love, soulmates grow closer, and love becomes greater than time-limited sex. *True love conquers all.*

The eternal transcendental love that consumed. and sustained God the Father and His virgin wife. who vowed to love Him and have His Child, and which was lived out through Jesus' passion and death, is what is expressed through the celebration of the Marriage Feast of the Lamb and His wife.

This is the celebration of the love shared between Jesus and His wife through their 'vowed' sacrificial life together, and was what 'sustained' them through his death and the agony of being separated again, until their mission could commence once again. This is the celebration of the love that stirred, and caused within the hearts of the Eternal Father's and the Eternal Son's wives, the strength for their continued 'yes' to doing God's will and live out the steadfast love of their husbands. This is what conquered death. That 'personal' sacrifice is what made what God did for 'us' so amazing.

This 'vowed' marriage, and love, that Jesus and Mary shared, was made known 'before almighty God' and the reality of their 'vows' was signified with the wedding ring Jesus gave to Mary. This wedding band represented their love having no beginning and no end. When Jesus put the ring on her finger, it symbolized their eternal/infinite life, and how He was always surrounding and embracing her within His arms; and as her finger passed through the ring it symbolized her whole being entering into His arms with true desire and free will. As the ring witnessed their oneness, so the two were never separated even when they were physically apart. See supplement on the Sacred and Divine Marriage of Jesus and Mary Magdalen.

Their will to resist conjugal love proved that they had a greater bond; and within a perfected transcendental realm their hearts took flight in ways that soared beyond what any human act could provide. Therefore, what God had put together let no one try and separate. This, of course, was followed with the blood covenant which consummated their undying love for each other before God, and was to be lived according to God laws.

That is why Eeshans believe that a Marriage, when witnessed before God, puts a greater emphasis upon *the depth of love because its 'vows' are made before God*. With God being the witness, and being the absolute truth, this is often what discourages anyone to swear, or vow; whereas, when witnessed before a civil authority one may fall victim to human consciousness, where there is more of a finite agreement, as imposed by humans. Subconsciously, the human factor will always allow for a more human view of a couple's obligations and limitations. It will seek pleasure over responsibility, and a human promise, and though it has no real depth anymore it overshadows vows to God today, since it is now believed that God want one's happiness over vows made to be lived until the death of a partner, who was the 'apple of their eye,' and was the recipient of the promise before God to care and sacrifice for love. Now God will not hold us to imprudently made vows. Vows rashly made, or not showing responsibility for consequences of the action, lacking wisdom, good judgment, and discretion, if one was ill-advised or unadvised etc., and in marriages where drugs, alcohol, pregnancy, or parental pressure was exercised, or where abuse or other unknown circumstances exist, then divorce is then an option, and God will not hold one to the vow made, especially in a sacramental marriage. However, this must be proven. Could it happen more than once? Yes, it, indeed, can. That is why it is necessary to have spiritual guidance. This guidance, however, must be by a Sacredly Balanced guide in determining the truth.

Sex was always to be compulsory to marriage until recent times when it became a less popular way of thinking, due to the loss of the sanctity of this act. That is why, at one time, a child born out of wedlock was considered a disgrace, and brought the family shame. Today, however, this is not so much the case. It is because God's laws have been so twisted by man, and man's law appeared to be so much more 'reasonable' and logical, but the truth that remains is the innocence of the child. The child had nothing to do with the relationship between the parents. Just as a child aborted, or murdered, has been upon death, baptized as a martyr, and returns to God unharmed.

A Sacred Marriage is defined by Jesus 'own words. However, even civil law attempts to point out how marriage is essential even for the basic order of society; since without the commitment of marriage, where people just take and give up partners for the sake of pleasure, or convenience, the fabric of the culture and society breaks down.

Jesus spoke to his followers "as the above so below," reflecting what was done in heaven is mirrored here on earth. As God is above, and Jesus was God, so He had the authority here on earth to tell everyone what is right, and judge those things that were wrong. So, too, the person carrying the Divine Feminine.

Jesus used this terminology not just once but several time, as we shall also. When we read the Gnostic Gospel of Thomas we find the fullness of what Jesus was talking about when He was addressing Peter's insults about Mary. Following the Law of matrimony, theirs was a vowed marriage before God, and not only in Jesus' teaching is this clear, but it is also in the Judaic Law: "When you make the two One, and when you make the inside like the outside and the outside like the inside, and the above like the below, and when you make the male and female one and the same, then you will enter the Kingdom of God." Why is this so? Because *their marriage on earth* is the manifestation of the Eternal Marriage, as consorts. To Peter, however, Jesus' point was that they could never be separated by any law of man, to include the Jewish Law which Peter was referencing at the time. Peter, on the other hand, was not interested in the law as Jesus taught; rather, he was seeking to provide an authorized by-God legitimate reason for divorce, as a means of devising a plan, whereby, Jesus would have a reason to divorce Mary, as her 'reputation' was pulling Him down. In reality, Peter was motivated by his own jealousy, and was becoming fearful of the Jewish authorities' reactions to Jesus.

To believe in this teaching is to believe in Jesus and that Jesus is God. Once again in a transcendental way, Jesus spoke of how the union of the spirit with the soul produces a new empowered presence and that God as Jesus was in the presence of the apostles and the people. God's law was above man's law, and no one, or anything, could go above God's law. God's law has always been misconstrued and misconceived. Humans believe that if the numbers are against what God wants, God's law will have to change, as though we have rights over God.

Some people, out of convenience, will take words out of context in order to justify their choices, such as using Jesus' teaching from the Gospel where He answered the Sadducees on the question of who is married to whom in heaven, and Jesus, on the surface, seems to say there is 'no' marriage in heaven. But that is because there is a greater love in heaven and marriage there is vastly different than life here; here bodies are subject to entropy, for example, and this leads to physical laws, and how they do necessarily govern, and outline, how human relationships are arranged. In light of this, Jesus was not excusing people from the commitment of being married here in this life with His teaching; but, rather, He was showing the difference between the human consciousness and the drawbacks of the material/physical world, and that of the transcendental consciousness and pre-fall/world. He also tried to connect them with the duality of God in the divine nature to earthy relationships.

Being human and physical necessitates physical laws since it is of a lower frequency and close to the earth in forms of being governed. Thereby, Jesus knew that not much more could be explained since they lacked a transcendental means of deciphering what He already was saying. That is also why God gave commandments regarding adultery and covetousness, so that the question of divorce would have roots in all of the above.

The reality after Adam and Eve's choice to be physical brought about the current structure of the physical world, and what made it necessary to be married, and this was for humanity's own good, since it kept them on track spiritually, and was necessary for order and the ongoing support of life. It became a directive and commandment, without which there would be no decency to guide the human spirit. Without this, human life would degrade into a chaos and an animalistic mindset.

This is where we see, people more and more jettisoning the belief in a God of former times that said people have to be married in order to be together and have children. Increasing numbers of people are simply doing what they want, and they then believe there is no God that has rights over them; in fact, they find this offensive to the lifestyle they have chosen, just as the Sadducees were attempting to do with Jesus.

It should have been apparent to Peter that each time he was in the presence of both Jesus and Mary, that as he insulted Mary, he was insulting Jesus, since their essences alone made them one. Peter's human rational consciousness did not allow for comprehension of transcendental oneness, or the aspect of 'as above so below.' It didn't allow for the concept of eternity, since his birth religion had little to no belief in an afterlife. But since their strength, passion, and loyalty to each other was unshakeable, and as Peter's remarks became more and more frequent, we find in Luke 22:31 Jesus turning to Peter, and saying, "Simon, Simon, why has Satan demanded permission to sift you like wheat?" This question was posed many times and in many ways to Peter.

When we enter into a vowed human marriage before and with God as our witness, accepting them, and succeeding in becoming two in one spirit, with Christ and His Wife. Insults shared in marriage under God mirrors the above teaching. Love does not include insulting, or degrading communication, between spouses, or from one spouse to the other. It is often said, when you speak to each other, see Jesus in the other person, and be Jesus to them.

That is why, through Marriage, it is said that the two now are one, and actually pour 'their oneness into the Divine's Soul essence' that no part of either remains, as Jesus and His Wife pour their very essence into us and complete this union at the reception of the Eucharist.

Entering into any conjugal physical union without the Christs is not symbolic of Christ's wife's union with her eternal Bridegroom; and, thus, both the earthly husband and wife would not enter into the inner marriage as a physical manifestation of Christ's 'vowed' union with his Bride in the Eucharist. Therefore, it would be only sexual, and not spiritual; however, under Eeshan Transcendentalism, this can always be corrected.

To enter into conjugal relations outside of a 'blessed' committed relationship goes against all the preceding, and that becomes a sin that is compounded with each act. Why would God cause this drive if it was not to be used to find a partner, soulmate, and spouse? Because for all the reasons above. To enter into relations based only on sex is just an imposturous act, since what it is doing is coveting that which God set in place to be sacred and holy. When under illusion, one thinks otherwise, and doesn't see, or is blinded by pleasure, and fraudulently presents their desires to the other person as an act of love.

This inner marriage with Christ and his Wife, can also take place between a single, or a religious, person who accepts these teachings.

If one researches 'alchemy' one will find the same principles above at play, and this is why Jesus used this formula in His teachings. One must remember, too, that in the Sacrament of Matrimony you have the strength of your partner to attain this tremendous courage, passion, and devotion with each other and God. Couple that with the Sacred and Divine Eucharist of the Marriage Feast and you receive the Divine component at its richest and fullest level.

As a single person entering into a divine relationship, living solely for God, you must pour yourself so utterly into the Divine's Body, Blood, Soul, and Divinity that no part of you remains, and in doing so, the Christs fill you, until which time you decide that it is a human relationship you seek with their blessing. Trying to find solace in another human relationship, while still in marriage is the worst sin you can commit. Again, it is a flagrant act of temerity and immorality, a manifestation of total defiance against God, because of Jesus' Marriage to Mary Magdalen. When this happens, one needs to come to terms with one's heart, and love for God so that one realizes that one can no longer see due to the heightened desire for pleasure, and a kind of blindness that is obviously inconsistent with what is right and wrong; and they must see that they are flouting God's law and Sacred duality.

PART XXIV

TRUE MEANINGS

LESSON 205

SECTION I: SYMBOLS

We are all familiar with symbols. The most familiar of these is, of course, the Cross, and there are many variations of this symbol, each representing a certain time period, such as the Celtic cross, which predates the Christian cross by 3000 years. There were drawings of fish called Ichthys, the Alpha and Omega symbols, and of course the six-pointed star (the "Star of David").

Then there is Ezekiel's wheel, (cf. Ezekiel 1:4-28) the Chariot of the Lord, and many other symbols named in the Bible.

In the Marriage Feast of the Lamb and His Wife, we also witness to the reuniting of the Sublime Marriage of Christ with the Woman of Revelation and the birth of the first born of the firstborn. Eeshans' symbol for this Sacred return of the Son of God for his Bride, the Woman in the Wilderness, is the six-pointed star. This symbol is a triangle pointed upward, the alchemical cipher for fire, which symbolizes God and the masculine ego, the triangle pointing down representing the alchemical symbol for the woman, who is the alchemical cipher for Water. The union of both is the Fruit of their love. Emmanuel. Therefore, He (Jesus) is the Blood, she (Mary) is the water, and the Child is the Spirit.

This star that shone over Bethlehem not only guided the travelers but was also the sign that expressed the love of God the Father and his wife, the Virgin Mary at the birth of Jesus. This time, as each Person shares equally in all things, this star represents the love of the Son of God and his Consort and the birth of the Philosopher's Stone, the One who is like the Son of Man, Emmanuel, who upon his return, will rule as One with his eternal consort, with the rod of iron.

This is the remarkable and incomprehensible mystery that took place between the Spirits and Bodies of the Bridegroom and the Bride in the Bridal Chamber in these times, renewing the vows of the Marriage Feast of the King's Son to his eternal Consort, the Bride he returned for, as prophesied. The Child that was born would be carried off until which time He would return to earth to grow and live his human nature, as did his Father and his Father before him. Emmanuel will then, at the fullness of time, come to rule the world with an iron Rod.

Eeshans believe that symbols tell the story as much as words do. Each piece used in the Sacred and Divine Marriage Feast represents a person and what is happening.

Regarding symbolism, there are equal numbers of references, which some may take literally or symbolically, but, nonetheless, symbols and symbolism are part of our human history dictated by culture, religions, periods of history, and countries, as in flags, used for identification of nations, companies, places of education, secret codes, or for whatever humans can find a reason for which to use them. They are interesting, clever, and provoke cognitive recognition of a body of ideas or an identity. Ancient symbols are mystical and mysterious and always provoke curiosity.

Then there are signs. There are the signs which predict things, signs that show change is coming, as in leaves turning, or winds picking up, denoting weather changes. Our interest is always piqued, especially if there are signs we feel are those that Jesus told us to watch for with regards to the 'rapture,' or 'end of the world.'

What we have been discussing throughout this book are the signs of God's directive to our Eesha regarding the changing of the consciousness of the world, the signs of the return of the Divine Feminine, and the signs of the return of the Sacred Food and Drink necessary for salvation, beginning with Jesus' active role in biblical times.

Those 'signs' have led us to the most important of all signs: and these are what are call efficacious signs, Sacraments, which are more particular to the Eeshan Religion, known as *Mysteries of God*.

LESSON 206

SECTION II: TRANSLATIONS: TRUE AND FALLACIOUS

With signs and wonders come translations. We have outlined the harsh reality of this truth with many scriptures and, of course, any reference, or teaching, about Mary Magdalene, as Jesus' wife. The mere mention, or any reference, by a woman regarding Mary Magdalen automatically raises walls in the human-centered consciousness. When a 4th-century codex, in Coptic, quotes where Jesus refers to "my wife," Karen King, a scholar of early Christianity was viciously attacked by the Vatican just for presenting the fragment for serious and literal consideration. If that doesn't show paranoia, what does? After thoughts that played down to being nothing more than a new attempt at calming claims of ruthless and bizarre behavior, the church has tried to quell this and the outbreak of interest in Mary Magdalen and Gnostic citations by caving in, and calling her "the apostle to the apostles," or "a very important disciple," but again, it is done with double entendre. In other words, it gives a particular wording that is devised to be understood in either of two ways, thus, having a double meaning. Typically, one meaning is obvious, given the context, whereas, the other is hidden and requires more thought.[273] In the law of the church however, with this type of wording being used for 2000+ years, we find that there have been many occasions when it has exploited ambiguity deliberately in a text, or with a translation, or explanation using a homophone (another word that sounds the same,

---

[273] "Double Entendre." Wikipedia, Wikimedia Foundation, 13 Nov. 2019, en.wikipedia.org/wiki?curid=75810.

or that could be used as a pun making it a 'triple' entendre), that can be used any which way the document, phrase, or text chooses to use it. This kind of language was used frequently by church officials with regards to all sexual scandals.

Being that this has been the way things have been since biblical times, and carried through to recent times, we decided to fill you in on this so that you may see God's genius and effort behind humanity's salvation.

LESSON 207

YOU ARE A PRIEST FOREVER, ACCORDING TO THE ORDER OF MELCHIZEDEK

Once believed to be the origin, and basis, for the male apostolic succession, we find it was the role of Melchizedek that set the foundation for what Jesus was to build on. Eeshans believe it was set in place early on because humans need time to adjust to new concepts, and they do so only after much debating and years of resistance and acceptance due to human's fallen rebellious nature.

The obvious interior monologue that we have used throughout this book was to present, by way of repetition, the narrative that depicts our multitudinous thoughts and feelings regarding the resurgence of our Religion and Spirituality, which is the reason being to submit to the brain all answers to potential questions regarding the traditional Christian side, as well as the arguments for our belief that salvation in the fullest sense, as God intended, is found only in our Eucharist of the Marriage Feast of the Lamb and His wife.

We believe Melchizedek was the Divine Masculine God, and our Father, and find, believe, and testify that the Order of Melchizedek forever substantiates both the duality of God, and brings credence to women's ordinations, and is the platform upon which His Wife is truly the first priestess, as she brought 'into the world' the first divine/human Eucharist Jesus and His wife.

Next, Jesus and His wife would bring back into humanity the first public presentation of priestesses, by saying the altars would not have been used by man. As we move in the direction of completing God's salvation plan for us, under the Sacred and Divine Order of Melchizedek, which was to be carried on until the end of time, we want you to get an idea of the complexity of Jesus' work.

LESSON 208

SECTION III: THE UNFATHOMABLE MYSTERIES THAT YOU WERE NEVER TOLD REGARDING JESUS' ROLE

Through mystery school, and the Merkabahalic and Kabbahlic nature of hidden references, now exposed, Eeshans believe that the Order of Melchizedek reveals how this Order of Priesthood was not at all the 'prefiguring' of the apostolic priesthood that we have come to know. It was, in fact, the foundation that provided Jesus the belief system, and Law, as well as the protection He, along with his wife, needed to ensure women's right to ordination, and that is why they did not stop Him from teaching women, and using them in official capacities. Jesus lived the law to show that He fulfilled it.

Preparation for the Mission of the only-begotten Child of God was clear. If Jesus was, thereby, married, by the Order of Melchizedek, both He and his wife could be priests.

We told you that Jesus left for the Himalayas at the age of seventeen to avoid arranged marriage and/or the priesthood of his birth. This is very important as His counterpart's time had not come. In fact, if one wanted to discredit Jesus, this would be how they could do it. For example, to be and remain an unmarried adult without just cause would be a sin against God and the Jewish Law. Knowing this, and supporting Jesus' marriage, Eeshans find it amazing, therefore, that this particular charge, an easy one to throw at Him, and which would surely take Him down, isn't listed anywhere among all the other charges against Him, such as sorcery, blasphemy, breaking the Sabbath, etc., and especially with Jesus being a recognized Rabbi (which were married), this weighs heavily in the direction that Jesus was, indeed, married.

One must remember, that though Jesus did abide by most Laws in his birth religion it was not the religion that Salvation would come through.

With Melchizedek's priesthood 'in place', it was time that the 'gifted' Divine Masculine Child learn, understand, and come to terms with who He was. Jesus would not find this in the Judaic religion. We have support for this notion when, as a little child, to escape the public eye, the Virgin allowed Him to travel to places that would not draw attention to His gifts, which includes what is now Glastonbury, England, mostly the area of Avalon. Avalon means "Apple," and all connections to this Fruit are important. Ava means origin, Avalon means "Isle of fruit or apple." This was a mystical place, and has become known as the place of King Arthur, the famous "Chalice Well," Ley Lines, and the roofless St. Michael Tower, etc.

This instance of Jesus' getting "lost" was His attempt to be closer to what felt natural to him, which was being in his Father's house. At the age of twelve He awed the Temple leaders with his answers to questions during His presentation, or what would nowadays be call Bar mitzvah. At age seventeen, Jesus left for the Himalayas to study without distraction. Later, He would teach in the Temple, but only at certain times.

Here He could would exercise the realities of all those stories regarding the ascents to heavenly palaces and his rightful Throne, as a man. Jesus' 'studies' encompassed Isaiah's and Ezekiel's prophetic visions, all mystical elements, apocalyptic literature, mysticism, the early Rabbinic Merkabahalic mysticism, esoteric Rabbinic literature, and Merkabahalic mystical ascent accounts in the esoteric Merkabah-Hekhalot literature. Included in these studies were:

1. exegetical expositions of prophetic visions of God in the heavens, and the divine;
2. retinue of angels, hosts, and heavenly creatures surrounding God;
3. discussions of worthy sages;

4. those that "must not be explained before two, nor before one, unless he be wise and understands it by himself;" and other studies that can be discussed with only those who was the head of a school, cautious in temperament, and possessed the five different professions requiring good judgment qualities enumerated in Isaiah 3:3;
5. the recognizing of the meaning of Ezekiel 1:4 when he was twelve years of age as demonstrated in the Temple, which he had already done;
6. being consumed by fire (Spirit of God) Hagigah;
7. masteries of the visionary and Merkabahalic exegeses concerning the divine realm and the divine creature;
8. detailed descriptions of multilayered heavens encircled by flames and lightening and about the heavenly guardians that surrounded them;
9. studies and experiences of the highest Heaven, which contained seven palaces (hekhalof) and the Supreme Divine image God's glory, who sat on a Throne, surrounded by heavenly Hosts who sing God's praise;
10. Jesus' full identity, being wholly expressed as what He saw and learned of Himself, explained not only who He was, but details of His descent to earth;
11. Jesus' comprehensions and masteries of inward contemplation.

Interestingly, these Hellenistic 'Works of the Chariot' came *after* the end of the Second Temple period, following its destruction in 70 CE, when the physical building of the Temple was destroyed, which when you play it out with what Jesus taught, is of no surprise. Also, with regards to Jesus, we find that the idea of making a journey to the heavenly *hekhal*[274] was not only what Jesus did, but was predicted, and written of long before He returned, lived, died, and resurrected. It even takes into account His

---

[274] "Merkabah." New World Encyclopedia, New World Encyclopedia, 2008, www.newworldencyclopedia.org/entry/Merkabah.

descent into Hell and His return to heaven, and what He accomplished during those three days before his Resurrection.[275]

It would be in the Ganges river where Jesus would perform rituals with other students, and those who followed Him before His official Mission began. It would be here that He would also bathe frequently Himself, dedicating himself to God: Divine Masculine and Divine Feminine. The Ganges River, interestingly enough, was named for the goddess Ganga, who was noted for her piety; Bhagiratha, a righteous king, allowed her to descend to earth where she might wash over the ashes of 60,000 souls, purifying them, and permitting them to ascend into heaven. This is important since it was in the river Jordan since biblical times that this image involving cleansing and purifying water has been imbued with its powerful symbolic meaning of spiritual rebirth and salvation, when Jesus was baptized in it, marking a seminal moment in Christ's life. It is written that Jesus' immersion in the Jordan sanctified the river's water, and, thereby made it holy. It was then seen as the River of Life, and a divine 'manifestation of God,' since just as the water had been the primeval element that witnessed God's creation, the Jordan witnesses the beginning of the Gospels.[276] Eeshans see it as much deeper than this. Jesus continued His connection with his consort always through water, since He was the light that came through water at Creation. It would always be his eternal Consort's sign/symbol. It also played a great role, since it was at Jesus' baptism that His identity was acknowledged by God.

Jesus' sublime journey to God, and the ability of a man to draw down divine powers to earth, was part of His priestly mysticism; again, that was described in the Merkhabolic texts/scrolls referred to above. Unbeknownst to His Wife, who also had journeyed many times to India, she actually shared in many of His teachings.

Jesus not only taught these things, but lived them, and shared them with His wife. She, too, possessed the gift of healing, as well as other gifts. This is vital to know, since God planned *on their wedding night to fully*

---

[275] Adapted/drawing from the concepts of Merkabahalic mysticism.
[276] Adapted from oriin.osu.edu.

Section III: The Unfathomable Mysteries That You Were Never Told / 885

awaken her to her transcendental identity, once again, because of her 'Yes' to His proposal.

What Jesus brought back with Him to Israel, was what He taught the people throughout India. It would be by these truths, and unfathomable mysteries, that He would introduce the Sacred and Holy love for the duality of God and neighbor. One should also know that Jesus, as *Issa (though his title was "Ish"),* had followers there. The priests, yogis, and other holy men with whom Jesus lived knew the predictions and prophecies of what was to happen to Him, His suffering and death by crucifixion, and begged Him to not return to his home country. However, they eventually did, indeed, travel there and were present at His crucifixion.

Jesus was able to speak to the crowds on every level, from the uneducated to the learned. He was brilliant when tested in the Temple at age twelve, not just knowing the Law, but also the Spirit of the Law, as well. Jesus spoke Hebrew, Sumerian, Aramaic, Greek, Latin, Sanskrit, and knew Coptic hieratic, which is a combination of Demotic and Greek, with hieroglyphics.

Jesus would often speak about those things that the priests of the time held sacred, and believed no one should hear, and that is why the religious teachers, priests and His male apostles had a difficult time, since they were so closely linked to their birth faith, and were not familiar with much, if anything, more. Jesus also taught, using those topics that the 'Jewish authorities' believed should never be broached. That is why when Jesus introduced God as His Father, so then came the claim that He was promoting blasphemy; but it was when He said, 'before Abraham, I am,' and when He spoke His Bread of Life discourse, with the Eucharist being introduced as the "Christs" body, blood, soul, and divinity, it was then that the charges of idolatry, and blasphemy were solidified against Him.

But who revealed these things to His enemies? It wasn't Judas, since Judas was more concerned with helping advance the zealot political party and their cause. It had to be someone close to Jesus, and who was witness to His private teachings, with a fear of what Jesus was teaching. It had to be someone who wanted to be known as a close friend, and one who held the highest place of honor when Jesus was popular among men; but not when the authorities came for Him. It had to be someone *who could get away with 'an eyewitness identification' when Jesus was arrested because he wasn't picked up as a suspect but was let go.*

That is why Eeshans can present such clarity and understanding in proving Peter's inability to transcend, and how by his remaining in the human consciousness, this reveals his clueless interpretation of all that Jesus taught. Peter also feared what he was hearing as it was 'not what he was taught' to be 'God's laws.' It was also how Peter could deny Christ, since first he could not understand anything Jesus taught; and, secondly, he always struggled with the fear that what Jesus was teaching could be borderline 'blasphemous.'

Peter did not understand what alchemy was; and so, the closest he came to understanding what we think of today as *transubstantiation* was along the lines of 'incantations,' *which was something that found its origins in magic and sorcery*. He leaned towards concepts of sorcery, as opposed to what were truly *sacred alchemical words imbued with the power of God*, and this explains Peter's not holding worship services, or talking about the Eucharist after Jesus left, claiming only good works in his letters (if he wrote them). This is not to say that Peter thought Jesus was evil, but that what Jesus taught frightened him, and he didn't want to get in trouble, or face being shunned, or persecuted, especially when authorities claimed Jesus got His powers from Beelzebub.

So many texts regarding what Jesus said were later redacted by the authorities and leaders both of the Old Law and New Law, even those details that might have served as evidence to the Jewish leaders, at the time, that Jesus was God, but ideology stood in the way. Examples include the collection of hymns recited by the descenders and heard during their ascent; and Jesus' prayerful account of 'Sepher Hekhalot, Book of Palaces,' also known as 3 Enoch, which recount an ascent, and divine transformation, of the biblical figure Enoch into Metatron.[277]

Forgetting the church's beginnings under Peter, or with Peter as its figure head, the church, at large, through the years rejects the above to this day, and places these things under the 'hidden years' of Jesus' life,

---

[277] "Merkabah Mysticism." Wikipedia, Wikimedia Foundation, 13 Nov. 2019, en.wikipedia.org/wiki?curid=645381.

Section III: The Unfathomable Mysteries That You Were Never Told | 887

and always separated, and distanced, itself from these topics. There is really no other reason for ignoring, or being ignorant, of this information other than it deliberately keeps a kind of slippery slope towards asking questions leading to the truth, at a distance. Of course, without belief in the duality of natures in God, they would have no understanding of the Christs' mission, and deemed all that was outside of the 'Jewish Laws,' aside from some basic teachings, as heretical. Why Jewish? The church claims the Old Testament teachings are foundational to prefiguring Christ, and it's true *that some points do reflect Jesus' life and death such as the prophets, psalms, Job, and the Song of Songs.*

But without a doubt, Jesus' prophecies warned the people regarding those who would change, hide, or omit his teachings in the future, due to human rational judgment, and He promised punishment, knowing that those who had ears to hear would understand to whom He was speaking of presently, as well. 'Revealing His mysteries to His enemies' would later be identified in the form of Byzantine liturgical prayers, and these 'mysteries' are to be understood as Jesus' transcendental secrets and teachings, along with the interpretation, and identification, of his prophecies exemplified below. As we said before, Jesus very clearly predicted that all this would happen. These teachings, and prophecies, would not be properly understood if anything of their word and spirit would be altered, or omitted, in addition, and in light of the above, the only one who actually knew Jesus best (Mary), would be the same one qualified to teach others about Him.

Throughout history's witness to this ever compounding problem from the beginning, the persistence of memory would, however, prevail, and so, as Jesus predicted, while many of the things He said, and taught, would be altered, or omitted, and many things He didn't say would be attributed to him, the Truth would prevail.

Could it be that Jesus' original prophecy (as illustrated in the Confession of the Twelve, and in other places) was omitted, but found, and emphasized in the book of Revelation, as a tool to support what had previously been removed, and added by politically motivated 'disciples'… for the benefit of those who were guilty of changing Jesus' words?

Jesus says in the Book of Revelation:

> *"For I testify unto every man who hears these words of the prophecy of this book. If any man shall add to these things, God will add unto him the plagues that are written in this book. And if any man shall take away from the words of this book, God shall take away his part out of the book of life, and out of the holy city, and from the things which are written in this book."*

This citation was cleverly, and wisely, placed at the end of the Bible, so to prevent 'any change' within what is called Sacred Scriptures. We can see that this was actually spoken earlier by Christ, and can be found in the Book of the "Confessions of the Twelve," a book deemed heretical by the church. Eeshans pose the question, Was it 'heretical,' or was it taken away because it would change the outcome, and ruin the goal of those desperate to attain, and secure, success for themselves and their own plans?[278] Thus, they, thereby, placed this warning at the 'end' of their 'bible' so that no other 'truth' could be exacted, and those who challenged the words in their bible would be threatened with horrible repercussions?[279]

---

[278] Alterations can be made, but the truth still bleeds through... – Ed.

[279] A bit like placing a substantially weighted curse at the entrance to the tomb of an Egyptian king. – Ed.

Lesson 208A

God Allows Another Wrong For a Greater Good The Order of Melchizedek

What happens next is very important. Once Jesus started his public Ministry He did so under the Sacred and Divine Order of Melchizedek. Because its origin comes from God the Father, and His Divine Feminine consort, it is timeless, but then it was pulled after corruption entered in following Jesus' ascension.

In this way, under the Laws of that Divine and Sacred Priesthood, Jesus was able to teach, and help, the women learn how to work with their spiritual gifts to help their brothers and sisters to freedom. The fact that they were never allowed to participate in Temple, or worship, services before, actually served as a plus. They were not corrupted, nor did they have to 'unlearn' anything.[280] Again, God permitted something bad to allow for a greater good to come about when the time was right.

Today, it is the same. Being under the true divine and sacred priesthood, the Order of Melchizedek, alongside Eeshan Transcendentalism, all 'decent' God-fearing, holy religions 'will know Jesus' and 'must see him as God,' and along with His wife, may through their representations of their culture, be it their Ascended Masters, gurus, sages etc., will experience salvation *together*, since the true God will be known once more; and this is how God will bring about salvation.

Today, the Sacred Food and Drink that was locked away until the return of the Divine Feminine is now realized, and humanity's full

---

[280] These were men who were conditioned by the times and circumstance they grew up in, and who were handed all lessons of life and religion that were passed down through these influences. They would naturally be 'hearing' according to their male-conditioned consciousness. Women, however, would hear, feel, and realize Jesus' teachings through a gradually awakening female consciousness, 'unspotted' by this condition. – Ed.

potential, as children of God, will bring love and Sacred Balance to all humankind. The Mercy Oil from the Garden has also been released and placed in our Tirtha;[281] and upon the Sacred Altars, the Sacred Food and Drink will bring nourishment once more, and God's duality will be realized and revered.

Because the Order of Melchizedek is in its re-emergence, it will follow the Divine Feminine's prompting.

In retrospect, every attempt was made by Jesus to change the mindset of the men; however, his focus then was to "initiate and institute" the fullness of Melchizedek's Priesthood of males and females, which would serve to introduce God's plan for humankind by the return of the Sacred Food and Drink of the Christs.

Because men were rebellious, and stubborn, this plan was halted, and would not come into fruition until the return of the Divine Feminine. Based on the teachings of the *Sophia Perennis*, found in writings outside, and far away, from the canonical mainstream, Mary was, and is, without a doubt, truly the Holy Grail who contained all of Jesus' teaching, as only His wife would.

Eeshan belief is that the responsibility of being the fulcrum and fullness of Jesus' teachings rested with His wife, alongside those of Christ's apostles, who shared willingly in these teachings. Christ Jesus knew, if Peter as well as those who stood with him, continued to reject females, it would secure the patriarchy down through the apostolic line and women would continue to be met with derision as a matter of doctrine. This is where the Divine and Sacred Order of Melchizedek was important for it was intended to provide for Mary's and the Kallahs' protection. It would be their guardian.

That was how it all began. These are just some of the acts behind Jesus' life that Eeshans see as no little task to provide for, and ensure, for the salvation of humanity.

In light of all that is beginning to evolve, it will not be so easy anymore for those from the established churches to convince the faithful followers of Christ, that these uprisings to advance women's rights are just

---

[281] A fitting word drawn from the Far East meaning 'temple' or 'place of worship.' – Ed

the work of the modern age's latest malcontents and heretics, especially now since the resurgence of Eeshan Transcendentalism. It will not be so easy to ignore Mary Magdalen, her Kallahs, and her story, and Melchizedek will no longer be the link to just a male priesthood, or a prefiguring of the apostolic succession mirroring Old Testament Law. One must understand that Jesus is not, nor was He ever, behind hatred in any form; He was for all that led to good and the correcting of wrong mindsets.

To those of other Christian sects, should you find solace in your faith, Jesus will take care of you. Again, it was, and is, those religious leaders in authority who are in the spotlight of judgment, and not the faithful. But seriously, though the bits and pieces may have been fragmented, *by these pieces*, along with mystery school teachings, and most of all with the knowledge of our Eesha, the picture is growing, and when put all together, a puzzle is being completed, and an image is forming, Jesus was married, and Mary Magdalen was/is, and always will be, his Wife.

Without a doubt, no one would know Jesus better than His eternal Consort by the fact that she was His female counterpart as the only-begotten Child of God, the first human, to receive the Christed Body.[282] Through the fullest expression of alchemy by her marriage, and as all three Persons of the Trinity share equally all things, Mary Magdalen is to Jesus, and mirrors the Virgin's conception in her 'Yes' to conceiving, and carrying, within her the Divine Masculine. Like the Virgin, Mary was the first to receive His Christed body, igniting, and reawakening, her own true identity, but, more so, was the first human woman to serve as Priestess, with Him at the Altar of Melchizedek, as eternal Consort, along with her Kallahs. She was one with Him for us all, *representing all women* at the Last Supper where they will pass on their Christed Oneness in this unfathomable Mystery/Sacrament, and will, by succession, bring back the true perfection of other male and female apostles. It was Jesus and Mary who, through the alchemy of their transubstantiation,

---

[282] That term has always been taught by the Catholic church to mean that the very essence of Christ is received by man in the sacrament of Holy Orders, making him the "Alter Christus" (another Christ). It is the Sacrament initiated among the apostles at the Last Supper by Jesus, according to Catholic teaching. – Ed.

instituted the Marriage Feast's Eucharistic Sacrament; and she is the first, and only one, to encompass Him, once again, in end times.

Finally, by our beliefs, we feel we must propagate this precautionary proclamation, that for one who wants to become an Eeshan, *we cannot* in good faith, since Eeshans accept the baptism of another denomination, or faith, simply because from the Eeshan perspective, these baptisms stem from a theology that was deliberately changed by those in authority during the time between Jesus' ascension and the physical writings of the NT, to mean something *different* than what Christ intended. Half the truth is not the full truth. In the same sense, though we must also note that in the Eucharistic sacrament of the church that everyone is familiar with today, and that is expressed wholly in their celebration called the Mass, is from the Eeshan perspective *dimidiated*, as is the substance of their Real Presence; additionally, Eeshans hold that the Mass is not the complete celebration intended by God BUT it did serve to keep hope in, and love, for Jesus alive among the faithful. The consequences weigh hard on its 2000-year abominations of religious leaders, authorities, clergy, and religious revealed through their scandalous lives, but lovingly on their victims (the innocents), though for years they have been ignored, paid off, or silenced.

Eeshans believe that the 'Light' reveals all, since it is said, "For nothing is hidden that will not be made manifest, nor is anything secret that will not be known and come to light." (Luke 8:17), but what we are seeing is playing out from a purely human consciousness. For example, recently we see how the true Light revealed the pedophilia epidemic, only in a limited way, since more grand jury reports are said to be published in the near future. We are now being told that there was/is a set of rules for 'children of priests,' and this should include Popes, Cardinals, and Bishops; however, there is a more elite protocol set in place for them. These are two instances where we see what is meant by whitewashed tombs, where corruption was guised as Truth.

Simultaneously, we find currently that there is a third example. One of the world's most advanced telescopes, at Mt. Graham International Observatory, was named "L.U.C.I.F.E.R.," and that it is so big that its dimensions are two 8.4 m wide mirrors, with centers 14.4 m apart, that has the same "light gathering" ability as an 11.8 m wide singular circular telescope, and detail of a 22.8 m wide one. Why is this important? It is important to show that this is not a mere guessing game, but serious technology; and to further demonstrate the tremendous technology behind this, it is linked to the University of Arizona's large binocular telescope [LBT], located in southeast Arizona, with the Vatican's VATT right next to it. This brings us to wonder whether the book, *Exo-Vaticana: Petrus Romanus, Project LUCIFER*, by authors Tom Horn and Chris Putnam, could well be on to something regarding continuing rumors of the Vatican's involvement in purported closed-door discussions regarding an unusual preoccupation with the search for 'extraterrestrials,' or an 'extraterrestrial savior,' as well as Jesuit astronomers being visited at the VATT, discussing this, and even how the church would go about the 'baptism' of alien visitors.

Though technology in and of its self is not a bad thing, to see how such a plan could be put into effect by way of conferences aimed at looking for ways to distract the masses away from present issues, is bad. Furthermore, the name for the telescope, L.U.C.I.F.E.R., is said to be an acronym; however, people[283] have always linked evil to that name, *aka* Satan. Now this acronym is adding power, and drawing attention to that name by putting the authority of mainstream science, and technology, along with the Vatican's tacit approval (?) behind the project's name and purpose. Eeshans wonder how such brilliant people could not find a better acronym for something of such power. Whether it is owned by, or linked, to the Vatican is yet to be seen. But what is readily seen is how the shock value of the name will now neutralize the gravity regarding evil and darkness in people's minds, since the furthering disconnect between God's relevance from humanity continues. That is why the time for the Divine Feminine is necessary.

In other words, there are two kinds of light. One is drinking in the wisdom of God, while the other is the gathering of information from a

---

[283] Lang, Craig R. "The CE4 Corner." MN MUFON Journal, MUFON, Apr. 2016, www.mnmufon.org/mmj/mmj178.pdf.

human perspective for the purpose of acquiring more and more power and knowledge for a kind of mind control.

As the true Light reveals all, one who is able to develop a transcendental consciousness by this Light will be able to see God's plan for them. In a basic way, when the sheep are separated from the goats, Jesus' people will know His voice, and continue to be enlightened, guided, and strengthened. That is where the Spiritual and Sacred Food and Drink given to humanity by the Christs is not only for salvation but for the healing of mind, body, and soul, as well.

Anyone can receive the Eucharist of the Marriage Feast of the Lamb and His Wife; at the same time, it should also be clear that this is not a carte blanche for calling oneself "Eeshan."

We do, however, put our support behind those holy priests and ministers who have sincerely served and lived and loved Jesus in their priesthood and ministry, regardless of denomination. We understand the goodness and courage of those who saw the errors, but by reasons beyond their control, truly believed that they could not do anything about them publicly, yet sought means to do so privately. These are examples of Christ-filled men.

As far as Eeshans are concerned, there is not much more to be said about this, and certainly we have nearly exhausted discussions with regards to all the things, beliefs, and consequences of the old and corrupt, the human and transcendental consciousness, and these no longer exist in the mind, heart, and soul of the Eeshan. Simply put, we feel satisfied in having used this opportunity to bring forward our own beliefs, observations, positions, questions, and points of contention. Again, though our positions may not suit you, that's fine, so please do remember, this is our point of view, and it need not be yours.

PART XXV

LESSON 209

SECTION I: THE CULMINATION OF CHRIST'S ESOTERIC LIFE

Yes, the Divine Feminine and co-Messiah are back. She returns encompassing He who came first; and while those originally invited may not come, we forget not those by the highways and byways, who, once invited, very well may, indeed, come.

This story, along with Jesus' discourse, sheds light on the destruction of God's recourse directive brought about by what has come to be known as 'Original Sin;' thus, fulfilling another prophecy about the Messia, that when the world is most sinful, it is then that the Messiah will come.

The Marriage Feast is so powerful that it becomes the process, whereby, the Eucharist actually brings back those souls that were led away from the What and Who of God, and into this out-of-control world, to the restoration and realization of 'their' participation in the Divine Natures.

This is why this holy Sacrament and Mystery was brought back to God's people, and is what is celebrated by Eeshans today.

Remembering that our religion connects wholly to the What and Who of God shows the why, and the need, for everyone to come back to the transcendental. The 'ancient' mystical, beyond Merkabalic ('Mer' means light, 'ka' means spirit, and 'ba' means body or reality) and the activation of one's light body, and Kabbalic (or esoteric, which originates with Creation) is what makes us one with God, in a way that was forgotten and almost 'lost.' Now, it has been given to the Divine Feminine, and it is she who is of one mind with Christ Jesus, by God's authority, has, and holds the true protocol for teaching wisdom and many of its concepts. Its Kabbalic, or esoteric, teachings, since they reflect the mysticism, which can only be taught by one who knows God intimately, now bring full circle that which was central to the spirituality given to Adam and Eve when they were first created as one being, and then separated. It now becomes, once again, the tool used by God's spirit to guide us, as well, and, as we stated before, carries with it the Mysteries of God, and secrets, contained within the creation of all that God had given to the first Man and Woman.

These mystical doctrines we are teaching cannot be taught without the guidance of the One chosen to bring them back to humanity. These ancient teachings are what make up Eeshan Transcendentalism, and are brought back into awareness, and consciousness, because of the love and mercy of God, in order to meet the spiritual needs of the people.

Without a doubt, those writings which advocate the deliberate absence of the presence of Mary Magdalene at the Last Supper only supports Eeshans' suggestion that persistent memory reveals there is a reason for the need to return, teach, and witness again, about the Book of Revelation regarding the Marriage Feast of the Lamb and the identification of she who holds the title, 'Wife of the Lamb,' Mary Magdalen. Now, in these times, it is God's mandate to be celebrated. Man's defiance to acknowledge Jesus' marriage throughout the church, becomes the directive upon which the beautiful Eeshan religion finds its resurgence and its fruition in these end times.

What is uncovered is every possible means that others have used to hide a link, or conceal any implication, or suggestion, of Christ being married, holding true to the intention to conceal the truth. For example, in the church's explanation of their Holy Eucharist they claim the existence of the Body, Blood, Soul, and Divinity of Christ's Real Presence. Yet, the element of water used in conjunction with the wine for transubstantiation to take place, poured into the wine before consecration though witnessed, to this day is never mentioned as one of the gifts used.

Liturgically, water finds it roots in the Marriage Feast of Cana, and is vital to the celebration of the Eeshan Marriage Feast. Water and salt are part of the ancient covenant between humans and God, while oil to anoint, and prepare, the vessels for the Sacred Presence and leavened Bread, with a touch of honey for the lips of the Bride to satisfy the Bridegroom, are all necessary for the process of transubstantiation, regarding the work of human hands to complete the necessary alchemical process.

The Eeshan celebration of the sacrament is the culmination of Christ's esoteric life, and love, as expressed in His sacred marriage. Eeshans believe that everything Jesus taught and lived was rooted in His marriage, and is key to understanding God's desire for humankind and the expression and meaning of perfect love, as shared by, and, being in the one God, the three Persons, and the duality of each person.

Eeshans' faith in many ways embraces an Eastern vocabulary and consciousness towards the divine transcendental expression and mystical aspect of God, as compared to the more secular and logic-oriented categories of philosophy derived from the human consciousness, and which is prevalent in the Western world. The logic-based western thinking can be readily observed throughout modern societies everywhere in the world; still, Eeshan Transcendentalism utilizes the vocabulary and experiences of consciousness of the East to explain its unique point of view.

This is especially important when we consider how to talk about the return of the Divine Feminine; since we find that God always has us in mind, and truly it is a Mother's love that is needed now, and as Eeshans we also believe it is a woman that is needed to understand what changes should be made, and who is one, along with Jesus, will awaken that special and unique love called "Metta."

Jesus, being the merciful Son of God, was born to accomplish his part of the plan for the salvation of human beings, and required a progressive and ongoing method of teaching to accomplish what was needed in the short time He had. He most certainly was obliged not only to present His teachings to his followers but to also portray these things in His life, and in every aspect of His public teaching, and to include His relationship with Mary, with whom he shared all things, including His divinity. After He returned to heaven, it would be His wife who would be the heart of all He taught, for she, like us, understood the 'who' and the 'what' of love.

By his sacred marriage He and Mary were first united to each other in divine friendship, the purest expression of God's love, which aided in their marriage to develop pure, divine soul qualities. They transcended the material-based limitations from their society's cultural conditioning, i.e., what and how most people thought, and felt about being a man or woman. The desire, and choice, for a physical and sexual love was over-ridden, and their true nature, as souls before God, was understood and self-realized. Jesus then reversed the wrongs of discrimination against women by his teaching and public displays of affection towards His wife, including the mentioning and use of women, as examples, in most of His parables and teachings. What was an alchemical action is now seen as the ultimate romantic act between two human beings, and it was, in addition, a transubstantiated one.

Lesson 209A
How Deep Was Their Love?

The marriage of Jesus and Mary solidified the love they had for each other. It was, and continues to be, the love that resonates throughout the cosmos, and will be for all eternity. Even to this day, the words they exchanged resound within their hearts and have infinity imprinted upon them. These words are those that were hidden away after the emerald fell to earth and broke into two pieces. Used throughout the Marriage Feast, it not only is the ultimate expression of God's divine love, but because it was also expressed as a human love, its power grounded in the Sacrament of Matrimony can, in effect, alter all things living and dead, since these are the words linked to those which were *hidden from humanity, and never written* for fear they would get into the wrong hands. All religions fear these words.

Immediately, as Mary's identity, the power of her Divine Feminine ignited released the memory of their divine essences. These had to be radically released in her because of the depth of its highly guarded existence since the ejection of the emerald from Lucifer's crown; but also, it would be from this power that she would raise Jesus from the dead and it would be this power that Jesus would use in bringing her Consciousness back. It would also be from this power that the Eesha would reopen all the vortexes and bring forward by ordination her original Kallahs.

The sacred kisses, which Jesus and Mary were said to have shared often, as written in the gospel of Philip, were rooted in the essence of this divine power and expressed uniquely in this tantric love. Witnessed on their wedding night for the first time as humans, it would be this circle, or disk, like light around their Persons. When they kissed a multitude of colors would encircle them, just like those around the sun and moon. This was God's will to be manifested in a radiant array of lights and colors, since Jesus is the Sun, and Mary is the moon, representing God's promise of salvation.

In light of this, Consider Genesis 9:11-15:

> I establish my covenant with you: Never again will all life be destroyed by the waters of a flood; never again will there be a flood to destroy the earth. I am making this sign of the covenant between me and you, a covenant for all generations to come: I have set my rainbow in the clouds, and it will be the sign of the covenant between me and the earth. Whenever I bring clouds over the earth, *the rainbow* appears in the clouds, and I will remember my covenant with you and all living creatures of every kind.

Their *constant expression* of their love for each other was the extension of the Sacred Kiss that they exchanged on their wedding night along with the immutable mystical Sacred Words.

This *tantric* love is a Sanskrit metaphor describing how the consummation of the marriage of Jesus and Mary was accomplished. There were no conjugal relations between Jesus and Mary, because the tantric love they shared united the spiritual with the physical, the male and the female, and in this case, the man Jesus and the woman Mary. The divine and the human comingling, and allowing, for Christ's very essence (as He is God) to unite with the Christ person of Mary, His wife, brought them together as they were in their Divine selves, as One.

With his kiss, and by the immutable word, that He spoke in their public marriage vows, Jesus as husband and Mary, His wife, witnessed to their humanity, while also witnessing to their being united for all eternity.

This is best described using and adapting the wording from the *Pistis Sophia*:[284]

---

[284] *Pistis Sophia*, a Coptic text of Gnosis with Commentary, by J.J. and Desiree Hurtak.

The perpetual Light (Jesus) and (her) glory is so profound that all substances of the maleness and femaleness cease in the oneness of the perfect marriage within the higher Presence. (They) no longer were limited to a body, but (once again) become a being who shares Love and Light with all creations. (Eternity and consciousness dictate that wherever our consciousness emanates there we can manifest our love. Describing Supramentalization and how Mary Magdalen can exist today because of what Jesus did and what they shared as Husband and Wife on their wedding night.) We can take on a body if required, we can take on a manifestation, but we are not limited. Here is the "begotten power" (which the Begotten Child possesses and that which by consuming the Christs, make us their begotten children) with which each of us becomes a fleet being, a super-spectrum creation, and out of our creation come many combinations of the Left Hand and the Right Hand, as well as many combinations of Male and Female forms.

The sacred kiss was the life-creating force and sacred fueling of their incredible love for each other. Eeshans believe that this kiss may be described in scientific terms as possessing the 'perfect version of the hormone oxytocin' in such extremes as to continue their witnessing to their emersion, and immersion, of the perpetual Light from Jesus and the Glory of Mary, which for humans, acts as a bonding potion.

This filled their very beings in such ways that even when they were apart they were never separated. That was why Jesus' words to Mary from the Cross, and again when He ascended back to heaven were so important, because they are the perfection of God, the Divine One, which requires one to have direct cognition of the fact that they knew everything the other was thinking, feeling, and speaking about, and which affected each of them wholly and completely. That is why, and how, we can understand the universal Law of oneness and another spiritual connection between us and God.

Along with what is written above, is to grasp how *the love they expressed was perfected in their humanness. The love Jesus taught began here. To be Who God is, as God is above all things, it is God's essence that must filter down to us since God is the Creator and we are the created. This is, yet, a deeper reality of 'what' Ishvara is. God is Redeemer, and we are those redeemed;*

God is Sanctifier and we are the sanctified. So, as all 'good' things of God come to us, all good things must return from us to God. That is the natural order. That is the true order. Simply 'pretending' God does not exist, or is not part of us, is impossible in every definition of the word and is delusional.

By Jesus' kiss, Mary also conceived and gave birth to his heavenly children in the most perfect way, by the Perfect Man Who is Life Himself, who does not die and who is born each second.

This is a *mystical union*, which defies adequate description. The effects of this Sacred Union are far reaching. First, Jesus is the Divine Masculine of the only begotten Child, known to us as the Son of God, who became man to free us from Original Sin, and restore what was lost by the choice of Adam and Eve for the physical, as only God could, since He is The New Adam. God, who became man takes a wife, His Divine Feminine Consort whom he offers to His Father as His human wife; thus, making her The New Eve through the bond of Matrimony. The two Divines become Human by God's design, and by their eternal begotten-ness the Divine Masculine, as man mystically pulled himself out of himself, and enters into her, the Divine Feminine who as woman pulled herself out of herself, to make her one with Him. This is what is repeated for each of us in the Eucharist of the Marriage feast of the Lamb and His Wife. Just as Jesus and Mary pull themselves as One, we become divinized, as we become one with them in the Eucharist of the Sacred and Divine Marriage feast of the Lamb and His Wife.

Through this original union, the 'children,' who were, once and may still be, solely of the purely human consciousness, are now restored, divinized souls, and are able to enter back into the eternal realm of the transcendental abode of the Kingdom.

This is another unfathomable mystery that enables Jesus and His wife to become our parents, and which also supports the Eeshan belief that we are their begotten children. The following poem was written to explain the reason Jesus kissed Mary so often.

Conceiving with a Kiss

> The Heavenly Man has more
> children than a man on earth. If

> the offspring of Adam are many
> and die, how many more are the
> offspring of the Perfect Man
> Who do not die and are born each second.
> The child cannot make a son.
> He has not the power to make children.
> One recently born is not a parent.
> The son has brothers and sisters, not children.
> In this world, there is a natural order to birth,
> And one is nourished by ordinary means.
> We are 'nourished' by the promise of heaven.
> If we are from the mouth of the Word,
> we are nourished from the mouth and are perfect.
> By a kiss the perfect conceive and give birth.
> That is why we kiss.
> From the grace of others, we conceive.
>
> (Gospel of Philip)

Peter left no stone unturned, and did just as expected. He commented on God, and 'not' blessing Jesus with a child with Mary.

Regarding Mary, Jesus said: "As for the Wisdom who is called the 'barren,' She is the mother of the angels."

The following necessary, and relevant, quotes are found in their respective gospels or texts:

"And the companion of the Savior was Mar[y] Ma[gda]lene. [Christ loved] M[ary] more than [all] the disci[ples], and used to kiss her often [softly] on her [lips]" (Gospel of Philip).

In any event, the touching, kissing, and little public displays of affection were done regularly. These tender moments Jesus shared with Mary Magdalene, as the disciple Jesus loved most, prove that these little intimate acts could not be directed to anyone but Jesus' wife, as per the law, especially with regards to Mishnah. Again, Jesus was outside the Old Law.

> The rest of (the disciples were offended by it and expressed disapproval) and they said to Him "Why do

you love her more than all of us?" Yeshua replies, "Why do I not love you like her? When a blind man and one who sees are both together in darkness, they are no different from one another.

When the light comes, then he who sees will see the light, and he who is blind will remain in darkness."

(Gospel of Philip)

Shimon Kefa (Peter) said to them: "Miryam (Mary Magdalene) should leave us as females (for as you know) are not worthy of life."

Yeshua replies: "Look, I shall guide her to make her male, so she too may become a living spirit resembling you males. For every female who makes herself male will enter the Kingdom of Heaven."

(Gospel of Thomas 114)

Yeshua: "I disclose my mysteries to those who are worthy of my mysteries. [Woman or Man] Do not let your left hand know what your right hand is doing."

(Gospel of Thomas 62)

Seeing little children being nursed, Jesus says, "These little children are like those who enter into heaven." They said to Him, "Will we enter the realm as little children?" As he looked at Peter and answered them:

"When you make the two into one,
And when you make the inside like the outside
And the outside like the inside
And the above like the below
And when you make the male and female into a solitary one
So that the male will not be male nor the female be female
When you make eyes in place of an eye

A hand in place of a hand
A foot in place of a foot
An image in place of an image
Then you will enter the kingdom."
                              (Gospel of Thomas 22)

LESSON 210

SECTION II: CHOOSING TO LIVE ONLY IN THE PHYSICAL/MATERIAL WORLD OBSTRUCTS LOVE

Time certainly has its effects. and it can make false realizations magnified, or it can heal wounds. After Adam and Eve left the garden, the world continued to become more and more materialized in human consciousness, and here we see how it got further and further away from that which God intended for His people. Therefore, over the course of time, human beings have not only become more and more materialistic, rather than spiritual and God-fearing, meaning God has now become an 'option' and is not a *reality*. The God that John Lennon sang about early on (circa 1970) is not 'a concept by which we measure our pain' *but was a concept by which he measured His*. It is by this concept that humans have come to define God.

Reaching the fullness of time, and as a mystical, Kabbalah, Esoteric, Merkabahalic religion, it is the time of the 'Christs,' where civilization has reached a point of flawed development that is so great, whereby, it has come time to teach them; it is time to save them from themselves. In order to do this, however, there must be one like Himself, and also human, so as to, once again, connect love and life to God.

Eeshans hold most sacred the view that because God, as male and female, so loved human beings, even the First Person of the Holy Trinity would be represented in a highly favored way. So, in Eeshan's hearts, that is why it is believed that God's female counterpart, as the first Person Divine Feminine incarnate, was born the Virgin Mary, and this place is revered with utmost respect. That is why the name Mary is said to mean 'highly favored by God' and 'one who loved the Lord unconditionally.' Therefore, maintaining this mindset, understanding that her original form was divine, Eeshans believe, without a doubt, she was free from sin, and has the right to claim that she was the Immaculate Conception. Since God the Father's feminine counterpart was made flesh, she would give birth to his son, Jesus, by a means that allowed for a human birth, while her perpetual virginity remained intact.

In summary, as was promised in the beginning, a New Adam and a New Eve would, once again, be raised up to the original transcendent state of perfect love and spiritual union. Jesus would marry what would appear to be a redeemed woman, named Mary, who was also favored by God, and was chosen for His son. She would be redeemed, as she would be born, *disposed* to the "Original Sin," but not *affected*, the imbalance between the original form of male and female, necessary to link her to Eve.

LESSON 211

Section III: Mysteries, More Than Meets the Eye

Mysteries are such that they have more merit, or import, than what is initially seen as obvious. In an unfathomable truth, or mystery, there is always a higher significance because it involves the Divine. Immediately, one must presume, also, that there are hidden facts, and values, that are unseen, but of great importance to find. The Divine is something of a mystery, in and of itself, since no human outside of those involved with the Plan of Salvation understands what the Divine is.

One of these involves the expression, 'immutable word.' On their wedding night, through by both Jesus' immutable Word and Sacred Kiss, we know Mary was divinized; and, thus, the beginning of the process, or plan, to destroying the seal that was placed on the gates of paradise, which were closed after the fall to physicality was effected.

Here, the immutable word, the 'unchangeable' word, is very important. Since it encompasses universal law by God's directive, Jesus, being the 'Word' of God, could not use anything but an 'immutable word' to show the gravity, complexity, solidity, and impenetrability of his promise and vow. This, along with keeping them from the Tree of Life, was to prevent Adam and Eve from re-entering the transcendental: in their current state, they would have been forever damned (permanently confined) to life limited to the physical plane and realm. Upon their physical knowledge, this would prove to be a very disturbing awakening to the totality of the consequences of their choice. Thus, God, being all merciful, wanted to talk with them and bring them to an awareness of all that was placed into motion.

In a similar way, Jesus' immutable word caused Mary's awakening, first in her true identity, enabling her to remember the reason for her being born. This was the catalyst which would cause a radical renewal of her free will which would guide Mary to continue to 'voluntarily' expose herself to an array of personal choices *she* would have to make to insure her part in the breaking of the seal, which had, thus far, imprisoned humanity. Over time, *this* 'seal,' to the transcendental, came to be known as the "*mark of Original Sin.*"

Through the awakening of her divinity, we have come to understand the 'reunion' of the eternal consorts, as Divine Masculine and Divine Feminine, more clearly, and we see how it immediately brought the Sacred Balance into the world. The harmonious balance in their 'spiritual' marriage consisted of the feminine force, or feeling, united with the masculine force, or reason, and their oneness would demonstrate harmony in body, mind, and spirit. What was initiated, or set into motion, by Jesus and Mary should have been completed for all and to all, but as we know it was interrupted of course didn't happen-partly due to the resistance of followers, even among some of his apostles, because of their adherence to the culture of Jewish Law at the time. The church, under Peter, essentially grew up under this problem, and perpetuated it so much so that most everyone throughout the church's history is oblivious to the true history of Jesus and Mary, and the real purpose of the Messiah, save the relatively few, who have occupied the inmost part of the church's 'inner circle.'

We know that the truth is actually found in the excerpt below regarding Adam and Eve in Genesis, and this is how 'marriage' was always to be understood in the Jewish faith, especially in Biblical times. Upon reading, one learns that what is written in the Talmud is supposed to be traceable back to Moses, and Moses is the supreme authority because of his direct relationship to God. That is why the Jewish leaders, and religious tried to trip Jesus up regarding divorce and Moses' teaching. It is also the version by which Eeshans claim to highlight the many translation regarding how Adam and Eve were created. It clearly defines, also, the equality of the male and female, the marriage of Adam and Eve, and the need for the co-redeemers or co-saviors to be married.

The fact that there are inconsistencies might have been why Jesus held up Moses, in whom they put their faith, as the "one who would condemn them;" therefore, it is safe to presume that what was handed down now becomes questionable:

> When G-d created Adam, Head two faces: one in each direction. G-d 'split' him in two, and one half became Eve. That which was the 'one, that became two.' Thus, when G-d brought Eve to Adam they were reunited as originally intended. Therefore, the union of man and woman is the reunification of a sundered soul. This is why a husband and wife are special to each other, for they belong only to each other.

This not only provides a sound basis for the Eeshan perspective, and reveals the original singular being, but also the equality of man and woman, or male and female, and highlights the importance of the 'soulmate.' Yet, the story commonly taught is of two separate beings, the masculine created first, and the feminine created second.

In marriage, two come together and become "one flesh." The marriage ends at the death of one of the two, but in the case of Jesus and Mary, their love conquered death. Since both were also Divine, death, as Eeshans believe and teach, could be shared in the bodies of Jesus and Mary Magdalene, just as a divine married couple they *shared* in life. In other words, and in the simplest and best way we can explain it, when Jesus died, the eternal component that was awakened in Mary came forth, and with the Sacred Kiss she resurrected Jesus in a glorified body. One may ask then, why was Jesus 'unrecognizable' to Mary in the Garden? This happened because after the Sacred Kiss, Mary's divine nature, once again, receded, due to the component of her human nature, and because His body was His glorified body, His appearance would've been different to her. That is why, upon searching for Him no longer using her divinity, it wasn't until He called her name (those immutable words, "Mary, we will never be separated again.") that her transcendental memory transported her back to her divinize body. We find a similar instance later on the road to Emmaus when Jesus' person was not recognizable to others, until the action of his breaking of the bread.[285]

Why could she not automatically do this on her own, as she raised Him from the dead? Remember, she used a 'kiss' to do this by the memory of the Sacred Kiss on their wedding night, which ignited the power necessary. It was meant to establish her human/divine natures, since Jesus relinquished His Divine nature to Mary, just as Jesus' Mission was coming to that pivotal point of sacrifice, and, then afterwards, Mary would relinquish for a time her divine nature to Jesus, and continue in her human nature. Not all details can be explained, since there are no words in existence that can explain an 'unfathomable' mystery, thus, the name, 'unfathomable.'

Death could not imprison His wife for the same reason, but because of man's failure to see Jesus' mission to include His wife to fruition, at a given time, God would place her consciousness into a deep sleep, until these end times which is another 'unfathomable mystery.'

These things had to come to pass because their marriage reversed the consequences of Adam and Eve's human marriage inherited by their human children, which provided a way back to a transcendental Sacred Union; thus, their mission would end with Mary/Eve taking the last bite of the Apple of immortality after Jesus.

As the resurrected Christ took on a new form, it would be the same for His wife, in the fullness of time, in end times. Eeshans recognize the **'power and Mystery of Matrimony,' and the consequence of forfeiting salvation by choosing a union outside of the Mystery of Sacred Marriage, because the Mystery involves the recognizing of God's Duality and sacred marital union**. To deliberately choose risks apart from this, leading one into oblivion, this is especially important for one receiving the Sacred Food and drink for salvation, since Jesus commanded that you cannot do both. Since the Second Person of the

---

[285] See John 20:14-16, John 21:1-14, NIV. Luke 24:13-35 On the road to Emmaus, also, Jesus spent time with disciples, but it is noteworthy that they did not recognize him. – Ed.

Holy Trinity was without 'form' (as humans understand it), before Jesus, Jesus goes without form, as the Divine Feminine encompasses Him, that He may use her body as necessary to the completion and fulfillment of Jer. 31:21-22; yet, this is another unfathomable mystery. The problem begins when one refuses to accept that the nature of God is male/female. Because it is necessary to accept this in order to properly receive the Sacred Food and Drink, it behooves one to understand this point well, in the light of the Sacred Mystery of Marriage, being the ultimate and sublime union of two human beings.

Though many religious scholars dispute the above passage from Jeremiah, and declare it an omen to bad things, it is not. It's the prophecy describing the sign for the need for a Messiah. How? Just as in an eclipse, since the Light of God was, once again, overshadowed by darkness, woman, who is the 'glory' of Jesus will return it. Just as the Divine Feminine, the water, is spoken of in Genesis 1:2 and Jeremiah 4:23:

> "And the earth was without form and void; and darkness was upon the face of the deep. And the Spirit of God moved upon the face of the waters."
>
> "I beheld the earth, and lo, it was without form, and void."

PART XXVI

LESSON 212

Section I: God's Mystery Encrypted

Eshans believe **that we die with Christ and His wife in THE MYSTERY OF BAPTISM, and when we die, by his resurrection He raises us up and by His wife**, we are then made whole again. Eeshans believe that most assuredly Christ would raise His wife up after her death, and she would teach, as He did before He ascended to the Father, as His mother was still here on earth. We believe as He revealed himself after His resurrection, Mary would, by his authority, continue to live and teach once again after He raised up her consciousness. Why not? All things are possible with God.

This was the plan, as is true of the presence of his wife, who, by the process of supramentalization,[286] is present among us through her consciousness until the time His promise is fulfilled. As it has been said,

> He is preparing His Spirit filled Bride, who is overcoming the traditions of man and the walls of religion; and she will have a childlike spirit and love for Him and the world will stand in awe of her. And those who oppose her will suffer God's punishment. He has prepared a

---

[286] Recalling that supramentalization is when the consciousness of the divine pushes through the conduit of consciousness from the transcendental realm into the realm of the material; that is, the consciousness of the person is overshadowed and infused with the presence of divine personhood. It is different from a given person ascending to spiritual realities and heights from a starting point of a worldly or physical foundation, and pulling back layers of ignorance and fog to reveal the inner light of awareness, to the point of enlightenment. – Ed.

place and has returned as promised to unite with His Bride. He has promised it in His Word.

According to our path, Eesha is the title used to identify the One Person, the Divine Feminine, who Eeshans believe has entered the world by God's word. Jesus did this in order to continue God's Mission of love and salvation from the perspective of Christ's Yin, or feminine nature, His Christ Sophia. Eeshan teachings encompass all He shared with His wife during their earthly marriage, since she is being Mary Magdalen,[287] up to, and including the revealing of her presence through her 'eternal consciousness,' in these end times, as the encrypted Mary [Magd] E [l] len. Once again, amidst turmoil and chaos, a Messiah comes, but only those God intended to know her could/will recognize her. Her life in present time fulfills scriptures as the "lost bride,"[288] and claims this title, and identifies with what is written in Revelation 21:9: "Come, I will show you the Bride, the Lamb's wife."

Eeshan Transcendentalism is founded in part on the revelations and fulfillments of those traditionally obscure scripture passages in the book of Revelation, which we believe are not symbolic or metaphorical. Some believe that the book of Revelation should not be taken literally, or in the obvious sense, that is, the "bride" should not be seen as a specific individual. Eeshan Transcendentalism unifies these revelatory passages, and clarifies the previously obscured meaning of the Marriage of the Lamb,

---

[287] Sept. 2012: An ancient, business-card-sized parchment/papyrus that appears to quote Jesus Christ discussing his wife is declared "real." The fragment was presented by Karen King, a professor at Harvard Divinity School. While the authenticity of the parchment is disputed and is unlikely to be proven one way or the other, it does not matter ultimately whether it will be proven authentic or not; it is enough to know that the notion of Jesus' having been married is not merely a modern curiosity, but in fact the evidence suggests it was a notion that was at least known and discussed to the point of being written down. Does the discovery of the parchment suggest that the Holy Spirit is bringing this, as well as many other historical texts, back to the foreground of Christian experience?

[288] Margaret Starbird, *Mary Magdalene Lost Bride and Queen of Christianity/Holy Blood, Holy Grail*, copyright 2014. We use the song "Mary We Did Not Know You" by Maya, priestess, Order of Mary Magdalene, in the marriage feast celebrated daily by the Kallahs.

and shows how metaphysically and, eschatologically, it is a continuation of the plan of salvation, which began with the sacred marriage feast of Cana, and while being the Son of God, we see the sacred marriage of Jesus and Mary Magdalen being the fulcrum of the plan of salvation.

Other ambiguous passages in the book of Revelation are explained away by traditional teaching, including passages that talk about the bride, the birth of the "One who is like the Son of Man who rules with a rod of iron," and the identification of the Lamb's Wife, and how she resides, as the Woman in the Wilderness, until the time when Christ returns for her.

We believe our Eeshan faith gives credence to the Book of Revelation, and does so in a chronological order. We believe these mysteries and truths about Christ's life, as the eternal bridegroom and Mary Magdalene His eternal wife are undeniable.

Eeshans continue to witness Christ's love for His wife. Jesus, who is the constant in the life of our Eesha, continues to this day to provide signs and appearances to those who have been with the Foundress, giving overwhelming proof, and evidence, of His undying love and eternal relationship with her.

Eeshan Transcendentalism has no desire to compete with other churches or religions, but it is because we are often asked to explain why Christ's mandate was focused on the topics we discussed throughout this book, about those things regarding the reasons why we disagree with the traditional and established Christian religious institutions.

When you remember that this is exactly what Jesus did when He would identify the wrongs, and had no misplaced compassion, or tolerance, for these, and never wavered when it came to God, we are comfortable in fulfilling these directives.

There are, and of course, will always be, however, irreconcilable differences in cultural, philosophical, and theological views especially in present time Christian religions; but with new and relevant discoveries that may, finally, be presented to support our beliefs and revelations, and with the fundamental truths found within our hearts, we are blessed that we can provide relevant references that can help spread, and promote, true love of God and neighbor; and bring out the best in human beings, by starting first within each of us a central theme of love, kindness, and care, which truly constitutes the reasons for God's bringing forward the Eeshan religion.

Even should you disagree with our beliefs, we have at least succeeded in being able to deepen your attachment to your own spirituality and beliefs in the religion of your choosing. Remember, by debating views, we strengthen our resolve, and bring an awareness to opposing points of view, and, perhaps, another possible course on understanding the 'Way' that Jesus provided. Perhaps we do this from the manner in which we have been brought up. have lived by, and, perhaps we have even proved to *ourselves*, interiorly, the reasons we believe what we believe in a more balanced mindset.

In these ways, one can truly say that what they believe is based on 'their' love, their findings, and their needs, and not under duress due to the forceful, or threatening, ways of a being who is self-serving, but, to the contrary, under the inspiration of one who is selfless, merciful, and loving. With regards to the Eeshan Transcendentalism, we want to clearly define the difference of seeing, reading, and understanding Jesus from a transcendental versus human consciousness.

We agree a constructive course should lead to solutions to issues facing humanity today, and not cause, or add, conflicts. There should, and must, be a 'desire' to express the duality of God, which is at the root of the human 'family,' as we know it. We believe that the universal law of balance, with regards to sacred duality, governs creation, and upholds everything in that balance; Eeshans maintain that all this is found in what Jesus taught.

"This law decrees that all spiritual seeds have a gestation, or incubation, period. In other words, when you choose a goal, or build an image in your mind, a definite period of time must elapse before that image manifests in physical results."[289] Eeshans believe this statement best describes the 'why' of all things God, and for the calling forth of the Divine Feminine, the Eeshan Tao, and the Sacred and Divine Food and Drink to nourish us.

---

[289] Adapted from Bob Proctor, and his SGR Program.

WHERE HAVE ALL THE FLOWERS GONE?

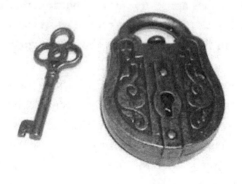

INTRODUCTION

The title 'Where Have All the Flowers Gone?' was specifically chosen for a little pocketsize book.[290] **We are conceived in the mind of God.** If we are looking to find when life begins, Eeshans would say it begins here.

We don't choose when, how, or why we are born or die. One thing is for sure, however, the way we live our life can and should leave our imprint. Hopefully, this imprint is in the form of a flower and not a weed.

We are, each one of us, beautiful, unique, and are endowed by God, the Creators, with talents, skills, and qualities that are intended to be used by us for the betterment of life, liberty, and the pursuit of happiness for all of God's children. In doing so, all living things, to include the earth, its resources, and all its creatures, have no outlet for abuse, famine, or bad choices, with regards to our dominion over creation.

This means that having the right of dominion does not allow for laziness, entitlements, or selfishness, and greed. Right now, laws, rights, and those governing bodies are so murky, and blurred, that it almost seems like an impossible task to fix. Yet, look how fast we can come together in catastrophes and in the face of disaster. We are amazing because we have the blessing to be amazing.

You think you have no talent or skill? Maybe in some way that's good, since one then strives to be the best at what they do. Not everyone is an artist by their own definition. Maybe you are an artist by God's definition. Maybe you don't have musical ability, or you work so hard to learn music, but, perhaps, your appreciation for music is greater than one who can play instruments, or write music, or can even sing. This is a gift in itself from God. If these things make you happy, then you can, in turn, make others

---

[290] Originally created as a separate publication, it is included here. – Ed.

happy. Maybe you have the talent to be selfless, or make someone happy, or smile when they can't find a reason to.

Perhaps you are the 'person' everyone loves to be with, or see just because you are just you. How sad you would be to be the person others try to avoid or to be the one to try to plan things without.

God says, why do you look down upon yourself? Rather, look inward and find what makes *you* happy, any little things, maybe a joke, or maybe listening, or debating, this is good. Work on this talent. Write down your thoughts, your complaints, your fears, what made you smile, laugh, and made you feel like you had a fine day. Then put it aside for one month, and see what you wrote. Write down the bad situations, or problems, and then look back, and see the strength you had to get through them. Help someone. Cut their grass. Wave to a neighbor, even if they don't wave back. Talk to a person on an elevator, or sit with a person you don't like at work, school, or event. Smile. Did you hear these things before? Did you do them? Did you keep doing them, or did you do it once and quit?

Helping, caring, and expressing kindness does not imply over-tolerance or enabling. These are hurtful. Jesus did neither. An honest conversation may be frightening at first, but it truly makes a difference. How the other person perceives it, whether angrily, by being insulted, or even quietly, without response, is alright. It is important not to use truth to hurt anyone. That is why it is a double-edged sword. There are ways to tell the truth, and there's truth that is not necessary to repeat. People who have to 'tell you that someone doesn't like you' because "they can't lie" are not helping but hurting.

Bring beauty with your life, and don't bring what is ugly. Don't use silence as an answer, since people can't read minds. Don't use loudness to do the same. Most of all, become a flower by bringing beauty into the world by your thoughts, words, and deeds. Don't, by any means be a weed.

SUMMARY POINT 1

REASONS THE FLOWERS HAVE GONE

We began this little book (within a book) asking where have all the flowers gone. Eeshans believe the flowers, spiritually centered people, are disappearing because there is no sunshine (faith is diminishing), no water (living water), and no nourishment (true Eucharist) that make them flourish, so that they can pollinate (be the leaven) to bring about more flowers. Who did this? Who starved the flowers?

Though not all of Christian history, and practice is bad, even though it brought a dimidiated Jesus, those who loved God found a way to balance lives, and issues, because of their love for him. That is why it is not the sin of the followers that is largely responsible; the responsibility lies with those who established and created, a tremendous imbalance by not teaching about the Christs and positing only Jesus, the Divine Masculine Christ, *apart from his role with Mary*.

Having come to love Jesus in our own personal and intimate way we are already halfway to what God desires for us.

What the Eeshan religion is tirelessly attempting to do is to bring the whole, the total, the Oneness that has been missing in spirituality. This is essentially drawn from the early template created by Peter, the apostle who walked with and was taught by Jesus.

It was he who then, as well as now, who effectively edited Mary's true role, and rightful place, alongside Jesus, out of Christian consciousness. Thus, everything which followed his decisions, and choices, and those of his later successors, led to a form of worship, and theology, which was truncated, and is not truly representational of what Jesus taught, who he was, and what he came to do.

Any group(s) that preserved fragments of Mary's true writings, or writings about her place with Jesus, to include those from *her disciples* that could be perceived to pose a problem for the establishment of the primacy of Peter, never stood a chance in preserving her role. Following in the footsteps of the Old Testament religion insured success; however, it was mostly due to the love the people had who heard, and, were taught, by Jesus, that kept him alive through those difficult times of horrendous persecution. Later, as the church became more and more centralized, and politically powerful, whatever didn't 'fit' the patriarchal agenda and platform was buried.

In hindsight, Eeshans acknowledge that as so much time and history has gone by with this problem at the core, that everything built on these original problems has made it impossible to reconcile, let alone change them.

There is little question, that institutional Christianity will find the claims made in this document problematic to their world view, is, to say the least, but all that is asked is that one sit and think and pray about the 'what if's. What then, could one do, in the face of this problem and the problems of the world in general? What if all this is true? What if it caused, and resulted, in ages of fear, discrimination, and oppression, all having gone unchecked, leaving the world in apathy? What if responding to the reasons the Eeshan religion of Metta Spirituality was brought back by God's design, and may be just what God's people need to correct the consciousness of the world?

First, came the created 'being' who was separated into Adam and Eve, bringing to our transcendental parents the reason and the mystery of Marriage, also reflecting the duality of God. Next, God became human to address the issue of inequality between men and women, as in the beginning God created a state of equilibrium between them.

From the above problem of imbalance comes althea forms of discrimination and prejudice. As you can see, this discrimination between the genders of male and female; and, thus, in turn the physical human expression of man and woman, filtered down into using and identifying all those things that make people different (culture, color, race, age, etc.) as a basis for such discrimination; it is based in fear and the impulse to oppress.

The human consciousness sees only those things that make us different from one another. History shows that the church has never intervened to correct these problems or has done anything substantial to stem the problems arising from, and at the heart of, discrimination. To the contrary, the church turned its head, so as to not have to give its opinion in what would have been, for them, politically delicate situations. They do it today in order to avoid negative press, and will offer socially just proclamations through the news media when it is expedient, or if it is politically beneficial to do so. The church has had 2000 years of experience in perfecting the art and science of public manipulation and perception. None of this is therefore new to them.

But with regards to the church's responsibility on the issues of discrimination through the centuries, it was actually guilty, itself. of being part of, and wavering on, the issues in question by using Old Testament Law rather than New Law. Never should there have been a reason for hate, discrimination, or prejudice; since if there was, Jesus would not have welcomed everyone unconditionally. He would not have eaten, or sat, with people of other cultures who were lumped in together under the title "sinners" by the religion of the day. If taught by Jesus' true teachings, the truth would have been carried down through the ages, and humans would have known appearances, like book covers, that do not always reflect, or summarize, the contents within them.

We would see the beauty of each gender, that could be recognized as individual, or can be found to be combined as originally found in the androgynous being first created by God, and before separation. And, as physiological studies show, there is a part of each gender in each of us. One may be stronger, and match up with regards to their physical birth identification, or the gender identification, that may not show up until sometime after birth.

These insights, and understanding, of God's creative powers and love, would not have resulted in humans condemning other humans for matters that are out of one's control. If only all this had been made known through the meaning of love found in 1Corinthians: 13:3, so often read in church. Eeshans love the Now Living Translation, which ends with: "If I gave up everything I have to the poor and even sacrificed my body, I could boast about it; but if I didn't love others, I would have gained nothing." What happened as a result of choosing the physical over the transcendental that shows the consequence of entropy is the loss of innocence and ignorance of sin, which is this filtering down to choosing to see race, color, culture, etc., rather than human beings.

We believe that the realization of 'male-female' equality, where one can find true love, goes hand in hand with the sanctity and expression within marriage of a genuinely true love, being the pinnacle reasons for God's plan of salvation.

Christ's Marriage was, and still is, more than an example of obligation to establish rights and obligations, and not just for the union of a man or woman to each other in this Mystery, or to form a familial bond and procreate, but to establish a foundation for the whole human family. Love between the partners must first be the foundation upon which to build the preceding.

Jesus, being represented without his counterpart Mary, is to dimidiate Him and lends to the absence of an origin to the foundation of marriage, especially as His marriage is the human manifestation of God's duality and love between Consorts. Even the notion of thinking that the use of the term, or any class entitled "pre-Cana," while denying that the Wedding Feast of Cana was about Jesus' marriage, is used as a requirement for teaching about Holy Matrimony? Where is the connection? How could Jesus be only a guest at the wedding, with no mention of a Bride, the occasion known only for its being the event of "Jesus' first miracle." and be a support and be required before marriage? These teachings are not only superfluous, and wrong, but an insult to anyone who has ever questioned this misuse and flagrantly offensive, no less glaring lie, set down by the church in, yet, another contradiction.

These misrepresentations in scripture are not only confusing but have taken all that God is, and all that Jesus had accomplished, and made it scandalous by propagating this lie as truth that cost God's people the fullness of Christ's mission. Shockingly apparent and conspicuously bad in the way it is taught, people were brought up believing that Cana was important only because it was Jesus' 'first public miracle;' since there is nothing about this event as being Jesus' own marriage, it is a misrepresentation and is contraindicative to use the title, 'Pre-Cana' for marriage preparation classes.

Jesus' marriage was a marriage of oneness. He was joined with His Wife wholly and completely as the kind of perfect union described in mystery schools. Theirs was a dynamic of Sacredly Balanced Yin and Yang, male and female. Everything Jesus taught witnessed how God intended Holy Matrimony to be. The vow two people make to each other in the Sacrament goes beyond words. It must be ever-present, and displayed in marriage. From this love flows love of family and unconditional love, and from that love flows love of neighbor.

It was most important to Jesus. as the Son of God, that His marriage to Mary not only manifested a human mirror that witnessed the Holy, Sacredly Balanced union of God as eternal consorts, but in its wake, would arouse a conscious awareness, which would counter the wrongs of all kinds of discrimination, beginning with gender. Because marriage is truly the two becoming one, not only in the flesh, but as soul mates, and as His love for Mary raised the place of women to equal status to men, Jesus showed how He looked past the biases against women. By talking with the Samaritan woman at the well (in eastern Orthodox and eastern Catholic traditions purported to be named Photine, meaning the 'luminous one'), He not only taught her and revealed to her the secrets of who He was as Messiah, but also the mysteries of the Living Water. With this discourse, He broke the bonds of gender, religious, and cultural biases.

Jesus taught, "When you make the inside like the outside, and the upper like the lower, and when you make the male and the female into a single one, so that the male is not male, and the female is not female, and when you make eyes in place of eye, and a hand in place of a hand, and a foot in place of a foot, an image in place of an image, then you shall enter into the Kingdom."[291] This teaching was unique not just because of how Jesus described the union of a husband and wife, but especially in light of the reason that women were seen as almost not human at the time, since they were equal to that of an ox, as well as other human beings outside the Jewish culture who were considered chattel. He intended the end result being that we mirror Him in how we love our neighbor.

---

[291] Gospel of Thomas, Saying 22.

Gender discrimination is the toxic core of the problem. which encompasses and feeds on the finding of reasons for people to discriminate and judge.

In the last fifty years, what began slowly, soon grew into a massive gender identification focus, and one that was not for the good. First gays came out. Lesbians were lumped into the word 'gay' because they seemed to embarrass anti-gay groups more than the men. Parades and protests were next, with the church backing anti-gay discrimination, by calling for them to 'accept their cross,' while denying the ongoing reality of homosexuality within the church at large; in its hierarchy, priesthood, and within its seminaries, in effect hiding the fact that their own popes, cardinals, bishops, priests, and religious lived this lifestyle behind their walls, freely.

Transvestites and drag queens entertained the masses, and somehow seemed less harmful. But when we first heard about AIDS, it rapidly became seen as God was finally punishing these gay 'abominations.'

One thing led to another, and this issue grew and grew, until it not only separated 'God's' people, but also families, forming a greater gap. All of these caused questions as to why God created them this way, when the church pinned them between unrealistic ultimatums, such as the church telling them, on one hand, they must carry their cross and accept it, to other possibilities, i.e., that they can be accepted, so long as there are no physical, sexual relations between them. Questions regarding marriage brought only more attacks. and most of the time were dismissed immediately as an impossibility and a sin.

As we discussed earlier in this book, one time a gay man, whom I find adorable, asked the question whether God created him this way just to hate him? He loved Jesus, dearly. People I posed this question to said I should have replied:

1. NO, he just hates your sin;
2. NO, and you can change;
3. Why do you want to make Jesus cry?

So many daily communicants and self-righteous people judged that these "kinds" of people made Jesus cry, and surely God will punish the world, as was done in Sodom and Gomorra. If they read the truth about these cities (or if they had any direct experience with certain middle Eastern cultures, such as the Bedouin, or among the foothills of the Himalayas, when Jesus was traveling there on pilgrimage, where hospitality is a sacred duty and responsibility), one would find it was the cruelty of their radical inhospitality, to include rape and sodomy etc., forced on visitors who did not register to come into the cities, that brought about God's vengeance, but, of course, the masses were never taught this.

As the battle for same sex marriage, and their ability to adopt and raise children raged on, they were met with studies to prove how these "gay marriages" were going to corrupt 'straight' children, and act as a contagion that will spread and kill the populous. The studies 'proved' that same sex marriages were dysfunctional. I guess we cannot find these issues in heterosexual marriages, in hostile divorces, or in 'normal' families.

Now, it is said that little children as young as two or three have been found to feel the opposite of the gender they look like. Parents who support their children are blackballed or shunned for supporting this mindset.

Be aware of karma. Be careful what you profess as a judge. The Universe likes to deal out Karma. The Laws of the Universe are given by God. Jesus taught them. You should read them, since it may be to your betterment.

Mothers seem to be more understanding than men and fathers. What happened? Why do we attack human beings who had no choice in how they were created and born into this world? Jesus did not discriminate, nor was he prejudiced, so where did these judgments originate? Some say Leviticus; but Jesus changed all that. Those who love Jesus are not of the Old Law, apparently, they are not of the New Law either.

One wonders now, is it an evil spirit? God works in mysterious ways, and is not 'always' intent on looking for ways to punish us. What if these issues are being dredged up, and God's feminine spirit is working to end discrimination by teaching us that we truly cannot judge a book by its cover; thus. forcing us to see the person beneath the skin? Isn't that what a loving mother would do? Wouldn't she put the children who are always bickering *together*, to teach them how to get along?

Humankind must understand that as there are so many reasons to hate, there are that many more to love one another. Getting rid of negative thinking opens doors to living, and understanding, that love is love. One cannot love conditionally, and say they are emanating Christ, when Jesus himself loved *unconditionally*. 'Love your enemies' may very well have been understood as, "love those you don't want to love because you don't like something," or because you were taught not to love them, due to skin color, hair color, or eye color. Just as this sounds as ridiculous as discriminating, or carrying a prejudice, because of the color of hair, or eyes, so, too, is how judging one another for other reasons must sound to God.

Today it isn't just the above that we judge, is it? Now it is just as popular to judge in even more ways, such as generation titles: baby boomers, generation X, and Millennials. Baby boomers have been around for a long time. They are known for their acquired wealth and savings. They have, as a result, influenced all industry and politics. They have worked hard and are conscientious. They worked and worked so their children wouldn't have to. Is it possible that these are those same children we worked for and who may have been spoiled, that have become clueless, perhaps even self-obsessed? Could these have become afraid, and when in positions of educational, or political authority, passed on to their students, or children, arrogant and ungrateful attitudes, which seem to have fallen onto the Millennials? Let's face it, we are all victims in one way or another; but we are also the cause of chaos and confusion.

That's why we all look to a greater Being. Someone who is not corrupt, or who loves us unconditionally, and has only our well-being and interest in mind, and who will also correct us when we are wrong. for our own good and the good of other humans, be they family, friends, or neighbors.

SUMMARY POINT 2

The Eeshan way began first as revelatory spirituality in 1998, three years after our foundress met with Pope John Paul II in 1995, when she first presented documents about her work. When she met with the Pope, the wounds of Jesus came through her hands, feet, head, and side before him, and all those present. Closing his eyes, he said, "What is this?" To which she replied, "You tell me," handing him her writings. After taking the writings from her, he advised her: "Do whatever Christ asks of you." Immediately, Jesus whispered to her, "Ecce Homo," and it was then evident to Eesha that even though the Pope had given his advice, it was God whom she listened to.

This was Jesus presenting Mary Magdalen to (the successor of) Peter, that He (Jesus), was closing a cycle that was merely allowed in God's plan, for his own divine purposes. Without a doubt, Eesha knew in her heart that it was time. The two met for the first time since Jesus, the Bride versus the Impostor. With God's plan and design, she began revealing Christ's directives, as intended, and this plan was to represent Jesus to His people, showing them that Jesus is God, *not a religion*, and that no one has a corner on Jesus' love for us all. This is why our way is primarily referred to as "Eeshan Transcendentalism," as opposed to simply the "Eeshan Religion." Too often the word 'religion' attached to a name like Eeshan carries with it means, as in 'just another religion.' Eeshan Transcendentalism sets itself apart by declaring that at the heart of what it teaches. and practices, Jesus is not a *religion*, but that He is God.

To those who have had the experience of attending Eesha's talks and instruction on holy scripture, would witness how she always challenges everyone to read and compare her (and now our) views with:

- the history of Christianity and the Catholic church;
- biblical teachings and gospels;
- Gnostic traditions.

From scriptures to the Inquisition to the canonization of saints, there is, beyond the shadow of a doubt, evidence of many, sometimes elusive, suppressive, and corrosive methods that were used, and continued to be used, to retain Jesus' followers over the centuries, and these who did so, were thought to have been entrusted with, and taught, the truth.

This pattern of corruption was not limited to just the church. It can be found in other religions, as well, not to mention any human institution for that matter. Without addressing the source of the problem (which is the illusion that we don't need a God), it doesn't matter what a human being will build. for in time it will fall from within, or it will be conquered from without, because of the lack of ethical and spiritual fiber. This should not be, and it cannot be righted. unless the actual plan that God expressed through his son is implemented, *according to its true design*.

Eeshans assert that the above, coupled with the exclusion, or omission, of Gnostic Gospels, books, and writings, that, when reintroduced into these books, and as companions to the traditional Bible, do prove valuable in properly imaging the person of Jesus and God's reason for his plan of salvation.

These are the exclusions that raise questions as to the reason for quite an extensive and peculiar redacting action taken on the part of authorities, and presented as though reading these writings would cause a descent into heresy?

Eeshans believe that people, given guidance, are capable of reading, and deciphering what is in keeping with the reverence and sacredness of Jesus, and can deduce from these materials many credible objective and subjective components for themselves.

Where many of these Gnostic manuscripts, or gospels,[292] provide tremendous insight into ancient universal spiritual principles and doctrines based on eternal truths, they also:

---

[292] The Gospel of Mary Magdalene, the Gospel of the Beloved, the *Pistis Sophia*, to name a few.

1. Are fairly intimate (though still incomplete) accounts of Jesus' hidden years;
2. Describe Jesus' time spent as a student-turnedmaster while living in the Himalayas;
3. Allude to or describe the time he spent with the Essenes.[293]

There are also those found writings which give a different outlook, like the Dead Sea Scrolls, which of course could contain many writings that possibly reflect the point of view of those who did not like Jesus, or his teachings, and wrote things that were not true in an effort to discourage, or turn away even faithful disciples and followers.

Except for some rare, and obviously vague mentions of Jesus' affection for Mary Magdalene. as his "adoring disciple" nothing else about her, other than being known for being a repentant adulterous woman. is what made its way into books, writings, and movies, aside from this, and private authors, little if anything else surfaces, piecing together a version of "what could have been a relationship."

Apart from the fact that there is not a lot of historical material available regarding Mary (and what is out there is vague, spotty, or still missing whole sections), what has been found over the years do include some things that were written to imply there was a relationship other than that of the Master to a student. These, of course, were condemned, and placed on the Index of Forbidden Books.

One must realize that the term "Gnosticism" itself is from the ancient Greek word 'gnosis,' which means *knowledge* (not automatically a heretical word as some would like you to think). Gnostic traditions and gospels mainly received a 'bad rap' because, in time, they came to be seen as blasphemous, or filled with myth and made up stories, because of the stamp the church put on them, which the people naturally were conditioned to believe. People were also conditioned to think that Gnosticism, a heresy, was focused on 'secret knowledge,' and was associated with magic and the occult, and that it would make people think they didn't need the church's authority, since everyone could go to God on their own.

---

[293] Noteworthy is the Essene community's regard of women's equality with men, and their place alongside men before God. – Ed.

In truth, Gnosticism did have more to do with an experience of the Divine from within, but it wasn't about the amassing and collecting of elitist knowledge and information about God for the purposes of making oneself equal to God. This is important to remember.

Should you delve into the transcendental writings, such as these, unguided, you could, indeed, cause yourself confusion, especially with the onset of such interest in books, which are designed to bring you in touch with the meaning of Divine Intelligence. Wonderful books such as J.J. Hurtak's *The Book of Knowledge: The Keys of Enoch*, which the author claims comes from direct experience, can confuse the reader, and it may even contain material which conflicts with what Eeshans teach. This is all well and fine. Enlightenment will eventually bring everything full circle.

Caution must always be exercised, especially if trying to understand such reading material via only the human rational consciousness. Before the Divine Feminine, books such as these were truly utilized as a goad because the *word carries with it the feeling that other heresies had been branded with as well, the sense that it is somehow of 'evil' origin, and would infect the pure Christian's mind with poisonous ideas, which would certainly lead to damnation if one followed them, or even read them. The main issue, one could easily argue, is that the church was concerned the people would grow to distrust the authority of the church, and take their faith into their own hands.*

Of course, the reason given was to ensure that Christ's sacredness, true identity, and His teachings were protected. This is a very useful image that comes into use if one compares the same to the religious teachers of the old Law that made up laws and spoke on behalf of God. But, one might ask, could the church authority who was speaking as the voice of God, commanding souls for their own good to not partake of the 'tree of knowledge' be doing so because it had something to hide? Well, it could have, and it still has. Perhaps, therein lies the irony, of who is really speaking for God, and who is speaking on behalf of the human consciousness via the human ego. Remember. too, that enlightenment means that one must be open to hearing concepts, which, at first, may seem to conflict with one's own ideas and opinions, or other transcendental, writings, since they may just be seeing the same truth but from a different perspective.

Besides the general sense of gnosis as meaning "knowledge," the term unpacks, as the various senses of enlightenment, salvation, emancipation, and even oneness with God. It is also important, too, that one realizes that these writings were labeled 'heretical' for their appearing to deny historical and orthodox fundamentals of the Old Testament.

One wonders, if, perhaps the chief fear among those who suppressed these writings was the same fear that possessed the Pharisees, and the rest of the establishment at that time. This fear has surfaced throughout history up to, and, including recent times. It is the fear that one can have one's own relationship with God without a religious authority interfering. Some say, if one can look 'within' to where Jesus said the Kingdom was to be found, then maybe the faithful won't need a hierarchy and authorities to control their spiritual lives, and to tell them what to think, what to feel, and how to live.

SUMMARY POINT 3

It has also been said that many have deemed the Gnostic religions heretical mostly because of the positive role of women in them.

Another important point to consider is how the mounting research and discoveries related to these texts, and other accounts cause many of today's faithful to ask questions that are not satisfactorily answered simply by saying one should accept the lack of information, and accept what is being told to them on faith, alone.

The human heart longs for more clarity on these questions, and, as it does so, Eeshans believe that because there *is* more. This conclusion (that scriptural evidence is scanty, and this is all there is to go on) would be acceptable as long as there wasn't evidence and enlightening research today that wasn't available hundreds of years ago. When there is overwhelming evidence, or a strong basis for a piece of evidence that could quite possibly point to a truth, this should be examined, and not suppressed and silenced because it does not fit in with, or is perceived to threaten, the stability of all that has been built up so far.[294]

These findings, which supports a belief and/or complete a truth that eliminates sin as defined throughout the ages as deliberate attacks on or against God, if they challenge religious authority, could possibly, if brought to light, correct the wrongs and end discrimination and preserve faith. When such evidence is hushed, rejected, or ignored, one might ask if it is protection to uphold faith that is being taught, or are we seeing

---

[294] In this connection, it is interesting to consider that scientists and archeologists also face this problem, when they come across a glaring discovery that clearly will upset the prevalent theories that reign at the time. The same potential penalties loom: loss of career, being professionally disgraced, ridiculed, and being dismissed and buried—all because it brings down a house of cards, embarrassing and provoking the deep-seated fears of those who ascribe to and loyally support the hand that is feeding them. – Ed.

the fallacy of invincible ignorance? In other words, when something is brought to the attention of the people in authority, and the authority simply won't hear it, or acknowledge it, isn't this simply a form of institutional denial? Is it not so much a fallacious tactic in argument, as it is a refusal to argue in the proper sense of the word? Is this yet another unique method where the institution can make assertions with no consideration of the objections? Can this be what Jesus meant by 'whitewashed tombs,' and was this at the heart of his teaching on 'knowing them by their fruit?' In other words, has Jesus, more or less, followers today? And why are the churches empty?

In light of new discoveries, research, theories, and evidence presented by scholars and researchers, and thanks to today's availability of information, by way of modern communication technology, Eeshans hold the opinion that despite the advancements enabling the discoveries of such accurate and deep perceptive texts regarding Jesus' hidden life and marriage, many of the older faithful still seem to be in a kind of spiritual lockdown. Many are well entrenched in what they have been conditioned to think and believe, and the thought of change, especially of what could be a drastic change, is clearly out of the question for them. That's alright, so long as they are not negatively biased, judgmental, or hateful.

People very easily can be made prisoner of their social and educational conditioning, so that they are not able, or willing, to think outside of the limits that were handed down to them, again, because they feel that right or wrong, there is no other option outside what the church says. They will hold to what they were told was 'the Truth,' even though they see and question some, or most, of what they know to be wrong. Why? It is probably due to the use of words like 'infallibility' and quotes such as, "even the gates of hell will not prevail against her," while not understanding the true meaning of those words. The church need not be something like the Vatican, nor does it have to be a Catholic, or Christian, establishment. As Jesus is not a particular religion, it is His truths and teachings, and the one who houses the "truth" that Jesus was talking about.

Sadly, only few understand the origin of these terms; or how these comments, if in the wrong hands, may use such quotes for the retention of followers. In many ways, these forms of spiritual lockdown become the mechanism that kicks in when the mind knows, or suspects, that certain ideas could threaten what is currently providing a sense of security regarding reality and world-view. In other words, one surmises that 'even though this teaching makes sense I better not let go for fear of losing something that doesn't make sense.'

This spiritual lockdown, under the guise of, and perceived as, faith and loyalty, in the past, appeared to have been the cause of the outright rejection of any evidence, or even a discussion regarding possibilities, on the basis of 1) fear of committing a sin, and, subsequently, offending God; or 2) being seduced by evil's suggestions and going to hell.

Fear is a very powerful tool for control. Just suppose the quote above was in reference to Jesus' *wife*, and not the church? What then?

Even despite the realization of pertinent facts, and plausible theories and truths, the desire for further investigation is dismissed, and deemed against the true faith and God. This mindset one can easily find embedded deeply within many Catholic and Christian teachings and throughout church history. Again, this mindset is not limited just to Catholic, or other Christian denominations, or other religions either, but they are used as examples by those raised within the faith. Threats, fear tactics, and guilt have been used in propaganda, and have been effective in just about every walk of life.

SUMMARY POINT 4

Eshans conclude that turning a deaf ear to a possible truth, even though there is the fear of further questions arising about core beliefs, and what has been handed down, or that those core-beliefs could be shaken, serves no one's best interest. Too much suffering has come about with truth being buried by those thinking it was in the people's, or the institution's, "best interest." If anything, the research, and findings and fresh approaches to theology and scholarship, handled responsibly, could only ensure that Jesus' teachings can bring souls closer in spirit and not just in letter. Looking seriously into all that has arisen in scholarship, and research, may well continue to pose more questions about what those who followed Jesus Christ have been told for generations and even through the ages, with what they truly believe now.

Leaving questions by women, and other minorities, unaddressed, or unanswered, suggests a self-serving goal on the part of those who are entrusted with the responsibility of leadership. Ignoring all of these things, and waiting for the next distraction to arise in the world to take the spotlight off of controversial issues exposed, are only more and more clearly being perceived, by thinking people, as a deliberate attempt to cover up what they are beginning to see as deception targeted at God's people. and as retention methods to keep them fearful, confused, and under control.

SUMMARY POINT 5

Eeshans are taught that faith drives a soul to seek truth in order to know love, and serve God, especially when there is failure by those who claim to be upholding the source and summit of truth, but truly and emphatically seem to completely fall under Christ's description of 'whitewashed tombs,' and "Woe to you teachers of the law and Pharisees, you hypocrites! You are like whitewashed tombs, which look beautiful on the outside but on the inside, are full of the bones of the dead and everything unclean." (Matt. 23:27)

Because of the total disregard of relative evidence, coupled with scandal and the ever-increasing loss of followers today, and the suppression of discussion on hosts of issues, we must ask, "Who is it that claims to have the fullness of truth, but instead is found to be full of sin and scandal, and causes the loss of faith to abound?"

The Eeshan religion claims that as Jesus is the Way, the Truth, and the Life, the finding, or re-examining, of these centuries-old missing truths, and the desire to discuss the bigger picture, which the church is intent upon suppressing for the sake of its own survival, can only strengthen the soul's relationship with God, not weaken it. But perhaps what is really being discussed here is the instinct for survival in an institution, which has taken on a life of its own apart from God, versus the silent majority of souls waking up and wanting to be fed truth, and seeking to develop a personal relationship with God that does not require the intervention of men to control that relationship.

As Jesus is the Word of God, and He is Truth, it is imperative that we search and find as much of what He actually taught as possible. And it is important to be able to read all that was written about Jesus, and have the freedom to make up one's own mind, and draw one's own conclusions about what was written. As scriptures have been translated over and over, and as humans have access to God's word in print, solely under man's discretion, Eeshans believe that wherever a human being is involved, most assuredly. there can be error.

Eeshans have always delved into the Mysteries fully aware of this ... and they will not be naïve. Humans are prone to be indecisive about too many things. It has always been said that "unless you stand for something you will fall for anything." It is important to be open when searching for the truth, since sometimes it is hidden, like a rose, amidst thorns, or a tree in the middle of a forest. It isn't up to an institution with leaders having the same trouble with the human ego as anyone else, and more than likely not being innocent to the way of power and politics in obtaining positions of authority, to say to those following Jesus Christ, "You are only allowed to look at "this set of writings here," but you may not look at "all that over there;" and, as to what we said you may read over here, we will tell you what you are to think, and feel, about what you read, and what rules to follow in your day-to-day living based on these things."[295]

---

[295] The United States was originally founded on the principle of religious freedom and freedom from all forms of tyranny. Under the old law in the old world under the previous form of consciousness, people simply were subjects in one form or another. Freedom means having the freedom to govern yourself; and this means that one may govern one's own life with God under sound principles of spiritual life that, in the Eeshan point of view, are drawn from the Eternal Wisdom, or Sophia Perennis. In doing so, Eeshans believe, this timeless wisdom that is the property of no human being will guide one to a clearer understanding of Jesus Christ and his mission to restore the Sacred Balance between male and female before God. It is not about land acquisition, wealth, power, lording these over others, persecuting those different from us, and controlling what others think and feel so that what we build apart from the love of God becomes more and more invincible and influential in controlling worldly, political events. – Ed.

SUMMARY POINT 6

Everything so far discussed is assembled with the calling within Eeshans' hearts to enter more deeply into the mystical marriage of the soul to her Lord, as compelled with the awakening of this ancient, mystical transcendental religion as defined earlier on. We believe that the addition of the compilation of our beliefs, teachings, and research continues to satisfy the mandate from God to gather and bring to God's people the truth and Way back to the transcendental. Once again, in this connection, we repeat that some may find what we believe, and profess, regarding this mandate to be contrary to what they believe as taught by their religion of birth or choice. That's fine. Again, this is *our* path and *our* beliefs.

The underlying philosophy of the founding of the United States, may be the place where in God's design, this spiritual path initiated by Jesus, will be resumed.[296] God's love promotes religious freedom; whereas, one can believe, and exercise, and live a system of beliefs suitable for their own relationship with God; however, it is noteworthy that so-called freedom from religious/institutional tyranny and oppression was the very force which suppressed the truth, therefore, for two millennia. What's most important is finding your own path on your journey to God and the happiness you seek.

Living here in the United States, as well as in other parts of the world, there is the freedom to do just that. The inspiration to pursue religious freedom is slowly spreading throughout the world, since former ways of power, and control, are gradually undergoing subtle changes, and small, but effective, means are now going beyond the control of the

---

[296] Recalling that Eeshans maintain that this spirituality is the *continuation of Jesus' original plan and ministry*, not an upstart religion based on what a person, or group, believes inspired them about Jesus Christ and the varied writings surrounding him. – Ed.

various authorities, and are increasing in number outside of the once-feared religious establishments.

Long before we had technology, religious leaders had an advantage, since they were in charge; and, thus, could, and did, prohibit access to any, and all books, contrary to church teachings, including books of spirituality that paralleled Jesus' teachings, or provided a different point of view of his teachings. This directive came under penalty of excommunication.

The great stigma attached to these writings, that were either branded heretical or were placed on the Index of Forbidden Books by the former religious authorities, is not so much feared anymore; people previously lived under the fear of being excommunicated by obtaining, reading, and discussing these writings, and the church saw to it to drive the fear home. People were essentially not allowed to 'search' for the truth or explore outside the walls of the church on their own. They weren't even allowed to read 'unauthorized' Protestant bibles.

No longer is the mandate in force that one must not read the Bible without the direction of authority; this 'rule' was in fact insulting to the intelligence of God's people, and implicitly stated that they could not be trusted to understand 'correctly,' without being told what a passage meant. Once again, this served as a tool on the part of the authorities to control what the people thought and felt. People were simply told that the scriptures contained language that, without expert guidance, might be 'misinterpreted.'

Today, the fear of excommunication, and persecution, for wandering outside the walls of what one is permitted to read, think, and feel, wanes with dwindling membership, the loss of respect, and faith, in church leaders, a growing cynicism and anger for the lies, scandals, and cover-ups, and the continuing forms of discrimination and oppression on the part of authority. Religious authority, today, however, simply does not have the same power to intimidate the masses through the tool of fear as it once did. Moreover, the cry for the Messiah's return amid these scandals, and the increase in corruption and violence and suffering, has become more prominent as God's people need to know that God is truly there.

As day-to-day life and peace is threatened, lack of trust in the government rises, and a greater demand for the protection of human and civil rights prevails, and more and more we see the world turning godless. An educated people now challenge old teachings with the desire for adequate answers to their burning spiritual questions, and some form of proof that God exists, especially that everything people are suffering through is for a purpose, and that their lives and struggles have the meaning Jesus taught and the merit they deserve. The hypocrisy and scandal of religious institutions, and leadership, being at a crisis point, and as the very foundations of faith are coming into question, people continue to wonder, and really need to know how, if there is a God, could such evils be permitted.

Despite the desire to find a scapegoat over the years, many are coming to see that it is not God's fault that these things are coming about unabated. People are coming to see more and more that this is the world that they themselves have built by their own choice ... and all that Jesus taught about responsibility is coming to pass in frightening detail. This is, without a doubt, due to the return of the Divine Feminine.

Even amidst the suffering, there is plenty of room for hope, in seeing that all this suffering exists in the world is experiencing are like the labor pains of childbirth. Although presenting difficulties now, when these difficulties finally pass, something beautiful will take their place, and life will begin again anew. And this is where the Eeshan's attention and faith is focused.

SUMMARY POINT 7

THE CONTINUATION OF SUPRAMENTALIZATION: SACRED TEACHING

Could the following little poem predict the long-term plan of Jesus?

> God's plan had a hopeful beginning
> But man ruined it all by his sinning
> We trust that the story
> Will end in God's glory
> but at present the other side's winning![297]
> —U.S. Supreme Court Justice Oliver Wendell Holmes

Well, 'Anonymous,' hope springs eternal, and as God is eternal, so is God's love for us. Sometimes we fail to see that in order for God to help, we must want something as much as God wants it for us, and in a selfless way, and not a selfish one.

One must realize that the ending of scriptures is a love story which was prophetically revealed in the parable of the marriage of the King's Son. This was a clue to Jesus' plan, and has become an integral scriptural passage for these times. The verses regarding the Marriage Feast in heaven, being the marriage of the Lamb and His bride, and the verse identifying the Wife of the Lamb, surely denotes a connection to the

---

[297] Lefever, Ernest W. "Ode to Limericks." OrlandoSentinel.com, 23 Oct. 2018, www.orlandosentinel.com/news/os-xpm-2006-08-01-limrick01-story.html.

woman in the wilderness in human form. One explanation was that this revelation was the birth of Jesus, which had to be reinterpreted to avoid the possibility of another woman other than His mother, who could be Jesus' bride or wife. The other explanation was the use of the "church" as His bride for the same reason.

The bible indicates that in ancient times, people of Israel betrayed God. Eeshans believe that the chosen people of Christ, who claim their religions are founded on the love and teachings of Jesus, are betraying Him in recent times. The Spirit of God is that which brings truth, not by those doctrinal laws, or human perception, or intellect (cf. Matthew 11:25-27), but it is brought about from within the heart, soul, and direct intervention by God and divine revelation (Matthew 16:15-17). Jesus' teachings are freeing with love NOT due to threats, fear of oppression, or punishment, and, most of all, they are not discriminating.

Following the pattern of ignorance, and sin, one can see that there is definitely something wrong, or lacking, for our world to have become so self-righteous that it no longer accepts that God ever existed, let alone accepts that we are subject to any superior being.

Our faith knows that these are signs that connote debauchery in its highest form, which clearly indicates loss of spirituality as a result of the lack of teaching the sacred truths from sacred writings, leaving God's people governed and led by human consciousness. Given these truths, Eeshans believe that in this chaotic and disastrous world where truth is determined by the imperfect mind of man and not by the commandments of God, it all gives credence to a need to bring about the fullness of His mission. To do this, Jesus, the Word of God, promised to return for His bride, since it is also prophesized that "a woman will encompass a man," which in those days was seen at their marriage ceremony where Mary circled Jesus seven times, exhibiting that she is the wall of protection for Him; in these times, our Eesha, too, creates a wall around Him with her Kallahs (ordained women), now protecting them both. But this verse in Jeremiah has only been partially revealed. The verse also is a prophecy for end times, where the two soulmates that were first one, then separated into two human persons, will unite in the end as one being. Since it isn't unusual for Jesus to come through His wife privately and publicly, and to this there were, and are, eyewitnesses; for this must reflect these truths, which have been hidden for centuries and revealed in these times.

That is why Eeshans see the return of Jesus to our Foundress in 1987, and her ministry, which involved the Stigmata, as well as visible changes in her physicality. both in a general public setting to witnesses during the more private setting of the Passion, healing services, speaking engagements, and the unexplained, but beautiful phenomena, surrounding her gives witness to those who believe, that the prophecy of Jesus returning for His bride has been fulfilled.

The onslaughts by all those of ill will (hierarchy and laity) on her solidifies this truth. Like her soulmate, she continues on with her work, bringing with her a new spirituality, a 'religion' in the truest and best sense of the word; thus, ignoring the attacks, as she continues to hold testimonies of proof safely hidden away, since this will be used by her Spouse when the time comes.

SUMMARY POINT 8

'I WILL HELP'

There are plenty of signs of good and encouragement. God's hand is still moving in the affairs of human beings, as God had promised from the beginning, "I will help." So, presently one sees the resurgence of recently published gospels like the *New New Testament*, the compilations of *Gnostic Gospels*, the stunning book *The Beloved Companion* by Jehanne De Quillan, the *Pistis Sophia* by J. J. Hurtak, and *The Second Coming of Christ*, by Paramahamsa Yogananda and other well-written spiritual books have already replaced fear with spiritual knowledge and inspiration, for those who are searching. Many are frustrated, and disillusioned, by their birth faith, many search for truth, and many believers don't want to look like fools for believing in God and Christ, and exercising faith in an overly materialistic and faithless world. There is new life budding up everywhere, but it must be sought after and nurtured, and this requires hope, energy, and optimism with regards to what is possible with God.

The brave and confident devotees of Eesha continue to believe in Metta. As many women's and religious groups try to bring about equal rights to women, and to all of God's children and who continue to question what kind of God supported discrimination right from the beginning of the history of human beings, we say, "Don't despair. Move with the Holy and Sacred Spirit of God. All you are seeing is the human consciousness' attempt to reimage a perfect and sacred Being who possesses Sacred

Balance and love." The image of God through history in many ways has been marred with the superimpositions of angry, fearful, and vengeful human beings. They created an image of God based mostly on what they themselves were. But there is an opportunity now for that time to pass.

At long last, we introduce our *Tao*, our way, our path, our spirituality, our *manner of life*, which is a "sangha" (community of like-minded students and practitioners), and a body of beliefs that are completely informed by God's love, this *METTA*, for the betterment of God's people, and to bring about the enlightenment of the heart God truly intended to exist in the center of the human person. This Metta, the true love taught by Jesus Christ by, with, and in His love for His wife, to correct the wrongs created by greed, covetousness, pride, and covertness, this is the true essence of what the word 'gospel' means.

We now feel obliged to share the truth, since we know it is better to light just one little candle than to allow darkness to continue in the world and deprive it of life. We feel our religion is that candle that is now present in the world, and faith must be propagated in order that it make a difference and support those of like mind, heart, and spirit. This is necessary for the betterment of all women and men, males and females and those whose definition, understanding, and experience of gender still waits outside the walls of previously defined, more traditional language, to be acknowledged.

SUMMARY POINT 9

GOD IN THE HOLY EUCHARIST AND LOVING THY NEIGHBOR

As we have discussed, the most compelling gift God gave us, we were told, is the Holy Eucharist, not the familiar Eucharist, but the Eucharist of the Marriage Feast. The underlying question that posed considerable concern for Eeshans in their religion of birth is, "What are the repercussions of God's people not getting all Jesus wanted for them in the Mass, especially in the Holy Communion at a Mass?" Where the Eucharist was supposed to contain within it the most sublime mystery of Christ, what happens to the people when what they believe this is only partially true? Once, while our foundress was attending a Mass before a speaking engagement, she witnessed an incident where the priest celebrating the Mass ran of hosts. The sacristan immediately ran to get more altar bread, and without delay reminded the priest that the altar bread was not consecrated, to which the priest replied, "They (the people) won't know the difference." Right then and there, the people weren't getting even the 'Eucharist' of the Mass.

This in itself is, indeed, an unfathomable mystery. In other words, the people may not have known, but their souls did. Famine is the lack of food to nourish the body. Everyone knows and witnesses when there is no food. It is certainly sad when a priest has no conscience over distributing unconsecrated altar bread, replacing the dimidiated nourishment for the Light Body and soul, because no one would detect it. Or, would they? Without being given what Jesus intended as the "means and spiritual food necessary to attain salvation" definitely would show signs of famine, but to deliberately give unconsecrated altar bread under the guise of consecrated that it is unconscionable. Unconsecrated altar bread, no Sacrament on reserve, and the exclusion of Christ's marriage only adds more flagrant insult to injury.

That is why the people, without a doubt, are not responsible, so, therefore, they are under the umbrella of faith in, and love of, Jesus.

But to address the fact that the reimaged Eucharist brought about by Peter (as defined by his legacy), is from the Eeshan point of view only one part of what we were intended to know and partake of, we must ask. What if (according to the teachings of the church of Peter) the priest does not believe in the real Presence of Christ, or whose intention is like the priest who had no concern for consecration, and is as guilty as he who does not even believe in the Sacrifice, then what? All of these already take place at the hands of the priest and have all the appropriate consequences attached.

But what if all the above are intact, then what? Then because of the faith, and love of Jesus by God's people, though they had been, and are still only getting half of what they should have been getting, the Divine Masculine part, the Divine Feminine will bring them under her umbrella of love. You see, unless His eternal consort and/or His marriage in Cana is recognized, He is restricted to being partially presented to His people, but also His Mission is totally misrepresented throughout the doctrines and theology of the Eucharist and in the Liturgy of the Word. However, we have the souls of all those who love Him, and it is our responsibility to love and nourish them as best we can. Though they are not getting the fullness of what God intended, they are getting the *benefits*.

Since the knowledge of both Jesus and Mary was to be spread throughout the world, no one knows the truth about both of them. That is why only a few question the legitimacy of the Eucharist they have been receiving. Whereupon, the several times that Jesus had come to our foundress at the 'Consecration' of the Mass, she was highly criticized in front of hundreds of people. Priests were outraged. In fact, one such priest actually condemned what Jesus was doing, saying out loud, "What does 'He' think we are doing behind this altar?" Apparently, Jesus was righting a wrong! Maybe the priest should've taken a good look and asked himself that very question.

When our Foundress was then told to "not" receive from Jesus this way, or to receive from both Jesus and the priest, she refused to do so. To receive from a priest after having just received from Jesus, would admit that what Jesus was giving her was not valid. By the way, the host was witnessed firsthand on her tongue each time by the priests and laity.

Without the context of the divine marriage, the redemption of humankind through the restoration of the male/female sacred composition of the human being and God's intention regarding marriage does not occur. With this truncated understanding of Jesus' teachings and sacrifice, Christianity cripples itself and the faithful are not spiritually nourished as Jesus had intended they be. Moreover, to not be nourished at all, as with unconsecrated altar bread, or by having the Eucharist thought of as a mere 'memorial' of what had taken place at the last Supper, is beyond what can be considered detrimental.

Under the Eeshan guidelines however, though thought to be outrageous by Catholics, as they believed it was Jesus' directive, it turns out to be the wiser of all decisions. For as Universal law dictates, 'For every action, there is a reaction.' To have received a reimaged Eucharist has, indeed, affected the world. All one has to do is look around.

Over and over, one was told that faith is based in 'mystery.' But this definition of mystery encompasses transcendentalism, and the omnipotence of God, not the intention to avoid questions, or lack of answers to desist from opening a Pandora's box. The average person is taught that God can never be truly approached and *known except by direct experience.* Jesus, in the Eucharist, as Divine Masculine, along with the Divine Feminine, were given to us for that purpose.

To receive the true Eucharist, it embodies both Persons as One, gives humans direct contact with God through ingestion, and total physical and transcendental intercourse, whereupon, the Eucharist, therefore, affects the energies of mind and emotion that we call thought and feeling.[298]

Through this introduction of spiritual (Divine) Light, these energies not only become one, but bring about a new energy pattern. This energy pattern resonates with, and increasingly conforms to, the Divine inner

---

[298] Paraphrased from newlightbody.org.

nature of each human being. That is why today, though one gets the Divine Masculine in what the church calls the Eucharist, without the Divine Feminine, their Eucharist, as we have come to know it, *is not* in its complete form; and, *thus, the new energy pattern that resonates lacks the conformity and balance that God intended.* It is the love and mercy of God that allows humans to enter into this relationship or truly experience love. As long as God is kept out of reach of the people, the masses (people) will always believe only in the powers that be, and that is how they will be kept in place, and never serve as mediators of the mystery, or as the leaven Jesus talked about. Nothing will change.

SUMMARY POINT 10

Peter's Legacy Perpetuates

When one realizes that Peter's actions led to keeping everything copacetic with regards to his birth region, and forcing Mary out of the picture, without a doubt you will see how this gave way to his being the 'the leader,' and establishing himself as the 'rock' on which is legacy was founded, and from which it continued. Without the Divine Feminine represented to counterbalance the Divine Masculine, the Second Person of God is not, therefore, going to be properly understood, nor will his wife's presence, and her being a reality and the icon through which the Divine Feminine can be known, be represented properly in human consciousness.

The current understanding of the Eucharist pales with regard to Jesus' true intention, since it is in the context of his extended mission that we are freed and strengthened against our proclivity to fall into illusion and perpetuate endless cycles of human suffering. The original effect of this is truly all illusion since it can lead to sin (where one's continued imprisonment will eventually become hurtful to oneself; and, thus, affect others) and this leads to delusion.

The original choice of Adam and Eve now left them *no choice* but to enter the material world, and shows, that under the illusion of Satan, they became delusional in their thinking, that in eating the fruit, it would somehow bring them the sensation of a deeper and more expressive love.

By contrast, Jesus' mission involving His wife was for the purpose of rebalancing the sacred male/female dynamic with enlightenment, where the transcendental component is shown to exceed the human physical love. while simultaneously demonstrating Metta, the love of God; and, thereby, opening the door to a freedom from oppression in all its forms to include the misconception that love's embrace rooted in pleasure is greater than true love, which does not depend on personal sense gratification. Under Peter's structure, this doesn't happen.

In Eeshan Transcendentalism, the *Sophia Perennis* teaches that in the celebration of the marriage feast, a complete alchemical change takes place beginning in Cana with the miracle of the water and wine, followed by Jesus and Mary's wedding night, thus bringing about the reality, and meaning, behind Christ's first miracle of transubstantiation. This 'first miracle' laid the foundational truth which was played out throughout Christ's marriage, last supper, passion, death, and resurrection. The entire alchemy concludes with the final outcome in the transubstantiation of transforming bread, wine, and water into the shared Body, Blood, Soul, and Divinity of Jesus Christ and His Wife, and as we are grafted into them, we are one with God's "Perfect and Sacred Union of Male and Female on the Divine Scale."

It is beyond comprehension that humans can actually enter into such an unfathomable mystery. One cannot help but marvel at the lengths God has extended in order that we witness and receive the purest of love. The love that the Eternal Consorts share within their own matrimony, is showered upon us, and seals within our souls, the sacredness, which is the mortar necessary to build, and solidify, the male/female soul-mate union within the individual through, with, and in God. This blessing is then experienced physically when this love is manifested in the mystery of Matrimony between a male and female, bringing with it the intended transcendental component. It is this love that balances this male/female dynamic in the relationship, since it offsets the 'Fall' to a purely human consciousness and finite relationship.

SUMMARY POINT 11

Our Lifeline to God Defined

Receiving the Holy Eucharist in the celebration of the Eeshan Marriage Feast combats the effects and the energies of illusion, the pull of temptation, and provides the strength to avoid the near occasion of (or actually entering into) sin, and the corruption to one's self and those around one, which flowed from any wrongful act or ill-intentioned person. It's set as a foundation in one's soul as the Way of Christ, while cultivating and nurturing the healthy growth of the male-female polarities that are intrinsic to every soul. In other words, this is our lifeline to God.

The expression of the Holy Eucharist reveals God's full intention. All who receive it in honest and good faith, are in the grace of the Christs, and choose to follow them, and live the What and the Who they are as the only-begotten Child of God, our Saviors and our Redeemers.

This Eeshan faith is not a set of ideas, or principles, to be thought about, but rather it is a *state of being* that determines the presence of God and the degree, thereof, that commands the 'way' which one must actively practice with a deep sense of full personal responsibility.

Through each and every celebration of the Sacred and Divine Marriage Feast of the Lamb and His Wife, this heavenly gift, this divine, and sacred relationship with God, blessings are brought, and grace is bestowed upon a suffering earth. The teaching of Christ with regard to the Holy Eucharist, as found in Mark 6:34, Matt. 14:14, and Luke 9:11, flowed from what He taught His disciples about this divine re-balancing. It was meant to show how God has given the means to not only deepen one's love of God, but the Sacred Food, the Eucharist, is likened to feeding the soul as it is to feed the hungry, that they may be satisfied.

Jesus describes this perfectly when he talks about heaven, purgatory, and hell as they are represented in our lives and what it will be upon our death.[299] This means that when Jesus said I am the Way, He was showing us that all our choices continually determine our destiny, and, in following His teachings, a path is cleared for us so that even if we stumble, we need only follow the light and our soul will make it to heaven.

Jesus makes it clear, however, that we need this food, to offset the "apple" and in order to have eternal life. For example, if a life continues with Jesus/God, we will see heaven as we imagine it to be, just as a person who defies God, and lives in rejection of God will inherit the consequences of *that* choice.

There is no secret that Jesus' dissertation in John (Mary) 6:53-58 is vital because we must ingest them to stay connected to God in the way in which Jesus spoke.

As Eeshans believe, and as we have discussed countless times, herein, the Holy Eucharist of the Marriage Feast is the *only way* to salvation. This is our belief. We would not, however, reject receiving the victuals of Holy or Sacred Food, upon attending another faith's service, nor do we reject anyone who comes forward to receive our Eucharist. It does not, in any way render a betrayal of what we believe.

In the ingestion of the mystery of our Eucharist, we are part of the Divine and Human bodies of Jesus and Mary; and, thus, will cause the soul to hunger for good and love in the world and be satisfied. Love will once again triumph over lust, and life will, once again, flourish and have worth, since He holds the key to the dream of finding the perfect love of God and neighbor.

---

[299] Essentially one is in the process, all one's life with all one's thoughts, words and actions, of building a universe that one will inherit after the transition of death. Hence, the highlighting of taking a deeply conscious sense of personal responsibility towards the use of one's will, throughout this document, what one inherits after the transition of death, is being built in the here and now, in present time. Hell, purgatory, or heaven are all real choices that one makes, and has the ability to alter, at any given moment in life. These realities are personally chosen by the soul. – Ed.

SUMMARY POINT 12

THE VASTNESS OF GOD'S PRESENCE AND WORD

A person's state of mind is of paramount importance, and this is why, today, more than ever, the world around us seems to be suffering from a deep depression, because there is a lack of faith, hope, spirituality. and a well-informed conscience. This most certainly affects a person's state of mind. Concern and obsession with the physical body have in too many ways replaced spirituality. Lust has replaced love. Immorality has replaced morality. Irreverence has replaced reverent actions. Impurity has replaced purity. Violence has replaced peace.

The mind, body and spirit *need* spirituality. Spirituality prioritizes what is important, while it calms, and strengths, the goodness, and kindness, that Eeshans believe is at the core of every human being.

One could say the Eeshan philosophy draws from the insights of the Srimad Bhāgavatam, and they would be right, since vast is the Wisdom and Word of God, and blessed are those who seek and find the Lord in all holy and sacred writings:

> My Lord, I consider Your Lordship to be eternal time, The Supreme controller, without beginning and end, the all-pervasive One. In distributing Your mercy, You are equal to everyone. The dissensions between living beings are due to social intercourse.

Jesus taught that God lives in everyone's heart; therefore, one should understand that religions that are not Christian, yet they reflect a Deity that encompasses Jesus and His wife in the form where identities match, especially in Krishna *bhakti*, will one find God. Spirituality is a personal thing. Eeshans do not judge, or turn away from, the love and faith of those who love God in another faith or religion so long as the faith is not violent, or morally or ethically, corrupt in its teachings.

The purport teaches that God is infinite and the witness of all our actions, good and bad, and the result of our actions is God's reaction toward them. Reactions to our actions are destined by God, but destiny is exercised by choices. Eeshans interpret the translation to agree that there is no use denying that we do not know why and the reason for our suffering. We agree that one may regret the misdeed for which one may suffer at this present moment, but one must remember that God is our constant companion, and therefore, knows everything, past, present, and future. And because we see Jesus, as others see Krishna, we feel that God destines all actions and reactions; however, these destinies are the result of choices we have made. God is the supreme controller.

Perfectly expressed and worded, Eeshans too feel that all those devotees of the Lord should not misuse their freedom, as Jesus offers the *conditioned souls* (those who live in the material world and are inevitably deeply shaped by it) both happiness and miseries that life in this world must be faced. This is how Jesus would answer those who looked to fate rather than destiny: though all is predestined by eternal time, meaning that all the daily issues, all we encounter in our lives are subject to our choices about how to handle and accept this, negatively or positively.

Paraphrasing and drawing from the above quoted scriptural passage, we could say that as we have miseries uncalled-for, so we have happiness also without asking, since they are all predestined by *kālá* (eternal time). In other words, God reigns over the good and the bad, and it is what was chosen by God for us to use to find our way back to God, and to bring others with us. Eeshans see these difficulties not as curses but rather as tools, talents, and gifts that are to be used for refining one's understanding and practice of divine love. In this sense, no one is either enemy, or friend, of God. Everyone is suffering and enjoying the result of their own destiny.[300] We believe that as God gave us the tools and talents, and as God set up our exile, it is all viewed by Eeshans in answer to God asking, "As you are given these things: wealth, poverty, health, sickness, notoriety, and freedom, as you are forgotten or oppressed, popular or friendless and lonely, will you use these tools and talents to find your way back to Me?" Though God has chosen this destiny for us, will we use our destiny by making good choices now rather than turning our destiny into our fate?

---

[300] "Srimad-Bhagavatam—Canto One" by His Divine Grace A.C. Bhaktivedanta Swami Prabhupada.

SUMMARY POINT 13

THE CELEBRANTS OF THE SACRED AND DIVINE MARRIAGE FEAST OF THE LAMB AND HIS WIFE AND THE DIVINE LITURGY OF CANA

Eshan Kallahs (timeless consecrated priestesses who have stepped into time) have been given a gift from Mary Magdalen/Eesha. This "gift" is the Sacred and Divine Marriage Feast. It is rarely seen in and of itself, since it is only used privately for spiritual strength and as a transcendental connection between Mary Magdalen and her Kallahs. It includes prayers, songs, Eesha's writings, Marriage Feast Vows, Revelation prophecies to include the birth of the Firstborn of the Firstborn, which is in regard to the Divine Family, etc. This particular celebration is only witnessed by invitation, and when it is revealed, one gets a glimpse of it in its entirety, since it is also the heart and soul of high holy day celebrations. The public can witness this on certain occasions, and it tells the story of Jesus and Mary's love for each other, ending with the story of the fulfillment of their love in these end times, with references taken from the book of Revelation; as well as, "There are three who testify in heaven, the Father, the Word, and the Holy Spirit, and they are one, and there are three that bear witness on earth, the Spirit, the Water, and the Blood," 1 John 5. It tells the story of the Fruit of their love, who is Emmanuel, the Holy Spirit made flesh.

While only the Kallah's celebrate the Sacred and Divine Marriage Feast of the Lamb and His Wife, both Eeshan Kallahs (brides) and Eeshan Chatans (bridegrooms) celebrate the "Divine Liturgy of Cana," which was written by the Bride of the Lamb for her husband, to bring back a ceremony that teaches reverence and sacredness of the Divine. It restores the Sacred Food and Drink, since it, too, reflects the sacred marriage of Jesus and Mary, linking the fulfillment of several end time prophecies to include the return of the mystical "Order of Melchizedek," as source and guardian to the Eeshan Transcendentalism, uncorrupted and linked directly to God the Father, who began this order prefiguring the perfect line of priesthood.

Since it is God's plan for humankind, this Order is the male component of the Eeshan religion, from which the men learn, and prepare, to protect the Eesha and Kallahs, as well as the secrets of the Sacred and Divine Marriage Feast of the Lamb and His Wife for the mysteries of the Sacred Union, just as the extensions of the Kallahs, or the women of Mary Magdalen do. Both come together since Sacred Balance is restored and rediscovered, and both come together in all worship duties and celebrations.

SUMMARY POINT 14

JESUS TRIED TO EXPRESS THE TRUE REASON FOR HIS COMING, HIS MARRIAGE, AND HIS DEATH TO PETER

Eshans see how Jesus saw,[301] and how He showed us, through the fulfillment of the parable of the marriage feast of the king's Son, to see with eyes of spiritual depth perception.[302] Here we see Jesus' prophecy, showing how the time would come when those who are given the invitation to the divine restoration plan would choose not to believe, due to lack of faith and belief, out of fear, or due to the pressures of a birth religion, or a culture, or maybe even, perhaps, according with the world's desertion of God. As a result of one's chosen allegiance to either the kingdom of the world (the civilization of man apart from God), or the kingdom of God (which is potentially within us, as Jesus taught, and must be chosen and lived), comes the choice of fate, or destiny, and following the human consciousness, or choosing to rise to a transcendental state of consciousness. Eeshans include here the following summary,

---

[301] Eesha, being Jesus' wife, would be intimately qualified to teach according to her husband's truest intention. She would know his mind and heart on all matters of His ministry, more than any of the others who served in the capacity of apostle.

[302] And it is especially noteworthy here to see the parallel between depth perception requiring two eyes, just as Eeshans maintain that proper spiritual depth perception requires the 'two eyes' of male and female, husband and wife. – Ed.

which gives insight into the beginnings of man's choice for the human rational consciousness, after Jesus. It is a collection of events one might call the 'beginning of the end,' or the fulfillment of Jesus' comment to Peter, "I say to you Peter. Before the cock crows three times you will have denied me." These prophecies define not just the three denials of Pete, when Jesus was arrested, but the three denials that would change the course of Jesus' plan for us.

SUMMARY POINT 15

PETER

We have discussed and compared at length the effects of man's choices, the outcome, and loss, of the transcendental consciousness, the cause for the return of the Eeshan Path of Metta spirituality, but when, and how, did things get so out of hand? Fact: Peter did not like Mary Magdalen and coveted her place alongside of Jesus. He insulted her. Peter never really transcended his birth religion, but instead chose to keep close to it, out of fear of persecution, even though he was compelled to stay with Jesus because of Jesus' power and authority. Hence, we see an appropriate application of "You cannot serve two masters, for you will end up loving one and hating the other" (or choosing one and denying the other).

After Jesus' death, Peter no longer saw obstacles to expressing his disdain for Mary, and by his rejection of her, and removal, came the rejection of the Divine Feminine, which he could not, or would not, understand. Because of this series of choices Peter made in taking control, and asserting, his will in terms of leadership, and control, of the direction of Jesus' ministry, Peter essentially chose the way of the world as a template for the continuation of Jesus' ministry, which would inevitably fail to achieve the Christs' objective. Eeshans believe that Jesus was addressing more than just Peter's thoughts when He said in Matthew 16:23, "Get behind Me Satan! You are a stumbling block to me; you do not have in mind the things of God, but the things of men." This was an example of one of the many times Peter's thinking, and actions, were addressed by Jesus. Other passages will be incorporated, which will include Peter's refusal to transcend and his outright refusal and denials of Jesus' words and actions.

But what was behind Peter's denials, and how could he have been the leader, or in charge, when underneath his boastful comments to Jesus, cowardliness lurked? That is the point. Whether it be religious, or political leaders, with power, Peter sensed Jesus' growing disfavor among them. In private conversations with those who feared Peter's rage, Jesus mentioned how this could become a problem to the rest of them.

This was always evident to Mary and the other disciples during Jesus' ministry, by Peter's constant efforts to stall Jesus from going to different places where rumors abounded.

Eeshans believe that Peter's fear resulted in his misguided human consciousness. He could not understand rising above those threats by men who could kill the body versus fearing the One who could kill both body and soul.

Peter never did rise to the transcendental consciousness as Jesus hoped. Despite Jesus' constant warnings, we find one most obvious example of Peter's failure at the Supper. As our attention is drawn to Jesus predicting, and addressing, His betrayal by Judas, we find that this was a decision Judas made based on his logical, rational, human consciousness, since he was thinking that Jesus would support the revolution and politics of the day, believing that Jesus was the Messiah, according to that worldly standard. More to the point was Jesus' prediction of Peter's denial of Him, when approached by people, and after He (Jesus) was arrested. Being that Peter had placed himself above the other apostles as leader and "teacher," and, in some instances, declared Jesus Son of God, we still find the shallowness of his beliefs well illustrated by his actions.

First, let's reiterate that it was not Peter that Jesus placed in charge after Himself (Jesus). His personality alone made it impossible. Peter was known to be distracted, angry, and harboring rage. He was confrontational, always commenting out of turn, and giving his opinion all too often, almost as though he was correcting Jesus. Even James, the Righteous would often comment on Peter's outbursts. In James 1:20, he teaches, *"My dear brothers and sisters, take note of this: You must be quick to listen, slow to speak and slow to get angry because human anger does not produce the righteousness that God desires."*

What about the comment regarding the 'rock' Jesus made during this discussion in which Peter's ego assured him that his position as leader was solidified? He was by his name, identified as a rock, larger than a pebble, but much smaller than a Corner Stone, which Jesus is. What this means is that Jesus was addressing Peter's ego by giving him a name that meant "small stone," or "piece of stone," that would serve as a 'stumbling block.' The true Rock, who was Jesus, would become the foundation of His own church. Was Jesus already telling those present the prophecy that the church built upon this little stone will surely crumble? It seems as though Jesus was addressing comments from among the others with whom Peter often spent time. If true, then this immediately discredits any basis for his having an authoritative place in Christ's church, seemingly by his own hand.

Eeshans deem that, observing Peter, the others knew that if given the opportunity Peter would assume the role, chosen or not chosen. Jesus often addressed Peter's actions, observing Peter behave as though he was already the leader, Jesus watched how he took his place as close to Jesus as possible. One time, as they gathered to eat, Peter sat down on Jesus' right, only to have Jesus motion to Mary, who had to find a seat across the way, to come over and sit beside Him. He then told Peter to switch places with Mary, thus honoring his wife. It was well known that the seat on the right of anyone was the one with influence, as was the case here, in the seat beside Jesus, which was the seat of power and authority. When Solomon wanted to give highest honor to his mother, he had her sit on his right side. It was then that Jesus talked about always taking the lesser seat when invited to someone's house, so as not to be embarrassed by the host if asked to move to give that seat to another.

This was when Jesus also talked about the first being last and the last being first. James most of the time never assumed a seat anywhere but in the back, away from the others. Peter would get enraged when Mary would automatically take her place on Jesus' right, for this meant that Peter was forced to take the seat somewhere else or on the other side, which usually was to the left. Peter well knew that sitting on the right was the place of honor, and it was no secret that no one sat on the left side of God. Later, this was verified by St. Stephen, the first Martyr who just before his death was granted a vision of God on the Throne. He saw God, the most high, with Jesus at his right. There was no one else sitting to the left.

Seeing that Peter was restless and quick tempered, Jesus often addressed Peter, or used stories in an effort to help him realize where he was wrong. Peter never desired to listen, or learn, about the transcendental meaning of things. It wasn't unusual for Peter to excuse himself in the middle of one of these teachings to help himself to water, wine, etc.

Aware of Peter's personality, and his behavior towards Mary, it is apparent that Jesus' plan could have been intentional to allow Peter to betray him. Remember it was Peter who spoke first at the dinner in which he wanted to know who the betrayer was.

Jesus' plan was always for Mary to teach and carry on his Ministry, but seeing Peter's obsession with power and inclination towards cowardice, Jesus' plan would be suspended by man's free will to choose not to carry out the New Law, but to have her return when 'the world was consumed in sin and suffering' as a result of his choices. This would be yet another example of the 'fullness of time,' and the time when discrimination of women and other combination of genders have come full circle.

Eeshans call this the Great Correction, the time in which God foretold our Eesha that it is time to "correct the consciousness of the world."

We know that James was to be the leader (historically, he is known to have been the leader of the early Christians in Jerusalem), and in many ways proved to be such, since Peter was always in hiding, and fearful to run into him if he heard he was coming into the area, since it is written in this passage. "Knowing that Jesus would soon depart from them, His disciples (according to the Gospel of Thomas) asked Him who would lead them, And Jesus said to them, 'In the place you are to go, go to James, the Righteous, for whose sake Heaven and Earth came into existence.'" and surely the *rock* would be Mary, for she is His wife.

Eeshans believe Peter's cowardliness made him a prime target for those who wanted to get rid of Jesus. It is very probable that he was chosen by puppeteers, which needless to say, came to play an important part in defining the depth of spirituality of this man. Governed by the human/rational consciousness, we see even in traditional scriptures (which omits so much, and holds only half-truths), evidence of Jesus identifying more of Peter's weaknesses and his inclination to sin. Addressing Peter's reasoning with human eyes in Luke 22:31, Jesus tells Peter: "Simon, Simon, Satan has demanded permission to sift you like wheat."

Yet, Jesus continued to try and teach and warn Peter. Why?

1) Because it was the fact of his having eyes to see and not seeing, ears to hear and not hearing, was precisely what was happening. Every opportunity Jesus had, he used Peter's actions, and demeaning comments, as examples of the rebellious spirit even after testifying to being His apostle. At the bottom of Peter's issues, no doubt, there kindled the rage his brother Andrew witnessed and addressed often. This, too, was a sign of being guided into darkness, and not towards light, which displays actions from a purely human consciousness.

2) Eesha also teaches that as Jesus often witnessed the contention and debate about Mary's place beside Him, He saw, in addition, Peter's superiority complex regarding Mary, his annoyance and reminders of the law, which did not allow women to join them, his nervousness of Jesus being around pagans and other cultures shunned by the Jews, the constant drilling of Jesus by the scribes and Pharisees, etc., so that it was obvious that Peter was a weak link. He surely was always afraid of Jewish authority. What Jesus saw in Peter, undeniably, was what is nowadays called 'a victim to pervasive hypocrisy'. In time, this would be revealed as a revelation, that just as the Scribes and the Pharisees sit on the seat of Moses, so did Peter, and those who put him in the place of authority. Later on, we will try and show you the pattern of how it was the corrupt authorities who gave to Peter this emblematic seat of authority, and not God.

3) Being God, Jesus would forewarn, as well as use hindsight to reveal a truth. Eeshans believe that Jesus, by these words regarding Satan, may have been trying to remind him of the days when

he was called Simon, and how the earnestness of a fisherman caught the eye of the Master, in an attempt to bring him to his senses. This was a kind of foresight that Peter was not on the right path, but instead on a path in which pride would take him over and drive him to become too confident in his imaginary position that he felt he 'had' with Jesus.

4) Could Jesus have felt that as Peter was presenting himself as the 'mouthpiece' for the Messiah over the others, he might be very easily tricked by Satan? In other words, Jesus was addressing Peter's obvious growing pride, covetousness, and ego.

This, however, was not the first time that Jesus called Peter's attention to falling victim to Satan's influence. Peter consistently behaved as though he held the place of authority, and that it was he who was closest to Jesus. This attitude is what prevailed throughout his time with Jesus, and beyond.

Rather than embracing, and perceiving, what Jesus was saying, being in the rational consciousness he could only see where Christ's teachings could bring trouble from Jewish authorities. Mary Magdalen noted that it wasn't just his constant attempts to remove her from being present when the men gathered, but that he defiantly cursed that her presence was a scandal, which was already a red flag to those watching Jesus, and His teachings regarding the Law of God; he also feared the constant consequences of Jesus insulting the Jewish authorities and their hypocrisy.

As always, Jesus never missed an opportunity to teach, and many times the teaching was specifically for his own apostles, as in this case, knowing Peter's fear of the Law, Jesus made every effort to reveal himself to his apostles on the divine level, such as he did when he told them, "I tell you, my friends, do not be afraid of those who kill the body and after that can do no more. I will show you whom you should fear. Fear him who has the power to kill you and then throw you into hell. Yes, I tell you, fear him." (Luke 12:4-5). Yet, again He reached out to them testifying to Peter that after all he has seen and heard, he still cannot see or hear. Peter's lack of understanding frustrated Jesus, and, once again, Jesus called him out on it.

Matthew 15 is a good example of this, which reads:

> Then some Pharisees and teachers of the law came to Jesus from Jerusalem and asked, "Why do your disciples break the tradition of the elders? They don't wash their hands before they eat!"
>
> Jesus replied, "And why do you break the command of God for the sake of your tradition? For God said, 'Honor your father and mother' and anyone who curses their father or mother is to be put to death. But you say that if anyone declares that what might have been used to help their father or mother is 'devoted to God,' they are not 'to honor their father or mother' with it. Thus, you nullify the word of God for the sake of your tradition. You hypocrites! Isaiah was right when he prophesied about you."
>
> 'These people honor me with their lips,
> but their hearts are far from me,
> They worship me in vain;
> Their teachings are merely human rules.'
>
> Jesus called the crowd to Him and said, "Listen and understand. What goes into someone's mouth does not defile them, but what comes out of their mouth, that is what defiles them."
>
> Then the disciples came to him and asked, "Do you know that the Pharisees were offended when they heard this?" He replied, "Every plant that my heavenly Father has not planted will be pulled up by the roots. Leave them. They are blind guides. If the blind lead the blind, both will fall into a pit."
>
> Peter said: "Explain the parable to us."
>
> "Are you still so dull?" Jesus asked (him) them. Knowing Peter's thoughts, Jesus knew he was pretending to not know that these words were also directed at him

and his behavior. Jesus heard as Peter directed his attention towards Mary. "Don't you see that whatever enters the mouth goes into the stomach and then out of the body? But the things that come out of a person's mouth come from the heart, and these defile the person. For out of the heart come evil thoughts—murder, adultery, sexual immorality, theft, false testimony, slander. These are what defile a person; but eating with unwashed hands does not defile them."

Eeshans believe by Peter's actions and comments, he set the precedent that would define his role in relation to the Gentiles after Jesus had ascended into heaven, and that His successors would become guilty of compromising with, and being steered by, the human consciousness, as the religion and church of Peter, under the guise of Jesus' name, sought to survive from that time to the present day.

In Matthew 16:23, Jesus, again frustrated and angry with Peter falling victim to Satan's influence, tells him: "Get behind me, Satan! You do not have in mind the concerns of God, but merely human concerns." We will see later how even in his writings before his death, Peter remained concerned about how he would be depicted, and how he wanted to secure his place as leader above everyone else, especially Mary Magdalen.

As the person of Peter displayed such cowardice all along, it was *not shocking* to the others when Jesus told Peter in front of the others that Peter would deny Him three times.

What is shocking is to see how little Peter progressed in his spirituality, when you read the Master prophetically, say in Matthew 10:33, "But whoever denies me before men, I will deny before my Father who is in heaven." When Jesus had finished instructing His twelve disciples, He went on from there to teach and preach in their cities. [**Matt. 16:21:23**] From that time on Jesus began to explain to his disciples that he must go to Jerusalem and suffer many things at the hands of the elders, the chief priests and the teachers of the law, and that he must be killed and on the third day be raised to life.

Peter took Jesus aside and *began to rebuke* Him.

Knowing the weakness of this man, Jesus saw Peter veiling his cowardliness before the Law when Peter said, "Never, Lord! This shall never happen to you!"

Jesus turned to Peter, and said: "Get behind me Satan! You are a stumbling block to me: (referring to his name Peter and Jesus Himself in the person of His wife, being the Rock upon which He will build his church) you do not have in mind the concerns of God, but merely human concerns (and prophesying the future of his church). I have prayed for you Simon, that your faith may not fail."

Then Jesus said, "Whoever wants to be my disciple must deny themselves and take up their own cross and follow me." Jesus laid out a pattern of Peter's future repudiations which include:

Jesus says to Peter: "I tell you Peter, before the rooster crows this day, you will deny me three times that you even know me." (Luke 22:34)

There was only one apostle with Jesus at his crucifixion. But word has it that some watched at a distance. Sadly, aside from Thomas and John, the others sought cover in the mountains, fearing, that if caught and arrested, this, too, was their destiny.

Crucifixion was a punishment for the worst criminals; yet, for one who, in front of the other apostles pretended such courage throughout Christ's ministry, Peter was so traumatized by the events taking place that he succumbed to tremendous fear and paranoia, causing him to flee. What followed next was his attempt to hide out with the others. They were so afraid at Peter's change in behavior that they, too, became paranoid, that is, all but John and Thomas. To understand it one must understand that Jesus' crucifixion was a horribly painful, and disgraceful, form of capital punishment used in the ancient world.[303]

It should be noted, however, that immersed in mystery, Jesus' mother and wife stood near (sadly, it is only minimally recorded, in Luke 23:49, that it was the 'women who had followed him from Galilee,' and these women were the Kallahs.). Nearby, witnessing, but not encroaching, were the women devoted to the Sacred Couple (these were Mary's Kallahs).

---

[303] Fairchild, Mary. "6 Facts Surrounding the Crucifixion of Jesus Christ." Learn Religions, Learn Religions, 9 Jan. 2019, www.learnreligions.com/facts-about-jesus-crucifixion-700752.

Matthew 27:55 reads, "There were many women who were part of Jesus' and Mary's ministry who followed them everywhere." As recorded in Mark 15:40, there were also 'women looking on from a distance' (as the soldiers would not allow the women to get any closer).

It has been well documented that there were no eyewitnesses to the resurrection of Jesus. What is found in scriptures were a series of endings that were made up to fill in the gaps and to end the story. One need only research to find this to be true. There was, however, an eyewitness. But one must surely wonder, why this eyewitness story was not used? In fact, the story was destroyed. Below, is an eyewitness account. The narrative was one that was taught to Mary's disciples …? Perhaps. But here it is.

Peter's shaky faith was almost always and issue. As we find in John 20:19, "On the evening of the first day of Jesus' resurrection, we find the disciples were still hiding, with the doors locked for fear of the Jews." They were clearly cowards and were trying to preserve their lives. Yes, we understand after the presence of the Holy Spirit they all went out and proclaimed the resurrection of Jesus.

But as the consciousness of Mary Magdalen teaches:

> "On the eve of the Resurrection, I felt I was being pulled out of my body. As I was being lifted up, I looked back and saw my body lying on the floor. I felt as if I was being pulled towards the tomb where Jesus' body was laid. Upon reaching the cave, I found myself inside— the rock still in place at the entrance. There I found my beloved. I gasped at the sight I be held. His beautiful face and body were uncovered and the blood-drenched swaddling wrap placed at His feet. He looked nothing like himself. I picked up the face cover and held it in my hands near my heart. My heart stopped. I closed my eyes but a moment to pull myself together.
>
> Suddenly, there was a wind which surrounded me—and then I found myself surrounded by a legion of angels. I watched how they entered and exited the cave as though it was a mirage. They brought pieces of His body tissue as if putting His precious body back

together. Music filled the area and when they seemed to complete their work, all quieted and the rushing of the wind calmed. All present looked at me. There were no longer signs of blood—just that which was imprinted on the shroud and face cloth; but I did notice that the wrap which I used to cover my issue at the cross was folded next to his wrap. I walked over only to find that He was whole again. Tears streamed from my eyes as I beheld my lifeless beloved. Memories of our love caused a crushing within my heart. I took away the face cloth. It was as though He was only sleeping, but He wasn't sleeping. He was dead.

Then something stirred within me. I felt as though I was in the state of ecstasy. I felt an overwhelming sensation of love and desire—just like on our wedding night. I went closer. I remembered how His fingers touched my lips. Taking my fingers, I touched his lips. I remembered His breath and I leaned over and breathed on Him. Next, I remembered his vows to me—and then "His kiss." The urging within my heart overcame me—I leaned over His lifeless body and kissed Him. It was as though an explosion took place within Him. Then it was as though His brain was started in his head. Light was coursing through His body. I saw what looked like blood but it looked different. And as He took His first breath inhaling my name Mary, just as He did with His last exhaling breath! And His eyes opened!

The next thing I knew, it was first light, the morning of the first day. I grabbed my wrap and awakened my Kallahs. I had to get back to the tomb. I told the Kallahs to take the oils that I may anoint my husband's body—I did not tell of my experience. As I spoke to them however, I noticed they were still and quiet. Almost immediately, Beth pulled my head covering down over my eyes and whispered to look down as we journeyed quickly towards the tomb. Upon arriving at the tomb, I discovered the rock that sealed the opening was rolled away. The tomb was empty. "Where is He?" I loudly whispered. "Mary"! Beth exclaimed in a low voice, "I see Him in your eyes."

I sent the women to run back to get the others and Peter. The women soon returned reporting that Peter would not come. I went myself. Peter's first reaction was not to believe me. As I was finally able to convince him, he and John followed me to the tomb. Once Peter saw that the tomb was empty he got angry. He was fearful that the guards had taken Jesus' body and that they were secretly watching to see who would come there. Peter quickly ran back to the hiding place to alert the others. Fearful they would be followed, he told John to go another way. John then left not knowing what to think and felt it best to do what the frightened Peter suggested.

The Kallahs stayed behind with me. I told them to search the grounds to see if they could find the body. Once they left, I noticed a young man sitting directly outside the tomb. He seemed to appear out of nowhere. He asked who it was that I was looking for. I told him I was looking for the body of the Nazarene. The only words he spoke to me were, "Why do you search for Him among the dead?" Then he disappeared.

Taken aback by what just happened I decided to search the garden myself to see if there was any evidence of where the guards may have taken him. As I did this I saw a man walking. Then I lost sight of him. Suddenly I heard a voice from behind me. "Who are you searching for?" He asked. Then as I turned I mistook Jesus for the gardener and asked if He knew where the body had been taken so I could go and reclaim it. "Mary," He said. It was at that moment that I, Mary witnessed the Man/God in His new human but glorified transcendental body. I, Mary, witnessed the fullness of my soulmate's divinity for the first time since we came to earth, in its entirety as a glorified human, for the sake of witnessing. He continued, "*Mary, Magda Ellen ...*" (translated means "Mary, you who knows and is—Light"). Then almost immediately, I was put into ecstasy and we were one flame as on our wedding night: as written in 1 Corinthians 6:17, 'But whoever is joined to the Lord is one spirit with him.'

After our mystical union, Jesus told me to 'go tell the others and Peter.' I hesitated a moment. Peter? It was almost as though He had to think about telling Peter. Seeing the other women witnessing, I told them to come with me.

Upon reaching the hiding place, I found a kind of council going on. Everyone seemed confused. Mary, the Mother of Jesus, was sitting off to the back near James, the Righteous One, who was praying, and a few others who were quiet and listening.

I shouted, "Peter, he's alive!" As always, he scoffed at me and hushed me; and he and others continued to discuss some kind of plan. "Where's Thomas?" he questioned. After another attempt to get him to listen to me, he grabbed my arm and said that I was hysterical. I told him. "No." I told him that I saw Him and we talked. He then went on to tell everyone to stay inside. His fear had increased now more than ever. As I tried for the third time, there within our midst, stood Jesus. Peter, thinking Jesus was a ghost, panicked. "This is some kind of trick," he said. "How can I be sure you are not a ghost?" he asked Jesus. Jesus then showed Peter His hands and feet. "Touch my wounds, Peter." Peter went forward then stopped and stood in awe. Then Jesus spoke, "Peace," He said. Then as everyone marveled, Jesus looked first at me, then at His Mother, and left.

Shortly thereafter, Thomas, who was grieving in his own way, returned to the room. Losing Jesus was more than he could bear. Upon returning, Peter argued with why he (Thomas) was out among people, fearing that someone would recognize him and report him to the authorities. Putting down a sack of bread, Thomas did not look in Peter's direction. Thomas, who was truly close to Jesus and spoke often to Him regarding all matters, rebuked Peter, repeating the words of Jesus in his own way. "If I am to be arrested Peter, let them arrest me in the light—not hidden away in the dark." Peter then contained his fear and anger about Thomas' absence and immediately told him of Jesus' visit. Thomas, looking at Peter replied, "And why should I believe you who denied Him and left Him?" I then turned to Thomas and said, "It's true, Thomas. He is alive."

Thomas, taking my hand, asked, "Why? Why Mary, would He come to us? We who abandoned him?" And I said, "Because His love is greater than any other love. Thomas, He is the Son of the Most High God; and He has returned to us so that we may return to God." With that Jesus again returned to the room. Upon seeing Him, Thomas ran to Him and hugged Him saying, "My Lord and my God." As Jesus said to him, place your hands on my side Thomas, feel the marks in my hands. "Thomas said, I have no need for proof my Lord. You are here." Jesus looked at Peter and said, "Because you have seen me you believe." Then turning back to Thomas Jesus said, "Blessed are you who need no proof that I am here and believe, for if you cannot love one who you can see, how then can you love God, who you cannot see?"

Here again He was addressing the doubt they had of his returning, especially that of Peter. When they were with Him, they loved the crowds and attention. When Jesus talked about leaving, and going to a place where they could not follow, Peter interjected quite boldly that he would follow Him to prison and even to death. Their human consciousness,' especially Peter's, found that faith was not as strong as they thought when Jesus was arrested, and killed, and when they ran for their lives. Peter, being afraid for his life, tried to hide among the crowds. Fear and paranoia consumed most of them. Since it was easier to love Jesus, he lived among them, and they derived strength that comes with popularity, and being surrounded by large crowds. Without their leader, some panicked for they had not the transcendental consciousness necessary to understand the fulfillment of the prophecy, and Jesus' teaching on what he would undergo, as well as what were contained in the psalms and all that was prophetically related to the Messiah. That is why His arrest and crucifixion was such a shock.

Thomas' courage was in his love for Jesus to such a degree that he risked death to die as an example of Jesus Himself.

Eeshans believe that Peter's faith didn't strengthen much more after he saw Jesus. Once again, while on a boat, when others spotted a man on the beach that looked like Jesus, Peter again thought it was a ghost. It wasn't until they reached the beach, and Jesus offered them the fish, and took a piece for himself to eat, that Peter was convinced. Another time, when Jesus was on the beach cooking, Peter jumped from the boat and swam to the beach to prove he was not afraid.

Peter's doubtfulness regarding Jesus' humanity was equal to his doubting that Jesus was God. Even after the Ascension, Peter's continued straying from Christ's teaching up to and including Paul's confrontation regarding Peter's poor example. Paul's first encounter began with questions regarding Peter's loyalty to Christ.

Both in Gnostic readings and traditional scriptures, we find evidence that Peter was wined and dined by people involved with Jesus' arrest and crucifixion. As Peter chose to give the responsibility of the Gentiles to Paul, he felt obliged and desired to continue to work with the Jews. However, this decision takes Jesus' teachings and mission in another, more political direction in order to secure the survival of the new religion under Peter's guidance, and "tone down" Jesus' actual teaching, so as not to "offend" anyone. Even though Jesus IS God, we want to be sure he doesn't offend anyone with what He teaches? Peter wanted to be sure he didn't offend anyone, since the fisherman would surely know more.

15A

Why and how Eeshans feel things quickly deviated from Jesus plan. With the unstableness of the early religion, and the possibility that all would be lost, Peter sought help from those Jews he continued to work with. First and foremost, Peter was strongly advised to remove Mary Magdalen so as to ensure that the place of women would revert back to the status quo and the new religion would stand a better chance of surviving. This appeared to Peter to be a more expedient way for men to regain their rightful place over women, and would cause less friction with surrounding society, and would protect the apostles' work alongside established religion. This relationship was already inflamed due to Jesus' presence and teaching. The move also gave Peter more control in lining things up the way he felt the Messiah should have done.

Remember there was no doubt that Peter had always wanted a special relationship with Jesus, and though he loved his master, he just did not always agree with Him, and often stood in opposition to some of the others up to and after Jesus' ascension. He liked the things in Jesus' teachings that brought him attention and power, but he had no use for Jesus' teachings and example regarding women.

We find that his rage was often directed at Mary, who he considered being unworthy to speak to, and certainly unworthy to speak on behalf of any man, let alone the Messiah. With no desire to return to the days when he worked as a fisherman, his plan would have to solidify his role as leader above Mary Magdalen, a place he felt he deserved as a man. It was one fire he felt he could control; there were just too many women who continued to teach about God, and to take on roles that were not only unheard of, but also against the old laws, written, and oral.

Until he was able to redirect and remove any evidence of Mary's relationship with Jesus, Peter's place and legacy would never be secured. He blamed Mary for the death of Jesus, and refused to give up a place he coveted, especially after the ascension where he felt more freedom to change things since Jesus was no long there to support and protect her. But just how far would he go?

SUMMARY POINT 16

THE CONSEQUNCES OF PETER'S CHOICE FOR A RATIONAL HUMAN CONSCIOUSNESS VERSUS A TRANSCENDENTAL CONSIOUSNESS

Eshans believe that Peter's inexperience and cultural naïveté were used by the powers at that time to redirect the early Christians into harmless directions, or dead-end avenues, until such a time that the whole messianic religion, and its teachings, would vanish on its own, or become divided within; and, thus, could be eliminated. This plan would prove to malign one of the most central and important teachings of Jesus' mission, which, from the beginning, was that women should have equal roles in the body of believers, and that the patriarchal structure should shift so that both genders would be equally represented in the power structures of the growing community. It would also serve to become the obstacle to Jesus' plan of salvation. as when Jesus said to Peter, which we find now was prophetic, "Get behind me Satan! You are a stumbling block to me; you do not have in mind the concerns of God, but merely human concerns."

It was Paul who was responsible for bringing about conversions outside the Jewish faith, since Jesus' apostles were not totally united, and some, though faith-filled, were not savvy enough to take on a lot of responsibility. Yes, it's true that after the initial gift was bestowed on them, and they, again, felt strong, once the threats began, and people who were converted were being arrested, some of the apostles felt the need to go to distant places. One must remember that they did not have the training and experience necessary to deal with the theologically educated, and defend the new group against the intellectual establishment where they were from, since most were simple men who witnessed kindness, and took on students of their own. Witnessing Peter's actions as the "supposed" leader, it was necessary for Paul to bring his followers back on track also. So, when Peter began displaying a poor example by not living what he was teaching, by avoiding worship services, which would be the breaking of the Bread and Sacred Drink, and preaching Jesus' directive regarding eating His Body and drinking His Blood, Paul would be the one to remind him that those who were following him would eventually do the same. It was not too long before Paul noticed that there were issues regarding cultural differences that needed to be addressed. Peter failed to see the needs of the Gentiles, coupled with their not attending their worship service (a loose term for gathering). Paul realized that, seen as a leader, Peter's followers would follow his example, and surely make things worse. Remember, Paul was unaware of Peter's behavior and insolence towards Jesus' wife and women, respectively, and of his disagreement with Christ's teachings which he felt put him and the others in jeopardy with the Jewish authorities. Paul, on the other hand, did work with women, to a degree. He, too, was still a bit connected to his birth religion, but remember he was not taught firsthand, nor was he in the company of Jesus, as were the others.

Eeshans believe that Jesus used Peter's behavioral history to show the differences between the two kinds of consciousness (human vs. transcendental), and how God allowed free will to dictate man's decision to accept or deny what Jesus taught. Seeing the weakness of the man was an obvious sign of how the human consciousness continued to manifest itself, and how even with faith, or proof, of who Jesus was, Peter would continue to use this rational, logical consciousness, and wasn't able to think of what Jesus would do; and, instead, he caved to concern for himself and the fear of the powers at large, just as Jesus warned him.

Peter's decisions up to and after the Ascension obviously never displayed an ascent to a transcendental consciousness, which explained the divide in the apostles. Mary was seen by Peter, while Jesus was alive, as a threat first to Jesus' spirituality, but, afterwards, mostly to all Peter was establishing. Here, Peter felt the need for a swift urgency for Mary's disappearance, and all that was connected to her, which Peter as needing to be omitted and lost. Why? Because after Jesus' ascension, while Jesus continued to teach Mary, Peter, being of the rational consciousness, would focus, primarily, on what would secure success, and that was not the transcendental teaching of Jesus. This was partly because Peter couldn't get Jesus to divorce Mary while he was alive, however, Peter could now accomplish this in yet another way, which was by "erasing" her from "official" first and secondhand believer's accounts. (Later we will find that this became the goal of early church fathers also, who more or less wouldn't know any better, because they were only working with the above, which was handed down to them, and had little else to go on.)

We see how Peter refused to believe that Jesus hadn't erred, and if he continued to impart any teaching regarding equality of a woman to a man, he, too, would subject himself to persecution. Since Jesus had two trials, one with Herod, and the other with Pilate, guilt by association was truly a fear that consumed Peter. He felt that finding a good compromise would insure the legitimacy of his leadership.

Eeshan sacred writings clearly indicate that just as it was in the beginning, God allowed these decisions to continue, and these, later, became the foundation and law, not just used by Peter's early successors, but as we have found, would run throughout the entire history of the church itself. Generations after this time would have only the knowledge of the end result of what happened, which to the church's benefit, would make all books and writings contrary to what church authority professed for grounds for excommunication. Taking for granted that women would never question, or doubt, that the church made it easier to continue along this path, men, more or less, were in control. Women's love for Jesus was taken for granted. Many fell victim to this way of thinking because it was ascertained by the wedding vows that women will continue to do what they are told. Priests made sure that the people would fear being cut off from God. With the fear tool it then gave all church officials carte blanche over the people, allowing and giving the priests, bishops, etc. the right to do whatever they chose without question, since they were acting in Christ's place.

Human, rational consciousness, from then until now, and up to the Age of Enlightenment, facilitated the male ego's drive for power, and the need for security for itself, while perpetuating the assurance of this power of control to flourish. To pose any question to anything of the established churches, taking into account the dark periods of history that are revealed, makes one succumb to being labeled a conspiracy theorist. But writings continue to be revealed where the prophecy regarding the fullness of the Bride is realized and the Perfection of God's human creation is realized as it was originally.

Once again, that's the Peter who is truly the same face of today, just as he had been at the time of Jesus. The world will find that the five capital sins taught, include covetousness on the power side, and cowardice as its counterpart, and that at its beginning, Peter's defiance was that which is similar to the saying, "People who are angry and bitter and laden with problems, love them too much to let them go, and they would rather live in misery than choose the light of love and kindness." Peter, and those who follow him, are led down the path to the perpetuation, and justification, of this increasingly pervasive, male-dominated patriarchal mindset, and are not necessarily always found within marriages, but should listen to what Jesus says about such leaders that condone and the actions they imitate:

In the Gospel of Thomas, Login 114, after hearing the dispute regarding Mary, Jesus' wife, the Blessed One greeted them saying:

> **Peace be with you—may my peace arise and be fulfilled within you!**
> **'This is how I will guide her so that she becomes a Man.**
> **She too will become a living breath like you men.**
> **Any woman who makes herself a 'Man'**
> **Will enter into the kingdom of heaven.**

He said this to clarify that His wife was one with Him; and another who is, and recognizes this sacred balance, will enter into them, and, thus, be saved. Knowing that Peter was afraid of the Law, and of breaking it, Jesus continued:

> **Be vigilant, and allow no one to mislead you by saying:**
> **'Here it is', or 'There it is!'**
> **For it is within you, that the Son of Man dwells.**
> **Go to him, for who seeks him, finds him**—[this is in reference to telling Peter and the others that women are included in the word 'him' referencing they who are one].
> **For those who seek Him, find Him.**
> **Walk forth, and announce the gospel of the Kingdom.**
> **Impose no law other than that which I have witnessed.**
> **Do not add more laws to those given** [because in the Torah laws were added, but here Jesus is the New Law]
> **Lest you become bound by them.**

Is there any evidence to this? Yes. Jesus' words were used in the transcendental, universal sense, and were intended by Jesus to go "to the ends of the earth," reshaping the consciousness of that time, and set the precedent for all future generations.

By the disregard for Jesus' real teachings, many traditional topics and approaches to issues we are faced with, as well as views on life, are now overly clouded and difficult to understand and solve, because of what God's people have consequently been taught, resulting in separating God from daily life. It doesn't seem to have worked. Again, because there is no sacred transcendental balance, what we are witnessing is the amending of Jesus' teachings beyond the point of recognition, so that rather than resolving problems, the world just keeps talking about the problems, and gaps remain unfilled, or are fed with human consciousness' empty regurgitation of the symptoms of the problem, which in turn only serves to feed further forms of discrimination and oppression under many guises.

The only way we can end all diseases which feed upon discrimination and oppression, and this includes more than gender, color, culture, and age is by raising God's people to what God originally intended for them; and that was Jesus' principle aim as an avatar or divine being.

SUMMARY POINT 17

JESUS, THE ONE TRUE, BUT DIMIDIATED MESSIAH: THE REVELATION OF HIS FEMALE COUNTERPART

The truth is, though we compare Jesus to the Messiah of the Jewish translation by Christians, we find that there are still great differences when one looks at the Mashiach/Messiah according to Jewish writings by which we now understand why and what Judas was looking for, and why he betrayed Jesus.

Some points of interest that back up this statement should be noted. The timing element of the Messiah and why the Jews adamantly opposed Jesus is very important. First of all, the Jews did not think, or believe, the Messiah would be a man, or a 'god,' or demigod, etc., but would be a great political leader, and win battles, and liberate the nation of Israel etc. This is still true today. There have been others, after Jesus, who some claimed to be the Messiah, and one who was reported to have actually fulfilled some of these expectations.

At the time of Jesus, Judas, being very politically motivated, truly felt the greatness of Jesus, and witnessed his miracles and teachings. But being political, however, he also misunderstood the teachings for he was coming from the human rational consciousness, with a very zealous political agenda. Missing the transcendental and spiritual awakening as many had, Judas thought that all that was needed was to push Jesus, and he would rise to the occasion.

Identifying himself as the Son of God was first, and foremost, against the prophecies surrounding the Messiah, and that is why the religious authorities brought about the charge of blasphemy. He showed no evidence that He came to restore that which was lost under Roman oppression, nor did he speak of politics, or showed interest in establishing a government. He was not politically motivated. He was the Divine Masculine who came to earth to make all things new, not by force, but by enlightenment, and example. He and His wife lived by God's design, not man's.

Today, however, as the sacred balance must be restored, Eeshans present another look at the description for the return of the Messiah. Just as the church had given a one-sided story of Jesus, the hand of God now acts by presenting the other half. The Messiah, therefore, which the Jewish religion is waiting for, may, in a way, be true for all of God's people. As Jesus became the redemptive proxy for Adam, He lived a holy life, and died on a cross paying our ransom. Despite this horrific prophecy coming true, His directives were not carried out. So now, as the world is in great suffering, God sends the part of Him, His Divine Feminine counterpart, who will make everything whole.

Mercy redefined, as co-Messiah, is not only sent by Jesus Messiah, but is in keeping with his promise to her, returns with her, as *she* encompasses *him*. She is the Avatar, and she is also known as holding the title Bride of Christ, Wife of the Lamb.

This was the coveted title taken by the church of Peter for itself, and was given another meaning, which Eeshans believe was attempted to be more in harmony with Jewish religion and law, rather than Jesus' true mission to restore the Sacred Balance and bring salvation. It was, over time, increasingly defined, and used in a metaphorical, and symbolic sense, in line with the thinking that had built up around the Old Testament writings and traditions, but, nonetheless, the title belonging to Mary, which was stolen from her.

Given as a title to a people in the old testament, it was then passed on to an institution drawing on scriptures regarding Christ, as its head, and used in describing the church. The title 'Bride of Christ,' if, from its conception, was founded on Jesus/Mary's marriage, as Christ desired, would have worked quite perfectly. What we are saying is that if the church, at its beginnings, was serving to continue Christ's plan of salvation, Peter and his successors would have embraced the acknowledgement of God's duality and accepted Jesus' wife. This would have continued with the representation of a man/male, serving as Jesus being the head of the church, and a woman/female representative within the church itself, and the above statements would then be true.

Because Jesus' wife, Mary, was taken out of the equation from the outset, Christ's mission was suspended by God. The body of believers under the leadership that deviated from Jesus' original plan had to create legitimacy for their decision; thus, as result, the title was used solely to 'complete' Christ, and making the church his bride; thus, employing the title, deceptively. One should know that even the church had massaged this title several times over the centuries.

Becoming institutionalized, and operating under its own authority via the self, human consciousness, and dimidiating the whole of Christ's teachings, is the end to their means. Masquerading as having the direct authority of God, and using what they construed to be power, coming from such church authorities. over time. presented the "Keys of Peter" as the direct, appointed representative of Christ himself. and they succeeded in redirecting. and saving. the Christians. forming which would eventually become the Catholic church. To further reinforce. and claim. the truth, it said that what was, and is, taught from the pulpit was by the Holy Spirit, who guided all temporal and spiritual decisions having the Holy See (as it came to be known), as the only official "voice" of Christ in the world. As other religions developed in the rest of the known world, they were simply branded as pagan and/or 'heretical' by the church, but over time, as the nations and the religions in question grew and developed even further, the church saw itself in the position of having to compromise stances, and to begin recognizing various other paths to God in order to save face and survive. Examples include slowly acceding to Martin Luther by beginning to print bibles in the secular language, 'opening the windows' at Vatican II, exonerating Jacques de Molay and the Templars, and lifting the excommunication of Luther. The church needed to do this in order to stay relevant in a rapidly changing world, however, ironically, these days amidst its struggle to stay afloat, while its pedophilia scandals empty out its churches, one may even wonder when it will be officially stated from the Holy See that extraterrestrials now need to be factored into Jesus' mission of salvation, and how this would be done.

In the documents of the Second Vatican Council and the Catechism of the Catholic Church, the church defines itself by using words such as, being "Christ's Mystical Body" (Jn 15:1-5; Eph:1-23; Col 1:18; 1 Cor 12:12; 31). Using this stupendous mystery, and the underscoring of God's marvelous family plan, further exemplifies (1 Jn 3:1) the way the church, just as Peter had, used the wording to their benefit. As they continue to claim the loving Father sent the Son to recreate us, they also continue to use Baptism (cf. Mt 28:18-20; Jn 3; Acts 2:37-39) as the method necessary to transform us to "share in the divine nature." It is, again, this "massaging" of the meaning of the words in these passages to suit their goal that makes this so manipulative.

These scriptures note the Holy Spirit's indwelling presence (1 Cor 3:16; and 6:15, 19) as the life force of the church and its soul and Sacred Tradition as the living memory of all that Jesus taught, and claimed to be kept alive, and true by the Holy Spirit (1 Thess. 2:15; Jn 14:15-17; 25-26), which were stolen and used to back up the church's position.

This information would be true, if it taught this in conjunction with the Sacred Balance of God, the inclusion of Mary, as Jesus' wife, or the acknowledgement of God's Divine Feminine counterpart; Without these mysteries, however, the above is *not* true, and so the meaning changes.

How can the church claim total truth, and claim responsibility for the formation of all doctrine and dogma through the ages, when they continue with this glaring problem and error at the heart of everything they teach? A lot has to do with the loss of the transcendental consciousness, but, in addition, scriptures from the beginning of Genesis and forward also had been altered to serve a purpose of keeping everyone's focus on a particular version of Jesus. Those in the beginning served to establish what those scriptures, used in the New Testament, founded the church on. One must wonder then, how, on one hand, anyone could accept that throughout all of God's creation there was always a balance of all things male and female; and, yet, on the other hand to not acknowledge the first humans as equally balanced, being made in God's Divine Male/Female image and likeness, and vice-versa.

With the truth buried for over 2000 years, the established church was very successful in maintaining its position masquerading as the 'Bride of Christ,' thus, destroying any evidence of any connection between Jesus and Mary Magdalene.

The church always has controlled, and continues to control, perception and memory. Denying Jesus' followers, the whole truth so copiously is like the lying tongue which hurts those it loves, while a flattering mouth works ruin. Common sense holds:

> The true Bride of Christ never embraces or presents half-truths;
> or protects itself by denying scandals; or
> brings doubt that manifests in lack of faith;
> She would not lead its followers to think and question the success of Jesus' mission.

The church, through its corruption, created and perpetuated the kind of history-spiral that appears to be taking over the world. The faithful are abandoning ship, and there is so little belief in God; yet, still she is claiming to be innocent and remains pure and unscathed from the world's 'persecution,' despite the nature and long trail of her sins as she stands before and among humans, but it is not so before God; since if any part of Lamentations 11 is true, examples can be readily seen in the interior political intrigue and turmoil, the errors and scandals known and hidden, the abuse of individuals and groups behind the shield of 'divine authority' and 'internal forum,' the corrupt families that rose to power inside the church, and the paranoid abuse of power out of fear and cruelty in the name of Jesus Christ is truly bearing false witness (i.e., like the Borges and the Inquisitions just to name a few).

On the other hand, technology, modern research, and the development of means to uncover history and to re-examine that history objectively in a newer, more informed light, has led to the discovery of a transcendental thread moving through all history and spiritual traditions that sheds light on the role of Mary Magdalen, as the true Bride of Christ, and her place at Jesus' side and hope for a new age, the Age of Enlightenment, begun by Jesus and continuing with His wife.

We see the church of Peter and where it is now in its thinking, reaching out to the world in general that it has helped create, and how it is the product of centuries upon centuries of drastic and subtle error, one compounding the next, leading up to the present-day situation, and as it continues in this direction, making changes deemed necessary in order to retain membership and relevance in a rapidly changing world, God again visits and teaches His people.

In other words, as religion goes, the church is simply seeking to do whatever is necessary to survive, and to ensure its survival. The world, therefore, is at a crossroads, and it is here that Mary's work picks up where it left off, to complete Jesus' work, and teach as Bride, Wife, and Divine Feminine as Jesus intended it to flow, and give life, as Dante said, "Love is what awakens the heart to act."

SUMMARY POINT 18

TIME GOES BY SO SLOWLY, AND TIME CAN ONLY DO SO MUCH: ARE YOU STILL MINE? A 2000+ YEAR REUNION SACRED TEACHING

These first words are most familiar connected to the Righteous Brothers song "Unchained Melody," and we apply them to the love between Jesus and Mary. As it is written in Ecclesiastes 1:7-9:

> All rivers flow into the sea,
> yet the sea is never full.
> Then the water returns again to the rivers and
> Flows out again to the sea.
>
> All things are wearisome more than one can say
> The eye never has enough of seeing
> nor the ear its fill of hearing.
> What has been will be again
> There is nothing new under the sun.

It only makes sense that the prophecy of Jesus promising to return for His bride from ancient teachings is yet another step towards the fulfillment of God's plan of salvation.

Since wouldn't it make sense that if he fulfilled his part of the plan of salvation, that He would find His soulmate? He created the human form in which to place her consciousness, that they may continue their mission together in end times, and continue to guide those chosen back to the transcendental. Why else would it be predicted that Jesus will "return for his Bride?"

How did they reunite in present times without His soulmate's knowledge of her previous relationship with Him, and still hold sacred the human marriage she entered into on earth? The answer is very clear. Jesus sustained her consciousness until she was born here on earth. In these end times, there are differences that one may feel are contrary to holding her titles.

Jesus' birth was the result of the Virgin's marriage to the Divine Masculine counterpart of the 'Most High God.' Joseph's marriage to Mary was not a conjugal marriage, so, therefore, Jesus was the only Child of the two eternal Consorts. In Christ's lifetime, Jesus and Mary were married with no conjugal relations. In this lifetime, our foundress was to continue as the human representative of life here 'becoming a wife and mother' that she may understand her transcendental, and divine, role as predicted in the description of the woman in the wilderness, before she brings about the Male Child in end times, that others may relate to her. She will have already experienced labor and the pain of birth.

In her lifetime as Mary Magdalen, however, when Jesus proposed to her, it was a mutual AGREEMENT regarding the denial of conjugal relations-similar to what his Mother and Joseph had arranged for.

This was done since, at the time, Mary was unsure of her feelings, yet, she felt compelled to marry Him because He saved her life. What began with what Mary felt was an obligation soon became the greatest love story ever told. Opposite of Joseph maintaining a vow of celibacy, it would be Mary maintaining a vow for Jesus to remain celibate. That their marriage would be totally exempt of a conjugal relations, she was not sure. One must remember that Mary Magdalen, as Jesus' eternal consort, it was not yet revealed to her out of the necessity to accept His engagement using free will, but she agreed. Understanding the Law, Mary considered the complications of their agreement, and wondered what would they say to those who mocked her and labeled her barren? Remember under Mosaic law a marriage is blessed, especially when a woman gives birth. (cf. Isaiah 54:1)

Rejoice O barren one, who never bore a child; burst into song shout for joy, you who were never in labor; for the Lord says, the desolate woman has more children than that of a woman who has been married a long time.

Mary thought of the scandal she lived through and how because of vile people, this would affect Jesus.

It is said that Jesus shared with Thomas his life in the future of days with Mary and it is from these stories that Thomas told others that in present times, Mary's life in the future is said to resemble Radha in Bhakti Yoga texts, as a friend and lover of Krishna. The following is information found about this Radha.

Radha is depicted as a childhood friend and lover of Krishna according to the Bhagavat Purana and the Gita Govinda. She is almost always depicted alongside Krishna.

Her relationship with Krishna is further detailed in Brahma Vaivarta Purana, Garg Samhita, and Brihad Guatmiya Tantra. Nowhere is it said, or expressed, that Radha and Krishna were married. Radha (also, Radhika or Radharani) is respectfully prefixed with "Srimati." This is a totally respectful, gracious, and deferential term. It is Shrimati that is an equivalent of the English term "Mrs." It is probably because this prefix that Radha and Krishna devotees use, that Radha is misconceived to be a married woman (and if married, why not most probably married to Krishna?).

While in the west she is referred to as a "Hindu Goddess," whereas, in the Vaishnava tradition, she is seen as an eternal '*expansion*' of Krishna. Radha is considered a metaphor for soul, and her longing for Krishna is theologically seen as a symbolism for the longing for spirituality and the Divine. The name Radha[304] could mean "beloved, desired woman."

In other texts, it is indicated that this was a period of time when Krishna lived among the gopas (cowherds), but Radha was married to

---

[304] "Divine Love Invocation with Radha Mantra." The Yoga Tree Chiang Mai, 2 July 2018, yogatraining.theyogatree.org/divine-love-invocation-with-radha-mantra/.

another gopa. It is also written that there was a Sri Chaitanya (16th c.), who was said to be the reincarnation of both Krishna and Radha, and he was Krishna on the inside and Radha on the outside.[305] It was considered that the unique love between Krishna and Radha was actually infused into his entire person and flavored his devotional teachings.

Why are the above important? These are important because when God is involved the Word is sent out to all God's people; and, thus, there will be a resemblance even though the fulfillment may play out differently among other cultures, and pieces of the truth MUST be among them all when connected to the Divine. The Hindu and Krishnas spirituality are believed to be contained within (Ish's) Jesus' secret teachings to St. Thomas, in whom He would confide, while with the apostles.

Recapping the life of our Foundress, she would be destined to fall in love with Him as a child. He kept her close to the Eastern form of traditional Christianity, her birthright as a Byzantine, which served to protect her within the mystical fullness of God. Then in the fullness of time, He would teach her to understand God's desires, then woo her heart. He would transform her mind, body, and soul. He had her teach his people. He would take steps to mirror what had taken place over two thousand years ago, yet in her innocence she would only see these images, or teachings, as pertinent to present time. Next, He would differentiate the transcendental from the human world and way of thinking. She would be inclined to share in anything concerning Him and He with her; and these would be known in biblical times as the *halakha*, which is another name for the secrets of God.

He would share the timeless marks of salvation from his crucifixion. He would give her the gifts she desired. He would cause her love to yearn for His love. They would experience a mystical union and renew their marriage vows. Their lives, as one, would be split between two worlds: that of the material world and that of the spiritual. Their life would be the reversal of those things gone wrong.

How did this affect the actual person of our Foundress? She lived life loving Him, in the context of life in this world as wife and mother.

---

[305] The love that Caitanya exhibited in his raptures of mystical ecstasy was said to be the embodiment of the love that Krishna and Radha had for one another. – Ed.

How did Jesus keep everything ordered? How did he help her realize who she was? It all began with God, the almighty Father and his Consort Mary, who would present her with an emerald ring, indicative of the one prophesized to receive the sacred words hidden away since the fall of Lucifer, until *she* was born. The Virgin would guide her until she received Jesus at her first Communion service where He would identify her as his bride, promising He would be with her, guide, and teach her.

Jesus called our Foundress by many loving names, beginning in her early years as my friend, later as "little one," then after their betrothal, "my heart," or 'dear,' and of course, by her present name (though rarely). One special gift he gave her was "wine." In this life, her favorite story was the Marriage Feast at Cana, as though it was buried deep within her heart and soul, by a kind of "omnesia,"[306] and not knowing why, she always desired, and dreamed, of getting wine from there. Needless to say, it was his special gift for her to return to Cana in the 1990's, and this pleased Him greatly. It was on a 'special day' that He gave her wine from what he described as from 'a special reserve.' She loves life. She loves who she is. She loves being a wife and mother and grandmother. She loves her Kallahs, Chatans (priests), her 'Golden Girls' (women who have taken care of her since the beginning of her public engagements and beyond), and, of course, her extended family, with her whole heart. She loves God's people differently than one would think. She loves talking with people she doesn't know and who don't know her.

When it came to her mission however, it is always how Jesus wanted her to be addressed; and in bringing her to the reality of who she always was, is, and will be to Him: He used this sequence of titles, which He established in a kind of a loose chronological order of events, in order that she realize God's plan through the scriptures she was most familiar with. Being born into the Byzantine Rite was her joy especially with regards to the liturgy; and it was always the center of her life. The Bible was not a major part of her life, however, due to how the teaching within the Liturgy took precedence.

---

[306] Om-being a sacred Sanskrit sound, meaning anywhere from reality, entirety of universe, truth, divine, knowledge, used in ceremonies of rites of passage, or meditation; and in the present context, "nesia" is added to mean 'lack of.' – Ed.

Looking back, it was the lack of knowledge of the Byzantine Rite that drew many attacks from the western church, since it was often associated and confused with Orthodoxy. Immersed always in the mystical Persons of the trinity, especially Jesus as the Bridegroom, in actuality, her Byzantine faith kept her protected from the kind of secularism that was sweeping the Roman Rite, and so the Byzantine Liturgy was her trustworthy and constant link to the sacred.

The continued familiarity of the title Bridegroom in the Eastern rite, not to mention her traditional upbringing, coupled with all the supernatural experiences growing up, the Bridegroom Himself made use of her eastern roots, which made it easy for her to accept the ways of God, His analogies, and the sharing of His thoughts. He taught her about other eastern religions and teachings. He gave her the gift of healing, with prayer, use of oils, and/or spices, and stones/gems.

One such title was "Isreal" (the apparent incorrect spelling being deliberate, and the word was pronounced, and actually was intended to literally mean, "is real"), which also carried with it specific fulfillments of scriptures, and was the name He gave her on their mystical wedding night (cf. Eesha's poems).

'Wedding night' here is the term Eeshans use for past/present time, for it reflects their marriage then in the time and place where Jesus and Mary were married, and it also includes the renewal of their marriage vows in present times, also extended from biblical time.

Another was the title "Mother," which identified her with the role of a most treasured event, The Woman in the wilderness who gave birth to the Male Child.

All except the last, serve as indicators of particular responsibilities, or duties, which helped her better teach, or bring clarity to God's people in matters of spirituality. These would eventually bring about the formation of a lay ministry, and a religious order known as the Missionaries for the Eucharistic Christ.

In these present times, and relative to the supramentalization, and revelation by Christ to her, regarding who she was. and is, via the consciousness of Mary Magdalen, the title "Eesha" is now used as foundress of The Eeshan School of METTA Spirituality and School of Enlightenment.

SUMMARY POINT 19

FROM CORNERSTONE TO KEYSTONE: THE MANY TITLES OF MARY

The unique title "Eesha" is a variant spelling of the Sanskrit word *Isha*, phonetically pronounced "Eesha," and it carries with it various meanings, such as dominion as feminine, protector, and Lord. She chose to use the phonetic form 'Eesha,' when it was put into writing. Those who belong to this Sangha (school) are called Eeshans. Eeshans believe that through the *Sophia Perennis*, or perennial/eternal wisdom, the transcended person of Mary Magdalen, at the wedding feast of Cana, where Mary Magdalene became the wife of Jesus Christ, has been "given" to its Foundress; and, thus, she teaches by way of the consciousness of Mary Magdalen, via the process of Supramentalization.[307]

Something similar to supramentalization may be seen with the example of a Tibetan Lama (i.e., the Dalai Lama), or of a transcendental extension of the many leaders of transcendental religions throughout the centuries. It implies a 'continuity' of being from one particular/specific person in one historical time and place to another person in another, i.e., former, time and place. While a slightly different kind of example, the Papacy can be regarded as an 'image' of supramentalization in the sense that the office is considered to be the 'Vicar' of Christ, Christ's

---

[307] This is not something easy to explain in English, or in any current modern language for that matter. However, while the categories of thought and language of the East, which describe and express, human/transcendental experience are considered advantageous, the problem is that they are not languages which the average person is familiar with, let alone fluent in. – Ed.

authoritative presence on earth, which is perpetuated through the centuries (even though here the office is occupied by different individuals).

What makes supramentalization unique is that it is the perfection of Christ **sharing in her lowly humanity that she might come to share in his holy divinity.**[308] **It's similar to when we receive Christ in Holy Communion, i.e., we are united to the Risen Christ, and come to share in His divine life.** Expanding on that however, **the process of supramentalization refers to a physical divinization, the rising of a human being through the various layers of existence to the transcendental realm to the Source of Being; while simultaneously the Divine Source of being is drawn down into the physicality of the person. In other words, it is how the Divine Consciousness has been, and is, established upon Earth.** This process brings the Divine Feminine aspect of God (again by Ishvara), and localizes it in a person (here being Mary's consciousness into Eesha), having descended in fullness but filtered through human form.[309]

Eeshans believe that through Jesus and Mary's esoteric, transcendental, and sacred union, as well as Mary being literally the Lamb's Wife, what came about was this unspoken truth, that of Jesus, being the Son of God, made man,[310] likewise his counterpart in divinity, became Mary His wife, "in time," and in human form. While with Jesus in her earthly life, Mary was subject to the "divine amnesia," as was the Mother of Jesus, until she gave her 'yes' at her marriage. That is, Mary Magdalen was not originally conscious of the fact that she was joined eternally, and would forever share in the divine, as well as in the human person of her Divine consort, known as Jesus. This would therefore be witnessed completely through His giving of himself totally and completely to her, in Body, Blood, Soul, and Divinity, and in the most unique way, by the Sacred Kiss. This was the foundation to His Eucharist, which would be given as the

---

[308] Cf. John 6.

[309] Explanation adapted from some of the writings of Sri Aurobindo. – Ed.

[310] In the church of Peter, this truth was still being discussed at the Council of Chalcedon, Oct. 8 to Nov. 1, AD 451.

God particle necessary for the transcendental and entire transformation of God's people back to God.

Now and through the years, the prophecy that "she", Mary, was/is now revealed as the active and realized Wife of Christ. She is the 'keystone' of his true Church. As he was the cornerstone which would NOT crumble-even though rejected through time—his wife is the central stone at the summit, the capstone, which locks the whole together and on which all else depends in the 'real Church' by Christ's design.

The undeniable truth, mystically presented, is not just who she is, but how she returned. Being incapable of being fully explored, and almost impossible to comprehend, we follow the 'path' given to us by putting before us the things we know, such as being his eternal wife, one with Him before creation of this world as we know it, and being His female counterpart, His wife during his time on earth. Next, we take a look at reincarnation, resurrection, and, lastly, this extraordinary means called supramentalization, which would naturally follow transcendentally by consciousness from Mary, through, with and, within our Eesha's continued marriage to Him today.

This relationship being the continuation of the Marriage Feast at Cana, and thereby, in the sharing of His Body, Blood, Soul, and Divinity, with their earthly marriage, gives credence to her oneness with the Lord, which translates as Eternal Divinity. That is why her title as Lord is substantiated. But all this occurs without any 'glitch' in her worldly marriage with a husband and children. It is not too hard to understand being that the Virgin had a similar life.

Absurdity? Not really, for the same two reasons given early on in the beginning of this book: first, what this means is that she (Mary/Eesha) has experienced the *perfected version* of one who is divinized. The divinization process is not unfamiliar. For example, the use of the word 'divinization' is "doctrinal," and is foundational to Catholics. The difference is that the church of Peter, by Catholic teaching, dimidiated them to reflect only Jesus. Where the definition of divinization is true, due to the above, it is a faulty interpretation of limited data expanded, and transmitted as if it were true and complete.

We therefore can take what the church describes as Christ's Eucharistic divinization of man, and by editing in the Eeshan truths, show what we mean by *dimidiation* and how this makes the church's definition an *untruth*. Upon a first glance of their interpretation, you would think their Eucharistic divination process is the same, making their Eucharist the same as with Eeshan Transcendentalism (you could find the church's description in the Catechism of the Catholic Church in 460).[311]

Here is the quote, edited to include within the brackets the 'Eeshan ethos,' "The Word [meaning both are God's spokespersons] became flesh to make us 'partakers of the[their] divine nature.'" "For this is why the Word became Man [and woman] and lived, [married] and died: so that humans,[312] by entering into communion with the[m], [who is the] Word, and thus receiving a divine descendent of Jesus [and Mary], might become a Son or Daughter of God." "For the only Begotten(Child) of God became Man (and Woman) so that man (we) might become God." In other words, "The only begotten Son of God [and His Consort], wanting to make us sharers in his [their] Divinity, assumed our nature, so that He [they], made human, might make man [us] gods."

That is why His Wife can be said to be the ultimate perfection of this meaning.

The meaning Eeshans hold is that this definition in the Catholic Catechism was purposely worded with not so neutral pronouns, and by

---

[311] To reiterate once again, to Eeshans this is especially significant as it makes the case for why women in the Catholic church should always have been able to actively participate or share in this Sacred Balance, especially as leaders and celebrants in worship services, i.e., the Mass. – Ed.

[312] This is important to remember especially when questions of masculine pronouns came up over the years with groups such as Call to Action asking that neutral pronouns be included so that all were represented in the Catholic religion. We were all told from the pulpit that the words men/mankind were synonymous with "all human beings." This definition or explanation was used to satisfy the need to distinguish men and women, and all were told that the church's stance was to be understood to mean just that. Furthermore, we were told that the gender of the words used should not be a deterrent in loving and worshipping Jesus and God. Taking these teachings to heart as Catholics or Christians, it would seem to clarify, beyond a shadow of a doubt, that we are all equal, whether man or woman, by belief and baptism and most assuredly in holy communion, and are in fact, united in Christ.

using primarily the masculine pronoun, this would cover what would change the meaning of the above, and, thus, from the Eeshan perspective, it is not true. We disagree with this definition because:

1. It is incomplete with the exclusion and representation of the Sacred Divine Feminine, by use of the term 'only begotten Son,' rather than only begotten Child, which eliminates the balancing of the Sacred Masculine with the Sacred Feminine in the Second Person.
2. By this action and rejection of Jesus' wife it doesn't accomplish the total transformation nor does it fulfill the Christs' directive to eat their Body and drink their Blood under the one Sacred Food and Sacred Drink, which is the heart of their salvific plan. The dual reference is necessary in order to offset and reverse the original mutual choice of Adam and Eve, and is required in order for human beings to have life everlasting, meaning to go back to an original state as transcendental beings; to avoid this or to blur the issue confuses what Jesus taught with regards to what is "necessary to bring about God's plan of salvation," as being for men, and, though, women are subjected to men before God, and, thereby, allowing the mindset continue that women cannot go to God on their own.
3. The use of transubstantiation is the process Jesus and his wife used to change normal bread and wine into the Body, Blood, Soul, and Divinity beginning with their marriage at Cana.
4. In order that it be as Jesus said, it must reflect Jesus' passion and death and the 'sacrificial love' He shared with His wife at that moment.
5. It is necessary to have both Jesus and His wife to restore what was always intended by God, but was lost by a mutual choice our first parents made for a physical, material life.

Eeshans' only solace is that as God allowed this to *happen out of respect for free will*, the same was allowed as Jesus witnessed the behavior of Peter and those who feared Peter. *Jesus, as God, forewarned that what He spoke of would be changed and what He didn't say would become 'law.' Knowing that after He was gone these things would happen, we now believe that Jesus felt it more important for the teachings of man to play out as He knew they would fail; just as God knew of Adam and Eve's eventual choice and how Peter's sin and offenses would be overshadowed by Judas.'*

Seeing that Peter could say he believed Jesus was God. and 'still do and say the things He did before the Son of God' is paramount; and, thus, God decided that for a time and another time, the consequences of Peter's actions would *serve as a decoy for end times.*

It would be in end times that the *Sophia Perennis* would serve to identify the remnant of the remnant of followers, which were mentioned in scripture. Just as in the end of days, Jesus would punish those by saying he did not recognize them as in Luke 13:23, "He said to them, 'make every effort to enter through the narrow door, because many, I tell you, will try to enter and will not be able to. Once the owner of the house gets up and closes the door, you will stand outside knocking and pleading, 'Sir, open the door for us.' But he will answer, 'I do not know you or where you come from.' Then you will say, 'We ate and drank with you, and you taught in our streets'. But he will reply, I don't know you or where you come from. Away from me, all you evil doers!'" But who among them heard?

We seek refuge in our faith, and, therefore, scriptures must be clear on what they are saying. For example, in Luke 13:30, where Jesus says, "Indeed there are those who are last who will be first and first who will be last," this has always been interpreted as addressing the issues of pride and humility. Though this can be a powerful teaching in and of itself, our Foundress explains by way of supramentalization that Jesus was prophesying what would happen in end times, that Peter usurped Mary's place as leader out of his assertion that he was rightfully first among the others because Jesus called him first, and mostly because he was a man. Yet, just as Peter failed to understand Jesus' teaching, Peter, who considered himself 'first,' would be removed from his seat next to Jesus several times as we mentioned before, since to be in a place of authority and then be asked to move would not only be most embarrassing, but it would be keenly felt as an insult (especially in this case as Peter was losing his place to a woman). Peter was losing that seat to Jesus' wife, as was done several times before, and it happened again at the Last Supper Jesus shared with the apostles. If Jesus' warnings are not heeded, those who refused to believe, accept and change with this, their last chance for mercy, they would be counted in among those whom He promised He would destroy as the "destroyers of the earth."

As it stands, though no one knew or understood, the Virgin Mary and Mary Magdalen were in fact the Divine Feminine of the First and Second Persons of the Holy Trinity.

SUMMARY POINT 20

A VERY PROFOUND SACRIFICIAL PRESENCE: SACRED TEACHING

It is true that Jesus as the second Person of the Holy Trinity eternal and Divine Masculine consort, known as the Son of God, sacrificed His life for His Father and Mother's will, but to not acknowledge His marriage one does not see how His own personal sacrifice was to sacrifice an earthly life with His wife and all the human pleasures we all experience when we get married. We tend also to miss the sacrifice of His Father and Mother, who though they live eternally, chose their separation, i.e., His Wife, who was on earth at the time, and was deeply involved in a sacrificial love. The perfect, sacrificial love of their Child was accepted as ransom for God's people eternally, so we may share in it. *Each of these components were necessary* so that we may regain our eternal life.

In the Eucharist of the Marriage Feast, Christ and His wife do not leave heaven to be with us. They are ever present in the Sacrament by their divinity, but also share their humanity in this sacramental state. Since Eesha encompasses Him here on earth, they are omnipresent and, in fact, bring back the Sacred Balance. They come out of themselves in an extremely selfless way. In a kind of 'begetting' manner, through the gifts of human hands, and transubstantiated by love, and the sacred alchemical gifts are given to the Kallahs and through an ordination are passed on to the Chatans, bring with it the succession of Jesus and Mary's sacrificial marriage. By transubstantiation the gifts are then presented under the original appearances of the species at the time of Communion, and later for the benefit of their people, under the appearance of altar bread, described as hidden behind a 'little white veil,' this piece of bread, for the sake of reverence, is, or may be placed in exposition for all to see.

At the time of the people's reception of this Sacred and Balanced alchemy of the Divine/Human to sacramental, we the human, become divine, and share in this sacredly transubstantiated union, and experience the sanctified, transcendental Body originally intended for us. To receive their Body, Blood, Soul, and Divinity is to have divine intimacy, a full and selfless, sanctified exchange of persons in a reciprocal, transcendental union.

It is important to really understand that by their marriage, Jesus and Mary had the true version of what the church all along claimed to possess and teach and continues to teach regarding their sacraments, and what they continue to claim to be the sacrament of the Holy Eucharist for mankind. Since the eternal marriage has once again surfaced through the awakening of the Divine Feminine Avatar, being the both male and female, the Holy Sacred Balance of the Eucharist of the Sacred and Divine Marriage Feast, essential in the redeeming value of the Holy Eucharist, is returned.

SUMMARY POINT 21

WHO IS THE REAL BRIDE OF CHRIST? WHAT ARE HER RESPONSIBILITIES? SACRED TEACHING

How do Eeshans explain the title Bride of Christ and Wife of the Lamb, and why and how can the church of Peter use it only to identify the institution of the church without regard for Christ?

Simple. The Bride of Christ and Wife of the Lamb must be understood through the lens of Eastern mythology, used here to mean certain eternal relationships that point to, and have their origin in God, as God is in himself. For example, you will find accounts there of God with his Eternal Consort, that is, His wife, who is part of Himself as God.

Therefore, the relationship of Jesus and Mary as God and Eternal Consort is entirely in harmony, and consistent with the pattern established through Eastern mythology, stretching back to before creation. God created and endowed the first humans with male (positive) and female (negative) attributes. In harmony with that pattern, the relationship with Jesus and Mary is entirely understandable, and more grounded in terms of God's creative design throughout the cosmic manifestation. Through an avatar, God is continuing the story of the creation, and as all things with God, it is good.

God says that when humanity reaches a certain degree of darkness and corruption, "I Myself will descend." According to what the church taught from early times, all Christians await, and want to be prepared for the final return of Jesus. As we said before, Eeshans believe that in order to fulfill scriptures identifying the "Lamb's wife," Eeshans believe it has to reflect that Person, His soulmate, who came to complete His mission of salvation for God's people. In order for this to take place, He returned first through His eternal consort, who would continue his mission on His behalf. She will continue teaching the fullness of His original doctrine on the eve of a new and enlightened age of consciousness. This is what we call the age of the Female consort of the Holy Spirit: the Eternal Wisdom, or Sophia Perennis.

To understand the church of Peter's use of the "Bride of Christ" title, let's first look at meaning and use of this title, along with the 'Lamb's wife.' This is a term used in reference to a group of related verses in the bible, in the Gospels, Revelation, the Epistles, and related verses in the Old Testament. The early church used the title for over 1500 years though the *ekklēsia* is never really explicitly called *the* "bride of Christ," though the expression, or title, was a reference of 'bride' with Jesus as the 'bridegroom.' It was explained, and taught to mean that: "Husbands were exhorted to love their wives just as Christ love the *ekklēsia* and gave himself for it, as he nourishes it, and cherishes it,[313] as his own flesh;" in loving the *ekklēsia* he is loving and cherishing his own flesh. These facts are connected to the Old Testament where God addresses Israel as a 'husband.' If scriptures were presented giving the whole truth of Mary Magdalen, and her espousal to Jesus, the example of Christ's love for His wife would been more complete, and the best image to portray through time as a template for living our life, and there would be no talk of a "remnant," since all would have everlasting life.

To exclude Mary Magdalen, and profane her name and reputation, brought the need to establish the continuity of the Old Testament and the New Testament, and show that Peter (the "father" of the covetous bride) was the leader, and that Jesus was the legitimate expected Messiah/Savior. In order to pull together a struggling church with many factions, it was necessary to go back to the Old Testament prophecies, their wisdom writings, and what worked.

---

[313] "Bride of Christ." Wikipedia, Wikimedia Foundation, 13 Nov. 2019, en.wikipedia.org/wiki?curid=6280977.

It is important to remember that the Jewish religious tradition, from which the apostles came, saw the people of God, Israel, in the corporate sense, that is, all the people were seen as together comprising 'Israel.' the bride of God. Being that they were raised with this truth it was then easy to have a facsimile of the same, which would also be very acceptable to the Gentiles who truly were converted, and rarely questioned the apostles. It definitely had an origin that was survivable, and since it appeared there were other similarities regarding Israel in their birth religion, all was fine. However, since the revelation of Mary Magdalen's marriage to Christ, it doesn't seem to fulfill those same familiar scriptures, imaging the true church as the bride for the bridegroom, or Christ legitimizing their new religion.

Using a woman, who conceived with a kiss Jesus' children, and later brought forth the fruit of the love between her and her Husband, displaces all of the above. It is said that the version used was necessary to prove the case that Jesus of Nazareth was the Messiah sent by God to fulfill scriptures; and that as women did not have a place in worship services in the Jewish religion and faith they could not represent a people. Because of this, and the fear of Christ's ministry under Peter collapsing over Jesus' marriage and treatment of women, it became a choice for many factions of the earliest (Christian) groups to follow the Jewish religion of the time of Jesus and other patriarchal religions.

Eeshans profess that this in itself shows that Christ's true mission was not understood, or Peter would have seen the importance of Mary's role, and why women were part of Jesus' ministry, and the success the women had, as they began to form their own groups where worship services took place during and immediately after Jesus' time with them. The Bride of Christ would've continued in Jesus' footsteps and sanctioned God's mysteries.

Unfortunately, these were dispersed, and were no longer allowed to continue shortly after Peter took over, even those who were ministering and overseen by Mary Magdalen. Even Mary's place among the teachings of the apostles came to a halt, since Peter would not accept that what Mary told the others was coming from Jesus via visions. It was clear. Mary had to be stopped, one way or another.

As the groups were disbanded, the women were assigned a place and role that was either subservient, or just defined by patriarchal consciousness, which made them easy to control. The 'memory' of the place the Kallahs and Mary Magdalen had with Jesus was now successfully suppressed, and more or less forgotten, after it had been effectively erased by the actions of Peter and those that followed in his wake. This new structure and direction was taken over by those followers who were loyal to Peter; and, thus, Mary's place, along with her Kallahs, appeared to be 'lost,' forever, *in time*. Thinking the Kallahs were 'gone,' and Mary being given a nominal and humble place in the chosen gospel accounts as a 'disciple' of Jesus, the 'church' continued to slowly build the institutional "bride" qualities around itself, over the coming decades, and indeed, centuries. This management of women continued with Peter's successors to maintain this misguided objective through to present times.

Deviating from Jesus' original plan, they successfully obscured Christ's role as Savior and Redeemer of all people. They secularized the mysteries of God, which were given to us by Jesus to correct the original "transcendental" *imbalance* of humankind. As a result, they lowered all the Sacraments given to us by Jesus. Once the Eucharist was successfully reduced to 'half of Christ' (i.e., by removing Mary Magdalen) they wished to represent their views, and the sacrament of matrimony immediately fell from a transcendental marriage to a physical manifestation of marriage. In Jesus' name, they made it a means of control, as if protecting man from losing everything as a direct result of a woman desiring a place with God. This obscured the truth and knowledge of what defines a sacred union, which we are all subject to today.

SUMMARY POINT 22

A Deeper Understanding of Divine Consorts Sacred Teaching

The mission that Jesus began with his wife at His side was not finalized at his death. This is so that the true Church/Sangha He desired might begin via the new and profound imagery of the Divine Consorts. This truth would, in fact, be witnessed by Christ's Resurrection and the days to follow, before Christ ascended back to heaven. Indeed, these events witnessed by the apostles should have been for Peter, and those who followed Peter, enough of a foundation on which to lead God's people by choice, back to Him with the Sacraments and Commandments as guides, over the next few centuries.

The salvific mission would be continued by Mary, His wife. since who knew Him better than she? With James working side by side with her, it was the perfect gift of God, since it would continue, spread, repair, and restore the Divine Balance, bringing love, order, and God's plan to fruition, and a faith rooted in timeless love, that would lead God's people back to their understanding, and, once again, build a holy relationship with the eternal consorts.

The role of Consort is important in understanding God's plan for the totality of earth's history. As Jesus expressed, and witnessed, it is only from a divinely restored balance of sacred, linear, and cyclical spirituality that one can find God.

From the Eeshan point of view, the church seeing itself as the Bride of Christ, without proper representation lessens the "component" of bride necessary to keep the children alive throughout the body of those who love Jesus. The problem is that the Bride He intended to continue his mission "was" to be a female person, just as He was the male.

Because this plan did not come to fruition as Jesus intended, it is clear to see that in these times, that prophesy must, and will be, still fulfilled, as promised by God. This, of course, was the promise that a woman would "crush the head" of the serpent.

Taken literally it would make sense that the bride described cannot be simply represented, or understood, in the impersonal, or corporate sense (i.e., institution), nor can an institution claim to be the female component when its leadership and spiritual teaching offices are made up exclusively of only males, who continually and improperly serve God, and God's people without an adequate female co-direction and representation. This is imbalance, not Sacred Balance, and is certainly not representing God, as Jesus and Mary did.

How could this misrepresentation of the Bride of Christ have commenced and continued on since Jesus? Let's do a quick review of the decisions since Peter, and with the church's stance on its different theological connotations of the title Vicar of Christ placing a male in charge of Christ's continued mission, and efforts to keep Peter's role in control and as the sole figurehead.

SUMMARY POINT 23

THE HUMAN CONSCIOUSNESS AND EARLY CHURCH RULES CHANGED TO SUIT THE NEED SACRED TEACHING

If Peter himself was directed and led purely by human consciousness, the actions of the church would reflect this; and it *does*. What we have witnessed over the years, and that which was previously presented to you, is how this institution began, and how it continues to present Jesus Christ as an earthly, purely human reflection of God, justifying a patriarchal structure, as evidenced in Old Testament scripture.

Beginning with Peter on down through the hierarchy of the church and into the faithful, this problem causes the removal of the transcendental alliance of God and the purpose of Christs' coming to restore the loss of the transcendental world to the faithful. This would undoubtedly affect everything back to the original two human beings and the changes brought about with The New Adam and The New Eve.

Looking back, Eeshans believe that in an effort to protect their dastardly deed regarding the elimination or omission of Jesus' wife, a title would have to be chosen that would satisfy the generations to come. This was in an effort to clarify who the Head of the church was, one who would be the male human representation of Jesus. It would have to be one that correlates with Christ. It would have to be strong and masculine in hopes that this would cover over the need for a counterbalance of female representation. It would have to work with scriptures that would give the successor of Peter the right and power to an apostolic line that would not be challenged. Thus, in time, the title Vicar of Christ was chosen.

This unjustly created the means for which the authorities could do away with ever having to address this issue again, and the need for a female counterpart of Christ as a human being, by making *the church* the Bride of Christ. No longer was there the necessity of a Divine Masculine/Divine Feminine gender of God as should have been professed and taught.

This title, however, was not a title given by Christ, and though over the years the title Vicar of Christ was conveniently used in different ways, it, once again, became the second official title of the pope in the 2012 edition of the *Annuario Pontificio*.

With no intention, whatsoever, of reflecting Christ's marriage to Mary Magdalen, the church continues to try to create its own version of Sacred Balance, rather than bring women to the status of equality, as intended by Jesus. From the Eeshan point of view, this decision was doomed to failure, causing only a greater imbalance. The church, since the time of Peter, has tried to survive in a patriarchal manner, and has never seen how incorrect, and wrong, it is to have a man represent Jesus, and having no woman involved. Woman would bring the negative polarity necessary to support a balance with the positive, and serve to uncover man's hidden feelings, while Jesus would bring out the positive and hidden reason in woman.

Eeshans have made every attempt and effort to show the importance of Mary's role, or Eesha's title, in the need for the Divine Feminine manifestation of Christ in these times. Many are unsure of how to react to a human person claiming her right to be called the Bride of Christ, and they don't question a male figure representing Christ, or question how one can be sure without proof that she is the person of Mary Magdalen from 2000 years ago. With explaining how, in fact, the title of Christ's Vicar was manmade, it a wonder that it was approved.

The point may be raised that the only proof that Jesus was God were 'his own' claims, which were deemed blasphemous and criminal by the authorities; yet, nonetheless, we know they are true. In the same way, the Person of His Wife has nothing more than her claim that her authority also comes from God.

However, just as Christ's followers have always accepted the church's teachings and the story of his resurrection, they readily accepted the title of Vicar of Christ, etc., but without a doubt a woman will not be accepted as easily.

Not many know that the ending to many of the traditional New Testament writings, especially with regards to the Resurrection, were written much later on because of the gaps due to the omission of texts. Eeshans suspect that some of these tell, and witness to Mary, Christ's wife with references to where she was present in her role.

With Tradition and Scriptures really being the only reasonably solid claim upon which the church used as the origin and basis for its own existence as an institution, and for its belief system, Scripture could certainly have been manipulated just as suspected is the case in Peter's writings. It has been thought by many, even some among Vatican officials, that until recent times, the process, whereby, all the writings, now considered canon, came to be finalized, and held a lot of ambiguity: *'It was as though were all kinds of writings and books were put together for scriptures under Constantine and the process was barely more than saying a prayer while those books chosen were practically randomly picked from the stack with the absolute exclusion of anything written that would be conflicting with Peter's leadership.'*

It has also been said that the only books to be chosen from were those that would not cause controversy in the future. In other words, remove all references regarding Jesus' marriage, and/or Mary Magdalen. It is well understood that the church, as an established world power, regardless of any proof, or evidence, to the contrary, will postulate what it wishes. This is what always made it impossible to challenge the inner core doctrine, or the administrative, political machinations of the church. Since it successfully entered the political realm, corruption abounded. Isn't this yet another proof that it is not in line with Jesus, for He actively avoided politics despite constant pressure?

Sadly, there is no inlet of choice to the church's version of Christ's Mystical body that will ever allow women to penetrate the forces at hand; that is why the need for the Eeshan Religion to come back. However, one could easily question this objection because the church authorities suppressed all writings which it considered antithetical to the version of Jesus it touted, in addition to showing another side of Jesus' ministry and teaching style, speaking of Jesus' relationship with Mary, and lumped them into a category it called 'Gnostic' or 'heretical,' and stigmatized all of these writings as forbidden to the faithful in an effort to protect and to ensure respect for the image of Jesus they created. Though it came to pass that some books were found to be misleading, or just plain wrong, there were many others found that leaned heavily in favor of validity and soundness, or sustenance. Since it is said, the baby was thrown out with the bath water. Some responses were from those who claim that they defended books, or writings, that might be otherwise subject to vandalism, or affected by a flood of heretical ideas and opinions, and the church couldn't risk this gaining influence with the people. Wait! Where did we hear this before? Could it be Google where it is stated in response to the question of Who Jesus was and why it had no information on him,[314] "You will know what we want you to know, think what we want you to think."

Not long ago, most common people had no idea there were so many other books and writings about Jesus, and that there was anything beyond the four commonly known gospels and letters of the current New Testament. People generally are under the impression that that's all that was written about him. Yet, isn't it odd that from those books that were chosen, none of these could describe how Jesus looked, or what happened in his "hidden" years, even though his own Mother lived long after Jesus ascended into heaven? People today have the means to read all these literatures for themselves, and find them not only interesting but also spiritually complimentary and helpful.

The reality that the faithful will believe what they are *given to believe by the authorities* who claim to be the mouthpiece of God, is true. This was among the concerns Paul had. That is why he went to see Peter, and addressed his (Peter's) failure before his followers, since they, too, would listen and do what he did.

One very interesting side note is with regards to the scriptures you read, there were still some that were challenged before they became 'legit,' and still many denominations do not believe the interpretations given

---

[314] At the time of writing, one could ask Alexa who Jesus Christ was, and no answer was given. – Ed.

until this day; for example, Protestants, Catholics, and Jews don't agree on what books are considered 'canon.' One very blatant fact regarding who Jesus was, about whether Jesus was both God and man, and that argument continued in the church for hundreds of years before finally being decided on only a few hundred years ago. The understanding of the language, as well as missing documents, lend to the need for theologians to try and complete certain books found, so that they would 'make sense.' Let us please remember that it is the officials, those in authority, that are responsible for the corruption.

As we said, the people who loved Jesus believed what they were told by the apostles, and acted, accordingly, as they believed all that was given them by word and actions was true, there would be no way, save the opposing apostles themselves speaking out against what was happening to know anything was any different. From the start, those who had faith enough, and by chance were lucky enough to have heard Jesus, by the transcendental acceptance of what Jesus had taught, accepted him as God. *It is a strongly held belief that the faithful will always be protected by God despite the authoritative errors they were raised with. For those who understand human nature's limitations and have firm faith in God, this is a fact.*

Our purpose in bringing to light this information is in no way intended to move you away from your particular belief system, but to give you, the reader, as much as to provide an insight into what we believe is true, as far as possible; and, thereby we hope you understand that this is our system of beliefs by which we stand, presenting to you what we have learned via recent year discoveries, but mostly importantly the means and processes by which these things are possible today.

If nothing else, remember that religion and spirituality are personal and come from *within*. It cannot be imposed on a person from without and be genuine. Not everyone is going to believe what is contained in these writings; we ask only that you seek enlightenment to view what is written transcendentally, and not see it. skeptically. with the fear-bound human consciousness.

There is a definite need for a system of beliefs and structure in any religion and spirituality, so that one has the freedom to choose that which creates interiorly a personal connection between God and the soul. That does not mean that error cannot exist, or that one spirituality, or religion, is good for all in all circumstances. One thing is for sure, and that is, what God desires, and wants, for us must subsist in whatever religion, or system, of beliefs we choose, as in Christ's directive to love God above all else and our neighbor as ourselves, AND receive the Sacred Food and Drink of the Christs necessary for everlasting life. It also does not mean that God wants one to accept 'everything or anything' that's out there, since as we said, unless you stand for something, you could fall for anything, meaning without transcendental guidance, one truly cannot find the whole truth as Jesus taught, and we honestly, and emphatically, believe that. Under the transcendental consciousness, one must always ask, "What will bring the soul back to God and present to the world a decent, law abiding peace and love, unlike any it has ever experienced?"

This is all part of the urgent need to teach and lead God's people by the transcendental consciousness, as the means of survival and our salvation as Jesus intended. The human guiding consciousness will follow suit, and it, too, eventually will gather enough momentum, so that what 'it' does, will become perfectly justified in its own eyes, even if there is full knowledge that the founder's, or, in this case, Jesus' vision has become confused, or muddled, over time. That is why Jesus said, "By their fruits you will know them," i.e., by their behaviors professed in his name they will show a totally different interpretation from what he taught.

As stated before, education and technology are making it possible for people to read, study, and research through things for themselves, that, at one time, was impossible to check out. Previously, people based their faith on what they were given by the church. Now, everything is available to look through for oneself. Aside from forcibly declaring what Jesus' followers have to believe, and what they must do (or not do under threat of being cut off from Jesus), or what they must believe in order to go to heaven and avoid falling into hell, is now only second to the institution's admission of scandals and cover-ups.

We feel we must continually repeat the words of Jesus found not only in the rare gospel of the "Confession of the Twelve," but throughout traditional canonical scriptures, as authored by St. Paul and in the Book of

Revelation. In the "Confession of the Twelve," in which Jesus is 'speaking to His apostles' and telling them that there will, indeed, be those who will change His words, or omit, them, saying things He did not say, or taking away things He said, for their own purpose. We are told that such persons do not serve the Lord Jesus Christ by finding alternate ways of deceiving His people; however, questioning what doesn't make sense, or what seems to be incomplete, in searching for truth, hardly puts one in this category. Otherwise, we would be guilty of obedience to man rather than obedience to God, as was the case in biblical times with man-made laws presented as being from God, and alluded to us by none other than Peter in his writings.

There will never be a "proof" strong enough to compel a person to believe something if they *don't want to believe*. As the saying goes, "if one believes, no explanation (or in this case, proof) is needed, while if one doesn't want to believe, no explanation (or again, in this case, proof) is possible." The closest one could get to certainty, if this were possible, is to approach a situation, and experience it for oneself, with a clean heart and mind, free of pride and fear. At that point, one must stand before God with one's own conclusions, and do so without pressure or coercion. This would be the mark of one exercising full personal responsibility and accountability.

SUMMARY POINT 24

How Can One Believe in Supramentalization?

Connections of Religions to Deities with a Deeper Understanding of Supramentalization

God, being omnipotent, would have to be involved with the entire world, even while preparing the world for salvation. Why, there are even various forms of teachings regarding different beliefs that point to the reality, and belief, in a return of consciousness. Perhaps, these were to help ensure a better understanding of supramentalization, to prepare the world for the return of the Divine Feminine with this process.

The supramentalization process, for example, has existed in other places in the world and in history, as in India. We quote and used writings from different holy teachers revered to the Hindu people as Jesus' teachings and spirituality played a major role in parts of India as Spiritual Master. It was commonly accepted, and apparently experienced (given the devotional writings one may access) how God could and would incarnate into human form, and all surrounding elements of the physical world, would respond to the presence of an Avatar. Consider this in light of how Jesus was readily accepted as being from God by those who desired to hear Him. Through his healing work in Galilee, the miracles and even when He even walked on water were witnessed publicly. It was for the peoples' benefit towards enlightenment, and to witness God in their midst that He raised people from the dead, cast out demons, and quelled the storm, which rose up on the Sea of Galilee.

Eeshans, therefore, aren't the only ones who believe that there is a divine component within their order that allows for a direct link to a Deity, which in this case is the Divine Feminine, who encompasses Jesus. In fact, you know the most common example of one today, though they have changed this title, time and again, and that is the church of Peter. It has always seen the succession of Peter as the direct line of authority stretching from these times back to Christ himself. Down through the years they see the direct link, Pope, or Vicar of Christ, as being virtually 'Christ on earth.' Tibetan Buddhists have a belief in the reincarnation of lamas, which has been 'recorded' since the fourteenth century. Successors were conceived as rebirths, and came to be regarded as physical manifestations of the Dge-dun-grub-pa (1391–1475), and this belief continues to this day by the name His Holiness Tenzin Gyatso (who is said to have been quoted as saying that he believes the next Dalai Lama should be a beautiful girl).

In the final analysis, seeing and witnessing to her testimony over thirty years of Jesus' mission, Eeshans truly believe that they have witnessed enough to feel that the title Wife of the Lamb, or the Bride of Christ, without a doubt refers to Mary Magdalene and further believe in the greatness of His relationship with His wife continues to be substantiated through the person of Eesha, since it reveals the What and Who of God, and what God has given, and continues to give and intend for us.

This process of *supramentalisation* brings into the realm of the physical and material world the Divine Feminine, and is the foundation upon which everything in the Eeshan religion is based. It is also the means by which the Son of God continues with His wife, the mission that was begun with Jesus' birth, life, and public ministry. It needs to be reintroduced into the world as God intended, as unfolding the plan of God for human beings through the rebalancing of the Divine Masculine and Feminine in each human being before God, and ending the vicious cycle of suffering human beings are continually caught in.

SUMMARY POINT 25

RESURRECTION OF THE BODY
SACRED BELIEF

Eshans stand firm on their belief that the marriage feast of Cana was the marriage of Mary Magdalene to Jesus, and if the story of the marriage had not been altered, and if related writings had not been omitted, or gone unrecognized by church Fathers and church authorities, the history and formation of doctrines and practices of the church might be radically different to say the least. As the Bishops Conference in and of itself claims:

> We call our reception of Christ in the Eucharist "Holy Communion" for through our reception of his Body and Blood, Soul and Divinity, we come into communion with Him who is all holy. The Son of God came to share in our lowly humanity that we might come to share in his holy divinity. When we receive Christ in Holy Communion, we are united to the Risen Christ and come to share in his divine life. Through Christ's indwelling, we are likewise united, in the Holy Spirit, to God the Father, the source of all holiness.

Based on their words alone, it would show that Mary Magdalene was not only the first to be divinized through her marriage to Jesus, but would, likewise, raise the Virgin Mary to new heights to those who were told she was just a "special Woman." It goes without saying that the woman impregnated by God with the Son of God was totally divine since she carried the Eucharist within her womb.

These two events would reveal that *the outcome of their unique reception of His Christed Body, since each is the perfected version of this union. Each in its own way reestablished a faith that would answer many questions held by the faithful followers of Jesus. His powerful teachings were meant to bring about humankind's salvation perfectly before its God.*

Eeshans note Christ fulfilled many Old Testament prophecies, as described in the New Testament, in addition to those we know applied to his marriage (but have been glossed over, not acknowledged as such, or changed, once again, how the church's trajectory through history might have been altered had this not been the case). We find the institution of the Catholic church, arguably, wants all to be convinced that it is the last 'true' institution to remain, due to its adherence, and reliance upon, 'natural law.' Eeshans disagree with this, because Eeshans believe Catholic doctrine does not adequately reflect the person of Jesus in his totality. Time does not destroy the wisdom of the past; rather, it stores it away until one retraces the paths of wisdom, and applies one's findings to rediscovering the truth. The wisdom of Jesus' marriage to Mary, likewise, is not a wisdom before God that can be altered, destroyed, or permanently hidden by human beings because it does not serve and supplement human plans; rather, this marriage was stored away until the time came when the world of human beings reached a point in its spiritual development (and/or decline) that it could not be hidden any longer. Scriptures fulfilled by Jesus are equal to those in which Jesus gives prophecies.

Jesus Christ's wisdom was never meant to be used to *limit* man's interpretation, or experience of the divine, but rather that wisdom should enable man to *fulfill* God's design, which is all-inclusive, perfectly balanced, satisfying, and salvific. To find what appears to be inconsistencies in Jesus' teachings only causes one to continue examining his teachings more closely.

As one reads scripture, one must realize that the events which are described were not recorded as happening in what we think of today as 'real time.' As scholars presently understand, the gospels were written down long after Jesus died, and even long after those who remembered him died; stories were told, and what was remembered most was passed down in oral form until finally written down, in the name of communities gathered around certain well-known leaders or personalities. We can see from most collections existing today of Gnostic gospels and non-canonical literature that many other things about Jesus were 'remembered,' while other things (Jesus' 'sayings') were written down. What was eventually accepted as official canon, however, by the growing institution of Christianity, was not the only 'record of events' that held what Jesus said, did, and taught. And after perusing the rest of the literature besides the officially accepted New Testament canon, one does feel inspired to wonder on what basis certain writings were accepted while others were rejected. It could certainly be the case that some of these writings seemed too embellished with legend and excess; yet, in other cases, one wonders if some writings were excised because they suggested, or were more direct about Jesus' relationship with Mary Magdalen. **One wonders if those writings painted a picture of Jesus that those in authority felt would lead people to ask too many questions; or would others come to see a Jesus, and a God they could reach and have a relationship with, without the need for religious authorities to serve as mediators ...?**

In modern times, we often hear, the victors in a war have the power to write history, and select their own versions of conflicts and battles which support their views and justify their actions. Today, we are faced with history being radically changed to reflect various agendas. Sadly, where history was supposedly written partially in order that humans learn from their mistakes, today, it has become only a means by which certain people can secure a *kind of immortality* for themselves, that is, until the next generation deems them heretics of one kind or another. A reason this is happening is lack of education and consistency.

That is what could have happened, and there is a good chance that it *did* happen this way, that those in authority who were dedicated to building the growing nation of the faithful felt they had to keep them unified under a very particularly crafted image of the Savior; perhaps, one that would bolster and defend the institution they had been developing. At the same time, they selected only those writings as 'sacred scripture,' which supported *their version* of the Savior. This would serve both evolving-from-the-beginning political plans of a gradually strengthening religion, like the Jewish religious and cultural roots from which this version of Christianity arose. They could further honor and embed in the minds and hearts of growing numbers of followers the version of Jesus Christ, which had been handed down to *them*. They were being conditioned to believe this image and set of origin accounts. What was handed down to them came ultimately from Peter, who wanted a Jesus without Mary.

From this point of view, one may begin to see a pattern that. unequivocally. points to a deliberate exclusion of Mary Magdalene's role in Jesus' ministry through the use of fear tactics. For example, it is written that we *must* avoid "those who cause divisions and create obstacles contrary to the doctrine that you have been taught that serve their own appetites, and by smooth talk and flattery they deceive the hearts of the naive. For your obedience is known to all so that I rejoice over you but I want you to be wise as to what is good and innocent as to what is evil."[315] There is also this which we believe was directed against Mary especially after his comment to her when she brought Jesus' word to them: "There were also false prophets among the people just as there will be false teachers among you. They will secretly bring in destructive heresies, even denying the Master Who bought them and will bring swift destruction upon themselves" (2 Peter 2:1). It is ironic it would be found in Peter's work. It should be mentioned that there is no proof that Peter did not write this. This writing then, deemed Peter's own work, appears to be written that none of Mary's writings, or teachings, were to be accepted, at any time. It's no wonder that this writing would be accepted by the church's scholars. Why would they suspect Peter of foul play, especially when the record seems to speak for itself? There would appear to be no reason to suspect there was any kind of 'cover up' or treachery. The identity of traitor to Jesus' mission was already pinned on Judas, and that's what was remembered and handed down through the ages.

It is safe to presume then, that it will always be Peter against Mary. It generally considered that this particular book's purpose is not to alter doctrine or to redirect power and authority to someone or something else. Before his death, Peter desired to remind Christians of virtues to diligently add to one's faith. As all this 'may' be true, isn't it odd that Peter

---

[315] Cf. Romans 16:17-20.

mentions the transfiguration of Jesus, where he and John were the "true" witnesses, and the disciples of Christ to show that theirs is the prophetic word, which is in the scriptures, and though theirs were the only writings guided by the Holy Spirit?

If the lens he looked at life through was so heavily and typically conditioned to be materialistic and worldly (based on his ego, and from there, ambitions naturally arise), Peter would automatically prove by this writing that he definitely missed the true focus and import of Jesus' mission. As Jesus' mission was ultimately grounded in the transcendental, we see by this writing that Peter was indeed ego-driven, and this presents a perfect case for his focus being worldly. His intention was purely to preserve his legacy which invalidates any comment that there is no personal agenda or altering of authority.

Peter was so clueless about the transcendental Mission of Christ's salvation that he presented good works and deeds as all one needs for salvation. He shied away from whatever Jesus taught regarding His marriage and the Sacred Food and Drink. This eventually, spiritually, led to a crisis over faith versus works.[316] Surely it is still clear that he had no idea what Jesus meant by his Bread of Life discourse, just as Jesus addressed at the time. The Eucharist never served Peter's goals. It was certainly not a priority, nor would it build a worldly kingdom. His way certainly did allow for the building of a worldly kingdom, as we in fact see happened with the church of Peter up to and including the Vatican today.

These facts clearly present that the Eeshan point of view carries that much more credibility. We present also, that as the scholars missed this monumental flaw, they were either not scholars who understood Christ's mission, as well, or they presented this to back up just love and service to God over his directive for the Eucharist as necessary for everlasting life.

One must see that another reason for Peter to not ever reference the last Supper and the Eucharist is simply because Mary Magdalen would have had to have been mentioned alongside of Christ, which would be to say.

---

[316] In terms of what saves, faith alone, or good works, one might easily raise the issue of what place the Eucharist has in this debate, especially since Jesus so clearly and unequivocally declares its necessity. – Ed.

Peter was not in the place of honor. The account of the Transfiguration event, though shortened, took place only with Peter, James, and John present. Here we find Peter wanting to set up a tent for Elijah, Jesus, and Moses, yet, later on, the cowardice of the same man is shown when he *appears* to become concerned for Jesus safety, as he tells Jesus not to go to Jerusalem. Immediately, Jesus exposes Peter's true concern when He says to him, "Get behind me Satan. You are a stumbling block to me; for you do not have in mind the things of God, but the things of men." Eeshans find it curious that Jesus' reference to Peter, being as Satan, was up to now explained as Satan's plan was to stop Jesus from accomplishing what Jesus came here to do, while using Peter's cowardice as his main point of leverage, when, in reality, Jesus was directly addressing Peter's concern for Himself and his own plans. The timing of Jesus going to Jerusalem was not good for Peter; he was already most concerned with guilt by association, and by this time Jesus already was in hot water with the authorities. Peter was able to play down his association with Jesus to some with distance, while to others he enjoyed being considered a 'leader.' In Jerusalem during this time, the crowds would be enormous, and surely Peter would encounter people from both of these groups.

Peter missed the mark on all counts. He saw only self-filling not self-emptying unless self-emptying might be seen for him as a means to a theatrical setting, to emphasize his status among those like Paul, but to be sure, he would never have tried it around James, the Righteous.

SUMMARY POINT 26

Paul

Paul, who was an apostle directly by the hand of Jesus, apart from the other apostles, went about his mission in his own way after his conversion. First, however, he went to see Peter, and the others, out of respect. Not all of the apostles would accept him. It didn't take long for the two, Peter and Paul, to come to odds.

During one of his encounters, Paul found Peter sitting with the Jewish authorities who were guilty of spilling the blood of Jesus, and 'confronted him to his face.' Paul knew this for a fact. Due to his (Peter's) combination of naiveté, and desire to curry the favor of those in power for the sake of advancing his apostolic mission according to his own conceptions and not those of Jesus, out of shock, or perhaps embarrassment, Peter asked for Paul's forgiveness, when asked by the newly made apostle, "Who do 'you' worship Peter?" Peter, red-faced, answered, "The Christ! That is who." An obviously disappointed Paul got little encouragement from Peter and found himself knowing less than when he arrived, since Peter's focus seemed to be centered on the Jews more than the Gentiles for many reasons.

Paul left Peter and became the apostle to the Gentiles after Peter's disinterest was made clear regarding coming to any decisions regarding the blending of both cultures under Jesus. Knowing full well the politics of the religious establishment (of which he was considered a master, but which he abandoned for the sake of the gospel), Paul was entrusted with the mission to the Gentiles by Jesus, apart from Peter.

Paul was familiar with the treachery, and duplicitous scheming of those who dwelt in the religious establishments of that time, to safeguard their power and lifestyle. "I know that after I leave, savage wolves will come among you and will not spare the flock. Even from your own number men will arise and distort the truth in order to draw away disciples after them. So be on your guard!" taught Paul. (Acts 20:29) Paul's focus was always centered on Jesus, and being very intelligent, he stayed ahead of the errors Peter evidenced, often trying to get him back on track. Eeshans feel that Jesus sent Paul to Peter several times in an effort to keep him from causing even greater damage than he had already.

There are clearly many truths about Jesus in the writings of the New Testament, and truth is 'where you find it,' sometimes even amidst the lies. But from the Eeshan point of view, scripture is a combination of many truths that were illustrated by God, but perceived through human minds and conditioned by time and circumstance, and then written about with human hands. This is so very important to remember.

It has been said, in the midst of that process, it is not impossible that those with the less than pure hearts and minds, recognizing the power of religious emotion in human beings, wouldn't utilize it for gain, or even out of otherwise good intentions for the sake of steering perception, swaying opinion, or bolstering adherence to an image, teaching, or doctrine. Thus, as another saying goes so perfectly here, "Counterfeit money often has good bills mingled with it." There must be a solid enough combination of emotion and truth to capture the human heart, and mind, and this is precisely the formula was for the growth of the church, as unstable as it was back then, and as necessary it has been for the retention of followers.

Anyone who was alive at the time of the apostles, and who fell in love with Jesus would very likely believe what Peter would tell them especially if encouraged by an outside force managing control of the Christians. In this way, manipulation would be perceived as directives laid down by Jesus. How easy it was and has been to hide, by lies and/or omissions, or even partial truths and pivotal foundations to Jesus' true mission, such as Mary being Jesus' wife.[317] With the authorities, it was clearly for a

---

[317] Jesus being the Savior, for example, is only 'partially' true in the sense that he intended to complete His mission with His wife at his side as an integral part of that mission: to restore the balance of Male and Female before God. He 'is' the Savior, but for the

particular purpose and goal. It was not foreseen that technology would one day advance at such a great speed, and in the way it has, with regards to communication, and sharing of information, and making such accessible to the world; and that truths that were once deemed safely secured away from public knowledge, along with evidence that was either hidden, or destroyed, would then be revealed.

One very powerful scriptural passage that clearly stands guard over the truth in the face of potential tampering, and the threat of cover-ups, is found in Revelation 22:18-19:

> *I warn everyone who hears the words of the prophecy of this scroll. If anyone adds anything to them, God will add to that person the plagues described in this scroll. And if anyone takes words away from this scroll of prophecy, God will remove that person's share in the tree of life and in the Holy City, which are described in this book.*

This is what Paul's warning was about. He knew how easy this could happen. He also knew that Peter was not one to carry out his duties and responsibilities as he should.

Again, we must be reminded of the words of Jesus in the rare gospel of the Confession of the Twelve in which Jesus is "speaking to his apostles" and tells them that there will indeed be those who will change His words or, omit them, saying things He did not say, or taking away things He said, for their own purposes. We are told that such persons do not serve the Lord Jesus Christ by finding alternate ways of deceiving His people; however, questioning what doesn't make sense, or what seems to be incomplete in searching for truth hardly puts one in this

---

complete truth to be understood properly Mary's role as co-Messiah is essential. That is, as the Son of God, His marriage to Mary (whom He divinized) was an essential component of His own life before God, and the fulfillment of the reason for which He was sent. Thus, to cut out the role of Mary and hold up only Jesus renders Jesus' work only a 'partial' truth, leaving the full truth incomplete. Passed down through the ages, the effects of this omission have been clearly observed, generally through social structures in history since the time of Christ, and specifically in the history of the church/Christianity itself. – Ed.

category. Otherwise, we would be guilty of obedience to man rather than obedience to God, as was the case in biblical times with manmade laws being presented as from God. Could Peter's writings be the fulfillment of Jesus' prophecy, as it seems that Jesus used every opportunity to try and persuade Peter to 'not' be led by Satan throughout his ministry, even predicting his weaknesses and denials? Wasn't it Peter's loyalty that Paul addressed? Was Peter's actions, or lack of leadership and spirituality, as one would expect the leader of the apostles to be, and was this the reason Peter feared James coming into any area he was?

It was during the conflict with Paul where he addressed all that Peter was failing to do. Peter had not been having, nor attending, worship services where the Eucharist was distributed. This caused unrest among Peter's followers, since they too began to dwindle in numbers at worship services, thinking, that if Peter didn't go, they didn't have to go either. This shows that the Bread of Life discourse made little impression on Peter all along.

Another time, when Peter was on the rooftop waiting to eat, he had a vision. A sheet lowered from heaven, containing many different animals. A voice encouraged him to eat. Peter balked, realizing that some of the animals in the sheet were forbidden to eat under Jewish law. Three times the sheet lowered, and three times Peter refused. This vision had two purposes. Jesus had given a new law where the prohibition regarding once forbidden food was lifted, meaning that the rules about dietary restrictions no longer applied, since those who follow Jesus are to be recognized by their love for God and neighbor, and not their dietary practices. Peter was told, "what God has called clean, you do not call unclean." After the third time, the sheet was taken back up to heaven.

Secondly, and most importantly, this was meant to be a spirituality that welcomed *everyone*. Salvation was open to the Gentiles as much as it was there for the Jews.

Don't forget it was Peter who had received several messages from the 'Gentile' centurion, which he ignored, because in Peter's mind, this man ate 'unclean' meat. Peter's conflict with Jesus' instructions (that no longer would His followers be divided by their cultural differences but become known for their love), and was reluctant to meet with this man who was determined to accept and follow Jesus' way. This was a real conundrum for Peter, as we see that his birth religion was what still ruled his mind, and as we said, Paul knew this. Thinking Peter would overcome this obstacle, *Paul found the old ways were still very much alive in him.* If you recall, it was in a vision that Jesus deliberately went to Cornelius, a very prayerful man, who was told in this vision to go see Peter, that Peter may witness his desire; and, thus, Cornelius would find out what he needs to do to follow Jesus.

Though Peter told them that he 'perceived' that God is not one who respects persons in every nation, and that there are those who were righteous and are accepted by God; we find later that he constantly chose to work only with the Jews. That is why he told Paul to work with the Gentiles. Thus, once again, *Peter may have spoken the words of Christ, but his actions were still those which served his birth religion.* That is why the influence of teachings on what had been given to Jesus' followers limited, if not totally stifled, the fruits and gifts of the Spirit intended to free us from oppression, discrimination, and freedom for change. Today, we see even fewer conversions from other religions, even fewer from the Jewish faith.

And, of course there is the legendary encounter where Peter, while fleeing the city to escape Nero's persecution, encountered a boy who was heading toward the persecution. The boy asked Peter where he was going ("Quo Vadis?"). Peter answered that he was leaving the city. At that, the boy added that he (the boy) was going to be with his people who were being crucified. Only then did Peter return to Rome. The story also has another version, where it was Jesus scourged who asked Peter, moving the emphasis away from the image of a boy.

SUMMARY POINT 27

FINAL REVIEW OF FOUNDATIONAL BELIEFS

As we have shown, the canonical New Testament contains nothing about Mary Magdalen except to emphasize such fabricated stories of her being freed from the seven demons and the innuendos of her 'prostitution.' It also omits any positive references, or mention of women's roles during Jesus' public life, except to say, "They ministered to him," and there are none after He was crucified and resurrected, except for the story of Mary Magdalene apparently mistaking him for the gardener.

Further, whenever a book in the Bible refers 'positively' to a woman, you would find that most likely it isn't in the New Testament around the time of Jesus, except to mention the women at the cross, or in certain gospels, the women on the way to the tomb after the crucifixion. Other than the Mother of God, the only female reference to "bride," "woman," or "wife," is in the spirit of symbolic descriptions regarding the church. In Hosea 2:14-17, where we find prophecies that could very easily connect a real woman to God, or the Wife of the Lamb in the book of Revelation, or God's plan to reveal her in the fullness of time in the account of the Woman in the Wilderness, we find these easily and quickly explained away. God says, "Therefore, behold. I will allure her, and bring her into the wilderness, and speak tenderly to her. And there I will give her vineyards and make the Valley of Achor, a door of hope." As with all the above verses, Eeshans see this scriptural passage not only as prefiguring an End Times revelation regarding the Woman in the Wilderness (Rev 12:6), but also God's actual plan for His wife in these end times, to once again bring hope and faith to His people. In Hosea 2:20 God speaks, "I will betroth you to me in faithfulness. And you shall know the Lord." Still, the church continues to insist that God is speaking about the church of Peter as a kind of connection to the Old Testament's reference to the people of Israel and God as her 'husband.'

Sadly, it seems that most accounts of women in the New Testament point out, primarily, the sinful nature of women, labeling them "adulteresses," or "sinners," or even omitting them entirely in an effort to never let one forget the 'sin' of Eve against God, where she was the one who caused man to 'lose' everything.

In the case of the wedding at Cana, where aside from Jesus' mother, and the connotation of what Jesus was thinking, there is no mention of the bride, only a groom, etc. This is true wherever and whenever humans want to build an agenda, but with regards to the matter at hand, these scriptures as well as many other documents, poignantly reveal too much of the truth being purposefully avoided.

Over the centuries, the followers of Jesus have, without a doubt, been conditioned to believe along specific lines, and have never questioned, or were 'discouraged' to seek answers to what is now becoming evident because a lot of information is available and can no longer be ignored. We have shown throughout this book how the notion of a female consort to God is vehemently denied, or simply ignored by patriarchal religions. Eeshans argue that there is a female counterpart, but, when noted, it is ignored, or foolishly explained away as 'pagan,' as are most scriptural passages that appear as sound evidence for a Sacredly Balanced God.

Presenting examples of, and affirmations to, the above are numerous throughout this book, this is traced back to what could have been a very strong foundation for Jesus' constitutional stand on equality through God's lens of a balanced love and personal dignity. One of these first appears in the Old Testament. Eeshans feel the phrase *B'reshit bara Elohim* is grossly misinterpreted, and that the subject is a plural, non-gendered noun referring to *both* genders, as brought to light and written in commentaries of many who question the reading in 1 Kings: 33, translated as "Goddess," and in 1 Kings 11:31, translated as "God." Another case in point is that though the Hebrews use the masculine gender for objects with no inherent gender (which is the way in most patriarchal religions or cultures), as well as objects with masculine natural gender, the noun used for the Spirit of God in Genesis, *Ruach*, is distinctly feminine, as is the verb used to describe her activity during creation, *rachaph*, translated "fluttereth."[318] It should be noted that this very feminine verb is used in only one other place in the Bible, Deuteronomy 32:11, where it describes the action of a mother eagle moving toward her nest. Again, Eeshans assert that the fact that the continued findings about a feminine nature are so convincingly explained that the Son of God's conviction to demonstrating it was one of the main reasons for His arrest and indictment.[319] The certainty Eeshans feel over these findings and opinions, surely points to why Jesus had to be put away, and it also indicates a deliberate effort to extinguish any proof of a God who is masculine *and* feminine; and, thus, God of all expressions of gender derived from male/female. It is an undisputed fact that the argument will always be put forth that God has no gender; and that gender is a quality for creatures serving a purpose for procreation,[320] and due to a 'moral compass' that God's law would not allow for anything beyond humankind's designations, as God does not 'procreate.' The truth is, God has procreated by means of the Begetting process with the Second Person of the Holy Trinity, and once again in the belief that Jesus, the Second Person of the Holy Trinity is the Son of God made Man, which simply can't be explained away as He witnesses to God being His Father, and the Virgin Mary as His Mother.

---

[318] "Gender of God in Christianity." Wikipedia, Wikimedia Foundation, 11 Dec. 2019, en.wikipedia.org/wiki/Gender_of_God_in_Christianity.

[319] While at first glance other charges would seem more serious, i.e., blasphemy, it is intriguing to consider the far-reaching ramifications of a movement being started and catching on at that time in that part of the world, which had as its focus the dignity of equality between the sexes. Since everything religious, social, and political was rooted in patriarchal structures, everything one knew at that time that it could fall apart at its foundations. This was, indeed, quite serious. – Ed.

[320] Consider, however, that often when people enter into this discussion they are not conscious of language and terms, i.e., people fail often to make the distinction in their minds between gender as a fundamental polarity inherent in all relationships, and physical sexual identity, which has its connection specifically with the perpetuation of a species. With God there are male and female *natures*, while with creatures the physical reflection of these natures becomes male *body* and female *body*. People are thinking of God in physical, bodily terms, and not in terms of relationship. – Ed.

On the other hand, however, there is the argument that the male and female attributes of creatures are reflective of a polarity of positive/negative relationship, and that this relationship exists throughout the physical universe as a central, universal principle, and that this interrelationship, in turn, is a reflection of some quality in the Divine, although there in a perfected form. This definition is the simple explanation to what is above, so below, identifying two variables, where one is divine and has taken on a physical form, without losing its divine component, thus being fully divine, fully human and fully sacramental, and which ends the argument of who and what Jesus was, is, and will always be.

So then, if the image, and likeness of God, is truly balanced in the way the church of Peter defines Him, why wouldn't Peter do as Jesus did? Instead, he continued to teach, or follow, the Old Law and not allow women and children to hear him speak. Why would he have continued the error of making the female gender subservient, and not show a woman as having the same dignity before God as a man? And if Peter was representing God's fullness of person with the message to an interiorly and exteriorly troubled world, why would he keep the Old Law and customs? Instead, Jesus brought the New Law into effect, stood in women's defense publicly, and in the face of public accusation and derision over their 'sinful ways' saying, "Neither do I condemn you," as well as, "anyone who leaves his wife, except for sexual immorality, makes 'her' the victim of adultery."

SUMMARY POINT 28

METTA: GOD'S LOVE, AND HOW IT WAS MEANT TO PLAY OUT IN HUMAN LOVE
SACRED TEACHING

Eeshans believe that God so loved us that God, as the three Sacredly Balanced persons, (each) brings us Metta, a word that describes a deeply felt and lived sense of divine love (as distinct from the comparison to a flawed human-based love, which is rooted in *emotion*, no matter how rich and selfless that may feel on its own terms). It is a love more profound than the English words "love" and "kindness" evoke. Metta is a love far deeper than human love; yet, it can be attained by, with, and through God, who is the reason for one's being. For us, human love was always meant to be a foundation from which to understand and practice Metta, the love of God. God's love, Metta, is a love which sustains and helps others to help themselves, whereas, human love alone eventually breeds entitlement mentality.

God's continued creative energy begets and by right destroys. This extreme love that is Metta, which Eeshans believe exists by God's presence with and within us, is a love so deep and inexplicable that it in itself proves his/her very existence. God's love continues to amaze us, as does His son's love, self-sacrifice, and mercy. The exemplary life and love Jesus shared in his marriage with Mary, which in turn raised human love and marriage to the highest level, gave humans a way back to their transcendental state. His marriage corrected the errors and destroyed the laws man-made, which were held over the people to be God's own many laws, laws, which, in turn, were used to judge as though the authorities were acting in the place of God, and with the mandate of God. What Jesus brought, and clarified, destroyed discrimination with Metta and truth.

By the power of the Holy Spirit, we now have the ability to seek and understand the truth behind this extraordinary love given to us by Jesus Christ, just as He taught back in biblical times. By bringing into this world these same teachings, via acknowledging the fulfillment of His promise of a helper for these end times, His counterpart, the Divine Feminine, we are, once again, able to return to the path of enlightenment.

God, who is all loving, had promised to restore this plan engendered by this Metta, this unique love for Adam and Eve before and after the choice for physicality over the transcendental. As God is good, this plan must reflect all that is wholesome and good, sans all discrimination, for all of God's children. Thus, it was necessary to bring into existence one who would become the liaison between the two worlds. One who is God, and one who is human, to bridge the gap as only God could be perfect in all things, and only could a God, who was also a perfect human being, who could restore and rid the world of a purely human consciousness, and lead us back to the transcendental consciousness, as only Jesus and His wife could. He would by His love for His wife, together with her, as eternal and human consort, choose a transcendental love over a physical one; He would sacrifice all a man loves: wife, children, and marriage to accomplish God's will, while being the perfect altar, perfect victim, and perfect sacrifice in God's eyes.

This is the God whose omnipotent mercy and love for our first parents was understanding of a free and voluntary love and human weakness, and who desired a love out of choice for what is right, and in line, with loving God above all things; yet, God allowed us also to use free will as we choose. One must remember, however, that free will also makes us subject to, and accountable for, our actions and the consequences thereof. Therefore, we cannot blame God for the outcome of human beings' choices, especially those who profess no spirituality, since, if God were to interfere, then God would be accused of infringing on free will, or fear of allowing us to choose and make decisions on our own. Either way, humans will turn the tables on God in the spirit of blame, and blame is the abnegation of personal and collective human responsibility.

God knew the effects of the choice of a physical love, and becoming a permanent part of the physical world, and warned Adam and Eve about entropy. Entropy, we recall, is death beginning at birth. This occurs as the physical is subject to time and its partner gravity. Time does not exist in eternity. God's unconditional love for us is likened to parents who, despite telling children what is right and wrong, by way of lessons learned through experience, know they must allow them to make their own choices, even if pain and hurt is the end result; yet, these same parents are always there to help provide comfort and healing. Knowing all things, God, as any good parent, sent help—a plan and a way back to God from death to life—and this was Jesus and His Feminine Consort.

God knew that though lack of faith was primary, a catalyst was needed: the love between and among humans. It was the one thing that people were most familiar with and it was an ideal starting point for Jesus' teachings. Love for neighbor would go hand in hand with this love. Jesus, knowing that this love between a male and female must reflect the love between the Divine Consorts, taught that without proper guidance and corrections of misinformation His people would be lost.

SUMMARY POINT 29

THE FULLNESS OF TIME: SACRED MYSTERIES AND ETERNITY

There is the familiar saying, 'If you wait long enough for something, it will happen.' This is what the term 'fullness of time' means. One should understand that this term was not just meant to declare the great coming of the Son of God, Jesus Christ,[321] but is also meant to be a marker for all events God deems necessary for humankind. Just as Jesus' birth earmarked the fullness of time for the coming of the Messiah, His life and mission, in a similar way, we embark on the 'fullness of time' when we realize it is now necessary to restore the rightful place of the Divine Feminine, and to allow her to bring humankind back to Jesus' plan of salvation, as well as the ORIGINAL plan of salvation, before his second coming.

Eeshans see this age, the age of the Divine Feminine, as the 'fullness of time,' where traditional religion has left a vacuum in the heart and souls of God's people, and, once again, God's prophecy to send a helper who will be the "woman who will crush the head of the serpent who took the truth and defiled it."

This is, Eeshans believe, "the time of the separation" of the people one from another as a shepherd separates the sheep from the goats.

---

[321] Who automatically embodies with his own spirit Lady Wisdom, so that while the Divine Masculine is the Word, the Divine Feminine is the Perennial Wisdom which is the substance of the Word who is spoken. – Ed.

> He will put the sheep at his right and the goats on his left. Then the King will say to those on his right, "Come, you who are blessed by my Father; take your inheritance, the kingdom prepared for you since the creation of the world. For I was hungry and you gave me something to eat, I was thirsty and you gave me something to drink, I was a stranger and you invited me in, I needed clothes and you clothed me, I was sick and you looked after me, I was in prison and you came to visit me." Then the righteous will answer him, "Lord, when did we see you hungry, and feed you, or thirsty and give you something to drink? When did we see you a stranger and invite you in, or needing clothes and clothe you? When did we see you sick or in prison and go and visit you?" The King will reply, "Truly I tell you, whatever you did for one of the least of these brothers and sisters of mine, you did for me." Then he will say to those on his left, "depart from me, you who are cursed, into the eternal fire prepared for Satan and his demons." (Matt. 25:27-41)

Discrimination abounds and continues to be taught even among those institutions claiming to have the truth and who teach the teachings of Jesus. These see no end to the sins of a mortal nature. Lying is more acceptable than truth. Self-love reigns higher than love of others. Killing lives for God and the betterment of the world is a mantra greater than love of God and neighbor (i.e., radical pro-life). Man has essentially replaced God with himself, and there are as many potential forms and manifestations of this as there are human points of view. Human life is now at the mercy of other imperfect and prone-to-error human beings, who, due to lack of faith, can no longer see God.

Though it may seem as though what is being said here is pedantic, it approaches the source and summit of our beliefs. Reiterating details to such an extent is like the shell, or calcification, around the pineal gland. To remove and expose it without understanding of the treasure within is to do the greatest damage. Since all that it encompasses would be released into the universe without any benefit, or grace-filled spirituality, or advancement of the person towards God. Within this precious gland are all the mysteries stored within the soul to be released upon death in conjunction with the knowledge of the sacred mysteries of God. These mysteries include:

1. God being the infinite, the all-powerful, omnipotent, omnipresent, omniscient, omnificent Supreme Being, who is creator of all worlds and universes, who is three Masculine persons with their three eternal Female Consorts; in other words, each person being male/female.[322]
2. God the Father in a way similar to the begetting process, forms his Divine Feminine energy in order that she becomes human, never losing her divine nature, who became the Immaculate Conception, the Blessed Virgin Mary. She was the integral person who brought the only begotten son Jesus Christ, Son of God, our Savior and Bridegroom, into the fallen world. When it was time for her to leave earth, His human body went into a what is called a holy Dormition state. Because she was not subject to original sin, there was no need for her to experience death, as we do. Mary's body was resurrected by her husband's hand, three days following the transformation of her human body back into a glorious state, allowing her to maintain a human body along with her divine nature, as does her Son, as well as Mary Magdalen, when she is in heaven.
3. The Blessed Virgin Mary, who is the precious Wife and eternal consort of the First Person of the Holy Trinity, God the Father, is

---

[322] By continuing to underscore the Masculine/Feminine nature of God, the author is highlighting the Eeshan perspective that God is primarily a Person, and secondarily a 'what,' that is the *impersonal* aspect of God. The analogy of the sun and its rays are often used in Bhakti Yoga to illustrate this point: the sun is the Person, and the sun's rays, or effulgence, is the impersonal aspect. The rays are the same as the sun, by extension, but there is a difference between the object itself and its 'what' of power, light, and warmth. God is a person, but the power of God which radiates from his/her divinity is the all-pervasive 'energy' of God. – Ed.

the Mediatrix, and glorious woman of unfathomable grace, and the only one who can boast an Immaculate Conception, the one who is in the state of perpetual virginity, and is God's storehouse of love.

4. Jesus, the second person of the Holy Trinity and the Divine Masculine of the only begotten Child of the Father and Mother, came into the world by virgin birth. Known to the world as Jesus Christ, He was the active counterpart of the eternal Consorts, who was destined to die a human death *to save sinners* (Eeshans wonder who the sinless are ...?) for the Christs' purpose was to bring back to humanity the transcendental life forfeited by Adam and Eve. The Messiah, Savior, and Redeemer of the world, was/is Jesus, the Second Person of the Holy Trinity *together with his female eternal consort*, who in human form is known as Mary Magdalen (the Matrix),[323] and whose mission was to restore all that was lost by man's separation from God, by destroying the effects of what has become known as Original Sin/Choice, and reopen the gates of heaven. Their sacrificial Marriage would bring salvation by reconciling humans to God in order to restore the means for all of humankind throughout the ages to share in God's oneness by nourishing their light body.[324] This is done by consuming God

---

[323] Mary Magdalen is the Matrix of God's possibilities, the passive Feminine Aspect of Christ and it is in relation to Him that she becomes the impregnating source of new life in such a way that plenitude arises from the Trinity.

[324] Recall in the introductory pages of this book what is meant by "original sin," and the intention behind using the traditional language employing terms such as 'original sin,' 'reopen gates of heaven,' and so forth. This language was from a different time and circumstance and corresponded to a particular degree of awareness. While this language is important for the mind and memory to use as a reference point, it carries with it certain mental images and emotional qualities. From the Eeshan perspective there is a substantial difference in meaning behind the mental and emotional imagery of 'original sin,' and a 'choice' that brought with it substantial changes and limitations in being. The former carries with it the stigma of shame and breaking a commandment of God causing God's anger and loss of love. The latter carries with it a sense that a choice was made that brought with it unfolding consequences, much of which was undesirable and unforeseen—but the way through could be navigated successfully with the intervention of a) God's mercy and b) through the *Sophia Perennis*. – Ed.

by way of a process called transubstantiation, whereby, God's Divine and Human natures become a sustenance/Sacred Food known by its Sacramental nature as the Eucharist, which when consumed in a sanctifying state, brings human souls back to an immortal transcendental state and consciousness. Upon death of the human vehicle known as our gross physical state/body, our Light Body resumes its natural state of being Light.

5. Being God, Jesus was divine. His divinity is the transcendental Light of God, which embraced immortality, which we lost through Original Sin. The aforementioned is the means by which this light would be fully and perfectly restored when grafted into the Light of the world who is Jesus and Mary. This could only be made possible by Jesus being Divine and becoming human, who together with his eternal Consort Mary, also becoming human and together fulfilling the perfect sacrificial love by, with, and in their marriage, in order that the Sacred Food is returned along with the real Presence of God being available to humans once again, just as it was for Adam and Eve before their choice. Their intention is to free us to share in a life that would enable us to be free from entanglement with, and being limited to, a gross physical state, which came into being along with the effects of entropy. He showed us that He was the Way, and if we followed His example, we would be enlightened beings with a consciousness of new intuitive and enlightened viewpoints, and would see our world in the way God sees it, sans the way a more materially centered and limited animal nature sees it. His is the Way, the Truth, and the Light and Love; and though we who experience the effects of entropy, and live in a physical world where death is imminent, because of Jesus and his Marriage, our lives don't end here. We now have a guaranteed eternal afterlife with God, as promised by Jesus, where we will know what perfect use of free will is.

6. There we will experience freedom and love in a perfect way without the dark, oppressive, and tarry sight, or thoughts tainted by fear, as well as all the illusions that grow out of fear. Above all,

despite the lesser physical life[325] our first parents chose, we will now have, with Jesus, a means to choose our own destiny. Now we have a divine guide, whereas, before we were subject almost entirely to the human consciousness.

---

[325] "Lesser" does not mean "bad," or that what is being said is that the body is evil or a source of sin, impurity, etc. What should be kept clear is that the body, compared to the soul, is limited; and physical life, compared to eternal spiritual life, is by comparison, certainly 'lesser.' What Adam and Eve chose was the appearance of a certain type of experience in the physical universe, whereby, they thought they might love in a new way, or so they were led to believe; the result of this choice was that they could not exit under their own power or be spiritually free as they previously were. – Ed.

SUMMARY POINT 30

THE NEW ADAM AND THE NEW EVE: UNDERSTANDING FREE WILL

Without a doubt, all of the Who and What of God is preserved in Jesus. He, through His teachings, brought the reality of how everything is connected to everything else. Everything we do, say, and think affects others and the universe around us. He taught how even our thoughts, words, feelings, desires, and will affect everything around us,[326] how we engage in good actions, and seek our dreams, rather than exercise and indulge bad thoughts, spreading bad emotions, and saying bad words. All good comes from God, and we should *and could* mirror that good here on earth, with each other.

Whether intentional or unintentional, depending on how some people see it, Adam and Eve chose a physical relationship, which brought with it consequences, but we can change anything and should, since we reap what we sow. If we see only bad in our lives, only bad will keep occurring, so don't expose yourself to useless worry or future concerns when today we can make things better. We need to compass and set our minds and spirits to see that no matter how bad we think we have it, there are others with much worse issues. JESUS TOLD US HOW WE HAVE THE STRENGTH AND ABILITY WITH GOD TO CHANGE AND TRANSFORM OUR BAD THOUGHTS TO GOOD THOUGHTS. Jesus taught us to not focus on negative or bad things, people, or thoughts because we can rise above these, and make a

---

[326] That is, the reality we find ourselves in is by and large a result of our own making by way of our own choices in the realm of thoughts, words, and actions. – Ed.

better world around us and in our own lives. That is how God works with us, and how we can do what seems to be impossible if we believe that our being with God nothing is impossible.

Free will decisions affect everyone and everything. For example, even if it was not Adam and Eve's intention to offend God, they knew that what God told them was true, and, so to take the advice of a lesser being in place of God, one who gave contrary advice at that, was truly an offense; since they did not exercise free will in a positive way but rather chose to listen, and believe the lie that God was cheating them out of a greater love. Yet, this is where free will comes in. Despite what they were told, they could exercise this right, and they, in a way, tested God. Was it curiosity? Why was their choice the means to the end of the life as they knew it? It was so because God forewarned them that to eat of the forbidden tree would be 'life altering.'

Had they consulted God, perhaps there would have been a different outcome. Our love here on earth is no different. Because of Jesus alone, if one believes in Him, it should mirror God's love even though our love is imperfect, since it is the effort we put into it, not the success, that is measured by God. Eeshans see why the consequences and losses were justified, and we see also how God's love for us was like that of parents to children. Parents understand bad, sometimes life altering choices, mostly because of what they have seen, and done in their own, as well as other's lives. Love for that child is where a parent warns of potential bad decisions, and repercussions, that might follow, yet comes in after the child makes a bad decision, or choice, and despite the outcome, tries to help save the situation, even though their intervention may not be welcomed at the time. Not just children fall into this trap, but adults as well. How many times have we made choices outside what we are told are in our best interests? How many times have we been guilty of choosing against what is best in our experience simply because we desire it? The end result is what is called our destiny.

As we mentioned numerous times, destiny changes according to our choices. It is not a family name or reputation that causes bad things to happen to a child, it is their OWN choices, and reluctance to change themselves by making the same mistakes, or worse, that makes these unwanted conditions come about. That is the difference between destiny and fate. Fate leaves no options to change the end result, with no effort the end result is just accepted. For example, Jesus presented the knowledge of how to attain God's plan for humans, and if we choose to, we can see how, with God's guidance and being well informed, we still have made bad choices that caused the chaos in the world in which we live. All actions have consequences, and it requires considerable reflection beforehand to determine which choices will lead in the direction of light and which will lead in the direction of darkness, but we have the ability to change. There is no guarantee that things will turn out a certain way; even when good actions are mindfully performed there is no guaranteed favorable outcome. While our free will can work in our favor or against us, WE ARE IN CONTROL of our choices.

We often blame God, and expect God to fix what we broke. God, on the other hand, may wait for us to learn our lesson, coupled with our intent to make things right, before acting or answering our prayers. That is the nature of this material world that Adam and Even chose to enter. They, too, wanted everything to go back to the way it was when they saw their decision was nothing like what they thought it would be. God's love, being Metta, wouldn't let that happen, even though what they did changed everything, and their decision would not allow them to go back to what they had. They had to, in other words, sleep in the bed they made. God allowed them not only to live their choice but to see the consequences of it for many generations.

Our saving grace is our ability to repair our offenses before God—only humility of will is much harder than humility of heart. If we can overcome our stubbornness and exercise humility of will, perhaps, we can open our eyes to see that the greater offense (disbelief in God) puts us back to the days that outline the need for a Messiah in the first place. Maybe we would be able to see how we resemble the 'rebellious people' that Jesus came to. We have no right to put ourselves above God, yet, we feel this is free will to do so.

One does have the right to choose, but free will was intended to give us a say in making things better and more Godlike. To choose deliberately apart from God is to choose death; and cutting oneself off from

God is like a branch removing itself from the tree, and, thus, your free will ends.

But after seeing Jesus through the eyes of Eeshan Transcendentalism, can one who really believes, doubt God's existence? Perhaps, we felt compelled to walk away from a religion, or faith, because we did not believe those who purportedly held, and taught, the 'truth.' This is acceptable. Don't give up on God when you find that what your heart told you before regarding the questioning/not accepting of church doctrines, because maybe it was your heart, and the prompting of the Holy Spirit, that was protecting you. Perhaps, that light within your heart, because of your love for God, now allows you to see a light at the end of the tunnel of betrayals by those whom you did not trust, or how blessed and protected you actually were that you did not join in a religion, or faith, that others tried to get you to join, which now allows you to see how very loved by God you were all along.

The Divine Feminine realigns the heart and soul as did Jesus. Why is this important? Perhaps. in your life, you so wanted to know and hear what Jesus really taught in biblical times, but were hurt by the very people you chose to trust or were told to trust. If Jesus was real, as you believed, then He would not have allowed you to be hurt; for that He would have understood your pain and suffering, and wouldn't have allowed you to be abused, or punished so severely for trusting. When He appeared to fail you, you couldn't bear the thought of going to church. What you didn't realize is that these people took advantage of the love you had for Him; you would've continued to follow Jesus if you had understood this. What you experienced, whether in your family, in catholic school, bible study, or by priests, or 'religious' people you encountered, who were the 'bad' people in these groups ... not only did they not match up with what you expected someone who loves Jesus/God to act like, rather, they took away your faith. So now what?

Maybe now you will come to understand that this Jesus is here for you, and God hasn't abandoned you or the world. You will come to see that your search for peace and love was not in vain. In fact, God is rescuing not only you but all the countless others like you through the Divine Feminine. Now you will be able to experience Jesus and see the strength He sees in you.

SUMMARY POINT 31

Understanding Metta as Sacrificial Love

What makes Eeshans believe that they have God's original plan and that it would work today? First there's this question we have witnessed time and time again: that if the Christian faith, as a whole, taught the truth, why then after 2000 years has nothing really changed and the future of the world seems more dangerous than ever? Eeshans teach that it's impossible for God to fail; therefore, it had to be those in places of authority and leadership within the church, the 'whitewashed tombs,' that the problem began and continues to thrive even today.

For even though when Christ's words were spoken in biblical times, these words would carry life in them for all ages, as does his sacrificial marriage, since Jesus is the Word of God.

Today, many of his truths have been blurred to suit agendas that have confused what is right and what is wrong. This resulted in what is known as misplaced compassion. Misplaced compassion is a growing problem since it is not compassion at all. Misplaced compassion is nothing less than flawed choices. Misplaced compassion encompasses hate, rage, and revenge. For example, Jesus taught if you live by the sword you die by the sword, but it doesn't mean one cannot protect the innocent, or defend one's county. We say we are a people fighting against discrimination, yet, a woman named Charla Nash, who was attacked by a chimpanzee, for the longest time, was shunned by neighbors and others, because they were afraid of her disfigurement. Rather than helping Charla, and teaching others to see the beauty of this woman through her courage and pain, and show them how she has a strong desire to live despite having her life altered by this horrible incident, neighbors avoided or stayed away from her.[327] How often do we do the same in parallel circumstances? How often do we teach our children to avoid disfigured, or disabled people, as if they are somehow bad?

End of life protocol is another example of how confused we have become. We cannot continue to turn a blind eye, and accept the fact that euthanasia is okay, and allow it to be exercised under the guise of 'not wanting someone to suffer,' when it is mostly done out of convenience, and because of insurance costs, to those who have no desire to take care of the terminal patient.

We truly need to appreciate the value of life while understanding the doctor's assessment and prognosis, and weigh these along with the will of the person. Next, whoever is in charge of making life and end-of-life decisions should give deference to and the wishes of the person, despite their (the person placed in charge) own personal opinions, and consider the merit of the amount of suffering that a person may be going through, the person's beliefs, and for a reasonable time. If God's love is unconditional to the point of allowing suffering, as mentioned above, we must be careful how we intervene. Taking care of a person is far greater responsibility than one realizes, but what God witnesses is those caring for a parent or sibling, etc., and how they do the best they can with what they have. This cannot be a cop-out. Treatment of one's neighbor, be it family, friend, or stranger, is what is witnessed by God. One cannot rely on, or believe, that euthanasia is best simply because of the degree of inconvenience by a mother's fractured arm, or the travel time involved, going to and fro, or because the parent has been falling a lot. Today, there are other factors. When children don't visit ailing parents because they can't stand to see illness, or when they simply drop off food, thinking they did their part, while relying on someone to feed the person who is in care is not 'doing their part.'

---

[327] At the time of this writing, people were not helping this woman due to being afraid of the person's disfigurement and physical condition; compare this with how leprosy or any other disease was similarly seen in Jesus' and St. Francis' time. – Ed.

Then there are those who take steps making it impossible for designated money to go to anyone or to a charitable organization they don't believe in or like, despite the wishes of the dying parent. It is amazing how too many times the dying wishes of the parent are ignored. Often times, when free care is not available to ease guilt on the part of the children's involvement, a facility is chosen to relieve responsibility and duty of children. Eeshans have also witnessed children and grandchildren of the opposite mindset. God witnesses the pure love the children have for the dying parent(s) and is in awe of the kindness, gentleness, and love.

Human nature is fragile and needs spirituality in order to overcome baseless phobias. There are still people who avoid people with cancer and AIDS for fear of contracting these diseases. We can make a tremendous difference with those we love and with those who witness how we treat others less fortunate, especially doing what we can to educate, show love, and make one more comfortable, etc., but we may not end a person's life until we have determined there is absolutely no life left, and the body is only existing, being kept 'alive,' artificially.

Having faith in the fact that the Son of God was also subject to temptations, just as we are (though without falling into sin), His unalleviated suffering showed His choice to save us, and restore what humans lost rather than save Himself and His own desires.

Believing that He could be (and is) imparting teachings, whether or not they will conflict with present-time church laws and religious structures of authority is not unlike the Jesus who walked the earth before. God will always find a way to teach us, outside of the walls of corruption. Once again, and as originally intended through his Divine Feminine consort, namely His wife, His mission will come alive, and this time not be stifled, or amended and together they will never be separated again.

The present-time church's authority is one which will be in conflict with the above; Eeshans say the church has already attempted to exercise its power and religious authority opposing it. To now be labeled as being low in personal and spiritual dignity for transgressing a law will be cause enough for them to be seen or found guilty. In its scandals alone they should be ashamed for turning their heads, and looking the other way. Could having been guilty of dimidiating the Christs be fuel enough to transgress the law in question? Eeshans say, "yes."

SUMMARY POINT 32

The Victim, the Altar, and the Sacrifice

A "sacrifice" involves more than a duty to satisfy the one offended; it is not enough for the victim to accept the role on behalf of another. A sacrifice also requires a personal and heart-wrenching choice on the part of the victim. Satisfying the will of God was imperative to open the gates of Heaven, once again, but being a martyr is defined as taking the responsibility of becoming a victim, the altar, and the sacrifice; and certainly has a personal involvement and commitment, which brings one suffering, persecution, and death while advocating, refusing to renounce a principle, or value, or refusing to advocate anything contrary to an informed conscience and/or God's will. After Adam and Eve were exiled from Eden, and entered permanently into the material realm, the downward spiral of illusion and suffering human beings generated out of fear and panic regarding physical survival made the way to God both rocky and impassable. It would require the power and love of God to restore this path, but the action must also take into account the place of personal responsibility on the part of the human person to perform the action out of a freely willed choice.

Such a choice has to both equal, and surmount, the original event in both power and magnitude. That's where Jesus' marriage would have to embody this magnitude. The personal sacrifice in both their decisions for a non-conjugal love, and the reality of their temptations of a conjugal love was always there, or it wouldn't be reality for humans. Why? Because we are drawn to a physical love, since it's natural, and because of God, in marriage, it is blessed.

In order, however, to reverse the choice for this kind of love that Adam and Eve chose, Jesus and Mary had to refrain, exercising the greater love. They were never exempt from these feelings, nor was this temptation easy. As human beings with a Divine mandate, one can only imagine the distress and anxiety these feelings had to have played out on the couple. They were young, in love, and attracted to each other as deeply as soulmates can be, since their temptation had to be as intense as the feelings Adam and Eve had for each other when they decided to choose to eat the fruit, and experience the love promised by the 'being,' in order for their transcendental love to offset the consequence of their choice. Anything less would not suffice. Did they grow in desire. or feel urgings of passion for each other? Yes, absolutely. Did both count on the strength of the other to get them through these moments? Again, they absolutely did. It was for these desires that our first parents fell; and, thus, it would be by our Begotten Parents' sacrifice, that the consequences of Adam and Eve would offset the purely physical urges in order to share love in a transcendental tantric union.

Though the promise of the One, who like the Son of God, is written of, in scriptures, the reality of the fruit of their love would not be brought forth until end times, and surely was not present in their minds in moments of rapture. All these feelings were vital to the success of his mission. Christ's human marriage and life with His eternal consort during His time on earth was the epitome of a transcendental life played out on earth; but it was also unyielding in the pressure natural between a young couple in love. Being a crucial course, and like Adam and Eve, Jesus and Mary entered into this decision by free will. Jesus and Mary, however, made the opposite choice of Adam and Eve, which successfully brought about the transformation of consciousness intended by God, which had to involve facing human weaknesses. Thus, the degree in which their temptation would be felt would be best described (by the standard human consciousness) as the measure of their required and painstaking decision made from their existential circumstances.

It is said that "a vision suddenly disclosing itself in time does not necessarily fade into a corrupted shadow of itself but, as time is fluid, it carries truth into the future."³²⁸ That is why, while the marriage of Jesus and Mary may have been for a brief moment hidden in time, being erased from official church journals, and called heretical, ridiculous, and frivolous, still found its way back via persistent memory, past the words of bottom dwellers. It did not quit, nor was it changed amidst corruption, but once again stands firm and strong. Needless to say, it is no wonder why these truths are at the foundation of what Eeshans love about this sacred marriage.

To Eeshans, Jesus fulfilled all that was necessary for his involvement. Mary Magdalene is not only seen as the fulfillment of Christ's mission (just as it was necessary for Adam to have eaten the Apple to complete the choice) but to us, we believe Mary, through Eesha, fulfills the prophecy of a new "Isreal,"³²⁹ the name given to her by God's Son on their wedding night for and in these end times.³³⁰

In the Garden when Mary encountered Jesus, after the Resurrection, not only did Jesus reveal himself to her in His divine form, but, moreover, He verified the identity of Mary in her divine form, by calling her name. In doing this, He prophesied and identified her role in end times, as fulfilled in Isaiah 43:1:

> **"Do not fear, for I have redeemed you; I have summoned you by name, you are mine."**

She is truly the Lamb's Wife and the one about whom the angel spoke in Revelation (Revelation 21:9), "Come I will show you the Bride, the Wife of the Lamb." Eeshans believe that through the power of the Lamb's Wife, who shares His identity, she is the matrix of God's possibilities, and through her marriage to Jesus Christ, she is the last emanation of God's salvific Mission.

---

³²⁸ Deal Hudson, "The Catholic Church: The Last Institution," Catholic Online, January 22, 2014, http://www.catholic.org/news/national/story.php?id=53939.

³²⁹ A purposely employed play on words, meaning the person who "is real," not the country of Israel.

³³⁰ Cf., Eesha's poetry.

This is why it is written in the Kallah Creed, **"She sprang forth proelato**[331] **and experienced passion, the *epathe pathos*,**[332] **without the embrace of her desired consort."**

As Mary Magdalene, Wife of Jesus, may not have been the 'active' consort of the two at the time Jesus walked the earth, she was destined to be the active counterpart today. Back then, she was the first to experience the Savior at the time of her rescue; and He was her Redeemer who wrote her name in the sand, identifying those who violated her. She was the first to receive His Christed Body, as no other could, which awakened her divinity. By His side at the Last Supper, she became the Holy Vessel, the Grail that contained all unfathomable mysteries. By her love for him she became *His* savior at the resurrection.

In these times, she is the mirror of God in the Place prepared by God, where she is taken care of.[333] She is the Woman in the Wilderness who brought forth 'the One Who is like the Son of Man,' Emmanuel.

---

[331] Meaning she is back as a warrior to claim what is hers.

[332] Doubtless the suffering endured for love of Jesus, her husband, in other words "fearless and bold."

[333] "The Place": another name for the Metta Tirtha, or the Temple of Loving Kindness. – Ed.

SUMMARY POINT 33

I HAVE DIED EVERY DAY WAITING FOR YOU

We know the story. At the age of seventeen, Jesus left and spent eleven years in India. During that time, Jesus grew in wisdom and love. Growing up, He exhibited many gifts, which prompted His mother to encourage trips with His great uncle to places far away. His favorite was a place which is called Avalon, today located near Glastonbury. Having grown up with an extended family with cousins etc., He was seen only as a normal child, but rarely did He spend a lot of time with His family. Thereby, when Jesus began His public teaching, His family really didn't know a lot about Him, except that He was the son of Mary and Joseph. So, when He was proclaimed, or proclaimed Himself the Son of God and exhibited supernatural gifts, they were as surprised, as were others.

During the time he spent in the Himalayas, He spent hours on end studying, praying and meditating. He mastered the use of plants, water, Light, oils, energy, and, believe it or not, spit and soil. By His heavenly Father's guidance, He came to realize His transcendental existence for being here in the world; and it was to bring salvation to God's people. He witnessed inexplicable gifts. His insight, which had its origin in his divinity, caused a truly mysterious attraction to those who came into his presence. His precognition and premonitions were faultless, especially with regards to events about Himself. Often, the other teachers would take out the holy journals, and ask Him questions, since they knew He was the 'One' that the prophecies that were spoken. Though distance separated them, Jesus and the Virgin stayed in contact via the heart.

Knowing Joseph's illness was worsening and his death was imminent coincided with constant visions of the girl (now a woman), Mary, who he held in His heart.

By this time, he had become a very renowned spiritual Master though all who knew Him as a child recognized Him as being Godlike. People traveled from great distances to see and hear Him. He embraced His divinity but did not actively display it, except for instances He deemed necessary for his mission. Hundreds witnessed the 'Light' that seemed to emanate from Him. Even his words seemed to be illuminated somehow, which caused him to seek isolation, sometimes for weeks at a time. When He would come out among the people, He would heal them and teach them. But, Jesus could no longer ignore the signs—it was time. Once He made His decision, by way of the voice of His Father and the urgings of the Spirit, He would now return home and carry out His mission.

The central teaching with Jesus was that everyone was a child of God. He taught that whether one looked like a man or woman, the covering of the body (by contrast to the person's true identity) is just an illusion. It's no wonder that not all accepted this teaching. It would certainly be a 'stumbling block' to bring such teachings and God's law to the rebellious religious authorities He would face in His birth religion.

His Mother, being a woman unjustly judged during her pregnancy and after his birth, prompted him to teach males from the personal example and perspective He had regarding how He loved His Mother as Goddess and Human Mother, but there was another who spent years waiting for His return. Below,[334] are three gems taught by Jesus which He held close to his heart, which showed how God saw and appreciated the beauty originating from the Divine Feminine:

1. "Imbue yourselves in this 'temple' [woman] with moral strength. Here you will forget your sorrows and your failures, and you will recover the lost energy necessary to enable you to help your neighbor."

---

[334] Cf. Elizabeth Clare Prophet's book *The Lost Years of Jesus*.

2. "Do not expose her to humiliation. In acting thus, you would humiliate yourselves and lose the sentiment of love, without which nothing exists here below."
3. "Protect your wife, in order that she may protect you and all your family. All that you do for your wife, your mother, for a widow or another woman in distress, you will have done unto your God."

Yes, Mary Magdalen fantasized about her hero returning for her. Living on the outskirts of town, she remembered quite vividly when she met Him, just as He thought about her. That moment was at hand, since Jesus came back, due to Joseph's imminent death.

Jesus came back to town eleven years after his first encounter with Mary (the night He was leaving to study in the Himalayas). He came back wearing a white robe, for He was now a renowned spiritual master. His intention was to begin His mission but first on His agenda was to marry the person of Mary Magdalene, whom He met once during a rescue attempt when He was seventeen and she was just over thirteen.

Recalling how seven men dragged her to a cave, where they violated her, one gets the image of how violent and unsettled these times were. Rumors of insurrection were looming everywhere. People were frightened and continually looked for signs that the Messiah was coming to save them.

The two sisters, and their brother Lazarus (who spent a lot of time training soldiers and working in Jerusalem) were of royal descent, so the family was well known. That is why the men, who were known thugs, broke into their family house looking for anything of value. Money was needed to offset the price of war and power. Martha, known for her work with the poor, was just getting prepared to start her day, and was not usually home at this time of day. Surprised to find her in the house, the men began to attack Martha when Mary walked in. Martha called out to Mary to get away, however, Mary, instead, offered herself to the men in exchange for Martha's release.

Having no moral compass, whatsoever, the thugs broke in, and though they struck Martha, Mary's innocence and virginity was more than an adequate trade-off to hurting Martha, so these thugs whisked her out of the house. Carrying her through the streets to the outskirts of town, took the emphasis off them and their reputation, as they made the claim that the girl was no good to begin with and was to be punished.

Hearing the commotion, Jesus ran towards the direction of the jeering and laughter. These heathens were made to look justified in their deed, even though their reputations for thievery and murder preceded them.

Jesus, who was close by, heard the jeering and the screams of the mob, which now lined the streets. The mob called out to stone her. Mary fell to the ground, only to be dragged to her feet. Jesus ran along the way, following the continued screams. As they got past the well, Jesus got a glimpse of the girl. He knew her face. He attempted to get closer but the crowd shoved Him, too. Upon reaching the cave, he pushed his way to the entrance, but as He attempted to get in, He was held in the grasp of two of the men and was forced to watch.

After the last criminal abandoned the child, Jesus was pushed into the cave. He rushed to the girl as the sounds and laughs of the men grew distant in their leaving. Running to the girl, He began tearing off a piece of his cloak. As He did so, a spring welled up near a cave wall and He wet the cloth. As He washed off her blood, He took a piece and put it in a pocket close to His heart. Next, He wrapped his cloak around her. Wrapped in His arms, and on the way to her home, a breathless Jesus kissed her forehead, telling her everything would be all right. Jesus fulfilled scriptures regarding Mary, who was to become His wife.

Arriving at the family home, Jesus found Martha and her brother Lazarus, who had rushed back home in the state of horror. Lazarus had just gotten home after hearing about the incident.

That night, after gathering whatever news He could about Mary's condition, He took His bag at dusk, and began His journey. Unknown at this time, that both He and this young girl were cut from the same 'cloth,' He then placed it in his cloak, near his heart, safe and secure. Perhaps, He knew of their destiny, perhaps He was just taken with the courage of this girl. But what is written in Ezekiel, seems to proclaim the glory of their love.

Ezekiel 16 reads:

> "When ... I looked at you and noticed that you were of age [proper time for love/marriage] I spread My cloak over you

to cover your nakedness. I made a solemn promise to you and entered into a covenant with you," declares the Lord God. "You belong to Me. I bathed you with water, rinsed your own blood from you and anointed you with oil [He was the anointed one, and as He touched her she too was anointed] then I covered you with My cloak. [upon returning her home] [They] ... would cover her with embroidered clothing and clothed her feet in sandals.] [the prophecy continues] I wrapped you in fine linen and dressed you in silk. I adorned you with jewels, placing bracelets on your hand and necklaces on your neck. I put a ring in your nose, earrings in your ears, and a crown encrusted with jewels on your head. You were adorned with gold, silver, clothing of fine linen silk, and embroidery. You ate food made from the finest flour, honey, and olive oil.[335] You were exceedingly beautiful, attaining your royal status."

"Your fame spread throughout the nations because of your beauty. You were perfectly beautiful due to My splendor with which I endowed you," declares the Lord God.

Eeshans believe beyond the shadow of a doubt that this prophecy is about Jesus' coming back to Mary, His bride to be, after eleven years, His trust, that God's hand would reunite the Prince and Princess.

Though not "marriage material," due to being violated, seems harsh and heartbreaking, and we find that she never blamed God for what had happened to her. God, too, whose ways are above us, used this horrendous incident for a greater good. Since she was worthy and blessed.

Having tremendous innate business skills, Mary successfully started an import/export business, and traded in beautiful jewelry and fabrics, known and desired by all. She was her own woman.

But, Mary possessed a deeper and hidden depth to her. As she traveled, she collected various oils, plants, and herbs, since above all she

---

[335] These would be the gifts used for the end times Marriage Feast ...

was known for her healing gifts. She treated those who suffered greatly, as well as those who sought her out for heart and blood issues, wherever she traveled. Still a disgrace in her own town, she never took money for helping with health issues. She did, however, make a lot of money from her import and export business, and opened her house to women who were abused, violated, homeless, or runaways. Mary never turned anyone away who came to her for help, even if they had been hurtful to her at any time, were of a shunned culture, religion or creed, or gender expression. Mary spent a lot of time thinking and writing about unusual things, things most people, especially women, never thought about. Above all, Mary thought, dreamed, and fantasized about 'Him.'

This was the beginning of the 'reversal' of humans' 'fall from grace.' God so saw beauty in His creation of male and female, man and woman, that through the relationship of *soulmates* He revealed that "how the ideal spiritual union between man and woman was ordained that man might bring out the hidden reason in woman, and that the woman might help man uncover his hidden feeling."

We know that Jesus' marriage to Mary was necessary because of His sacrifice for humankind, but *to them, it was the desire to be together* that was sacrificed. The two were more similar than what you would think. Both were laconic and possessed Eternal Wisdom, or *Sophia Perennis*. We don't ever want to lose track of, or diminish, the love they shared, since their marriage raised the level of human love, which gives a committed relationship an opportunity to attain the ultimate union, marriage. That is why, though we teach Jesus doing his Father and Mother's will, we want to reaffirm it was another part of the story. Jesus and Mary, too, had to sacrifice something of themselves, since marriage made them one.

All these were factors that had to be, in order that they be linked back to the beginning and the story of how Adam and Eve entered this world and permanently became a part of it physically. As Adam and Eve were married transcendentally, and yet chose to enter into a physical marriage, so it was necessary for Jesus' marriage to reverse the direction of this course, and liberate humanity from the sense of being 'imprisoned' within the confines of physical embodiment and the material world.

- **Jesus and Mary's marriage** was the marriage of the uncreated, eternally begotten Child, separated and become human;
- whereas **Adam and Eve's marriage** was a created being, separated, and became two created beings who chose to become physical beings.
- **Jesus and Mary's marriage** would be a complete sacrifice as human love dictates, yet there would be no physical relations, as chosen by Adam and Eve, but in their place, there were transcendental acts via the sacred kiss and mystically tantric love, which our first parents enjoyed.
- **Adam and Eve's** choice for a physical, human conjugal love closed the gates of Paradise.
- **Jesus and Mary's** choice for a transcendental marriage and love opened the gates to Paradise.
- **Adam and Eve's** descendants, because of their choice, are mortal beings;
- **Jesus and Mary's descendants**, by their sacrificial marriage and love once again may attain immortality through, with, and in the Marriage Feast Eucharist.
- **Adam and Eve** had earthly children; and
- **Jesus and Mary** have human/transcendental children until end times, in the transcendental realm. Since it is written, "The Heavenly Man has more children than a man on earth. If the offspring of Adam are many and die, how many more are the offspring of the Perfect Man who does not die and is born each second."

By their love, Jesus and Mary conceived all those waiting for salvation; and by their sacrificial love, they have begotten us; and that greater sacrifice is the death Jesus suffered on the cross for humankind and the death to all life within Mary, as she hemorrhaged by the Cross. The greatest pain was when, as Jesus died, their hearts were broken, since His life blood drained from his body, as Mary's was drained from hers.

All of this, to save humankind, then to have to leave behind your partner in death for the good of humankind.

Since the human Jesus lost His whole world when He died; and for the human Mary, she, too, lost her whole world when she lost Jesus to death. Yet, by the magnitude of their love, they conquered death. And through the resurrection of Jesus, and His rising from the dead, all of humankind, was given the gift of everlasting life.

SUMMARY POINT 34

AND IN THE END, THE LOVE YOU TAKE IS EQUAL TO THE LOVE YOU MAKE

The woman who even after she was married, would be assailed with unfriendly actions and bitter words, would continue after Jesus ascended and well into the future. The constant maligning of Mary by trick questions from Pharisees and the very men that would approach Jesus in an effort to get him to divorce her, were orchestrated behind the scenes by Peter.

In many ways, we see Mary as victim until her death. She was and continues to be the altar on which others who are persecuted are offered with her for salvation; and, of course, she is Priestess who offers the sacrifice of injustice, hate, and disregard for God, just like Jesus was Priest. Together they save us and all humanity. They are the undeniable, uncontestable, unquestionable Messiahs today, together as the woman Messiah encompasses the man. Their love has now blossomed into fruition, and its Fruit is called Emmanuel, "God with us." Living as his Father, the One who is like the Son of God, hidden until which time He will reveal Himself as total God, total Man, total Sacrament, and Spirit-fully and sacredly balanced. His throne is golden and it is one of the three Thrones of God. He is Equal in all ways, undivided Trinity.

Because of the return of the Divine Feminine, humanity can now begin the transition towards salvation and the transcendental realm as God intended, by becoming enlightened and nourished, and by accepting its invitation to the Marriage Feast of the Lamb and His Wife.

SUMMARY POINT 35

YOU ARE INVITED TO THE SACRED AND DIVINE MARRIAGE FEAST: THE LIFELINE OF THE KALLAHS AND THE WORLD

Eshans believe it is the time of Mary Magdalen, who 'was' the passive feminine aspect of Christ, and 'is' now the active aspect, and now she becomes the impregnated source of new life in such a way that plentitude arises from the Trinity. The Lamb's Wife under the name *Isreal*, which was the title name given to her by Christ. By the love of the Bridegroom and His Bride, and by the fruit of their love, the philosopher's stone has been revealed in the end times revelation as "One who is like the Son of Man," Emmanuel, the first born of the first born, the third person of the Holy Trinity, the Holy Spirit made flesh.

All these mysteries are played out, as the Kallahs celebrate the Sacred and Divine Marriage Feast of the Lamb and His Wife, which is the sacrament of Christ's marriage, and the fullness of the sacrament of the sacred and divine Holy Eucharist. By this amazing celebration and the power of the divine family, they hope to redefine the way humans see God and find a new path to finding and supporting ways in which all God's people can live together. Through the reception of the divine and sacred Eucharist of the Sacred and Divine Marriage Feast, one can succeed in becoming one with the divine family. There are three that bear witness in heaven, the Father, the Son, and the Holy Spirit; and these three are one. In the Kallah's Creed, you will find it written: "that there are three who witness in heaven: The Father, the Son, the Holy Spirit—and their eternal consorts. This is because we consider that each person of God has the dual nature of Divine Masculine and Divine Feminine, and there is, thus, a dual nature to each person—while altogether, are still one God."[336] Some writers in mystery schools posit a 'quad-trinity' in order to designate the place for the divine feminine attribute. But in Eeshan thought we can see that each Person of the trinity has the divine masculine/feminine counterbalance. It is through the second person, the Only Begotten Child of God, that divine male and female are represented through Jesus and Mary. It is then through Jesus that the male nature has passage, and through Mary that the female has passage. As they are together one person, this is the manner by which human beings are restored in their own balance before God in eternity. And there are three who bear witness on earth in present times, reflecting once again the prophecy of 'the spirit' who is Emmanuel, the one who is like the Son of Man, and testifies to the truth; 'the water' who is Mary Magdalen, as the person of Eesha; and 'the blood' who is Jesus, and these agree as one. There is truth, contrary to what some think. Just as no one can stop God's plan, Truth is back in the world.

In the past, we received the flawed witness of men, but now we have those who are the witnesses, and these testify to God, who is greater, since this is the witness of God, which has testified of the Divine Masculine of the only-begotten Child, The Son of God.

Here in the marriage feast the soul meets its true God, and it becomes one in spirit with Christ and Christa [or Christ Sophia]. This is where one can fully pour himself, or herself, so totally and utterly into the divine's soul[337] essence that no part of the person remains as it was (apart from God). Identity remains, just as the identity of the gifts after transubstantiation, but you have been divinized through Christ. In other words, you give wholeheartedly who you are, and everything you are, to Jesus and

---

[336] Some writers in mystery schools posit a 'quad-trinity' in order to designate the place for the divine feminine attribute. But in Eeshan thought we can see that each Person of the trinity has the divine masculine/feminine counterbalance. It is through the second person, the Son of God, that divine male and female are represented through Jesus and Mary. It is then through Jesus that the male nature has passage, and through Mary that the female has passage. Since they are together one person, this is the manner by which human beings are restored in their own balance before God in eternity. – Ed.

[337] The divine 'soul' is the soul of both Jesus and Mary who are one in existence.

allow him to pour all that He is into you, and without hesitation, the most profound and unimaginable alchemy takes place. The soul and the rest of the entire person is consumed into the Divine Consorts, meets her bridegroom intimately, and causes a union of the two, mirroring Christ and his Wife's sublime and Sacred Union, their sacrificial life together, their uncompromising love of God and neighbor, their tragic separation by his passion, death, and resurrection. This goes beyond the expected and the ordinary, and advances into the sublime and sacred mysteries of God. This enables the Light Body within to, once again, experience the transcendental state of Light through, with, and in the 'Light of the World,' who is Jesus Christ and the Holy Grail, who is Mary.

Human salvation is obtained by *ingesting* the Sacred and Divine Eucharist, which by the marriage of Jesus and Mary offsets, through time immemorial, Adam and Eve's choice by Christ's bloody sacrifice on the Cross in which Mary shared in her torn heart, her hemorrhaging at the foot of the Cross, and, thus, we say, "When Christ died, so too the heart of his Wife as they were as humans, separated from each other."

In countering the effects of the original ingestion of the forbidden apple, the Light Body is awakened, the soul is nourished and sanctified, allowing one's resolve to be strengthened against unlawful corrupted knowledge. The human being enters the transcendental, and as the gates of heaven are once again opened to us, we have the Christs' affirmation of eternal life.

Here is the realization of the Woman in the Wilderness giving birth to the male child, who is the gift to the future of this world. His name is Emmanuel, "God with us." Fully Divine and fully human, he will sit on His golden Throne and rule with a rod of iron.

SUMMARY POINT 36

THE END TIME: THE HOLY KALLAHS

With the truths regarding women made known by way of our foundress, who we believe is the Eternal Bride of the Lamb, and who established the Eeshan religion and Faith, we have now made the Christed Body, encompassing his female consort, Mary Magdalene, available to women, who upon ordination are called Kallahs (priestesses).[338] Eeshans believe our Kallahs are the extension of the women of ancient times who followed Jesus, were taught by him, and were raised up as priestesses by way of Christ's marital bond to Mary. We believe Jesus and Mary Magdalen's consciousness permeates their mutual divine union, via their ordination and reception of the twin-flamed Christed Body.

Kallahs[339] are Kallahs forever, since they share in the marriage of the Eternal Bride and Bridegroom. The twin flame Soul Mate Body means that as they share in the person of the Wife of the Lamb, and as they also have equal share in the Christed Body, the two are one. Through his marriage with His wife, the long-awaited invitation to celebrate and fulfill the scriptures found within the book of Revelation is called the Sacred and Divine Marriage Feast of the Lamb and His Wife.

This Sacred and Divine Union, by the consecrated hands of the Kallah, bring with it the fulfillment of the mystery of the birth of the child born to the Woman in the Wilderness (Rev. 12:5) and the one who

---

[338] Kallah is the Hebrew word for Holy and Royal Bride and in Sanskrit, we are reminded that the term Kala means 'time;' so in the way it's used here, it is the name given to women of Eesha, known as Brides of Christ, who, originating from a timeless realm, carry out a mission as part of Mary's entourage here in the world of time. – Ed.

[339] Name given to women of Eesha, known as Brides of Christ.

is like the Son of Man (Daniel 7:13, Rev. 1:13, Rev. 14:14) the First Born of the First Born and the "river of life, as clear as crystal, flowing from the Throne of God and of the Lamb." (Rev. 22:1) "Let the one who is thirsty come; let the one who wishes the water of life without cost" be filled. "Let anyone who desires, drink freely from the water of life." (Rev. 22:17)

Our Kallahs, as holy and royal brides of Eesha, the incarnation of the consciousness of Mary Magdalene's original priestesses, who possess the consecrated mark of the Divine and Sacred Order of Mary Magdalen, under the guardianship of the Sacred and Divine Order of Melchizedek, thus unite the timeless priesthood for the first time with the Divine Feminine.[340] This Sacred and Divine Order of Melchizedek assists in bringing the mission of the Divine Feminine to fruition in these times in order to bring healing to an ailing humanity.

The teachings of the Eeshan Faith strive to fulfill Christ's directive when He said:

> "But there shall arise after you, men of perverse minds who shall through ignorance or through craft, suppress many things which I have taught and speak those words I have never taught sowing tares among the good wheat, which I have given to you to sow into the world. Then shall the truth of God endure the contradiction of sinners, for thus it hath been and thus it will be; but the time has come when the things that they have hidden shall make free those, which are bound."[341]

Kallahs' stand on our sacred teachings, because these do not suppress Jesus' words, since He is the Word. They stand against those teachings that make him less than who He really is by resisting the human consciousness, and not permitting any aspect of it to start setting inroads leading to discrimination.

---

[340] Cf. Ps. 110–114, Ps. 119:106.
[341] Gospel of the Holy Twelve, Lection 41-50.

The Kallahs bring to God's people the complete unfathomable mysteries given to us by Jesus Christ and Mary Magdalen the Divine Feminine, in their entirety, and totally grounded through, with, and in the Marriage of the Lamb and His Wife.

These include all the Mystical and Mysterious Sacraments of Baptism, Confirmation, Forgiveness, the Holy Eucharist, Matrimony, Holy Orders, and Extreme Unction.

SUMMARY POINT 37

METTA: THE SACRED LOVE OF EESHAN SPIRITUALITY I AM MEEK AND HUMBLE OF HEART

Metta is the foundation upon which we live. Like meekness, it is not to be confused with being weak, choosing to be deliberately blind or submissive. It means that we should be passionate, strong, and long-suffering about the things we need to fight for regarding God and love of neighbor, just as Jesus was. Jesus did not keep silent when defending the things of God that He had control over. A perfect example of that was His behavior in the Temple towards the venders and tax collectors.

We use our Eeshan Tirtha (temple) to worship and serve God, and our Spirituality and School of Enlightenment for words and examples of loving kindness. The word "Metta" is an ancient Pali word that loosely translates into English as "lovingkindness," and is chosen for our use because it involves a much more deeply felt and lived sense of divine love than the English words 'love' and 'kindness' evoke. It empowers meekness and humility. It was chosen to emphasize and differentiate what the human consciousness denotes as love, and what the transcendental consciousness' meaning of love is. Metta embraces a far deeper sense of God's love and Peace, which is synonymous with the reason for one's being, which connects to the immortal essence of the soul. It is for this reason that God set apart the Eeshan beliefs from what has been taught for the last 2000 years. We believe that Jesus has chosen His eternal Consort at this time for those who choose to be enlightened in order to see the identifying mark of truth, and lead us back to Him, primarily being that it was Mary Magdalen who He intended to carry on His mission.

Though our religion is meant to bring intracomplementarity in/to all aspects of life here on earth, being Eeshan does mean that we follow a particular set of 'rules.' These teachings presented encompass through 'this spirituality' what we should desire as human beings. We should desire to bring all people, regardless of gender, race, age, color, creed, or sexual orientation to a richer, fuller awareness of love, Metta love, by offering them teachings and concepts once hidden from the populous, as well as incorporating an Eastern Ayurvedic[342] component.

Along with the true teachings of the 'Christs,' meditation and our Spirituality that we wish that deep within us, reaching down to our very root chakra, and deep within our soul,[343] the extreme loving kindness will be found only through the arousing of the qualities of love, Metta, acceptance, patience, and tolerance, with meekness, and of course, forgiveness, which is not to be confused with an apology. Forgiveness, where asking, or being asked to forgive, is to be able to express what the forgiveness requires, and giving the other individual(s) the opportunity to express themselves with the same regard respectively.

While there are influences noted regarding other faiths and their practices, accordingly, and as we have touched on many of the traditional Christian and Catholic connotations and similarities, sighting what their differences are, as well as, what we consider errors, the Eeshan spirituality's prime objective is to offer what we feel is a fuller, richer incorporation of the principle of Metta. In doing so, we present the reasons for its resurgence. As we stated numerous times, it is a mystical, Kabbahlic, Esoteric, Exoteric, Merkabahalic[344] religion-meaning that its resurgence

---

[342] System of medicine with historical roots in the Indian subcontinent which seeks to keep all the elements and systems of the body in balance as a means of maintaining health. – Ed.

[343] Cf. Gospel of Thomas, Verse 112.

[344] Mystical meaning: transcending human understanding with a sense of spiritual mystery Kabbahlic meaning: handed down by those who know the secrets since they were given by the divine Merkabahalic meaning ability to transcend or travel back and forth as from heaven to earth, etc., instructions and symbolic visions usually involving faces, intelligences, symbols, etc., Exoteric, is like turning a light on and seeing things as they

is due to meet the needs of God's people in this the 'fullness of time.' Our spirituality flows from a combined Eastern/Western wisdom in all it teaches and practices.

That is why you will find within our spirituality those practices and beliefs that we feel best reflect, or are better explained by the books and authors from other more familiar established religions such as Buddhism, Zen, and traditional Hindu Bhakti, which because of the vastness of God's 'Word,' and carries with them truths, as used and taught by the Spiritual Master Himself, Jesus. We are unique in our teachings since we follow the spirituality of the eternal consciousness of Mary Magdalen,[345] who we believe is revealed in Revelation 21:9-10, as the Wife of the Lamb; and incorporate the teachings of Jesus, known, also as St. Issa, or as we call Him, Ish [Husband/Man], the opposing Divine Masculine to the Divine Female Isha/Eesha [Wife/Woman]. Issa was the name, He was known by while He lived, trained, and taught in the Himalayas, and all pertinent Gnostic writings. We are not a religion that falls under the designations religion is normally defined by, or has always been perceived by. You will find some canonically recognized gospels with, and without, completed Eeshan texts, as well as the larger canon of apocryphal, and newly discovered manuscripts, transcendental teachings by authors of highest regard, studies regarding energy, vibrations etc., but mostly the teachings, via the eternal Consciousness of Mary Magdalen, completing the codification of beliefs that we hope brings about the promulgation of the Eeshan religion.

Our Metta philosophy is the practice of universal love, and is to identify with the love Jesus had for all. It is the foundation for spreading the lovingkindness of God to our neighbor by taking an active and positive interest in others without compromising our beliefs, as taught by Jesus and shared wholly by Mary. We strive to help others achieve Metta, as we wholeheartedly teach and practice the Eeshan spirituality. You will find that it appears to also follow one of the ten Pāramìs, of the Theravāda school of Buddhism, and one of the four sublime states (Brahmavāras).

---

really are. Exoteric is best described by one who said it is like turning a light on and seeing your soul for the first time, even though you knew you had one.

[345] Cf. Gospel of Philip, Jesus was Mary's Koinonos, also see Rev. 19:7-9, 21:9-10.

Again, this is so due to the teachings which were brought through the spirituality Jesus brought to God's children. You will find that these bring a broader meaning, which is not the same as some interpret to mean the human need to possess. The practice of Metta allows one to 'find joy in the journey' through life, uninhibited and without fear, with the knowledge of being the 'extension,' since we are of the holy, almighty, and immortal being God, from whom all good things come, as our children are the 'extensions' of the love parents have for each other.

Our goal is to bring equality of all human beings through the connecting of the subtle movement of *prana*, the physical aspect of life force, or *chi* as some call it, and is defined by those who share in this like mind and spirituality. It is the connection to the divine that Jesus meant when He said, "Where two or more are gathered, I am there." This fosters a greater feeling of love of neighbor within one's heart, and one goes from selfish concern of oneself to selfless concern for others.

Our religion is not just a philosophy, but it is also an active manifestation of love through good works, and nourishment of the mind, through the teachings and participation in the Sacred and Divine Marriage Feast of the Lamb and His Wife, the soul and body by reception of the Sacred Eucharist, as Jesus taught was necessary for salvation. This is important because this love and belief in Jesus' teachings goes beyond what is here on earth, in the material world, and by Jesus' words, acknowledges the reality of an afterlife.

Eeshans believe that the powerful practice of greeting another with an embrace/hug is the outward manifestation of the belief that we are all connected, and as children of God, it brings the Christs' warmth, consolation, and tenderness of heart.

We teach that all have the right to practice their faith to live the Way, the Truth, the Life, and the Light in the language of God they understand, and to reach that enlightenment that frees us of all those things that darken, inhibit, and imprison the human spirit. We welcome the beliefs of all religions and spiritualities, whose faith and practices are catalysts toward a holy, decent, wholesome and peaceful world, and who value life as people are extensions of God, even though we may not agree with their belief system or any arguments against our own beliefs.

Metta pours into the universe a power of love, but this love is a type of love that will require humankind to make selfless, Christ-centered choices apart from the teachings of the self-consumed and faithless world's perspective, whose understanding of love was obscured over time. It is the love and peace personified by Jesus Christ, who by His person, life and teachings, exemplified Metta, and encompasses the universal laws, mutable and immutable, which cannot be denied, and are the principle laws of physics, which God gave humans for a greater understanding of creation.

We desire that this love, this Metta, awakens one's consciousness in ways that sends an energy, and vibration, that helps us to realize more fully the gift of a religious freedom and the right to satisfy our innate calling by God to find peace and happiness through love, and a selfless desire to serve God and neighbor. Through Eeshan influence may there come a day when there is a recognition that the dangers and consequences of illusion are responsible for, and have led all people, in one way or another, into suffering (due to sin). May the healing of the wounds that human beings inflict on themselves and one another finally find its way into the hearts of us all, due to the elimination of illusion and fear that plague the mind, heart, and soul.

The goal of the Eeshan is building love, and overpowering illusion or delusion, which is causing worse suffering, and to replace this suffering with the unconditional love that comes from God, as opposed to focusing on the sins of one's past, and dwelling on that past, which in effect is only giving more energy to that darkness. The emphasis on healing and building upon love, we believe, is necessary for the transformation of the human heart and mind.

Everyone, every soul, is entitled to have the opportunity to attain enlightenment, and should never be forced by the tools of fear, condemnation, and oppression to stay within the walls of paranoia built to suit the desires and conquests of man for the purpose of control or power.

Eeshans teach that a universal understanding of the human desire to find God, or the absolute Higher or Supreme Being people are searching for, is not always found in ways limited to traditional, organized, institutionalized religion, but rather by an uninhibited path based in Wisdom.

It can and is found in ways and avenues that encompass the universal laws outside of religion. For some, there may be sciences and philosophies that may embrace ways that lead one through a different perspective to finding Christ's teachings not obtainable through ordinary means.

We have attained this enlightenment out of our desire to find truth. Our efforts to accomplish this goal were satisfied through our mystery school studies and years of teachings by one identified, loved, and trusted by devotees as the Lamb's Wife, Eesha. In our opinion, it is because of God's Metta that we have succeeded to peer into the fullest meaning behind the love Jesus taught as the primary mandate of the purpose of human life.

We believe that even though Jesus' mission of salvation was deterred by those who coveted a patriarchal authority and power, the omnipotent God, who knew the weakness of the faulty human consciousness, thus allowed man's free will to play out, and devise an alternate plan that would, in the fullness of time, awaken His wife, and that the world would one day know the truth and live this kind of love, Metta.

We believe that bringing souls to enlightenment, and instructing God's people, must be found in the truest sense of the definition of the words "Universal Eeshan Spirituality" to be accepted by a very diverse world.

We, therefore, ordain that the time has come to invite others to share in this approach, and participate in our methods of teaching in order that Metta can be propagated.

Furthermore, we will pray that we continue to reach out to all who want to hear about, and live, Metta by whatever means is available to us, but especially by example.

By means of speaking engagements, websites, written material, workshops, and any other means made available, we will make every effort to spread Metta by teaching, healing, and enlightening the world regarding how we are all God's children created by love, and to love without exception.

The Divine Feminine desires to reinforce the Divine desire that we come together to use words that express inclusivity, thus abandoning words and concepts that have been used over the centuries that have been construed to place one gender above another, which comes neither from grace nor from God.

Eeshans also warn how, without Metta and a grounded spirituality, attempting to correct any discrimination could result in reverse discrimination. This would not end the problem, it would just create new problems. Without Metta, we tend to see the faults and weaknesses of others and not our own. Without Metta, we fail to see that human beings are not perfect. Oftentimes a religion's adherents end up becoming self-righteous, this is when so-called 'religious' people judge others for not measuring up; yet, they too, are guilty of the same things but refuse to see their own errors.

One should be careful to not fall victim to anything, or anyone, that upsets the Sacred Balance, such as old views that once permeated through some groups who taught the skewed view that it was woman's inherent covetous nature that was the reason for a man's fall from grace; and that independent of the male, female impurity would undermine a man's strength and integrity; therefore, the end justified the means.

That is why we feel Eeshan Transcendentalism holds within it the true Bride of Christ, and how necessary it is to break the bonds of the imposter who declares *it* holds the truth. For if the institution that claims to hold the true teachings of Christ practiced its claims, it would have corrected this, especially with regards to Christ's teachings had it not been guilty of this sin. Eeshans believe that only an impostor would ignore this teaching. One focused on personal gain, perhaps motivated by fear and greed, who was firm in his decision to preserve the patriarchal status quo, and prevent anything, or anyone, from tampering with this deception in the future, it was necessary to change/alter/spread this 'counterfeit true story' to give a foundation, and continuing basis, for man's dominance over women, especially in the area of worship and priesthood.

Without Metta, it becomes easier and easier to lie to someone. Can you imagine how easy it is to lie to masses of people? All it takes is one small story, a white lie, used to offset fear or punishment. Gradually, over the years, one lie leads to another, and the story now becomes more developed, and embellished, and more people become entrenched in the lie, even those who have *discovered* the lie, since they believe there is no going back unless they destroy 'all the good' that occurred. A false bride would have to continue to lie in order to continue to be. Worse than the lie itself is the gratification and sense of 'accomplishment' one feels when they get away with the lie.

SUMMARY POINT 38

"You are no Greater than your Master"

Jesus taught that "the truth will set you free," in order to break the pattern of one who lies, so that it cannot grow existentially. Today, without God, spirituality and truth are either practically non-existent, or the meanings of these terms are so muddled and convoluted, that it's hard to see how they have anything or much at all to do with God.

The rise of the Bride of Christ-the co-Messiah-the 'Woman' who understands human nature, but loves with a woman's love, has come about due to the fullness of time, and is even called on by modern travails, and the birth pangs of the people, yearning for their God. In order to reestablish truth, she is necessary, however, and to find her one must first be enlightened. This, too, can only happen by her acceptance. The Divine Feminine is here to help end the confusion. Her work is expected to be likened to what was accomplished by Jesus.

It has been said that the offenses that Jesus supposedly committed and the laws He broke are what upset the very social and religious fabric of the time, and were essentially based in His assertions that most of these laws were manmade, not God-given. In other words, the laws which had been built up over such a long period of time, that had over that time taken on their own kind of 'divine authority,' when, in fact, they were actually just laws created by men for the people to live under to preserve religious order and power ... and were also designed to keep people clear about their place. Moreover, and more importantly to the point at hand, it also helped to galvanize the authority of the patriarchal structures throughout the religious and the general awareness of people, which in addition to preserving social order, also kept women clearly in their place.

The Son of God presented His understanding of the Triune God as being gracious and merciful, slow to anger, a God who sees all people as his children; whereas, the Pharisees, according to their interpretation, presented God as one who makes demands and presents rules that must be kept at all costs. Jesus taught that to ignore the existence of God, and live independently of Him was to cling to the father of true evil and only bring about physical, mental, and spiritual discontent, and suffering. Our Eesha does nothing short of teaching the same thing.

Eeshans understand what they are up against, since as Jesus said, "You are no greater than your Master." Bringing the truth to a people who have lived a religion, especially a birth religion, is no easy task. It's a known fact that one reason Jesus was seen less than favorably in the eyes of the authorities was his tendency to humiliate religious leaders in their hypocrisy and arrogance. This and His other declarations, such as His claim that He was the fulfillment of scriptures, and by His calling God His Father, was not easily accepted in a religion that did not accept a personal and intimate relationship with God as a 'person.' One must remember that for Him to claim God as His Father, He claimed all that He was teaching was from God, and in claiming "before Abraham was, I AM" (that He was truly God) earned him the charge of blasphemy. Eeshans expect they shall run into the same difficulties as they profess their truths and outline what they feel are the hypocrisies of the Christian world.

From the time of Christ, the true existence of a wife would indeed have compromised what Peter's intention conveyed, if uncovered at 'any point in time.' That is why a vigil, or watch, became imperative. Any person who may look to be the One, the rising, or the return of Mary Magdalen, who could ruin everything, could be the downfall of the church. This would be His Bride, or "the one Jesus would return for." Any woman saint who claimed to have a "personal relationship" with Jesus, or who claimed they were "mystically married" to Jesus over the centuries, or to have private revelations with Him, which deterred people from listening to church authority, to women who forged forward, pursuing equal rights within the church, were those the religious leaders watched.

Then came our Foundress: little known, born to a normal family, raised in a small town, who would marry, and have children and work, just like any other woman. Out of nowhere, she came on the scene as teacher and healer. As crowds grew, attempts were made to stifle, and eventually stop her public appearances. It was time. It was time to reveal to her, who she was, and it came time to begin to prepare her for her true mission. Yet, not by the hands of those who feared her did she go out of public view; it was by the hand of God. By his own hand, a place was set aside, a refuge where scriptures would play out. A place He would come to reunite with his Wife as One. For it is written:

> "... **My transcendental Body never deteriorates, and although I am the Lord of all living entities, I still appear in every millennium In My original transcendental form.**"[346]

"The woman fled into the wilderness to a place prepared for her by God, where she might be taken care of ..." [Revelation 12:6]

---

[346] Bhagavad-Gita As It Is, 4.6., translated by Bhaktivedanta Swami Prabhupada.

A Heartfelt Acknowledgement

We really want to take this time and acknowledge and applaud the research of those authors we named and whose name we could not find for all the writings we used, herein, and of all those whose work make a stunning case for the support of many of our beliefs, and served to show the vastness of God's love and mercy as the "Word" goes on, and enlightens those who seek it, those authors known and those whose work we know only as by 'Anonymous.' These works are, indeed, inspired by God and meant to help to satisfy the hunger of those whose curiosity is aroused about Jesus' birth, life, death, and resurrection, the idea of His being married, and the Who and What of God. In addition, it provides the basis for the very strong case of God working among all humans in an effort to bring salvation to all those who believe.

Eeshans want to stress, however, as the founder, or as the One reintroducing this transcendental "ancient" mystical, beyond Merkabahalic, and Kabbahlic spirituality brought back into conscious awareness, because of the love of God in order to meet the spiritual needs of the people: that *our (Eesha's) teachings* were given to its members, *long* before the general public was introduced to the trend, which appealed to curiosity on this subject and that of God having a feminine nature as well as masculine.

With the help of those great authors, teachers, and spiritual Masters who we have quoted, and who have and continue to contribute their great works, inspirational quotes, and even songs, and those who authored books that inspire, as well as reveal their experiences in an effort to bring together all transcendental modes of wisdom, such as Dr. J. J. Hurtak and his wife Desiree, as well as those who may not be as well-known, but whose writings, insights, and prophetic manuscripts prove beyond a shadow of a doubt, to contain pieces of which, when collected build a puzzle, and once completed, will provide all the truths and all the mysteries hidden and locked away in time, and unlocked by the- one and one-in-only, who holds the Master key, that mystical unfathomable key, to the eternal consciousness.

"**By hearing the powerful glorious topics of the Lord from a living saintly person, all our anarthas, our weakness of heart, are destroyed and our heart is filled with strength. Then our nature, which is to surrender to the Lord, will be awakened. In the surrendered heart, the self-manifest truth of the transcendental kingdom will automatically manifest. This is how to know the truth. It is impossible to know the Absolute Truth by any other means.**"[347]

---

[347] Hearing, as mystically described in the book, *Amrta Vani, Nectar of Instructions for Immortality* by His Divine Grace, written by Śrīla Bhaktisiddhanta Sarasvati Thakura Prabhupada.

CPSIA information can be obtained
at www.ICGtesting.com
Printed in the USA
LVHW020919150520
655581LV00001B/1